Clinical Laboratory Science Review

Second edition

Robert R. Harr
Chair, Department of Medical Technology
Bowling Green State University
Bowling Green, Ohio

F. A. DAVIS COMPANY • Philadelphia

F. A. Davis Company
1915 Arch Street
Philadelphia, PA 19103

Copyright © 2000 by F. A. Davis Company

Printed in the Unites States of America

Last digit indicates print number: 10 9 8 7 6

Publisher: Jean-François Vilain
Developmental Editor: Christa Frantantoro
Production Editor: Elena Coler
Cover Designer: Louis Forgione

As new scientific information becomes available through basic and clinical research, recommended treatments and drug therapies undergo changes. The author(s) and publisher have done everything possible to make this book accurate, up to date, and in accord with accepted standards at the time of publication. The authors, editors, and publisher are not responsible for errors or omissions or for consequences from application of the book, and make no warranty, expressed or implied, in regard to the contents of the book. Any practice described in this book should be applied by the reader in accordance with professional standards of care used in regard to the unique circumstances that may apply in each situation. The reader is advised always to check product information (package inserts) for changes and new information regarding clinical laboratory practice.

Library of Congress Cataloging in Publication Data

Clinical laboratory science review / [edited by] Robert R. Harr.—
    2nd ed.
        p.   cm.
    Includes bibliographical references.
    ISBN 0-8036-0443-2 (pbk. : alk. paper)
    1. Medical laboratory technology Examinations, questions, etc.
I. Harr, Robert R.
    [DNLM: 1. Laboratory Techniques and Procedures Examination
Questions. 2. Chemistry, Clinical—methods Examination Questions.
3. Technology, Medical Examination Questions. QY 18.2 C6415 1999]
RB38.25.C574 1999
616.07'56'076—dc21
DNLM/DLC
for Library of Congress   99-23448
                                                                         CIP

Preface

The primary purpose of the *Clinical Laboratory Science (CLS) Review* is to assist candidates who are preparing for certification or licensure examinations in clinical laboratory science. This review can also be used by those who wish to update their medical laboratory knowledge and renew their theoretical skills. In addition, educators in clinical laboratory science and medical technology programs may wish to recommend this review as a study guide for their students in various courses.

A potential user of the *CLS Review* may ask, "Why should I purchase this review book when several other review books are available?" The answer lies within the unique organization and explanation found with each question. Over 1500 multiple choice questions in seven major content areas appear together with answers, short explanations, test item classifications, and taxonomy levels ranging from 1 (recall) to 3 (problem solving). The questions of each section comprise a thorough review of the discipline and are ordered to facilitate the coherent understanding of the subject. Regardless of certification examination format or sponsor, the *CLS Review* provides a rapid and efficient review and self-assessment for the computer adaptive examinations for medical technologist (MT), medical laboratory technician (MLT), categorical exams given by the American Society of Clinical Pathologists (ASCP), clinical laboratory scientist (CLS), clinical laboratory technician (CLT), categorical examinations given by the National Certification Agency (NCA) for medical laboratory personnel, and certification exams sponsored by the American Medical Technologists (AMT) and the International Society for Clinical Laboratory Technology (ISCLT).

The review begins with the Introduction section, which includes detailed information on the design of the questions, use of this book to prepare for an examination, and test-taking skills. The introductory section is followed by questions arranged within the seven major content areas. Each section contains a list of references, which are also recommended for further review. A comprehensive certification examination is given at the end of the question sections using questions selected from the book. This exam will help the students to determine their levels of retention and learning from the book. A disk that contains a mock computerized certification exam is also supplied. The questions on the disk are different from any that appear in the book. The computerized exam will help the students identify their levels of preparation and give them experience in taking an examination by computer.

The materials in the *CLS Review* were prepared by educators and clinical experts who have national recognition for their accomplishments in clinical laboratory science. Materials from recent developments in practice as well as major textbooks were used in formulating these questions. Peer review of the questions was performed as part of the publication process. Many new questions have been added in the new edition. The number of problem solving questions and color plates has been greatly expanded, and more complete explanations are provided for the more important and difficult questions.

The *CLS Review* has been designed as an individual guidebook for measuring personal knowledge and test-taking skills. It should prove to be a valuable tool for ensuring the success of the student preparing for a national certification exam, course exams, or licensure, and for the practitioner updating theoretical skills.

Reviewers

Karen S. Long, MS, CLS(NCA), MT(ASCP)
Associate Professor
Medical Technology Program
West Virginia School of Medicine
Morgantown, West Virginia

Sharon Martin, EdD, MT(ASCP)
Coordinator of Instructional Technology Design
Central Virginia Community College
Lynchburg, Virginia

Susan King Strasinger, DA, MT(ASCP)
Visiting Assistant Professor
Medical Technology Program
West Florida University
Pensacola, Florida

Contributors

Barbara Caldwell, BS, MT(ASCP)SH
Assistant Professor
Betty Ciesla, MS, MT(ASCP)SH
Assistant Professor
Denise M. Harmening, PhD, MT(ASCP), CLS(NCA)
Professor and Chair
Mitra Taghizadeh, MS, MT(ASCP)
Assistant Professor
   All from the Department of Medical and Research Technology
   School of Medicine
   University of Maryland at Baltimore
   Baltimore, Maryland
Chapter 1   Hematology

Sharon M. Martin, EdD, MT(ASCP)
Coordinator of Instructional Technology Design
   Central Virginia Community College
   Lynchburg, Virginia
Chapter 2   Immunology
Chapter 3   Immunohematology

Robert R. Harr, MS, MT(ASCP)
Associate Professor and Chair
   Department of Medical Technology
   Bowling Green State University
   Bowling Green, Ohio
Chapter 4   Clinical Chemistry
Chpater 5   Urinalysis and Body Fluids
Chapter 8   Photomicrographs and Color Plates
Chapter 9   Sample Certification (Self-Assessment) Examination

Pamella Phillips, MEd, MT(ASCP)SM
Education Coordinator
   Department of Medical Technology
   Bowling Green State Technology
   Bowling Green, Ohio
Chapter 6   Microbiology
Chapter 7   Education and Management

Lynn Shore Garcia, MS F(AAM), CLS(NCA)
Manager of Clinical Microbiology
   University of California at Los Angeles Medical Center
   Los Angeles, California
Chapter 6, Unit 11   Parasitology

Contents

Introduction

The *Clinical Laboratory Science (CLS) Review* has been planned to provide a challenging personal assessment of practical and theoretical knowledge needed by clinical laboratory scientists. The *CLS Review* has been designed to help you identify strengths, weaknesses, and gaps in your knowledge base. Because taxonomy level is a part of the assessment, you will also be able to concentrate on the type of question that causes the most difficulty. The suggested approach to maximizing the use of the *CLS Review* is to read all the introductory materials thoroughly, especially the test-taking skills sections, before attempting to answer the questions.

This *CLS Review* was developed as a tool to facilitate both self-assessment and new learning. The units are arranged in a logical sequence corresponding to the organization of a textbook and follow the pattern of presentation used in clinical laboratory science lectures. The questions within a unit are related and can be used by students as they progress through their courses in order to improve understanding. The sections are comprehensive and suitable for all certification levels, although some questions may be more appropriate for one certification level, for example, MT (CLS) than another. The *CLS Review* is intended to supplement courses in the curriculum and to assist technologists and technicians who are reentering the laboratory. In addition, it is designed to improve performance on generalist, categorical, and specialist certification exams.

Design of Questions

All the questions in this book are multiple choice. Each question is followed by the correct answer, a brief explanation, and a test item classification. The test item classification consists of the subject category, task, and taxonomy level of the question. A question in Blood Banking, for example, which asks for an interpretation of an ABO problem, may have the test item classification "Blood Bank/Evaluate laboratory data to recognize problems/ABO discrepancy/3." The test item classification places the question in the major category of blood banking; the question asks for an evaluation of data; the subcategory is ABO discrepancy; and the taxonomy level classifies the question as problem solving. Taxonomy level 1 questions address recall of information. Taxonomy 2 questions require calculation, correlation, comprehension, or relation. Taxonomy 3 questions require problem solving, interpretation, or decision making.

This question design allows you to compute a score, which helps to identify weaknessess and strengths in various content areas and tasks. You may then focus study time on a particular content area or on practice of a specific taxonomy level. For example, if several mycology questions are answered incorrectly, then extra time should be devoted to studying this content area. If, however, several fact recall questions (taxonomy 1 level) are missed over several different content areas such as hematology, chemistry, and immunology, then repetitive review is indicated for all of these sections. A weakness revealed in questions that require mathematical solutions (taxonomy 2 level) may require you to seek additional practice in answering questions requiring calculation. If interpretation or problem solving (taxonomy 3 level) has been identified as a weakness, then the best approach may be to study the explanation that follows each question to understand the logic or reasoning behind the development of the solution.

Using This Book to Prepare for an Examination

During your professional education, you have received an enormous amount of information from both classroom and practical experiences. National certification examinations are similar to comprehensive tests and are designed to evaluate your knowledge over a wide range of content areas. The practice questions given in the book are a starting point to refresh and assess your knowledge as you prepare to take these certification exams. Although the review book is comprehensive, it cannot review every aspect of clinical laboratory science and is not a substitute for thorough study and review of your class notes and texts.

Carefully answer the questions in this book, and read each explanation whether you answered the question correctly or not. Make a separate list of notes about troublesome questions or difficult content areas. Take the comprehensive exam in the book, then take the computerized exam. Compare your scores by content area for the two exams. Begin studying the area in which your score was best and progress to the other areas from the next best score to the worst. Class notes and old tests may serve as the best initial source of review material, but we recommend that you also use the textbook references found in the *CLS Review*. Repeat each chapter in the *CLS Review* a second time, then take both tests again. Your score for both tests should improve significantly. You should see more improvement in the comprehensive exam score because those questions come right from the review book chapters. If your score for this test does not improve significantly, try studying at a different time and place in order to improve your concentration. Leave enough time to review your class notes and texts thoroughly at least one more time before the certification exam date.

National certification examinations are criterion-referenced. This means that examination performance is scored passing or failing independently of the performance of other candidates taking the examination. Candidates, therefore, are tested against a specified knowledge base. The minimum passing score for certification examinations is normalized to minimize the variance between examinations. However, the minimum passing score usually falls within the range of 60%–70% correct responses. A score below 65% on any content area in the *CLS Review* is an indication that you have not mastered the material in this area, and that further study is required.

The *CLS Review* questions are meant to stimulate and refresh your knowledge of an entire content area, not just the specific point addressed by a given question. Therefore, the explanations are as important to the review process as the question and correct answer. Please remember that the questions in the *CLS Review* are intended to represent only sample examination questions. Do not memorize these questions!

Test-Taking Skills

BEFORE THE EXAM

First, make a study plan. You may choose to review your study materials first, then take the examinations in this book. You may want to take the examinations first and then focus your study time on weak areas. You may even choose to answer the questions by using your study materials as a reference. There is no "right" or "wrong" strategy for exam preparation. Use whatever approach works best for you, but be sure to give yourself sufficient time.

Manage your study time wisely. You may be preparing for a 4-hour written examination or a 2½ hour computer examination covering material that has been introduced over a 1- or 2-year period. You cannot expect to review all of this material in only a few days. Allow yourself ample time to study all areas completely and carefully. Try to set aside an allotted time period every day.

Assemble all of your study materials before you begin your review. Searching for old notes or textbooks may become time consuming and frustrating. You may have a tendency to "give up" looking for needed materials, if you do not have them readily available. Therefore, a major content area may be neglected or unstudied.

Provide a study environment. Choose a quiet, comfortable area for your study. Find a place where you will not be distracted or disturbed.

Simulate test conditions. Regardless of your study plan, some portion of the review process, for example, the mock examination, should be taken under simulated test conditions. Examinations should be timed, uninterrupted, and designed to observe other realistic testing practices.

ON EXAM DAY

Get sufficient rest before the exam day. Eat properly and, if possible, engage in some light physical activity such as walking. Dress comfortably; layered clothing may provide some alternatives if the examination room is too hot or too cold.

Wear a watch so that you can keep track of time. Do not take notes or books with you. If you have not prepared prior to the examination day, you cannot cram last-minute facts. You should bring along a calculator that is familiar.

Relax for a few minutes before the exam begins. Close your eyes and breathe deeply. Perhaps focus on a special activity that you may have planned as a reward for yourself after the examination.

Have confidence in your abilities. At this point, you have successfully completed a rigorous course of classroom and clinical training and the examination represents merely the last step in this long process. Tell yourself that you have adequately practiced and prepared for the examination and that you are ready.

DURING THE EXAM

Read all directions. Make sure you understand how to take the examination.

Read questions carefully, and note key words. Accept the question as you first read it; do not read your own thoughts into the question and do not look for hidden meanings.

Quickly look at all of the answers. Next, carefully read all choices. You may wish to mentally place a *T* for true and an *F* for false beside each alternative, or to reject outright obviously wrong choices.

Select your first choice and do not change your answers. Answer all the questions. There is no penalty for quessing on certification examinations. Always answer to the best of your ability the first time. The computer-adapted exam selects the next question based on your previous answer.

Apply a few simple rules to those questions you cannot answer. Consistently choose the same letter on those questions. Use the first, last, or a middle alternative. *B* is the most common correct answer. Choose the longest answer. Select the alternative with the most repeating parts. Pick items that are more specific or detailed than the others. On combination answers, try to figure out which combinations are not related and do not logically belong together.

Do not overlook words such as "not," "never," always," "most," "least," "best," "worst," or "except." Statements that contain unqualified absolutes ("ways," "never") are usually incorrect. In contrast, alternatives that are worded to contain exceptions ("usually," "generally") are often true.

Do not panic if you do not know an answer. Continue the test and do not allow anxiety to make you forget items that you know.

Work steadily and do not spend too much time on questions you do not know; keep an eye on the time. Four hours are usually allotted for a 200-question written test or 2½ hours for a 100-question computer exam. Try to pace yourself so that sufficient time remains after completing the test to review all of your answers. Do not change your original answer unless you are certain that you made a mistake when you answered the question initially.

CHAPTER ONE

Hematology

Basic Hematology Concepts/Laboratory Procedures

1. When performing a peripheral smear differential examination, the battlement scan pattern is employed:
   A. To compensate for the fact that small lymphocytes are concentrated in the feathered edge
   B. To compensate for the fact that larger leukocytes are found more frequently in the feathered edge
   C. To compensate for the fact that eosinophils are found more frequently in the center of the film
   D. Because leukocytes are distributed evenly throughout the film

   Hematology/Apply principles of basic laboratory procedures/Microscopic morphology/Differential/1

2. Erythrocytes that vary in size from the normal 6–8 μm are described as exhibiting:
   A. Anisocytosis
   B. Hypochromia
   C. Poikilocytosis
   D. Pleocytosis

   Hematology/Apply knowledge of fundamental biological characteristics/Microscopic morphology/RBC/1

3. Which of the following is the preferable site for bone marrow aspiration and biopsy in an adult?
   A. Iliac crest
   B. Sternum
   C. Tibia
   D. Spinous processes of a vertebra

   Hematology/Apply knowledge of fundamental biological characteristics/Bone marrow/1

Answers to Questions 1–3

1. **B** Blood films that have been prepared by the wedge push technique have an uneven distribution of leukocytes in different areas of the slide. There are more segmented neutrophils, monocytes, and eosinophils in the feather and side edges. Small lymphocytes will be more plentiful in the center of the film. The battlement scan pattern is used to review each slide in a standardized fashion, thus minimizing distributional abnormalities (see diagram).

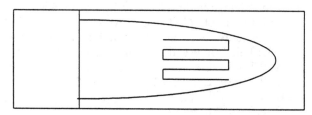

2. **A** A mature erythrocyte is approximately 7 μm in diameter. Changes in normal size are denoted by the term *anisocytosis*. *Hypochromia* is a term that indicates increased central pallor in erythrocytes, and *poikilocytosis* denotes a change in red cell shape.

3. **A** The iliac crest is the most frequently used site for bone marrow aspiration and biopsy. This site is the safest and most easily accessible, with the bone just beneath the skin and neither blood vessels nor nerves in the vicinity.

4. Mean cell volume (MCV) is calculated using the following formula:

A. $\dfrac{\text{Hgb}}{\text{RBC}} \times 10$

B. $\dfrac{\text{Hct}}{\text{RBC}} \times 10$

C. $\dfrac{\text{Hct}}{\text{Hgb}} \times 100$

D. $\dfrac{\text{Hgb}}{\text{RBC}} \times 100$

[handwritten: MCV = $\dfrac{\text{Hct}}{\text{RBC}} \times 10$]

Hematology/Calculate/RBC Indices/2

5. What term describes the change in shape of erythrocytes seen on a Wright's stained peripheral blood smear?

A. Poikilocytosis
B. Anisocytosis
C. Hypochromia
D. Polychromasia

Hematology/Apply knowledge of fundamental biological characteristics/Microscopic morphology/ RBC/1

6. Calculate the mean cell hemoglobin concentration (MCHC) using the following values: Hgb: 15 g/dL (150 g/L); RBC: $4.50 \times 10^6/\mu\text{L}$ ($4.50 \times 10^{12}/\text{L}$); Hct: 47% (0.47).

A. 9.5% (.095)
B. 10.4% (.104)
C. 31.9% (.319)
D. 33.3% (.333)

Hematology/Calculate/RBC Indices/2

7. A manual white blood cell (WBC) count was performed. A total of 36 cells were counted in all 9-mm² squares of a Neubauer-ruled hemacytometer. A 1:10 dilution was used. What is the WBC count?

A. $0.4 \times 10^9/\text{L}$
B. $2.5 \times 10^9/\text{L}$
C. $4.0 \times 10^9/\text{L}$
D. $8.0 \times 10^9/\text{L}$

Hematology/Calculate/Manual WBC/2

8. When an erythrocyte containing iron granules is stained with Prussian blue, the cell is called a:

A. Spherocyte
B. Leptocyte
C. Schistocyte
D. Siderocyte

Hematology/Apply knowledge of fundamental biological characteristics/RBC Microscopic morphology/Stain/1

9. A 7.0-mL etheylenediaminetetraacetic acid (EDTA) tube is received in the laboratory containing only 2.0 mL of blood. If the laboratory is using manual techniques, which of the following tests will most likely be erroneous?

A. RBC count
B. Hgb
C. Hematocrit
D. WBC count

Hematology/Apply knowledge to identify sources of error/Specimen collection and handling/ Hematocrit/2

10. A 1:200 dilution of a patient's sample was made and 336 red cells were counted in an area of 0.2 mm². What is the RBC count?

A. $1.68 \times 10^{12}/\text{L}$
B. $3.36 \times 10^{12}/\text{L}$
C. $4.47 \times 10^{12}/\text{L}$
D. $6.66 \times 10^{12}/\text{L}$

Hematology/Calculate/Manual RBC/2

Answers to Questions 4–10

4. **B** MCV is the average "volume" of the red cells. This is obtained by dividing the hematocrit (Hct) or packed cell volume (PCV) by the red blood cell (RBC) count in millions per microliter of blood, and multiplying by 10. The MCV is expressed in cubic microns (μm^3) or femtoliters.

5. **A** *Anisocytosis* refers to a change in size. *Hypochromia* is an increase in central pallor in erythrocytes. *Polychromasia* describes the bluish tinge of the immature erythrocytes (reticulocytes) circulating in the peripheral blood.

6. **C** MCHC is the average concentration of hemoglobin (Hgb) in red cells expressed in percent. It expresses the ratio of the weight of Hgb to the volume of erythrocytes and is calculated by dividing Hgb by the hematocrit, then multiplying by 100. A decreased MCHC indicates that cells are hypochromic.

7. **A** The formula used for calculating manual cell counts using a hemocytometer is: Number of cells counted $\times$ dilution factor $\times$ depth factor (10) divided by the area. In this example, $36 \times 10 \times 10 = 3600 \div 9 = 400/\text{mm}^3$ or $0.4 \times 10^9/\text{L}$.

8. **D** Occasionally erythrocytes in pathological conditions may contain iron in the form of hemosiderin. These granules can be stained with Prussian blue, and the red cells are then termed *siderocytes*.

9. **C** Excessive anticoagulant causes shrinkage of cells; thus the hematocrit will be affected. RBC and WBC counts remain the same, as does the Hgb content.

10. **B** RBC count = number of cells counted $\times$ dilution factor $\times$ depth factor (10), divided by the area. In this example, $336 \times 200 \times 10 = 672,000 \div 0.2 = 3.36 \times 10^{12}/\text{L}$.

11. What phagocytic cells produce lysozymes that are bacteriocidal?
A. Eosinophils
B. Lymphocytes
C. Platelets
D. Neutrophils

Hematology/Apply knowledge of fundamental biological characteristics/Leukocytes/1

12. If a patient has a reticulocyte count of 7% and a hematocrit of 20%, what is the corrected reticulocyte count?
A. 1.4%
B. 3.1%
C. 3.5%
D. 14%

Hematology/Apply principles of basic laboratory procedures/Calculate/Reticulocyte/1

13. A decreased osmotic fragility test would be associated with which of the following conditions?
A. Sickle cell anemia
B. Hereditary spherocytosis
C. Hemolytic disease of the newborn
D. Acquired hemolytic anemia

Hematology/Apply principles of basic laboratory procedures/RBC/Osmotic fragility/2

14. What effect would using buffer at pH 6.0 have on a wright-stained smear?
A. Red cells would be stained too pink.
B. White cell cytoplasm would be stained too blue.
C. Red cells would be stained too blue.
D. Red cells would lyse on the slide.

Hematology/Evaluate laboratory data to recognize problems/Microscopic morphology/Stain/2

15. Which of the following erythrocyte inclusions *can* be visualized with supravital stain, but *cannot* be detected on a Wright's stained blood smear?
A. Basophilic stippling
B. Heinz bodies
C. Howell-Jolly bodies
D. Siderotic granules

Hematology/Apply principles of basic laboratory procedures/Microscopic morphology/RBC inclusions/2

16. A falsely elevated hematocrit is obtained using a defective centrifuge. Which of the following *calculated* values will *not* be affected?
A. MCV
B. MCH
C. MCHC
D. Red cell distribution width (RDW)

Hematology/Evaluate sources of error/Microhematocrit/2

17. A Miller disc is an ocular device used to facilitate counting of:
A. Platelets
B. Reticulocytes

C. Sickle cells
D. Nucleated red blood cells (NRBCs)

Hematology/Apply knowledge of standard operating procedures/Reticulocytes/1

Answers to Questions 11–17

11. **D** Eosinophils migrate to sites where there is an allergic reaction or parasitic infestation, releasing peroxidase, pyrogens, and other enzymes including an oxidase that neutralizes histamine. They are poorly phagocytic and do not release lysozyme. Neutrophils are highly phagocytic and release lysozymes, peroxidase, and pyrogenic proteins.

12. **B** In anemic states the reticulocyte percentage is not a true measure of reticulocyte production. The following formula must be applied to calculate the corrected (for anemia) reticulocyte count. Corrected reticulocyte count = reticulocytes (%) $\times$ Hct $\div$ 45, the average normal Hct. In this case, $7 \times (20 \div 45) = 3.1$.

13. **A** Spherocytes are a prominent feature of hereditary spherocytosis (HS), hemolytic disease of the newborn, and acquired hemolytic anemia. The osmotic fragility test is increased in the presence of spherocytes, whereas this test is decreased when sickle cells, target cells, and other poikilocytes are present.

14. **A** The pH of the buffer is critical in Romanowsky's stains. When the pH is too low (<6.4), the red cells take up more acid dye (eosin), becoming too pink. Leukocytes will also show poor nuclear detail when the pH is decreased.

15. **B** Heinz bodies are irregular, refractile, purple inclusions that are not visible with Wright's stain but show up with supravital staining. The other three inclusions can be detected with Wright's stain.

16. **B** The MCV = Hct $\times$ 10/RBC count, and MCHC = Hgb $\times$ 100/Hct; therefore, an erroneous hematocrit will affect these parameters. The MCH = Hgb $\times$ 10/RBC count and is not affected by the hematocrit. Centrifugal force for microhematocrit determination should be 12,000 g for 5 minutes in order to avoid error caused by trapped plasma. The RDW is a Coulter counter parameter that reflects the variance in the size of the red cells.

17. **B** The traditional reticulocyte count involves the counting of 1000 RBCs. The Miller disc is a reticle that is placed in the ocular and divides the field into two squares, one being nine times larger in size than the other. Reticulocytes are enumerated in both the squares as the red cells are counted in the smaller one.

18. **SITUATION:** Cell indices obtained on a patient are as follows: MCV 88 μm^3 (fL); MCH 30 pg; MCHC 34% (.340). The RBCs on the peripheral smear would appear:
    A. Hypochromic, microcytic
    B. Normochromic, microcytic
    C. Normochromic, normocytic
    D. Hypochromic, normocytic

    Hematology/Evaluate laboratory data to recognize health and disease states/RBC Indices/2

19. All of the following factors may influence the erythrocyte sedimentation rate (ESR) *except:*
    A. Blood drawn in a sodium citrate tube
    B. Anisocytosis, poikilocytosis
    C. Plasma proteins
    D. Caliber of the tube

    Hematology/Apply principles of basic laboratory procedures/ESR/2

20. What staining method is used most frequently to stain and count reticulocytes?
    A. Immunofluorescence
    B. Supravital staining
    C. Romanowsky staining
    D. Cytochemical staining

    Hematology/Apply knowledge of standard operating procedures/Reticulocytes/1

21. The Coulter principle for counting of cells is based upon the fact that:
    A. Isotonic solutions conduct electricity better than cells do.
    B. Conductivity varies proportionally to the number of cells.
    C. Cells conduct electricity better than saline does.
    D. Isotonic solutions cannot conduct electricity.

    Hematology/Apply principles of basic laboratory procedures/Instrumentation/Cell counter/2

22. A correction is necessary for WBC counts when nucleated RBCs are seen on the peripheral smear because:
    A. The WBC count should be higher.
    B. The RBC count is too low.
    C. Nucleated RBCs are counted as leukocytes.
    D. Nucleated RBCs are confused with giant platelets.

    Hematology/Evaluate laboratory data to take corrective action according to predetermined criteria/Leukocytes/2

23. Using a Coulter counter analyzer, an increased RDW should correlate with:
    A. Spherocytosis
    B. Anisocytosis
    C. Leukocytosis
    D. Presence of NRBCs

Hematology/Correlate laboratory data with other laboratory data to assess test results/RBC Microscopic morphology/2

24. Given the following values, which set of red blood cell indices suggests spherocytosis?
    A. MCV 76 μm^3 MCH 19.9 pg   MCHC 28.5%
    B. MCV 90 μm^3 MCH 30.5 pg   MCHC 32.5%
    C. MCV 80 μm^3 MCH 36.5 pg   MCHC 39.0%
    D. MCV 81 μm^3 MCH 29.0 pg   MCHC 34.8%

    Hematology/Evaluate laboratory data to recognize health and disease states/RBC Indices/3

Answers to Questions 18–24

18. **C** The MCV, MCH, and MCHC are all within the reference interval (normal range); hence, the erythrocytes should be of normal size and should reflect normal concentrations of Hgb.

19. **A** EDTA and sodium citrate can be used without any effect on the ESR. Anisocytosis and poikilocytosis may impede rouleaux formation, thus causing a low ESR. Plasma proteins, especially fibrinogen and immunoglobulins enhance rouleaux, increasing the ESR. Reference ranges must be established for different caliber tubes.

20. **B** The reticulum within the reticulocytes consists of ribonucleic acid (RNA), which cannot be stained with Wright's stain. Supravital staining with new methylene blue is used to identify the reticulocytes.

21. **A** Coulter cell counters use the principle of electrical impedance. Two electrodes suspended in isotonic solutions are separated by a glass tube having a small aperture. A vacuum is applied, and as a cell passes through the aperture it impedes the flow of current and generates a voltage pulse.

22. **C** The automated hematology analyzers enumerate all nucleated cells. NRBCs are counted along with WBCs, falsely elevating the WBC count. To correct the WBC count, determine the number of NRBCs per 100 WBCs. Corrected WBC count =
$$\frac{\text{WBC count} \times 100}{100 + \# \text{NRBCs}}.$$

23. **B** The Coulter counter's RDW parameter correlates with the degree of anisocytosis seen on the morphologic examination. The reference range is 11.5%–14.5%.

24. **C** Spherocytes have a decreased cell diameter and volume, which results in loss of central pallor and discoid shape. The index most affected is the MCHC, usually being in excess of 36%.

25. Which of the following statistical terms reflects the best index of precision?
A. Mean
B. Median
C. Coefficient of variation
D. Standard deviation

Hematology/Correlate laboratory data with other laboratory data to assess test results/QC/Statistics/3

26. Which of the following is considered a normal hemoglobin?
A. Carboxyhemoglobin
B. Methemoglobin
C. Sulfhemoglobin
D. Deoxyhemoglobin

Hematology/Apply knowledge of fundamental biological characteristics/Hemoglobin/1

27. Which condition will shift the oxyhemoglobin dissociation curve to the right?
A. Acidosis
B. Alkalosis
C. Multiple blood transfusions
D. Hgb Kansas

Hematology/Correlate laboratory data with other laboratory data to assess test results/RBC/Metabolism/2

28. What is the major type of leukocyte seen in the peripheral smear of a patient with aplastic anemia?
A. Segmented neutrophil
B. Lymphocyte
C. Monocyte
D. Eosinophil

Hematology/Correlate clinical and laboratory data/Leukocyte/Aplastic anemia/1

29. What is the normal WBC differential lymphocyte percentage (range) in the adult population?
A. 20%–50%
B. 10%–20%
C. 5%–10%
D. 50%–70%

Hematology/Correlate basic lab values/Differentials/1

30. In which age group would 60% lymphocytes be a normal finding?
A. 40–60 years
B. 11–15 years
C. 6 months–2 years
D. 4–6 years

Hematology/Evaluate laboratory data/Differentials/2

31. Which of the following results on an automated differential suggests that a peripheral smear should be reviewed manually?

A. Segs = 70%
B. Band = 10%
C. Mono = 15%
D. Eos = 2%

Hematology/Correlate lab data/Instrumentation/2

Answers to Questions 25–31

25. **C** *Standard deviation (s)* describes the distribution of a sample of observations. It depends upon both the mean (average value) and dispersion of results and is most influenced by reproducibility or precision. Because *s* is influenced by the mean and expressed as a percentage of the mean, the coefficient of variation $\left(\dfrac{s}{\text{mean}} \times 100\right)$ can be used to compare precision of tests with different means (e.g., WBC and RBC count or low vs. high controls).

26. **D** Deoxyhemoglobin is the physiological Hgb that results from the unloading of oxygen by Hgb. This is accompanied by the widening of the space between β chains and the binding of 2,3-diphosphoglycerate (2,3-DPG) on a mole-for-mole basis.

27. **A** Acidosis is associated with a shift to the right of the oxyhemoglobin dissociation curve and, therefore, increased oxygen release (decreased affinity of Hgb for oxygen). The other three conditions will result in a left-shifted oxyhemoglobin curve.

28. **B** The bone marrow in aplastic anemia is spotty with patches of normal cellularity. Absolute granulocytopenia is usually present; however, lymphocyte production is less affected. Consequently, lymphocytes constitute the majority of the nucleated cells seen.

29. **A** The normal adult percentage of lymphocytes in a white cell differential is between 20% and 50%. This range is higher in the pediatric population.

30. **C** There is a relative neutropenia in children from age 4 months–4 years of age. Because of this, the percentage of lymphocytes is increased in this population. This is commonly referred to as a reversal in the normal differential percentage (or inverted differential).

31. **C** A relative monocyte count of 15% is abnormal, given that the baseline monocyte count in a normal differential is between 1% and 8%. An increased monocyte count may signal a myeloproliferative process such an chronic myelomonocytic leukemia, an inflammatory response, or abnormal lymphocytes that may have been counted as monocytes by an automated cell counter.

32. In which stage of erythrocytic maturation does Hgb formation *begin*?
A. Reticulocyte
B. Pronormoblast
C. Basophilic normoblast
D. Polychromatic normoblast

Hematology/Apply knowledge of fundamental biological characteristic/Microscopic morphology/1

33. The binding and dissociation of oxygen are monitored by the oxygen dissociation (OD) curve. When a hypoxic condition exists, which two of the following conditions are ideal for increased oxygen delivery?
A. 2,3-DPG is ($\downarrow$) OD curve shifts right.
B. 2,3-DPG is ($\uparrow$) OD curve shifts left.
C. 2,3-DPG is ($\uparrow$) OD curve shifts right.
D. 2,3-DPG is ($\downarrow$) OD curve shifts left.

Hematology/ Evaluate lab data to recognize health and disease states/O_2 Dissociation curve/3

34. Which of the following Hgb configurations is characteristic of Hgb H?
A. γ_4
B. $\alpha_2\text{-}\gamma_2$
C. β_4
D. $\alpha_2\text{-}\beta_2$

Hematology/Apply knowledge of fundamental biological characteristics/Hemoglobin/2

35. What is the most likely explanation of the following results from an EDTA sample?

WBCs $4.9 \times 10^3/\mu$L	Hgb 12.2 g/dL	MCV 113 μm^3
(4.9×10^9/L)	(122 g/L)	(fL)
RBCs $2.80 \times 10^6/\mu$L	Hct 31.5%	MCH 43.6 pg
(2.80×10^{12}/L)	(0.315)	MCHC 38.7%
		(.387)

A. Macrocytic anemia
B. High reticulocyte count

C. Hereditary spherocytosis
D. High titer of cold agglutinins

Hematology/Correlate laboratory data with other laboratory data to assess test results/CBC/3

Answers to Questions 32–35

32. D In normal erythrocytic maturation, Hgb formation begins in the polychromatic normoblast and is seen as a pink coloration of the cytoplasm. The red cell is programmed for the sequential development of a full complement of Hgb by the time the precursor cells lose their nucleus and become the mature red cell.

33. C At a basal metabolic rate, there is an equilibrium between oxygen delivery and use. As conditions of anemia develop, the body attempts to compensate by shifting the OD curve, thereby making fewer cells more efficient. This is accompanied by an increased level of 2,3-DPG—the molecule that controls hemoglobin's affinity for oxygen.

34. C The structure of Hgb H is β_4. Hgb H disease is a severe clinical expression of α thalassemia in which only one α gene out of four is functioning.

35. D Autoagglutination at room temperature may cause a low RBC count and high MCV from an electronic counter. The hematocrit will be low because it is calculated from the RBC count. Low RBC count and hematocrit cause falsely high calculations of MCH and MCHC.

Normocytic/Normochromic Anemias

1. Hypersplenism is characterized by:
   A. Polycythemia
   B. Pancytosis
   C. Leukopenia
   D. Myelodysplasia

   Hematology/Correlate clinical and laboratory data/ WBC/Hypersplenism/2

2. Which organ removes erythrocyte inclusions without destroying the cell?
   A. Liver
   B. Spleen
   C. Kidney
   D. Lymph nodes

   Hematology/Apply knowledge of fundamental biological characteristics/Physiology/1

3. Spherocytes differ from normal red cells in all of the following *except:*
   A. Decreased surface to volume
   B. Decreased central pallor
   C. Decreased resistance to hypotonic saline
   D. Increased deformability

   Hematology/Apply knowledge of fundamental biological characteristics/RBC microscopic morphology/2

4. Which of the following is *not* associated with hereditary spherocytosis?
   A. Increased osmotic fragility
   B. An MCHC greater than 36%
   C. Intravascular hemolysis
   D. Extravascular hemolysis

   Hematology/Correlate clinical and laboratory data/Hereditary spherocytosis/2

5. Osmotic fragility and autohemolysis tests are performed on a patient with hereditary spherocytosis. Which of the following results is most likely?
   A. Initial hemolysis at 0.35% NaCl—complete hemolysis at 0.20% NaCl
   B. Initial hemolysis at 0.45% NaCl—complete hemolysis at 0.35% NaCl
   C. Initial hemolysis at 0.60% NaCl—complete hemolysis at 0.55% NaCl
   D. Initial hemolysis at 0.65% NaCl—complete hemolysis at 0.45% NaCl

   Hematology/Evaluate laboratory data to recognize health and disease states/Special test/Osmotic fragility/2

Answers to Questions 1–5

1. **C** Hypersplenic conditions are generally described by the following four criteria: (1) cytopenias of one or more peripheral cell lines; (2) splenomegaly; (3) bone marrow hyperplasia; (4) resolution of cytopenia by splenectomy.

2. **B** The spleen is the supreme filter of the body, pitting imperfections from the erythrocyte without destroying the integrity of the membrane.

3. **D** Spherocytes lose their deformability due to the defect in spectrin, a membrane protein, and are therefore prone to splenic sequestration and hemolysis.

4. **C** Classic features of intravascular hemolysis such as hemoglobinemia, hemoglobinuria, or hemosiderinuria do not occur in hereditary spherocytosis. The hemolysis seen in hereditary spherocytosis is an extravascular rather than an intravascular process.

5. **D** Spherocytic cells have decreased tolerance to swelling and, therefore, hemolyze at a higher concentration of sodium salt as compared to normal red cells.

6. The anemia seen in sickle cell disease is usually:
   A. Microcytic, normochromic
   B. Microcytic, hypochromic
   C. Normocytic, normochromic
   D. Normocytic, hypochromic

Hematology/Apply knowledge of fundamental biological characteristics/RBC microscopic morphology/Hemoglobinopathy/1

7. Which is the major Hgb found in the RBCs of patients with sickle cell trait?
   A. Hgb S
   B. Hgb F
   C. Hgb A_2
   D. Hgb A

Hematology/Apply knowledge of fundamental biological characteristics/Anemia/ Hemoglobinopathy/1

8. Select the amino acid substitution that is responsible for sickle cell anemia.
   A. Lysine is substituted for glutamic acid at the sixth position of the α chain.
   B. Valine is substituted for glutamic acid at the sixth position of the β chain.
   C. Valine is substituted for glutamic acid at the sixth position of the α chain.
   D. Glutamine is substituted for glutamic acid at the sixth position of the β chain.

Hematology/Apply knowledge of fundamental biological characteristics/Hemoglobinopathy/1

9. All of the following are usually found in Hgb C disease *except:*
   A. Hgb C crystals
   B. Target cells
   C. Lysine substituted for glutamic acid at the sixth position of the β chain
   D. Fast mobility of Hgb C at pH 8.6

Hematology/Apply knowledge of fundamental biological characteristics/Anemia/ Hemoglobinopathy/1

10. Which of the following hemoglobins migrates to the same position as Hgb A_2 at pH 8.6?
   A. Hgb H
   B. Hgb F
   C. Hgb E
   D. Hgb S

Hematology/Correlate clinical and laboratory data/Hemoglobin electrophoresis/1

11. Which of the following electrophoretic results is consistent with a diagnosis of sickle cell trait?
   A. Hgb A: 40%   Hgb S: 35%   Hgb F: 5%
   B. Hgb A: 60%   Hgb S: 38%   Hgb A_2: 2%
   C. Hgb A: 0%   Hgb A_2: 5%   Hgb F: 95%
   D. Hgb A: 80%   Hgb S: 10%   Hgb A_2: 10%

Hematology/Evaluate laboratory data to recognize health and disease/Special test/Electrophoresis/2

12. In which of the following conditions will autosplenectomy most likely occur?
   A. Thalassemia major
   B. Hgb C disease
   C. Hgb SC disease
   D. Sickle cell disease

Hematology/Apply knowledge of fundamental biological characteristics/Anemia/ Hemoglobinopathy/1

13. Which of the following is most true of paroxysmal nocturnal hemoglobinuria (PNH)?
   A. It is an acquired hemolytic anemia.
   B. It is inherited as a sex-linked trait.
   C. It is inherited as an autosomal dominant trait.
   D. It is inherited as an autosomal recessive trait.

Hematology/Apply knowledge of fundamental biological characteristics/PNH/1

Answers to Questions 6–13

6. **C** Sickle cell disease is a chronic hemolytic anemia classified as a normocytic, normochromic anemia.

7. **D** The major hemoglobin in sickle cell trait is Hgb A, which comprises 50%–70% of the total. Hgb S comprises 20%–40%, and Hgb A_2 and Hgb F are present in normal amounts.

8. **B** The structural mutation for Hgb S is the substitution of valine for glutamic acid at the sixth position of the β chain. Because glutamic acid is negatively charged, this decreases its rate of migration toward the anode at pH 8.6.

9. **D** Substitution of a positively charged amino acid for a negatively charged amino acid in Hgb C disease results in a slow electrophoretic mobility at pH 8.6.

10. **C** At pH 8.6, several hemoglobins migrate together. These include Hgb A_2, Hgb C, Hgb E, Hgb O, and Hgb C_{Harlem}, which are located nearest the cathode.

11. **B** Electrophoresis at alkaline pH usually shows 50%–70% Hgb A, 20%–40% Hgb S, and normal levels of Hgb A_2 in a patient with the sickle cell trait.

12. **D** Autosplenectomy occurs in sickle cell anemia due to repeated infarcts to the spleen as a result of the overwhelming sickling phenomenon.

13. **A** PNH is an acquired hemolytic anemia with an insidious onset, resulting in a chronic hemolytic state. It most often occurs in middle-aged adults.

14. Hemolytic uremic syndrome(HUS) is characterized by all of the following *except:*
A. Hemorrhage
B. Thrombocytopenia
C. Hemoglobinuria
D. Reticulocytopenia

Hematology/Correlate clinical and laboratory data/HUS/2

15. An autohemolysis test is positive in all the following *except:*
A. Glucose-6-phosphate dehydrogenase (G-6-PD) deficiency
B. HS
C. Pyruvate kinase (PK) deficiency
D. PNH

Hematology/Correlate clinical and laboratory tests/ Special test/2

16. Which antibody is associated with paroxysmal cold hemoglobinuria (PCH)?
A. Anti-I antibody
B. Anti-i antibody
C. Anti-M antibody
D. Anti-P antibody

Hematology/Apply knowledge of fundamental biological characteristics/Anemia/PCH/1

17. All of the following are associated with hemolytic anemia *except:*
A. Methemoglobinemia
B. Hemoglobinuria
C. Hemoglobinemia
D. Increased haptoglobin

Hematology/Correlate clinical and laboratory data/Anemia/Hemolytic/2

18. Autoimmune hemolytic anemia is best characterized by which of the following?
A. Rouleaux formation
B. Spherocytes
C. Stomatocytes
D. Helmet cells

Hematology/Correlate clinical and laboratory data/Anemia/Hemolytic/2

19. "Bite cells" are usually seen in patients with:
A. Rh null trait
B. Chronic granulomatous disease
C. G-6-PD deficiency
D. PK deficiency

Hematology/Correlate clinical and laboratory data/RBC microscopic morphology/1

20. The morphologic classification of anemias is based on which of the following?
A. M:E (myeloid:erythroid) ratio
B. Prussian blue stain
C. RBC indices
D. Reticulocyte count

Hematology/Correlate clinical and laboratory disease/RBC microscopic morphology/1

21. Which of the following is a common finding in aplastic anemia?
A. A monoclonal disorder
B. Tumor infiltration
C. Peripheral blood pancytopenia
D. Defective DNA synthesis

Hematology/Apply knowledge of fundamental biological characteristics/Aplastic anemia/1

Answers to Questions 14–21

14. **D** The anemia seen in HUS is multifactorial, with characteristic schistocytes and polychromasia commensurate with the anemia.

15. **D** The autohemolysis test is positive in G-6-PD and PK deficiencies and in HS but is normal in PNH because lysis in PNH requires sucrose to enhance complement binding. Addition of glucose, sucrose, or adenosine triphosphate (ATP) corrects the autohemolysis of HS. Autohemolysis of PK can be corrected by ATP.

16. **D** PCH is caused by the anti-P antibody, a cold autoantibody that binds to the patient's RBCs at low temperatures and fixes complement. In the classic Donath-Landsteiner test, hemolysis will be demonstrated in a sample placed at 4°C that is then warmed to 37°C.

17. **D** Haptoglobin is a protein that binds to free Hgb. The increased free Hgb in intravascular hemolysis will cause depletion of haptoglobin.

18. **B** In autoimmune hemolytic anemias, production of autoantibodies against one's own red cells will cause hemolysis or phagocytic destruction of RBCs. A positive direct antiglobulin (DAT or Coomb's) test identifies *in vivo* antibody-coated red cells.

19. **C** In patients with G-6-PD deficiency the red cells are unable to reduce nicotinamide adenine dinucleotide phosphate (NADP) to NADPH; consequently, Hgb is denatured and Heinz bodies are formed. "Bite cells" appear in the peripheral circulation as a result of splenic pitting of Heinz bodies.

20. **C** Anemias can be classified morphologically by the use of laboratory data, physiologically, and clinically based upon an assessment of symptoms. RBC indices are critical in assessing an anemia morphologically.

21. **C** Aplastic anemia has many causes, such as chemical, drug, or radiation poisoning; congenital aplasia; and Fanconi's syndrome. All result in depletion of hematopoietic precursors of all cell lines, leading to peripheral blood pancytopenia.

22. Congenital dyserythropoietic anemias (CDAs) are characterized by:
A. Bizarre multinucleated erythroblasts
B. Cytogenetic disorders
C. Megaloblastic erythropoiesis
D. Elevated M:E ratio

Hematology/Apply knowledge of fundamental biological characteristics/Anemia/Characteristics/2

23. Microangiopathic hemolytic anemia is characterized by:
A. Target cells and Cabot rings
B. Toxic granulation and Döhle bodies
C. Pappenheimer bodies and basophilic stippling
D. Schistocytes and nucleated red blood cells

Hematology/Correlate clinical and laboratory data/RBC microscopic morphology/Anemia/2

24. Which antibiotic is most often implicated in the development of aplastic anemia?
A. Sulfonamides
B. Penicillin
C. Tetracycline
D. Chloramphenicol

Hematology/Correlate clinical and laboratory data/Aplastic anemia/1

25. Sickle cell disorders are:
A. Hereditary, intracorpuscular RBC defects
B. Hereditary, extracorpuscular RBC defects
C. Acquired, intracorpuscular RBC defects
D. Acquired, extracorpuscular RBC defects

Hematology/Apply knowledge of fundamental biological concepts/2

26. Which of the following conditions may produce spherocytes in a peripheral smear?
A. Pelger-Huët anomaly
B. Pernicious anemia
C. Autoimmune hemolytic anemia
D. Sideroblastic anemia

Hematology/ Evaluate lab data to recognize health and disease states/Morphology/3

27. A patient's peripheral smear reveals numerous NRBCs, marked variation of red cell morphology, and pronounced polychromasia. In addition to a decreased Hgb and hematocrit values, what other CBC parameters may be anticipated?
A. Reduced platelets
B. Increased MCHC
C. Increased MCV
D. Decreased RDW

Hematology/Correlate lab data with clinical picture/Complete blood count/2

28. What red cell inclusion may be seen in the peripheral blood smear of a patient post-splenectomy?

A. Toxic granulation
B. Howell-Jolly bodies
C. Malarial parasites
D. Siderotic granules

Hematology/ Correlate clinical lab data/ Inclusions/1

Answers to Questions 22–28

22. **A** There are four classifications of CDAs, each characterized by ineffective erythropoiesis, increased unconjugated bilirubin, and bizarre multinucleated erythroid precursors.

23. **D** Microangiopathic hemolytic anemia is a condition resulting from shear stress to the erythrocytes. Fibrin strands are laid down within the microcirculation, and red cells become fragmented as they contact fibrin through the circulation process.

24. **D** Chloramphenicol is the drug most often implicated in acquired aplastic anemia. About half of the cases occur within 30 days after therapy and about half of the cases are reversible. Penicillin, tetracycline, and sulfonamides have been implicated in a small number of cases.

25. **A** Sickle cell disorders are intracorpuscular red cell defects that are hereditary and result in defective Hgb being produced. The gene for sickle cell can be inherited either homozygously or heterozygously.

26. **C** Spherocytes may be produced by one of three mechanisms. First, spherocytes are a natural morphologic phase of normal red cell senescence. Secondly, spherocytes are produced when the cell surface-to-volume ratio is decreased as seen in hereditary spherocytosis. And lastly, spherocytes may be produced as a result of antibody coating of the red cells. As the antibody-coated red cells travel through the spleen, the antibodies and portions of the red cell membrane are removed by macrophages. The membrane repairs itself, hence the red cell's morphology changes from a biconcave disk to a spherocyte.

27. **C** This patient's abnormal peripheral smear indicates marked red cell regeneration. Because so many reticulocytes were being released from the marrow, and reticulocytes are larger than the normal RBCs, the MCV will be slightly elevated.

28. **B** One of the main functions of the spleen is the pitting function, which allows inclusions to be removed from the red cell without destroying the cell membrane. As a result of splenectomy, Howell-Jolly bodies may be seen in great numbers.

29. Reticulocytosis usually indicates:
   A. Response to inflammation
   B. Neoplastic process
   C. Aplastic anemia
   D. Red cell regeneration

Hematology/ Correlate lab data for clinical condition/Morphology/2

30. Hereditary pyropoikilocytosis (HP) is a red cell membrane defect characterized by:
   A. Increased pencil-shaped cells
   B. Increased oval macrocytes
   C. Misshapen budding fragmented cells
   D. Bite cells

Hematology/Evaluate lab data to recognize health and disease states/Red cell membrane/1

Answers to Questions 29–30

29. **D** The bone marrow's appropriate response to anemia is to deliver red cells prematurely to the peripheral circulation. In this way, reticulocytes and possibly nucleated red cells may be seen in the peripheral smear. Reticulocytes are polychromatophilic macrocytes, and the presence of reticulocytes will indicate red cell regeneration.

30. **C** HP is a membrane defect characterized by a spectrin abnormality and thermal instability. The MCV is decreased and the red cells appear to be budding and fragmented.

Hypochromic/Microcytic Anemias

1. The osmotic fragility test result in a patient with thalassemia major would most likely be:
   A. Increased
   B. Decreased
   C. Normal
   D. Decreased after incubation at 37°C

   Hematology/Correlate clinical and laboratory data/Microscopic morphology/Osmotic fragility/1

2. All of the following are characteristic findings in a patient with iron deficiency anemia *except:*
   A. Microcytic, hypochromic red cell morphology
   B. Elevated platelet count along with small platelets
   C. Decreased total iron-binding capacity (TIBC)
   D. Increased RBC protoporphyrin

   Hematology/Correlate clinical and laboratory data/Anemia/Iron deficiency/2

3. Iron deficiency anemia may be distinguished from anemia of chronic infection by:
   A. Serum iron level
   B. Red cell morphology
   C. Red cell indices
   D. Total iron-binding capacity

   Hematology/Evaluate laboratory data to recognize health and disease states/Anemia/3

4. Which anemia has red cell morphology similar to that seen in iron deficiency anemia?
   A. Sickle cell anemia
   B. Thalassemia syndrome
   C. Pernicious anemia
   D. Hereditary spherocytosis

   Hematology/Correlate laboratory data with other laboratory data to assess test results/Anemia/RBC microscopic morphology/2

5. Iron deficiency anemia is characterized by:
   A. Decreased plasma iron, decreased % saturation, increased TIBC

   B. Decreased plasma iron, decreased plasma ferritin, normal RBC porphyrin
   C. Decreased plasma iron, decreased % saturation, decreased TIBC
   D. Decreased plasma iron, increased % saturation, decreased TIBC

   Hematology/Evaluate laboratory data to recognize health and disease states/Anemia/Iron deficiency/2

Answers to Questions 1–5

1. **B** Numerous target cells are present in thalassemia major patients. Because target cells have increased surface volume, the osmotic fragility is decreased.

2. **C** Morphologic characteristics of iron deficiency anemia include a microcytic, hypochromic blood picture. Platelets are usually small and increased in number. There is an increase in TIBC and in RBC protoporphyrin due to a decreased level of iron.

3. **D** In iron deficiency anemia, the serum iron is decreased and the total iron-binding capacity is increased. In chronic disease the iron is trapped in reticuloendothelial (RE) cells and therefore is unavailable to the red cells. Serum iron and TIBC are both decreased.

4. **B** Iron deficiency anemia and thalassemia are both classified as microcytic, hypochromic anemias. Iron deficiency anemia is caused by defective heme synthesis, whereas thalassemia is caused by decreased globin chain synthesis.

5. **A** Iron deficiency occurs in three phases: iron depletion, iron deficient erythropoiesis, and iron deficiency anemia. The latter is characterized by decreased plasma iron, increased TIBC, decreased % saturation, and microcytic, hypochromic anemia.

6. Storage iron is usually best determined by:
   A. Serum transferrin levels
   B. Hgb values
   C. Myoglobin values
   D. Serum ferritin levels

   Hematology/Apply knowledge of basic laboratory procedures/Iron/1

7. All of the following are associated with sideroblastic anemia *except:*
   A. Increased serum iron
   B. Ringed sideroblasts
   C. Dimorphic blood picture
   D. Increased RBC protoporphyrin

   Hematology/Evaluate laboratory data to recognize health and disease states/Anemia/Sideroblastic/2

8. What is the basic hematologic defect seen in patients with thalassemia major?
   A. DNA synthetic defect
   B. Hgb structure
   C. β Chain synthesis
   D. Hgb phosphorylation

   Hematology/Apply knowledge of fundamental biological characteristics/Hemoglobinopathy/1

9. Which of the following is the primary Hgb in patients with thalassemia major?
   A. Hgb D
   B. Hgb A
   C. Hgb C
   D. Hgb F

   Hematology/Correlate clinical and laboratory disease/Hemoglobin/Hemoglobinopathy/1

10. Skeletal abnormalities and marrow hypertrophy are present in thalassemia major patients due to:
   A. Depletion of calcium
   B. Unbalanced globin chain production
   C. Erythropoietin deficiency
   D. Hypersplenism

   Hematology/Evaluate laboratory data to recognize health and disease states/Hemoglobinopathy/Characteristics/3

11. In which of the following conditions is Hgb A_2 elevated?
   A. Hgb H
   B. Hgb SC disease
   C. β-Thalassemia minor
   D. Hgb S trait

   Hematology/Correlate lab results with disease state/2

12. Which of the following parameters may be similar for the anemia of inflammation and iron deficiency anemia?
   A. Normocytic indices
   B. Decreased serum iron
   C. Ringed sideroblasts
   D. Pappenheimer bodies

   Hematology/Correlate lab data to recognize health and disease states/2

Answers to Questions 6–12

6. **D** Ferritin enters the serum from all ferritin-producing tissues and therefore is considered to be a good indicator of body storage iron. Because iron stores must be depleted before anemia develops, low serum ferritin precedes the fall in serum iron associated with iron deficiency anemia.

7. **D** The defect in sideroblastic anemia involves ineffective erythropoiesis. The failure to produce RBC protoporphyrin occurs because the nonheme iron is trapped in the mitochondria and is unavailable to be recycled. This leads to decreased red cell protoporphyrin.

8. **C** In thalassemia major there is little or no production of the β chain, resulting in severely depressed synthesis of Hgb A. Severe anemia is seen, along with skeletal abnormalities, and marked splenomegaly. The patient is usually supported with transfusion therapy.

9. **D** Patients with thalassemia major are unable to synthesize the β chain; hence little or no Hgb A is produced. However, γ chains continue to be synthesized and lead to variable elevations of Hgb F in these patients.

10. **B** Unbalanced chain production in thalassemia major leads to excess, unpaired α chains. These chains will precipitate in immature erythroid cells, causing ineffective erythropoiesis and/or hemolysis. In compensation, the bone marrow will be chronically overactive resulting in skeletal abnormalities.

11. **C** Hgb A_2 is part of the normal complement of adult Hgb. This Hgb is elevated in β-thalassemia minor because the individual with this condition has only one normal β gene; consequently, there is a slight elevation of Hgb A_2 and Hgb F.

12. **B** Thirty to fifty percent of the individuals with the anemia of chronic inflammation demonstrate a microcytic hypochromic blood picture with decreased serum iron. Serum iron is decreased because it is unable to escape from the RE cells to be delivered to the pronormoblast in the bone marrow.

Macrocytic/Normochromic Anemias

1. Which morphologic classification is characteristic of megaloblastic anemia?
A. Normocytic, normochromic
B. Microcytic, normochromic
C. Macrocytic, hypochromic
D. Macrocytic, normochromic

Hematology/Correlate clinical and laboratory data/Microscopic morphology/RBC/2

2. A Schilling test gives the following results: Part I: 2% excretion of radioactive vitamin B_{12} (normal = 5%–35%); Part II: 8% excretion of radioactive B_{12} after intrinsic factor was given with vitamin B_{12} (normal = 7%–10%). These results indicate:
A. Tropical sprue
B. Transcobalamin deficiency
C. Blind loop syndrome
D. Pernicious anemia

Hematology/Evaluate laboratory data to recognize health and disease states/Special test/3

3. All of the following are characteristics of megaloblastic anemia *except:*
A. Pancytopenia
B. Elevated reticulocyte count
C. Hypersegmented neutrophils
D. Macrocytic erythrocyte indices

Hematology/Correlate clinical and laboratory data/Anemia/Megaloblastic/2

4. A patient with a vitamin B_{12} anemia is given a high dosage of folate. Which of the following is expected as a result of this treatment?
A. An improvement in neurological problems
B. An improvement in hematologic abnormalities

C. No expected improvement
D. Toxicity of the liver and kidneys

Hematology/Select course of action/Anemia/Therapy/2

Answers to Questions 1–4

1. **D** Megaloblastic anemias are a group of asynchronized anemias characterized by defective nuclear maturation due to defective deoxyribonucleic acid (DNA) synthesis. This abnormality accounts for the megaloblastic features in the bone marrow and the macrocytosis in the peripheral blood. These anemias are normochromic because there is no defect in the Hgb synthesis.

2. **D** Pernicious anemia is caused by a lack of intrinsic factor, which prevents vitamin B_{12} absorption. An abnormal excretion in Part I indicates that B_{12} was not absorbed through the intestine. Normal excretion of labeled B_{12} after administration of intrinsic factor in Part II of the Schilling test indicates pernicious anemia.

3. **B** Megaloblastic anemias are associated with an ineffective erythropoiesis and therefore a decrease in the reticulocyte count.

4. **B** Administration of folic acid to a patient with vitamin B_{12} deficiency will improve the hematologic abnormalities; however, the neurological problems will continue. This will help confirm the correct diagnosis of B_{12} deficiency.

5. Which of the disorders below causes ineffective erythropoiesis?
A. G-6-PD deficiency
B. Liver disease
C. Hgb C disease
D. Pernicious anemia

Hematology/Evaluate laboratory data to recognize health and disease states/RBC physiology/2

6. A 50-year-old patient is suffering from pernicious anemia. Which of the following laboratory data are most likely on this patient?

WBC	PLT
A. 12,500/μL(12.5 × 10⁹/L)	250,000/μL(250 × 10⁹/L)
B. 6,500/μL(6.5 × 10⁹/L)	80,000/μL(80 × 10⁹/L)
C. 5,000/μL(5.0 × 10⁹/L)	750,000/μL(750 × 10⁹/L)
D. 2,500/μL(2.5 × 10⁹/L)	50,000/μL(50 × 10⁹/L)

Hematology/Correlate clinical and laboratory data/Microscopic morphology/RBC/2

7. Which of the following may be seen in the peripheral blood smear of a patient with obstructive liver disease?
A. Schistocytes
B. Macrocytes
C. Howell-Jolly bodies
D. Microcytes

Hematology/Apply principles of basic laboratory procedures/Microscopic morphology/1

8. The macrocytes typically seen in megaloblastic processes are:
A. Crescent-shaped
B. Teardrop-shaped
C. Ovalocytic
D. Pencil-shaped

Hematology/Apply principles of basic laboratory procedures/Microscopic morphology/Differential/1

9. Which of the following are most characteristic of the red cell indices associated with megaloblastic anemias?
A. MCV 99 fl, MCH 28 pg, MCHC 31%
B. MCV 62 fL, MCH 27 pg, MCHC 30%
C. MCV 125 fL, MCH 36 pg, MCHC 34%
D. MCV 78 fL, MCH 23 pg, MCHC 30%

Hematology/Correlate clinical and laboratory data/Megaloblastic anemia/2

10. A patient has 80 nucleated red cells per 100 leukocytes. In additon to increased polychromasia on the peripheral smear, what other finding may be present on the CBC?

A. Increased platelets
B. Increased MCV
C. Increased hematocrit
D. Increased red cell count

Hematolology/Correlate clinical and laboratory data/Megaloblastic anemia/2

Answers to Questions 5–10

5. **D** Ineffective erythropoiesis is caused by destruction of erythroid precursor cells prior to their release from the bone marrow. Pernicious anemia results from defective DNA synthesis; it is suggested that the asynchronous development of red cells renders them more liable to intramedullary destruction.

6. **D** Patients with pernicious anemia demonstrate a pancytopenia with low WBC, PLT, and RBC counts. Because this is a megaloblastic process and a DNA maturation defect, all cell lines are affected. In the bone marrow, this results in abnormally large precursor cells, maturation asynchrony, hyperplasia of all cell lines, and a low M/E ratio.

7. **B** Patients with obstructive liver disease may have red cells that have an increased tendency toward the deposition of lipid on the surface of the red cell. Consequently, the red cells are larger or more macrocytic than normal red cells.

8. **C** Macrocytes in true megaloblastic conditions are oval macrocytes, as opposed to the round macrocytes that are usually seen in alcoholics and obstructive liver disease.

9. **C** The red cell indices in a patient with megaloblastic anemia are macrocytic and normochromic. The macrocytosis is prominent with an MCV ranging from 100 to 130 fL.

10. **B** The patient will have an increased MCV. One of the causes of a macrocytic anemia that is not megaloblastic is an increased reticulocyte count, here noted as increased polychromasia. Reticulocytes are polychromatic macrocytes; therefore, the MCV wil be slightly increased.

Qualitative/Quantitative WBC Disorders

1. Which of the following is an unusual complication that may occur in infectious mononucleosis?
   A. Splenic infarctions
   B. Dactylitis
   C. Hemolytic anemia
   D. Giant platelets

   Hematology/Evaluate laboratory data to recognize health and disease states/Infectious mononucleosis/3

2. In a patient with human immunodeficiency virus (HIV) infection one should expect to see:
   A. Shift to the left in WBCs
   B. Target cells
   C. Reactive lymphocytes
   D. Pelgeroid cells

   Hematology/Evaluate laboratory data to recognize health and disease states/AIDS/Microscopic morphology/1

3. Which inclusions may be seen in leukocytes?
   A. Döhle bodies
   B. Basophilic stippling
   C. Malarial parasites
   D. Howell-Jolly bodies

   Hematology/Apply knowledge of fundamental characteristics/WBC inclusions/1

4. Which of the following is contained in the primary granules of the neutrophil?
   A. Lactoferrin
   B. Myeloperoxidase
   C. Histamine
   D. Alkaline phosphatase

   Hematology/Apply knowledge of fundamental biological characteristics/WBC kinetics/2

5. What is the typical range of relative lymphocyte percentage in the peripheral blood smear of a 1-year-old?

   A. 1%–6%
   B. 27%–33%
   C. 35%–58%
   D. 50%–70%

   Hematology/Evaluate laboratory data to recognize health and disease states/Differential normal values/2

Answers to Questions 1–5

1. **C** Occasionally patients with infectious mononucleosis develop a potent cold agglutinin with anti-I specificity. This cold autoantibody can cause strong hemolysis.

2. **C** HIV infection brings about several hematologic abnormalities seen on peripheral smear examination; most patients demonstrate reactive lymphocytes and have granulocytopenia.

3. **A** Döhle bodies are RNA-rich areas within polymorphonuclear neutrophils (PMNs) that are oval and light blue in color. Although often associated with infectious states, they are seen in a wide range of conditions and toxic reactions including hemolytic and pernicious anemias, chronic granulocytic leukemia, and therapy with antineoplastic drugs. The other inclusions are associated with erythrocytes.

4. **B** Myeloperoxidase, lysozyme, and acid phosphatase are enzymes that are contained in the primary granules of neutrophils. The contents of secondary and tertiary granules include lactoferrin, collagenase, NADPH oxidase, and alkaline phosphatase.

5. **D** The mean relative lymphocyte percentage for a 1-year-old is 61%, compared to the mean lymphocyte percentage of 35% for an adult.

6. Qualitative and quantitative neutrophil changes noted in response to infection include all of the following *except:*
A. Neutrophilia
B. Pelgeroid hyposegmentation
C. Toxic granulation
D. Vacuolization

Hematology/Apply knowledge of fundamental biological characteristics/WBC microscopic morphology/2

7. Neutropenia is present in patients with which absolute number of neutrophil counts?
A. $<1.5 \times 10^9/L$
B. $<5.0 \times 10^9/L$
C. $<10.0 \times 10^9/L$
D. $< 15.0 \times 10^9/L$

Hematology/Evaluate laboratory data to recognize health and disease states/Differential normal values/2

8. The morphologic characteristic(s) associated with the Chediak-Higashi syndrome is/are:
A. Pale blue cytoplasmic inclusions
B. Giant lysosomal granules
C. Small, dark staining granules and condensed nuclei
D. Nuclear hyposegmentation

Hematology/Recognize morphologic changes associated with disease/WBC inclusion/2

9. The familial condition of Pelger-Huët anomaly is important to recognize because this disorder must be differentiated from:
A. Infectious mononucleosis
B. May-Hegglin anomaly
C. A *shift-to-the-left* increase in immature granulocytes
D. G-6-PD deficiency

Hematology/Recognize morphologic changes associated with disease/WBC inclusion/2

10. What is the expected laboratory finding in a patient with a cytomegalovirus (CMV) infection?
A. Heterophile antibody: positive
B. Epstein-Barr virus (EBV)–immunoglobulin (IgM): positive
C. Direct antiglobulin test (DAT): positive
D. CMV–IgM: positive

Hematology/Evaluate laboratory data to recognize health and disease states/Differential normal values/2

11. Neutrophil phagocytosis and particle ingestion are associated with an increase in oxygen utilization referred to as *respiratory burst.* What are the two most important products of this biochemical reaction?

A. Hydrogen peroxide and superoxide anion
B. Lactoferrin and NADPH oxidase
C. Cytochrome b and collagenase
D. Alkaline phosphatase and ascorbic acid

Hematology/Apply knowledge of fundamental biological characteristics/WBC kinetics/2

Answers to Questions 6–11

6. **B** Neutrophil changes associated with infection may include neutrophilia, shift to the left, toxic granulation, Döhle bodies, and vacuolization. Pelgeroid hyposegmentation is noted in neutrophils from individuals with the congenital Pelger-Huët anomaly, and as an acquired anomaly induced by drug ingestion or secondary to conditions such as leukemia.

7. **A** Neutropenia is defined as an absolute decrease in the number of circulating neutrophils. This condition is present in patients having neutrophil counts of less than $1.5 \times 10^9/L$.

8. **B** Chediak-Higashi syndrome is a disorder of neutrophil phagocytic dysfunction due to depressed chemotaxis and delayed degranulation. The degranulation disturbance is attributed to interference from the giant lysosomal granules.

9. **C** Pelger-Huët anomaly is a benign familial condition reported in 1 out of 6000 individuals. Care must be taken to differentiate Pelger-Huët cells from the numerous band neutrophils and metamyelocytes that may be observed during severe infection or a *shift-to-the-left* immaturity in granulocyte stages.

10. **D** If both the heterophile antibody test and the EBV-IgM tests are negative in a patient with reactive lymphocytosis and a suspected viral infection, the serum should be analyzed for IgM antibodies to CMV. CMV belongs to the herpes virus family and is endemic worldwide. CMV infection is the most common cause of heterophile-negative infectious mononucleosis.

11. **A** The biochemical products of the respiratory burst that are involved with neutrophil particle ingestion during phagocytosis are hydrogen peroxide and superoxide anion. The activated neutrophil discharges the enzyme NADPH oxidase into the phagolysosome, where it converts O_2 to superoxide anion ($\cdot O_2^-$), which is then reduced to hydrogen peroxide (H_2O_2).

12. Reactive lymphocytes may best be distinguished from blasts by which of the following morphologic characteristics?
A. Fine chromatin
B. High nuclear:cytoplasmic (N:C) ratio
C. Prominent nucleoli
D. Basophilic cytoplasm

Hematology/Recognize morphologic changes associated with disease/WBC morphology/2

Answer to Question 12

12. **A** Both reactive lymphocytes and blasts may have basophilic cytoplasm, a high N:C ratio, and the presence of prominent nucleoli. Blasts, however, have an extremely fine nuclear chromatin staining pattern as viewed on a Wright's-Giemsa's stain.

Acute Leukemias

1. Auer rods may be seen in all of the following *except:*
   A. Acute myelomonocytic leukemia (M4)
   B. Acute lymphoblastic leukemia (L1, L2, L3)
   C. Acute myeloblastic leukemia (M1, M2)
   D. Acute promyelocytic leukemia (M3)

   Hematology/Apply knowledge of fundamental biological characteristics/Acute leukemia/1

2. Which type of anemia is usually present in a patient with acute leukemia?
   A. Microcytic, hyperchromic
   B. Microcytic, hypochromic
   C. Normocytic, normochromic
   D. Macrocytic, normochromic

   Hematology/Correlate clinical and laboratory data/RBC microscopic morphology/Anemia/2

3. Select the term describing a peripheral blood finding of leukocytosis with a shift to the left, accompanied by occasional nucleated red cells.
   A. Myelophthisis
   B. Dysplasia
   C. Leukoerythroblastosis
   D. Megaloblastosis

   Hematology/Apply knowledge of fundamental biological characteristics/WBC differential/1

4. The basic pathophysiological mechanisms responsible for producing signs and symptoms in leukemia include all of the following *except:*
   A. Replacement of normal marrow precursors by leukemic cells causing anemia
   B. Decrease in functional leukocytes causing infection
   C. Hemorrhage secondary to thrombocytopenia
   D. Decreased erythropoietin production

   Hematology/Correlate clinical and laboratory data/Leukemia/2

5. Which French-American-British (FAB) designation is called the *true* monocytic leukemia and follows an acute or subacute course characterized by monoblasts, promonocytes, and monocytes?
   A. FAB M1
   B. FAB M3
   C. FAB M4
   D. FAB M5

   Hematology/Evaluate laboratory data to make identifications/Leukemia/3

Answers to Questions 1–5

1. **B** Auer rods may be seen in myeloblasts, promyelocytes and monoblasts, but are not seen characteristically in lymphoblasts.

2. **C** Anemia in acute leukemia is usually present from the onset and may be severe; however, there is no inherent nutritional deficiency leading to either a microcytic, hypochromic, or megaloblastic process.

3. **C** The presence of immature leukocytes and nucleated red cells is denoted *leukoerythroblastosis. Myelophthisis* refers to replacement of bone marrow by a disease process such as a neoplasm. The development of abnormal tissue is called *dysplasia.*

4. **D** The accumulation of leukemic cells in the bone marrow leads to marrow failure, which is manifested by anemia, thrombocytopenia, and granulocytopenia. A normal physiological response to anemia would be an increase in the kidney's production of erythropoietin.

5. **D** M5 leukemia has an incidence of between 1% and 8% of all acute leukemias. It has a distinctive clinical manifestation of monocytic involvement resulting in skin and gum hyperplasia. The WBC count is markedly elevated, and prognosis is poor.

6. In which age group does acute lymphoblastic leukemia occur with highest frequency?
A. 1–15 years
B. 20–35 years
C. 45–60 years
D. 60–75 years

Hematology/Correlate clinical and laboratory data/Leukemia/1

7. Disseminated intravascular coagulation (DIC) is most often associated with which of the following FAB designations of acute leukemia?
A. M1
B. M3
C. M4
D. M5

Hematology/Evaluate laboratory data to recognize health and disease states/Leukemia/DIC/2

8. An M:E ratio of 10:1 is most often seen in:
A. Thalassemia
B. Leukemia
C. Polycythemia vera
D. Myelofibrosis

Hematology/Evaluate laboratory data to recognize health and disease states/Leukemia/M:E/2

9. Which of the following is a characteristic of Auer rods?
A. Composed of azurophilic granules
B. Periodic acid-Schiff (PAS)-positive
C. Predominantly seen in chronic myelogeneous leukemia (CML)
D. Nonspecific esterase-positive

Hematology/Apply knowledge of fundamental biological characteristics/Leukocytes/Auer rods/1

10. SITUATION: The following laboratory values are seen:

WBCs 6.0×10^9/L	Hgb 6.0 g/dL
RBCs 1.90×10^{12}/L	Hct 18.5%
Platelets 130×10^9/L	Serum B_{12} and folic acid: normal

WBC Differential	**Bone Marrow**
6% PMNs	40% myeloblasts
40% lymphocytes	60% promegaloblasts
4% monocytes	40 megaloblastoid
50% blasts	NRBCs/100 WBC

These results are most characteristic of:
A. Pernicious anemia (PA)
B. Acute myeloblastic leukemia (M1)
C. Erythroleukemia (M6)
D. Myelomonocytic leukemia (M4)

Hematology/Evaluate laboratory data to make identifications/Leukemia/3

11. A 24-year-old man with Down syndrome presents with a fever, pallor, lymphadenopathy, and hepatosplenomegaly. His CBC results are as follows:

	WBC differential
WBCs 10.8×10^9/L	
RBCs 1.56×10^{12}/L	8% PMNs
Hgb 3.3 g/dL	25% lymphocytes
Hct 11%	67% PAS-positive blasts
Platelets 2.5×10^9/L	

These findings are suggestive of:
A. Hodgkin's lymphoma
B. Myeloproliferative disorder
C. Leukemoid reaction
D. Acute lymphocytic leukemia

Hematology/Evaluate laboratory data to recognize health and disease states/Leukemia/3

Answers to Questions 6–11

6. **A** Acute lymphoblastic leukemia (ALL) usually affects children from age 1–15 and is the most common type of acute leukemia in this age group. In addition, ALL constitutes the single most prevalent malignancy occurring in pediatric patients.

7. **B** The azurophilic granules in the leukemic promyelocytes in patients with M3 (acute promyelocytic leukemia), contain thromboplastic substances. These activate soluble coagulation factors, which when released into the blood cause DIC.

8. **B** A disproportionate increase in the myeloid component of the bone marrow is usually the result of a leukemic state.

9. **A** Auer rods are a linear projection of primary, azurophilic granules, and are present in the cytoplasm of myeloblasts and monoblasts in patients with leukemia.

10. **C** Pernicious anemia results in pancytopenia and low B_{12}. In M6, more than 50% of nucleated bone marrow cells are erythroid and more than 30% nonerythroid cells are blasts.

11. **D** Common signs of acute lymphocytic leukemia are hepatosplenomegaly (65%); lymphadenopathy (50%); and fever (60%). Anemia and thrombocytopenia are usually present and the WBC count is variable. The numerous lymphoblasts are generally PAS-positive.

12. **SITUATION:** A peripheral smear shows 75% blasts. These stain positive for both Sudan Black B (SBB) and Peroxidase (Px). Given these values, which of the following disorders is most likely?
    A. Acute myelocytic leukemia (AML)
    B. CML
    C. Acute undifferentiated leukemia (AUL)
    D. ALL

    Hematology/Evaluate laboratory data to recognize health and disease states/Leukemia/Cytochemical stains/3

13. In myeloid cells, the stain that selectively identifies phospholipid in the membranes of both primary and secondary granules is:
    A. PAS
    B. Myeloperoxidase
    C. SBB
    D. Terminal deoxynucleotidyl transferase (TdT)

    Hematology/Apply principles of special procedures/Leukemia/Cytochemical stains/1

14. Sodium fluoride may be added to the naphthyl ASD acetate (NASDA) esterase reaction. The fluoride is added to inhibit a positive reaction with:
    A. Megakaryocytes
    B. Monocytes
    C. Erythrocytes
    D. Granulocytes

    Hematology/Apply principles of special procedures/Leukocytes/Cytochemical stains/2

15. Leukemic blasts reacting with anti-CALLA (Anti-CD10) are characteristically seen in:
    A. B cell ALL
    B. T cell ALL
    C. Null cell ALL
    D. Common ALL

    Hematology/Evaluate laboratory data to recognize health and disease states/Leukemia/Immunochemical reactions/2

16. Which of the following reactions are often positive in ALL but are negative in AML?
    A. Terminal deoxynucleotidyl transferase and PAS
    B. Chloroacetate esterase and nonspecific esterase
    C. Sudan Black B and peroxidase
    D. New methylene blue and acid phosphatase

    Hematology/Apply principles of special procedures/Leukemia/Special tests/2

17. A patient's peripheral blood smear and bone marrow both show 70% blasts. These cells are negative for SBB. Given these data, which of the following is the most likely diagnosis?
    A. Acute myelogeneous leukemia
    B. Chronic lymphocytic leukemia
    C. Acute promyelocytic leukemia
    D. Acute lymphocytic leukemia

    Hematology/Apply principles of special procedures/Leukemia/Cytochemical stains/2

Answers to Questions 12–17

12. **A** Usually less than 10% blasts are found in the peripheral smear of patients with CML, unless there has been a transition to blast crisis. The organelles in the cells of AUL are not mature enough to stain positive for SBB or Px. Blasts in ALL are characteristically negative with these stains.

13. **C** Phospholipids, neutral fats, and sterols are stained by SBB. The PAS reaction stains intracellular glycogen. Myeloperoxidase is an enzyme present in the primary granules of myeloid cells, and to a lesser degree in monocytic cells. Terminal deoxynucleotidyl transferase is a DNA polymerase found in thymus-derived and some bone marrow-derived lymphocytes.

14. **B** NASDA stains monocytes (and monoblasts) and granulocytes (and myeloblasts). The addition of fluoride renders the monocytic cells (and blasts) negative, thus allowing for differentiation from the granulocytic cells, which remain positive.

15. **D** The majority of non-T, non-B ALL blast cells display the common ALL antigen (CALLA) marker. Lymphoblasts of common ALL are TdT-positive and CALLA-positive but do not have surface membrane IgM or μ chains. Common ALL has a lower relapse rate and better prognosis than other immunological subtypes of B-cell ALL.

16. **A** Both terminal deoxynucleotidyl transferase and PAS are negative in AML. PAS is positive in about 50% of ALL with L1 and L2 morphology but is negative in L3 (B-cell ALL). Terminal deoxynucleotidyl transferase is positive in all types of ALL except L3.

17. **D** SBB stains phospholipids and other neutral fats. It is the most sensitive stain for granulocytic precursors. Lymphoid cells rarely stain positive for SBB. As 70% blasts would never be seen in CLL, the correct response is ALL.

Lymphoproliferative/ Myeloproliferative Disorders

1. Repeated phlebotomy in patients with polycythemia vera (PV) may lead to the development of:
   A. Folic acid deficiency
   B. Sideroblastic anemia
   C. Iron deficiency anemia
   D. Hemolytic anemia

   Hematology/Evaluate laboratory data to recognize health and disease states/Anemia/2

2. In essential thrombocythemia, the platelets are:
   A. Increased in number and functionally abnormal
   B. Normal in number and functionally abnormal
   C. Decreased in number and functional
   D. Decreased in number and functionally abnormal

   Hematology/Evaluate laboratory data to recognize health and disease states/CBC/Platelets/2

3. Which of the following cells is considered *pathognomonic* for Hodgkin's disease?
   A. Niemann-Pick cells
   B. Reactive lymphocytes
   C. Flame cells
   D. Reed-Sternberg cells

   Hematology/Evaluate laboratory data to recognize health and disease states/Lymphoma/1

4. In myelofibrosis, the characteristic abnormal red cell morphology is that of:
   A. Target cells
   B. Schistocytes
   C. Teardrop cells
   D. Ovalocytes

   Hematology/Correlate clinical and laboratory data/RBC microscopic morphology/1

5. PV is characterized by:
   A. Increased plasma volume
   B. Pancytopenia
   C. Decreased oxygen saturation
   D. Absolute increase in total red cell mass

   Hematology/Evaluate laboratory data to recognize health and disease states/RBC/Leukemia/2

Answers to Questions 1–5

1. **C** Iron deficiency anemia is a predictable complication of therapeutic phlebotomy because approximately 250 mg of iron is removed with each unit of blood.

2. **A** In essential thrombocythemia the platelet count is extremely elevated. These platelets are abnormal in function, leading to both bleeding and thrombosis diathesis.

3. **D** The morphologic common denominator in Hodgkin's lymphoma is the Reed-Sternberg (RS) cell. It is a large, binucleated cell with a dense nucleolus surrounded by clear space. These characteristics give the RS cell an "owl's eye" appearance.

4. **C** The marked amount of fibrosis, both medullary and extramedullary, accounts for the irreversible red cell morphologic change to a teardrop shape. The red cells are "teared" as they attempt to pass through the fibrotic tissue.

5. **D** The diagnosis of PV requires the demonstration of an increase in red cell mass. Pancytosis may also be seen in about two-thirds of PV cases. The plasma volume is normal or slightly reduced and the arterial oxygen saturation is usually normal.

6. Features of *secondary* polycythemia include all of the following *except:*
A. Splenomegaly
B. Decreased oxygen saturation
C. Increased red cell mass
D. Increased erythropoietin

Hematology/Evaluate laboratory data to recognize health and disease states/RBC disorder/2

7. The erythrocytosis seen in *relative* polycythemia occurs because of:
A. Decreased arterial oxygen saturation
B. Decreased plasma volume of circulating blood
C. Increased erythropoietin levels
D. Increased erythropoiesis in the bone marrow

Hematology/Correlate clinical and laboratory data/RBC disorder/2

8. In PV, what is characteristically seen in the peripheral blood?
A. Panmyelosis
B. Pancytosis
C. Pancytopenia
D. Panhyperplasia

Hematology/Apply knowledge of fundamental biological characteristics/Polycythemia/1

9. The leukocyte alkaline phosphatase (LAP) stain on a patient gives the following results: 10(0); 48(1+); 38(2+); 3(3+); 1(4+). Calculate the LAP score.
A. 100
B. 117
C. 137
D. 252

Hematology/Calculate/LAP score/2

10. SITUATION: Observe the laboratory values shown in the accompanying table.

WBC Differential

WBCs 76 × 10^9/L	55% PMNs	RBC morphology Normocytic/ normochromic
RBCs 4.2 × 10^{12}/L	15% bands	
Platelets 398 × 10^9/L	12% lympho- cytes	WBC morphology Moderate toxic granulation Occasional Döhle body
Hgb 12.5 g/dL	7% monocytes	
Hct 26.7%	2% eosinophils 1% basophil 8% metamyelocytes	

Which test is most helpful in establishing a diagnosis?
A. LAP stain
B. Nonspecific esterase stain
C. Acid phosphatase
D. SBB stain

Hematology/Evaluate laboratory and clinical data to specify additional tests/Leukemia/3

Answers to Questions 6–10

6. **A** The red cell mass is increased in both primary polycythemia (polycythemia vera) and secondary polycythemia. Splenomegaly is a feature of the former but not the latter. Erythropoietin is increased and oxygen saturation is decreased in secondary polycythemia.

7. **B** Relative polycythemia is caused by a reduction of plasma rather than an increase in red cell volume or mass. Red cell mass is increased in both polycythemia vera and in secondary poly-cythemia, but erythropoietin levels are high only in secondary polycythemia.

8. **B** PV is a myeloproliferative disorder character-ized by uncontrolled proliferation of erythroid precursors. However, production of all cell lines is usually increased.

9. **C** One hundred mature neutrophils are counted and scored. The LAP score is calculated as: (the number of 1+ cells × 1) + (2+ cells × 2) + (3+ cells × 3) + (4+ cells × 4). The reference range is approximately 20–130.

10. **A** These results may be caused by CML or a leukemoid reaction. CML causes a low LAP score, whereas an elevated or normal score occurs in a leukemoid reaction.

11. A 62-year-old man with fatigue and vague abdominal pain for 1 month had the results shown in the accompanying table.

WBCs	21.0×10^9/L
Platelets	780×10^9/L
Hgb	9.0 g/dL
Hct	26.7%

WBC Differential	20 NRBCs/100 WBC
53% PMNs	**RBC Morphology**
16% bands	Moderate anisocytosis
12% lymphocytes	Marked poikilocytosis
8% monocytes	Few bizarre agranular,
6% metamyelocytes	giant platelets
3% myelocytes	**Bone Marrow**
2% blasts	Marked fibrosis
	Increased megakaryocytes

These values are most suggestive of a diagnosis of:
A. Essential thrombocythemia (ET)
B. Idiopathic myelofibrosis (IMF)
C. CML
D. AML

Hematology/Evaluate laboratory data to recognize health and disease states/Leukemia/3

12. What influence does the Philadelphia (Ph¹) chromosome have on the prognosis of patients with chronic myelocytic leukemia?
A. It is not predictive.
B. The prognosis is better if Ph¹ is not present.
C. The prognosis is worse if Ph¹ is not present.
D. The disease usually transforms into AML when Ph¹ is present.

Hematology/Evaluate laboratory data to recognize health and disease states/Genetic theory and principle/CML/2

13. Which of the following is/are commonly found in chronic myelogenous leukemia?
A. Many teardrop-shaped cells
B. Intense LAP staining
C. Marked myeloid metaplasia
D. An increase in basophils

Hematology/Evaluate laboratory data to recognize health and disease states/CML/2

14. Multiple myeloma and Waldenström's macro-globulinemia have all the following in common *except:*
A. Monoclonal gammopathy
B. Hyperviscosity of the blood
C. Bence-Jones protein in the urine
D. Osteolytic lesions

Hematology/Evaluate laboratory data to recognize health and disease states/Myeloma/Characteristics/2

15. What is the characteristic finding seen in the peripheral smear of a patient with multiple myeloma?
A. Microcytic hypochromic cells
B. Intracellular inclusion bodies
C. Rouleaux
D. Hypersegmented neutrophils

Hematology/Apply knowledge of fundamental biological characteristics/Myeloma/RBC microscopic morphology/1

16. In which of the following conditions does LAP show the *least* activity?
A. Leukemoid reactions
B. Idiopathic myelofibrosis
C. Polycythemia vera
D. Chronic myelogenous leukemia

Hematology/Correlate clinical and laboratory data/LAP score/CML/1

Answers to Questions 11–16

11. **B** Anemia, fibrosis, myeloid metaplasia, thrombocytosis, and leukoerythroblastosis occur in idiopathic myelofibrosis.

12. **C** Ninety percent of patients with CML have the Philadelphia chromosome. This appears as a long arm deletion of chromosome 22, but is actually a translocation between the long arms of chromosomes 22 and 9. Often, a second chromosomal abnormality occurs in CML before blast crisis.

13. **D** CML is marked by an elevated WBC count demonstrating various stages of maturation, hypermetabolism, and a minimal LAP staining. An increase in basophils and eosinophils is a common finding. Pseudo Pelger-Huët cells and thrombocytosis may be present. The marrow is hypercellular with a high M:E ratio (e.g., 10:1).

14. **D** Destruction of the bone as evidenced by radiography is seen in multiple myeloma but not in Waldenström's macroglobulinemia. In addition, Waldenström's gives rise to a lymphocytosis that does not occur in multiple myeloma and differs in the morphology of the malignant cells.

15. **C** Multiple myeloma is a plasma cell dyscrasia that is characterized by an overproduction of monoclonal immunoglobulin. Rouleaux is observed in multiple myeloma patients due to increased viscosity and decreased albumin/globulin ratio.

16. **D** Chronic myelogenous leukemia shows the least LAP activity, while the LAP score is slightly to markedly increased in each of the other states.

17. A striking feature of the peripheral blood of a patient with CML is a:
A. Profusion of bizarre blast cells
B. Normal number of typical granulocytes
C. Profusion of granulocytes at different stages of development
D. Pancytopenia

Hematology/Evaluate laboratory data to recognize health and disease states/WBC/CML/2

18. Which of the following is often associated with CML but *not* with AML?
A. Infections
B. WBCs greater than 20.0×10^9/L
C. Hemorrhage
D. Splenomegaly

Hematology/Correlate clinical and laboratory data/CML/Characteristics/2

19. All of the following are associated with the diagnosis of multiple myeloma *except:*
A. Marrow plasmacytosis
B. Lytic bone lesions
C. Serum and/or urine M component (monoclonal protein)
D. Philadelphia chromosome

Hematology/Correlate clinical and laboratory data/Myeloma/2

20. Multiple myeloma is most difficult to distinguish from:
A. Chronic lymphocytic leukemia
B. Acute myelogenous leukemia
C. Benign monoclonal gammopathy
D. Benign adenoma

Hematology/Apply knowledge of fundamental biological characteristics/Myeloma/2

21. Franklin's disease is also known as:
A. μ Heavy chain disease
B. γ Heavy chain disease
C. α Heavy chain disease
D. α Light chain disease

Hematology/Apply knowledge of fundamental biological characteristics/Immunologic manifestation of disease/Immunoglobulins/1

22. Waldenström's macroglobulinemia is a malignancy of the:
A. Lymphoplasmacytoid cells
B. Adrenal cortex
C. Myeloblastic cell lines
D. Erythroid cell precursors

Hematology/Apply knowledge of fundamental biological characteristics/Immunologic manifestation of disease/Plasma cell dyscrasia/2

23. Cells that exhibit a positive stain with acid phosphatase and are not inhibited with tartaric acid are characteristically seen in:
A. Infectious mononucleosis
B. Infectious lymphocytosis
C. Hairy cell leukemia
D. T-cell acute lymphoblastic leukemia

Hematology/Apply principles of special procedures/Leukemia/Cytochemical stains/1

Answers to Questions 17–23

17. **C** The WBC count in CML is often greater than 100×10^9/L, and the peripheral smear shows a granulocyte progression from blast to segmented neutrophil.

18. **D** Splenomegaly is seen in more than 90% of CML patients, but it is not a characteristic finding in AML. Infections, hemorrhage, and elevated WBC counts may be seen in both CML and AML.

19. **D** Osteolytic lesions, monoclonal gammopathy, and bone marrow infiltration by plasma cells comprise the triad of diagnostic markers for multiple myeloma. The Ph[1] chromosome is a diagnostic marker for CML.

20. **C** Benign monoclonal gammopathies have peripheral blood findings similar to myeloma. However, a lower concentration of monoclonal protein is usually seen. There are no osteolytic lesions, and the plasma cells comprise less than 10% of nucleated cells in the bone marrow. About 30% become malignant, and therefore the term monoclonal gammopathy of undetermined significance may be more appropriate.

21. **B** Franklin's disease is demonstrated by an anomalous serum M component that reacts with an anti-IgG but not with antiserum against light chains. γ Chains are present in both serum and urine. Patients have a mixed cell lymphoma usually without bone marrow involvement or lymphocytosis.

22. **A** Waldenström's macroglobulinemia is a malignancy of the lymphoplasmacytoid cells, which manufacture IgM. Although the cells secrete immunoglobulin, they are not fully differentiated into plasma cells and lack the characteristic perinuclear halo, deep basophilia, and eccentric nucleus characteristic of classic plasma cells.

23. **C** A variable number of malignant cells in hairy cell leukemia (HCL) will stain positive with tartrate-resistant acid phosphatase (TRAP+). Although this cytochemical reaction is fairly specific for HCL, TRAP activity has occasionally been reported in B-cell, and rarely T-cell leukemia.

Coagulation/Fibrinolytic Systems

1. Which of the following is the anticoagulant of choice for most coagulation studies?
   A. Sodium oxalate
   B. Sodium citrate
   C. Heparin
   D. EDTA

   Hematology/Select methods/reagents/media/ Specimen collection and handling/Hemostasis/1

2. Which ratio of anticoagulant to blood is correct for coagulation procedures?
   A. 1:4
   B. 1:5
   C. 1:9
   D. 1:10

   Hematology/Select methods/reagents/media/ Specimen collection and handling/Hemostasis/1

3. Which results would be expected for the prothrombin time (PT) and activated partial thromboplastin time (APTT) in a patient with polycythemia?
   A. Both prolonged
   B. Both shortened
   C. Normal PT, prolonged APTT
   D. Both normal

   Hematology/Correlate clinical and laboratory disease/Coagulation test/2

4. What reagents are used in the PT test?
   A. Thromboplastin and sodium chloride
   B. Thromboplastin and potassium chloride
   C. Thromboplastin and calcium chloride
   D. Actin and calcium chloride

   Hematology/Select methods/reagents/media/ Coagulation tests/1

5. Which test(s) will be abnormal in a patient with Stuart-Prower factor deficiency?
   A. PT
   B. APTT

C. Thrombin time
D. Two of the above

Hematology/Correlate clinical and laboratory data/ Hemostasis/2

Answers to Questions 1–5

1. **B** The anticoagulant of choice for most coagulation procedures is sodium citrate (3.2%). Because factors V and VIII are more labile in sodium oxalate, heparin neutralizes thrombin, and EDTA inhibits thrombin's action on fibrinogen, these anticoagulants are not used for routine coagulation studies.

2. **C** The optimum ratio of anticoagulant to blood is one part anticoagulant to nine parts of blood. The anticoagulant supplied in this amount is sufficient to bind all the available calcium, thereby preventing clotting.

3. **A** The volume of blood in a polycythemic patient contains so little plasma that excess anticoagulant remains and is available to bind to reagent calcium, thereby resulting in prolongation of the PT and APTT. For more accurate results, the plasma:anticoagulant ratio can be modified by decreasing the amount of anticoagulant in the collection tube.

4. **C** Thromboplastin and calcium chloride (combined into a single reagent) replace the tissue thromboplastin and calcium necessary *in vivo* to activate factor VII to factor VIIa. This ultimately generates thrombin from prothrombin via the coagulation cascade.

5. **D** Stuart-Prower factor (factor X) is involved in the common pathway of the coagulation cascade; therefore, its deficiency will prolong both the PT and APTT. Activated factor X along with factor V, in the presence of calcium and platelet factor III (PF3) converts prothrombin (factor II) to the active enzyme thrombin (factor IIa).

6. The following factors are measured by either the PT or APTT *except:*
A. Factor VIII
B. Factor IX
C. Factor V
D. Factor XIII

Hematology/Apply principles of basic laboratory procedures/Coagulation tests/1

7. A modification of which procedure can be used to measure fibrinogen?
A. PT
B. APTT
C. Thrombin time
D. Fibrin degradation products

Hematology/Apply principle of basic laboratory procedures/Coagulation tests/2

8. All of the following are characteristics of vitamin K *except:*
A. It is required for biologic activity of some coagulation factors.
B. Its activity is enhanced by heparin therapy.
C. It is required for carboxylation of glutamate residues of some coagulation factors.
D. Its deficiency is caused by prolonged antibiotic treatment.

Hematology/Apply knowledge of fundamental biological characteristics/Hemostasis/Vitamin K/2

9. Which statement about the fibrin degradation product test is *false?*
A. Detects early degradation products
B. Elevated in disseminated intravascular coagulation
C. Evaluates the fibrinolytic system
D. Detects late degradation products

Hematology/Apply principles of basic laboratory procedures/Hemostasis/FDP/2

10. Which of the following platelet aggregating agents demonstrates a monophasic aggregation curve when used in optimal concentration?
A. Thrombin
B. Collagen
C. Adenosine diphosphate (ADP)
D. Epinephrine

Hematology/Apply knowledge of fundamental biological characteristics/Hemostasis/1

11. In a vitamin K-deficient patient, which of the following coagulation tests would be abnormal?
A. PT and APTT
B. Bleeding time
C. Fibrinogen level
D. Thrombin time

Hematology/Correlate clinical and laboratory data/Hemostasis/2

12. Which of the following *is not* correct regarding the international normalized ratio (INR)?
A. Uses the International Sensitivity Index (ISI)
B. Standardizes PT results
C. Standardizes APTT results
D. Is valuable information for patients receiving oral anticoagulant

Hematology/Apply knowledge of fundamental biological characteristics/Hemostasis/2

Answers to Questions 6–12

6. **D** Factor XIII (fibrin stabilizing factor) is a transamidase. It creates covalent bonds between fibrin monomers formed during the coagulation process to produce a stable fibrin clot. In the absence of factor XIII, the hydrogen bonded fibrin polymers are soluble in 5M urea or in 1% monochloroacetic acid.

7. **C** Fibrinogen can be quantitatively measured by a modification of the thrombin time, because the thrombin clotting time of diluted plasma is inversely proportional to the concentration of fibrinogen.

8. **B** The activity of vitamin K is not enhanced by heparin therapy. Vitamin K is made by the organisms in the intestine, and is essential for synthesis of vitamin K-dependent clotting factors (II, VII, IX, X) and proteins C and S. This activation is accomplished by carboxylation of glutamic acid residues of the inactive clotting factors.

9. **A** The fibrin degradation product (FDP) test detects the late degradation products (fragments D and E), but not early degradation products (fragments X and Y).

10. **B** Collagen is the only agent that demonstrates a single-wave (monophasic) response preceded by a lag time.

11. **A** Patients with vitamin K deficiency will exhibit decreased production of functional prothrombin proteins (factors II, VII, IX, and X). Decreased levels of these factors will prolong the PT and APTT.

12. **C** INR is used to adjust for the difference in thromboplastin reagents made by different manufacturers and used by various institutions. The INR calculation uses the ISI value and should be reported in patients who have been on and responding to an oral anticoagulant for at least 2 weeks. INR is not used in APTT testing.

13. Which of the following is necessary for endogenous activation of plasminogen?
A. Streptokinase
B. Transamidase
C. Tissue plasminogen activator
D. Stuart-Prower factor

Hematology/Apply knowledge of fundamental biological characteristics/Hemostasis/1

14. Which of the following proteins is the primary inhibitor of the fibrinolytic system?
A. Protein C
B. Protein S
C. α_2-Antiplasmin
D. α_2-Macroglobulin

Hematology/Apply knowledge of fundamental biological characteristics/Hemostasis/Plasmin/1

Answers to Questions 13–14

13. **C** Tissue plasminogen activator (TPA) is an endogenous activator, released from the endothelial cells by the action of protein C. It converts plasminogen to plasmin. Streptokinase is an exogenous activator of plasminogen.

14. **C** α_2-Antiplasmin is the main inhibitor of plasmin. It inhibits plasmin by forming a 1:1 stoichiometric complex with any free plasmin in the plasma and, therefore, prevents the binding of plasmin to fibrin and fibrinogen.

Platelet/Vascular Disorders

1. All of the following are characteristics of thrombotic thrombocytopenic purpura (TTP) *except:*
   A. Renal dysfunction
   B. Thrombocytosis
   C. Microangiopathic hemolytic anemia
   D. Neurologic abnormalities

   Hematology/Correlate clinical and laboratory data/Anemia/2

2. All of the following physiological conditions may be associated with thrombocytopenia *except:*
   A. Decreased platelet production
   B. Abnormal platelet distribution
   C. Increased platelet destruction
   D. Increased proliferation of pluripotential stem cells

   Hematology/Apply knowledge of fundamental biological characteristics/Hemostasis/2

3. Aspirin prevents platelet aggregation by inhibiting the action of which enzyme?
   A. Phospholipase
   B. Cyclooxygenase
   C. Thromboxane α_2 synthetase
   D. Prostacyclin synthetase

   Hematology/Apply knowledge of fundamental biological characteristics/Hemostasis/1

4. Which of the following factors is essential for normal platelet adhesion?
   A. Fibrinogen
   B. Glycoprotein Ib
   C. Glycoprotein IIb, IIIa complex
   D. Calcium

   Hematology/Apply knowledge of fundamental biological characteristics/Hemostasis/2

5. Which of the following test results is normal in a patient with classic von Willebrand's disease?
   A. Bleeding time
   B. Activated partial thromboplastin time
   C. Platelet count
   D. Factor VIII:C and VWF levels

   Hematology/Correlate clinical and laboratory data/Hemostasis/3

6. All of the following laboratory results support the diagnosis of von Willebrand's disease *except:*
   A. Increased bleeding time
   B. Decreased factor VIII assay
   C. Decreased platelet retention
   D. Normal platelet aggregation to ristocetin

   Hematology/Apply principle of basic laboratory procedures/Coagulation tests/2

Answers to Questions 1–6

1. **B** Thrombotic thrombocytopenic purpura is a rare disorder that has severe clinical manifestations. Thrombocytopenia is always present due to intravascular platelet aggregation.

2. **D** Increased proliferation of pluripotential stem cells is associated with thrombocytosis and not thrombocytopenia.

3. **B** Aspirin prevents platelet aggregation by inhibiting the activity of the enzyme cyclooxygenase. This inhibition prevents the formation of the precursors of thromboxane α_2 (TXA2), a potent platelet aggregator.

4. **B** Glycoprotein Ib is a platelet receptor for von Willebrand's factor (VWF). Glycoprotein Ib and VWF are both essential for normal platelet adhesion.

5. **C** Von Willebrand's disease is an inherited, qualitative platelet disorder resulting in an increased bleeding time, prolonged APTT, and decreased factor VIII:C and VWF levels. The platelet count is usually normal.

6. **D** Von Willebrand's disease is associated with an increased bleeding time test, and decreased results of both factor VIII assay and platelet retention tests. Von Willebrand's disease is a disorder of platelet adhesion caused by deficiency of VWF. Platelet aggregation in response to ristocetin is decreased in von Willebrand's disease.

7. When performing platelet aggregation studies, which set of platelet aggregation responses would most likely occur in a patient with Bernard-Soulier syndrome?
   A. Normal platelet aggregation to collagen, ADP, and ristocetin
   B. Normal platelet aggregation to collagen, ADP, and epinephrine; decreased to ristocetin
   C. Normal platelet aggregation to epinephrine and ristocetin; decreased to collagen and ADP
   D. Normal platelet aggregation to epinephrine, ristocetin and collagen; decreased to ADP

   Hematology/Correlate clinical and laboratory data/Hemostasis/3

8. Which set of platelet responses would most likely be associated with Glanzmann's thrombasthenia?
   A. Normal platelet aggregation to ADP and ristocetin; decreased to collagen
   B. Normal platelet aggregation to collagen; decreased to ADP and ristocetin
   C. Normal platelet aggregation to ristocetin; decreased to collagen, ADP, and epinephrine
   D. Normal platelet aggregation to ADP; decreased to collagen and ristocetin

   Hematology/Correlate clinical and laboratory data/Hemostasis/3

9. Which of the following is a characteristic of acute idiopathic thrombocytopenic purpura (ITP)?
   A. Spontaneous remission within a few weeks
   B. Found predominantly in adults
   C. Nonimmune platelet destruction
   D. Insidious onset

   Hematology/Apply knowledge of fundamental biological characteristics/Hemostasis/1

10. TTP differs from DIC in that:
    A. APTT is normal in TTP but prolonged in DIC.
    B. Schistocytes are not seen in TTP but are present in DIC.
    C. Platelet count is decreased in TTP but normal in DIC.
    D. PT is prolonged in TTP but decreased in DIC.

    Hematology/Correlate clinical and laboratory data/Hemostasis/3

11. Several hours after birth, a baby boy develops the following symptoms and laboratory value: petechiae and purpura, hemorrhagic diathesis, and a platelet count 18×10^9/L. The most likely explanation is:
    A. Drug-induced thrombocytopenia
    B. Secondary thrombocytopenia
    C. Isoimmune neonatal thrombocytopenia
    D. Neonatal DIC

    Hematology/Correlate clinical and laboratory data/Hemostasis/2

Answers to Questions 7–11

7. **B** Bernard-Soulier syndrome is a disorder of platelet adhesion caused by deficiency of glycoprotein Ib. Platelet aggregation is normal in response to collagen, ADP, and epinephrine but is abnormal in response to ristocetin.

8. **C** Glanzmann's thrombasthenia is a disorder of platelet aggregation. Platelet aggregation is normal in response to ristocetin, but abnormal in response to collagen, ADP, and epinephrine.

9. **A** Acute idiopathic thrombocytopenic purpura is an immune-mediated disorder found predominantly in children. It is characterized by abrupt onset, and spontaneous remission usually occurs within several weeks.

10. **A** Thrombotic thrombocytopenic purpura is a platelet disorder in which platelet aggregation increases and therefore results in thrombocytopenia. Schistocytes are present in TTP as a result of microangiopathic hemolytic anemia; however, the PT and APTT are both normal. In DIC, PT and APTT are both prolonged, the platelet count is decreased, and schistocytes are seen in the peripheral smear.

11. **C** Isoimmune neonatal thrombocytopenia is a congenital disease that occurs in infants whose mothers lack a specific platelet antigen(s) that is present on the fetal cells. The mother develops the alloantiplatelet antibodies through exposure to the offending platelet antigen during pregnancies or transfusions. The passive transport of the antibody is responsible for the thrombocytopenia in these infants.

Coagulation System Disorders

1. The APTT is sensitive to a deficiency of:
   A. Factor VII
   B. Factor X
   C. PF3
   D. Calcium

   Hematology/Evaluate laboratory data to recognize health and disease states/Hemostasis/Factor deficiency/2

2. Which test result is anticipated to be normal in a patient with dysfibrinogenemia?
   A. Thrombin time
   B. APTT
   C. PT
   D. Immunologic fibrinogen level

   Hematology/Correlate clinical and laboratory data/Hemostasis/3

3. A patient with a prolonged PT is given intravenous vitamin K. The PT corrects to normal after 24 hours. What clinical condition most likely caused these results?
   A. Liver disease
   B. Factor X deficiency
   C. Fibrinogen deficiency
   D. Obstructive jaundice

   Hematology/Correlate clinical and laboratory data/Hemostasis/Vitamin K deficiency/3

4. **SITUATION:** The PT and APTT are corrected with aged serum, but *not* with absorbed plasma. What factor is deficient?
   A. V
   B. VII
   C. X
   D. XI

   Hematology/Evaluate laboratory data to recognize health and disease states/Hemostasis/Factor deficiency/3

5. A prolonged APTT is corrected with factor VIII-deficient plasma but *not* with factor IX-deficient plasma. What factor is deficient?
   A. IX
   B. VIII
   C. V
   D. X

   Hematology/Evaluate laboratory data to recognize health and disease states/Hemostasis/Factor deficiency/3

Answers to Questions 1–5

1. **B** The APTT is sensitive to the deficiency of coagulation factors in the intrinsic pathway (factors XII, XI, IX, VIII) and common pathway (factors X, V, II, I).

2. **D** In a patient with dysfibrinogenemia, fibrinogen is not polymerized properly, causing abnormal fibrinogen-dependent coagulation tests. However, the level of plasma fibrinogen determined immunologically is normal.

3. **D** Obstructive jaundice contributes to coagulation disorders by preventing vitamin K absorption. Vitamin K is fat-soluble and requires bile salts for absorption. Parenteral administration of vitamin K bypasses the bowel, and hence, the need for bile salts.

4. **C** Absorbed plasma contains factors I, V, VIII, XI, and XII. Aged serum contains factors IX, X, XI, and XII. Correction of both tests with aged serum but not absorbed plasma suggests factor X deficiency.

5. **A** Because the prolonged APTT is not corrected with a factor IX-deficient plasma, factor IX is suspected to be deficient in the test plasma.

6. All of the following are characteristics of classic hemophilia A *except:*
A. Normal bleeding time
B. Sex-linked inheritance
C. Severe hemarthrosis
D. Decreased VWF:Ag

Hematology/Correlate clinical and laboratory data/Hemostasis/Hemophilia/2

7. In DIC, which test result is *unlikely?*
A. Prolonged thrombin time
B. Decreased platelet count
C. Decreased APTT
D. Prolonged APTT

Hematology/Correlate clinical and laboratory data/ Hemostasis/DIC/3

8. Which of the following is a predisposing condition for the development of DIC?
A. Adenocarcinoma
B. Sepsis
C. Liver disease
D. All of the above

Hematology/Correlate clinical and laboratory disease/Hemostasis/DIC/1

9. Factor XII deficiency is associated with:
A. Bleeding history
B. Epistaxis
C. Decreased risk of thrombosis
D. Increased risk of thrombosis

Hematology/ Apply knowledge of fundamental biological characteristics/Hemostasis/2

10. The following results were obtained on a patient: prolonged bleeding time, normal platelet count, normal PT, and prolonged APTT. Which of the following disorders is most consistent with these results?
A. Hemophilia A
B. Hemophilia B
C. Von Willebrand's disease
D. Glanzmann's thrombasthenia

Hematology/Correlate clinical and laboratory data/ Hemostasis/3

11. The following lab results have been obtained from a 40-year-old woman: PT = 20 seconds; APTT = 50 seconds; thrombin time = 18 seconds. What is the most probable diagnosis?
A. Factor VII deficiency

B. Factor VIII deficiency
C. Factor X deficiency
D. Hypofibrinogenemia

Hematology/Correlate clinical and laboratory data/Hemostasis/3

Answers to Questions 6–11

6. **D** Hemophilia A is a sex-linked disease, characterized by hemarthrosis and visceral bleeding due to deficiency of VIII:C and not VWF:Ag.

7. **C** In DIC there is a diffuse intravascular generation of thrombin and fibrin. As a result, coagulation factors and platelets are consumed, resulting in a decreased platelet count and an increased PT, APTT, and thrombin time.

8. **D** Adenocarcinoma can liberate procoagulant (thromboplastic) substances that can activate prothrombin intravascularly. Sepsis can directly produce DIC through several mechanisms. DIC may also occur as a consequence of liver disease.

9. **D** Factor XII is a contact activator of the intrinsic pathway. Hemorrhagic manifestations are not associated with factor XII deficiency because thrombin can activate factor XI to XIa, and factor VIIa can activate factor IX to IXa. Factor XII-deficient patients commonly present with thrombotic episodes due to a decrease in their fibrinolytic activity.

10. **C** Von Willebrand's disease is a disorder of platelet adhesion associated with decreased VWF and factor VIII causing prolonged bleeding time and APTT. Hemophilia A and B are factors VIII and IX deficiencies, respectively, in which bleeding times are normal and APTTs are prolonged. Glansmann's thrombasthenia is a platelet aggregation defect in which the APTT is normal.

11. **D** Fibrinogen (factor I) is a clotting protein of the common pathway and is measured by the thrombin time. In hypofibrinogenemia (fibrinogen concentration <100 mg/dL), the PT and APTT are both prolonged because the deficiencies of the common pathway proteins would affect both tests. In factor VII deficiency the APTT is normal, in factor VIII deficiency the PT is normal, and in factor X deficiency the TT is normal.

Inhibitors and Thrombotic Disorders

1. All of the following are characteristics of antithrombin III *except:*
   A. It is synthesized in the liver.
   B. It is an α_2 globulin.
   C. It is a cofactor of heparin.
   D. It is a pathologic inhibitor of coagulation.
   Hematology/Apply knowledge of fundamental biological characteristics/Hemostasis/AT3/2

2. All of the following tests are affected by heparin therapy *except:*
   A. Thrombin time
   B. APTT
   C. Whole blood clotting time
   D. Reptilase time
   Hematology/Apply knowledge of fundamental biological characteristics/Hemostasis/Heparin/2

3. An abnormal APTT seen with a pathologic circulating anticoagulant is:
   A. Corrected with aged serum
   B. Corrected with absorbed plasma
   C. Corrected with normal plasma
   D. Not corrected with any of the above
   Hematology/Correlate clinical and laboratory data/Hemostasis/Special test/2

4. The lupus anticoagulant is directed against:
   A. Factor VIII
   B. Factor X
   C. Factor IX
   D. Phospholipid
   Hematology/Apply knowledge of fundamental biological characteristics/Hemostasis/1

5. All of the following statements regarding warfarin sodium (Coumadin) are true *except:*
   A. It is a vitamin K antagonist.
   B. It needs antithrombin (AT) as a cofactor.
   C. PT is used to monitor its dosage.

   D. It is not recommended for pregnant and lactating women.
   Hematology/Apply knowledge of fundamental biological characteristics/Hemostasis/1

Answers to Questions 1–5

1. **D** Antithrombin III (heparin cofactor) is the most important naturally occurring physiological inhibitor of blood coagulation. It carries about 75% of antithrombotic activity and is an α_2 globulin made by the liver.

2. **D** Reptilase is thrombinlike in activity. The reptilase time is used to evaluate the conversion of fibrinogen to fibrin. Reptilase time is not affected by heparin; therefore, it can be used to distinguish the cause of an abnormal thrombin time.

3. **D** In the presence of a pathologic circulating anticoagulant, mixing tests will not correct the abnormal APTT. These anticoagulants are pathologic substances and are endogenously produced. They are either directed against a specific blood factor or against a group of factors.

4. **D** The lupus anticoagulant reacts with phospholipids rather than clotting proteins and, therefore, interferes with the assays of the phospholipid-dependent coagulation tests.

5. **B** Coumadin is a vitamin K antagonist drug that retards synthesis of the active form of vitamin K-dependent factors. The PT and INR are used as monitoring tests. Because Coumadin crosses the placenta and is present in human milk, it is not recommended for pregnant and lactating women. Antithrombin is the heparin (not Coumadin) cofactor.

6. All of the following are characteristics of protein C *except:*
   A. It is a vitamin K-dependent zymogen.
   B. It is activated by thrombin.
   C. It inhibits cofactors Va and VIIIa.
   D. Its activity is inhibited by protein S.

   Hematology/Apply knowledge of fundamental biological characteristics/Hemostasis/1

7. ε Aminocaproic acid (EACA) is an inhibitor of:
   A. Platelet activation
   B. Stabilization of the fibrin clot
   C. Collagen attachment
   D. Fibrinolysis

   Hematology/Apply knowledge of fundamental biological characteristics/Hematology/1

8. Which of the following is most commonly associated with activated protein C resistance (APCR)?
   A. Bleeding
   B. Thrombosis
   C. Epistaxis
   D. Menorrhagia

   Hematology/Correlate clinical and laboratory data/Hemostasis/2

9. A-30-year-old woman develops signs and symptoms of thrombosis in her left lower leg following 3 days of heparin therapy. The patient had open heart surgery 3 days ago and has been on heparin since. Which of the following would be the most useful to investigate the cause of her thrombosis?
   A. Monitor the APTT.
   B. Monitor the PT.
   C. Monitor the platelet count.
   D. Increase the heparin dose.

   Hematology/Correlate clinical and laboratory data/Hemostasis/3

10. The following lab results were obtained on a 25-year-old woman with menorrhagia after delivery of her second son. The patient has no previous bleeding history.

   Normal platelet count; normal bleeding time; normal PT; prolonged APTT

   Mixing of the patient's plasma with normal plasma corrected the prolonged APTT upon immediate testing. However, mixing followed by a 2-hour incubation at 37°C caused a prolonged APTT. What is the most probable cause of these laboratory results?

   A. Lupus anticoagulant
   B. Factor VIII deficiency
   C. Factor IX deficiency
   D. Factor VIII inhibitor

   Hematology/Correlate clinical and laboratory data/Hemostasis/3

11. A 50-year-old white man has been on heparin for the past 7 days. Which combination of the following tests is expected to be abnormal?
   A. PT and APTT
   B. APTT, TT
   C. APTT, TT, fibrinogen assay
   D. PT, APTT, TT

   Hematology/Correlate clinical and laboratory data/Hemostasis/3

Answers to Questions 6–11

6. **D** Protein S functions as a cofactor of protein C and as such enhances its activity.

7. **D** Fibrin deposition is accelerated with the use of ε aminocaproic acid.

8. **B** Activated protein C resistance is the single most common cause of inherited thrombosis. In 90% of individuals, the cause is gene mutation of factor V (Leiden factor V). Affected individuals are predisposed to thrombosis, mainly after age 40. Heterozygous individuals may not manifest thrombosis unless clinical conditions predispose them to thrombosis.

9. **C** The platelet count should be checked every few days in patients receiving heparin therapy for the first time because heparin-induced thrombocytopenia and thrombosis (HITT) may develop. HITT should be suspected in patients who are not responding to heparin therapy and/or are developing thrombocytopenia and thrombotic complications while on heparin therapy.

10. **D** Factor VIII inhibitor is found in 10%–20% of hemophiliac patients receiving replacement therapy. It may also develop in patients with immunologic problems, women after child birth, patients with lymphoproliferative and plasma cell disorders, or it may develop in response to medications. Factor VIII inhibitor is an IgG immunoglobulin with an inhibitory effect that is time and temperature dependent. The presence of factor VIII inhibitor causes elevated APTT in the face of a normal prothrombin time. Mixing studies in factor VIII and IX deficiencies will correct the prolonged APTT both at the immediate mixing stage and after 2 hours' incubation. The APTT would not be corrected by mixing studies if lupus anticoagulant were present. In addition, lupus anticoagulant is not associated with any bleeding.

11. **D** Heparin is a therapeutic anticoagulant with an antithrombin effect. It also inhibits factors XIIa, XIa, Xa, and IXa. PT, APTT, and TT are all prolonged in patients receiving heparin therapy. Quantitative fibrinogen assay, however, is not affected.

Hematology Problem Solving

1. A 19-year-old man presented to the Emergency Room with severe joint pain, fatigue, cough, and fever. Review the following lab results:

WBCs	21.0×10^9/L
RBCs	3.23×10^{12}/L
Hgb	9.6 g/dL
PLT	252×10^9/L

   Differential: 17 band neutrophils; 75 segmented neutrophils; 5 lymphocytes; 2 monocytes; 1 eosinophil; 26 NRBCs

   What is the corrected WBC count?
   A. 8.1×10^9/L
   B. 16.7×10^9/L
   C. 21.0×10^9/L
   D. 80.8×10^9/L
   Hematology/Calculate/WBC corrected for NRBCs/2

2. A manual WBC count is performed using the Unopette system. Eighty WBCs are counted in the 4 large corner squares of a Neubauer hemocytometer. The dilution is 1:100. What is the total WBC count?
   A. 4.0×10^9/L
   B. 8.0×10^9/L
   C. 20.0×10^9/L
   D. 200.0×10^9/L

   Hematology/Calculate/Cell Count/2

3. A manual RBC count is performed on a pleural fluid using the Unopette system. The RBC count in the large center square of the Neubauer hemocytometer is 125 and the dilution is 1:200. What is the total RBC count?
   A. 27.8×10^9/L
   B. 62.5×10^9/L

C. 125.0×10^9/L
D. 250.0×10^9/L
Hematology/Calculate/Cell Count/2

Answers to Questions 1–3

1. **B** The formula for correcting the WBC count for the presence of NRBCs is:

   $$\frac{\text{Total WBC} \times 100}{100 + \#\,\text{NRBCs}} \text{ or } \frac{21.0 \times 100}{126} = 16.7 \times 10^9/\text{L}$$

   where total WBC = WBCs $\times 10^9$/L

2. **C** The formula for calculating manual cell counts using a hemocytometer is:

   $$\frac{\#\,\text{cells} \times 10\,(\text{depth factor}) \times \text{dilution factor}}{\text{area}} \text{ or}$$

   $$\frac{80 \times 10 \times 100}{4} = 20,000 \text{ or } 20.0 \times 10^9/\text{L}$$

3. **D** Regardless of the cell or fluid type, the formula for calculating manual cell counts using a hemocytometer is:

   $$\frac{\#\,\text{cells} \times 10\,(\text{depth factor}) \times \text{dilution factor}}{\text{area}} \text{ or}$$

   $$\frac{125 \times 10 \times 200}{1} = 250,000 \text{ or } 250.0 \times 10^9/\text{L}$$

4. Review the Coulter VCS scatterplot of white blood cells. Which section of the scatterplot denotes the number of monocytes?

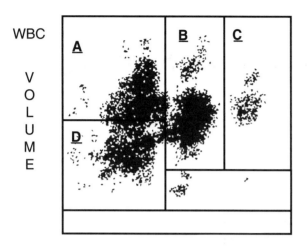

WBC

V
O
L
U
M
E

DF 1

A. A
B. B
C. C
D. D

Hematology/Apply basic principles to interpret results/Automated cell counting/2

5. Review the following automated CBC values.

WBCs 17.5 × 10⁹/L (*flagged*) MCV 86.8 fL
RBCs 2.89 × 10¹²/L   MCH 28.0 pg
Hgb 8.1 g/dL   MCHC 32.3%
Hct 25.2%   PLT 217 × 10⁹/L

Many sickle cells were observed upon review of the peripheral blood smear. Based on this finding and the above results, what automated parameter of this patient is most likely *inaccurate* and what follow-up test should be done to accurately assess this parameter?
A. MCV/perform reticulocyte count
B. Hct/perform manual Hct
C. WBC/perform manual WBC count
D. Hgb/perform serum:saline replacement

Hematology/Apply knowledge to identify sources of error/Instrumentation/3

6. Review the following CBC results on a 2-day-old baby girl:

WBCs 15.2 × 10⁹/L   MCV   105 fL
RBCs 5.30 × 10¹²/L MCH   34.0 pg
Hgb   18.5 g/dL   MCHC 33.5%
Hct   57.9%   PLT   213 × 10⁹/L

These results indicate:
A. Macrocytic anemia
B. Microcytic anemia
C. Liver disease
D. Normal values for a 2-day-old infant

Hematology/Apply knowledge of fundamental biological characteristics/Normal values/2

Answers to Questions 4–6

4. **A** White blood cell identification is facilitated by analysis of the impedance, conductance, and light-scattering properties of the WBCs. The scatterplot represents the relationship between volume (x axis) and light scatter (y axis). Monocytes account for the dots in section A, neutrophils are represented in section B, eosinophils in section C, and lymphocytes are denoted in section D.

5. **C** When an automated WBC count is performed using a hematology analyzer, the RBCs are lysed to allow enumeration of the WBCs. Sickle cells are often resistant to lysis within the limited time frame (less than 1 minute) during which the RBCs are exposed to the lysing reagent and the WBCs are subsequently counted. As a result, the nonlysed RBCs are counted along with the WBCs, thus falsely increasing the WBC count. When an automated cell counting analyzer indicates a *review flag* for the WBC count, and sickle cells are noted on peripheral smear analysis, a manual WBC count must be performed. The manual method will allow optimal time for sickle cell lysis, and to thereby accurately enumerate the WBCs.

6. **D** During the first week of life an infant will have an average hematocrit of 55%. This value drops to a mean of 43% by the first month of life. The mean MCV of the first week is 108 fL; after 2 months the average MCV is 96 fL. The mean WBC count during the first week is approximately 18 × 10⁹/L, and this drops to an average of 10.8 × 10⁹/L after the first month. The platelet count of newborns falls within the same normal range as adults.

7. Review the following Coulter VCS scatterplot, histograms, and automated values on a 21-year-old college student.

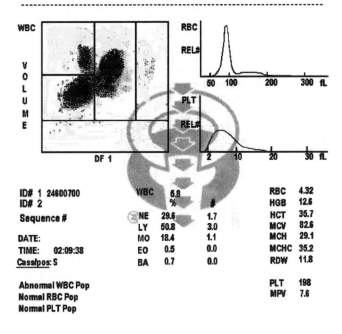

ID# 1 24600700	WBC	5.8		RBC	4.32
ID# 2	%	#		HGB	12.6
Sequence #	NE	29.6	1.7	HCT	35.7
	LY	50.8	3.0	MCV	82.6
DATE:	MO	18.4	1.1	MCH	29.1
TIME: 02:09:38	EO	0.5	0.0	MCHC	35.2
Cass/pos: S	BA	0.7	0.0	RDW	11.8

Abnormal WBC Pop
Normal RBC Pop   PLT   198
Normal PLT Pop   MPV   7.6

SUSPECT FLAGS:

--------WBC----------------RBC---------------PLT----------
                    DEFINITIVE FLAGS:
Monocytosis %

WBC Differential: 5 band neutrophils; 27 segmented neutrophils; 60 atypical lymphocytes; 6 monocytes; 1 eosinophil; 1 basophil

What is the presumptive diagnosis?
A. Infectious mononucleosis
B. Monocytosis
C. Chronic lymphocytic leukemia
D. β-Thalassemia

Hematology/Apply knowledge to identify sources of error/Instrumentation/3

8. Review the following Coulter VCS scatterplot, histograms, and automated values on a 61-year-old woman.

WBC Differential: 14 band neutrophils; 50 segmented neutrophils; 7 lymphocytes; 4 monocytes; 10 metamyelocytes; 8 myelocytes; 1 promyelocyte; 3 eosinophil; 3 basophil; 2 NRBC/100 WBC

What is the presumptive diagnosis?
A. Leukemoid reaction
B. Chronic myelocytic leukemia

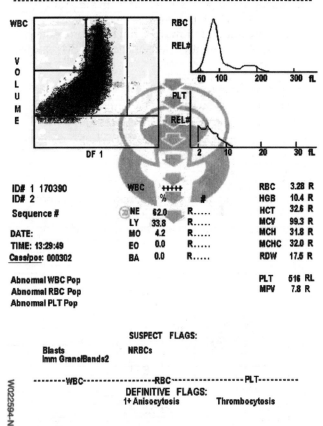

ID# 1 170390	WBC	++++		RBC	3.28 R
ID# 2	%	#		HGB	10.4 R
Sequence #	NE	62.0	R.....	HCT	32.6 R
	LY	33.8	R.....	MCV	99.3 R
DATE:	MO	4.2	R.....	MCH	31.8 R
TIME: 13:29:49	EO	0.0	R.....	MCHC	32.0 R
Cass/pos: 000302	BA	0.0	R.....	RDW	17.5 R

Abnormal WBC Pop
Abnormal RBC Pop   PLT   516 RL
Abnormal PLT Pop   MPV   7.8 R

SUSPECT FLAGS:

Blasts   NRBCs
Imm Grans/Bands2

--------WBC----------------RBC---------------PLT----------
                 DEFINITIVE FLAGS:
           1+ Anisocytosis   Thrombocytosis

C. Acute myelocytic leukemia
D. Megaloblastic leukemia

Hematology/Evaluate laboratory data to recognize health and disease states/Instrumentation/3

Answers to Questions 7–8

7. **A** The automated results demonstrated abnormal WBC subpopulations, specifically lymphocytosis as well as monocytosis. However, on peripheral smear examination 60 atypical lymphocytes and only 6 monocytes were noted. Atypical lymphocytes are often misclassified by automated cell counters as monocytes. Therefore the automated analyzer differential must not be released and the manual differential count must be relied upon for diagnostic interpretation. Lymphocytosis with numerous atypical lymphocytes are a hallmark finding consistant with the diagnosis of infectious mononucleosis.

8. **B** The ++++ on the Coulter VCS printout indicates that the WBC count exceeds the upper linearity of the analyzer (>99.9 × 10⁹/L). This markedly elevated WBC count, combined with the spectrum of immature granulocytic cells seen on peripheral smear examination, indicates the diagnosis of chronic myelocytic leukemia.

9. Review the automated results from the previous question. Which parameters can be released without further follow-up verification procedures?

    A. WBC and relative percentages of WBC populations

    B. RBC and PLT

    C. Hgb and Hct

    D. None of the automated counts can be released without verification procedures.

Hematology/Apply knowledge to identify sources of error/Instrumentation/3

10. Refer to the following Coulter VCS scatterplot, histograms, and automated values on a 45-year-old man. What follow-up verification procedure is indicated before releasing these results?

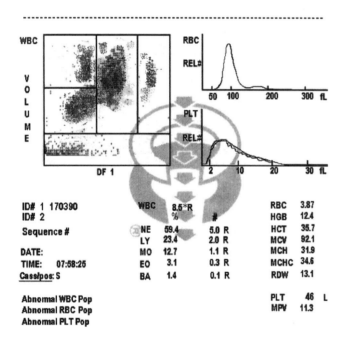

ID# 1 170390
ID# 2
Sequence #
DATE:
TIME: 07:58:25
Cass/pos: S

	WBC	8.5*R	#		RBC	3.87
		%			HGB	12.4
NE	59.4	5.0 R		HCT	35.7
LY	23.4	2.0 R		MCV	92.1
MO	12.7	1.1 R		MCH	31.9
EO	3.1	0.3 R		MCHC	34.6
BA	1.4	0.1 R		RDW	13.1
				PLT	46 L
				MPV	11.3

Abnormal WBC Pop
Abnormal RBC Pop
Abnormal PLT Pop

SUSPECT FLAGS:
NRBCs

--------WBC----------------RBC----------------PLT---------
DEFINITIVE FLAGS:
                Thrombocytopenia

    A. Redraw using sodium citrate tube; multiply PLT × 1.11.

    B. Dilute the WBC 1:10; multiply × 10.

    C. Perform plasma blank Hgb to correct for lipemia.

    D. Warm specimen at 37°C for 15 minutes; rerun specimen.

Hematology/Apply knowledge to identify sources of error/Instrumentation/3

Answers to Questions 9–10

9. **D** All of the automated results have *R* or *review* flags indicated. The specimen must be diluted to bring the WBC count within the linearity range of the analyzer. When enumerating the RBC count, the analyzer does not lyse the WBCs and actually counts the WBCs in with the RBC count. As such, the RBC count is falsely elevated because of the increased number of WBCs. Therefore, after an accurate WBC has been obtained, this value can be subtracted from the RBC count to obtain a true RBC count. For example, using the values for this patient:

Step 1: Obtain accurate WBC count by diluting the sample 1:10.

$$WBC = 41.0 \times 10 \text{ (dilution)} = 410 \times 10^9/L$$

Step 2: Convert this value to million units of measure in order to subtract from RBC count.

$$410 \times 10^9/L = 0.41 \ (\times 10^{12}/L)$$

Step 3: Subtract the WBC count from the RBC count to get an accurate RBC count.

$$3.28 \text{ (original RBC)} - 0.41 \text{ (true WBC)} = 2.87 \times 10^{12}/L = \text{accurate RBC}$$

The hematocrit may be obtained by microhematocrit centrifugation. The true MCV may be obtained using the standard formula.

$$MCV = \frac{Hct}{RBC} \times 10$$

where RBC = RBC count in millions per microliter. Additionally, the platelet count must be verified by smear estimate or performed manually.

10. **A** Platelet clumps will cause a spurious decrease in the platelet count by automated methods. The WBC value has a R (review) flag due to the platelet clumps being falsely counted as WBCs; therefore, a manual WBC count is indicated. The platelet clumping phenomenon is often induced *in vitro* by the anticoagulant EDTA. Redrawing the patient using a sodium citrate tube will usually correct this phenomenon and allow accurate platelet enumeration. The platelet count must be multiplied by 1.11 to adjust for the amount of sodium citrate.

11. Refer to the following Coulter VCS scatterplot, histograms, and automated values on a 52-year-old woman. What follow-up verification procedure is indicated before releasing these results?

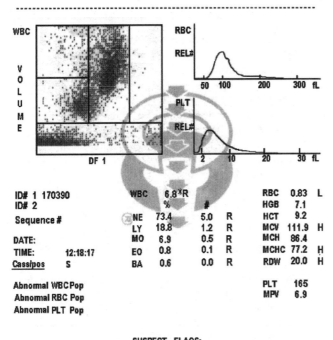

ID# 1 170390
ID# 2
Sequence #
DATE:
TIME: 12:18:17
Cass/pos   S

	WBC	6.8 *R				RBC	0.83	L
		%	#			HGB	7.1	
NE	73.4	5.0	R		HCT	9.2	
LY	18.8	1.2	R		MCV	111.9	H
MO	6.9	0.5	R		MCH	86.4	
EO	0.8	0.1	R		MCHC	77.2	H
BA	0.6	0.0	R		RDW	20.0	H

Abnormal WBC Pop
Abnormal RBC Pop
Abnormal PLT Pop

PLT   165
MPV   6.9

SUSPECT FLAGS:

Imm Grans / Bands 2   NRBCs   Platelet Clumps
                       RBC Agglutination

--------WBC------------------RBC------------------PLT----------
DEFINITIVE FLAGS:
Anemia
2+ Anisocytosis
3+ Macrocytosis

A. Redraw using sodium citrate tube; multiply PLT × 1.11.
B. Dilute the WBC 1:10; multiply × 10.
C. Perform plasma blank Hgb to correct for lipemia.
D. Warm the specimen at 37°C for 15 minutes; rerun the specimen.

Hematology/Apply knowledge to identify sources of error/Instrumentation/3

12. Refer to the following Coulter VCS scatterplot, histograms, and automated values on a 33-year-old woman. What follow-up verification procedure is indicated before releasing these results?
A. Redraw using sodium citrate tube; multiply PLT × 1.11.
B. Dilute the WBC 1:10; multiply × 10.
C. Perform plasma blank Hgb to correct for lipemia.
D. Warm the specimen at 37°C for 15 minutes; rerun the specimen.

Hematology/Apply knowledge to identify sources of error/Instrumentation/3

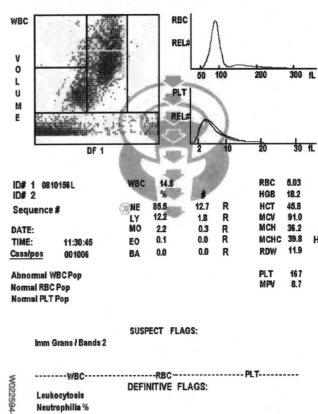

ID# 1 0810156L
ID# 2
Sequence #
DATE:
TIME: 11:30:45
Cass/pos   001006

	WBC	14.8				RBC	5.03	
		%	#			HGB	18.2	
NE	85.5	12.7	R		HCT	45.8	
LY	12.2	1.8	R		MCV	91.0	
MO	2.2	0.3	R		MCH	36.2	
EO	0.1	0.0	R		MCHC	39.8	H
BA	0.0	0.0	R		RDW	11.9	

Abnormal WBC Pop
Normal RBC Pop
Normal PLT Pop

PLT   167
MPV   8.7

SUSPECT FLAGS:

Imm Grans / Bands 2

--------WBC------------------RBC------------------PLT----------
DEFINITIVE FLAGS:
Leukocytosis
Neutrophilia %

Answers to Questions 11–12

11. **D** The presence of a high titer cold agglutinin in a patient with cold autoimmune hemolytic anemia will interfere with automated cell counting. The most remarkable findings are a falsely elevated MCV, MCH, and MCHC, as well as a falsely decreased RBC count. The patient's red cells will quickly agglutinate *in vitro* when exposed to ambient temperature below body temperature. To correct this phenomenon, incubate the EDTA tube at 37°C for 15–30 minutes and then rerun the specimen.

12. **C** The rule of thumb regarding the Hgb/Hct correlation dictates that Hgb × 3 ≅ Hct (± 3). This rule is violated in this patient; therefore, a follow-up verification procedure is indicated. Additionally, the MCHC is markedly elevated in these results, and an explanation for a falsely increased Hgb should be investigated. Lipemia can be visualized by centrifuging the EDTA tube and observing for a milky white plasma. To correct for the presence of lipemia, a plasma Hgb value (baseline Hgb) should be ascertained using the patient's plasma, and subsequently subtracted from the original falsely elevated Hgb value. The following formula can be used to correct for lipemia.

$$\text{Whole blood Hgb} - \left[(\text{Plasma Hgb})\left(1 - \frac{\text{Hct}}{100}\right)\right] =$$

Corrected Hgb

13. Refer to the following Coulter VCS scatterplot, histograms, and automated values on a 48-year-old man. What follow-up verification procedure is indicated before releasing the five-part WBC differential results?

A. Dilute WBC 1:10; multiply × 10.

B. Redraw using sodium citrate tube; multiply WBC × 1.11.

C. Prepare buffy coat peripheral blood smears.

D. Warm specimen at 37°C for 15 minutes; rerun specimen

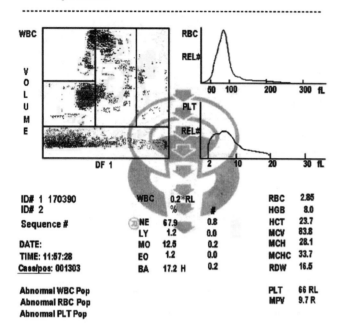

ID# 1 170390	WBC	0.2*RL		RBC	2.85
ID# 2		%	#	HGB	8.0
Sequence #	NE	67.9	0.8	HCT	23.7
	LY	1.2	0.0	MCV	83.8
DATE:	MO	12.5	0.2	MCH	28.1
TIME: 11:57:28	EO	1.2	0.0	MCHC	33.7
Case/pos: 001303	BA	17.2 H	0.2	RDW	16.5

Abnormal WBC Pop
Abnormal RBC Pop
Abnormal PLT Pop

PLT 66 RL
MPV 9.7 R

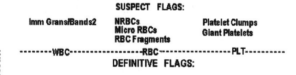

SUSPECT FLAGS:

Imm Grans/Bands2 | NRBCs | Platelet Clumps
| Micro RBCs | Giant Platelets
| RBC Fragments

--------WBC--------------RBC------------------PLT----------

DEFINITIVE FLAGS:

W022594-N

Hematology/Select course of action/Instrumentation/3

14. Review the following CBC results on a 70-year-old man:

WBC	58.2 × 10⁹/L	MCV	98 fL
RBC	2.68 × 10¹²/L	MCH	31.7 pg
Hgb	8.5 g/dL	MCHC	32.6%
Hct	26.5%	PLT	132 × 10⁹/L

Differential: 96 lymphocytes; 2 band neutrophils; 2 segmented neutrophils; 25 smudge cells/100 WBCs

What is the most likely diagnosis based on these values?

A. Acute lymphocytic leukemia

B. Chronic lymphocytic leukemia (CLL)

C. Infectious mononucleosis

D. Myelodysplastic syndrome

Hematology/Evaluate laboratory data to recognize health and disease states/Leukemia/1

Answers to Questions 13–14

13. **C** The markedly decreased WBC count (0.2 × 10⁹/L) indicates that a manual differential is necessary and very few leukocytes will be available for differential cell counting. To increase the yield and thereby facilitate counting, differential smears should be prepared using the buffy coat technique.

14. **B** CLL is a disease of the elderly, classically associated with an elevated WBC count, relative and absolute lymphocytosis. CLL is twofold more common in men, and smudge cells (WBCs with little or no surrounding cytoplasm) are usually present in the peripheral blood smear. CLL may occur with or without anemia or thrombocytopenia. The patient's age and lack of blasts rule out acute lymphocytic leukemia. Similarly, the patient's age and the lack of atypical lymphocytes make infectious mononucleosis unlikely. Myelodysplastic syndromes may involve the erythroid, granulocytic, or megakaryocytic cell lines, but not the lymphoid cells.

15. Refer to the following Coulter VCS scatterplot, histograms, and automated values on a 28-year-old woman who had preoperative laboratory testing. A manual WBC differential was requested by her physician. The WBC differential was not significantly different from the automated five-part differential; however, the technologist noted 3+ elliptocytes/ovalocytes while reviewing the RBC morphology. What is the most likely diagnosis for this patient?

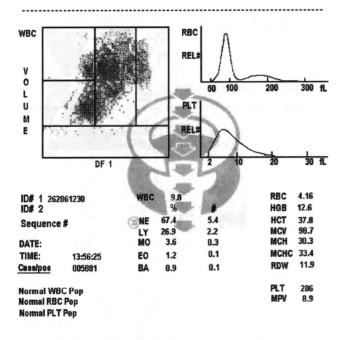

ID# 1 262861230
ID# 2
Sequence #
DATE:
TIME: 13:56:25
Cass/pos   005881

WBC 9.8
          %   #
NE 67.4   5.4
LY 26.9   2.2
MO 3.6   0.3
EO 1.2   0.1
BA 0.9   0.1

RBC   4.16
HGB   12.6
HCT   37.8
MCV   98.7
MCH   30.3
MCHC 33.4
RDW   11.9

PLT   286
MPV   8.9

Normal WBC Pop
Normal RBC Pop
Normal PLT Pop

SUSPECT FLAGS:

--------WBC----------------RBC----------------PLT----------

MANUAL DIFFERENTIAL

Neutrophil 64.6%	Lymphocyte 27.4%
Monocyte 4.8%	Eosinophil 2.2%
	Basophil 1.0%

A. DIC
B. Hereditary elliptocytosis (ovalocytosis)
C. Cirrhosis
D. Hgb C disease

Hematology/Evaluate laboratory data to recognize health and disease states/2

16. A 25-year-old woman presented to her physician with symptoms of jaundice, acute cholecystitis, and an enlarged spleen. On investigation, numerous gallstones were discovered. Review the following CBC results:

WBC	11.1×10^9/L	MCV	100 fL
RBC	3.33×10^{12}/L	MCH	34.5 pg
Hgb	11.5 g/dL	MCHC	37.5%
Hct	31.6%	PLT	448×10^9/L

WBC Differential: 13 band neutrophils; 65 segmented neutrophils; 15 lymphocytes; 6 monocytes; 1 eosinophil

RBC morphology: 3 + spherocytes, 1+ polychromasia

What follow-up laboratory test would provide valuable information for this patient?
A. Osmotic fragility
B. Hgb electrophoresis
C. G-6-PD assay
D. Methemoglobin reduction test

Hematology/Evaluate laboratory data to recognize health and disease states/2

Answers to Questions 15–16

15. **B** The finding of ovalocytes as the predominant RBC morphology in peripheral blood is consistant with the diagnosis of hereditary elliptocytosis (HE) or ovalocytosis. This disorder is relatively common and can range in severity from an asymptomatic carrier to homozygous HE with severe hemolysis. The most common clinical subtype is associated with no or minimal hemolysis. Therefore, HE is usually associated with a normal RBC histogram and cell indices, and will go unnoticed without microscopic evaluation of the peripheral smear.

16. **A** The MCHC is elevated in more than 50% of patients with spherocytosis, and this parameter can be used as a clue to the presence of HS. Spherocytes have a decreased surface-to-volume ratio, probably resulting from mild cellular dehydration. The osmotic fragility test is indicated as a confirmatory test for the presence of numerous spherocytes, and individuals with HS will have an increased osmotic fragility.

W022594-N

17. Refer to the following Coulter VCS scatterplot, histograms, and automated values on a 53-year-old man who had preoperative laboratory testing. What is the most likely diagnosis for this patient?
A. Iron deficiency anemia (IDA)
B. PV
C. Sideroblastic anemia
D. β Thalassemia minor

Hematology/Evaluate laboratory data to recognize health and disease states/2

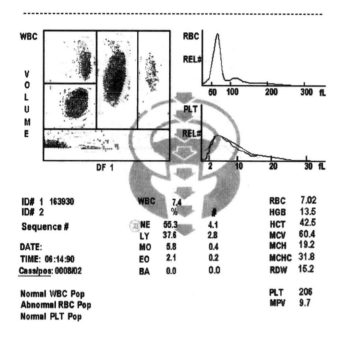

ID# 1 163930
ID# 2

Sequence #

DATE:
TIME: 06:14:90
Cassipos: 0008/02

	WBC	7.4	#		RBC	7.02
	%				HGB	13.5
NE	55.3	4.1		HCT	42.5
LY	37.6	2.8		MCV	60.4
MO	5.8	0.4		MCH	19.2
EO	2.1	0.2		MCHC	31.8
BA	0.0	0.0		RDW	15.2
				PLT	206
				MPV	9.7

Normal WBC Pop
Abnormal RBC Pop
Normal PLT Pop

SUSPECT FLAGS:

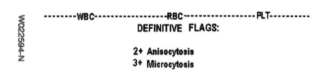

DEFINITIVE FLAGS:

2+ Anisocytosis
3+ Microcytosis

18. Review the following CBC results:

WBCs	11.0×10^9/L	MCV	85.0 fL
RBCs	3.52×10^{12}/L	MCH	28.4 pg
Hgb	10.0 g/dL	MCHC	33.4%
Hct	29.9%	PLT	155×10^9/L
	12 NRBCs/100 WBC		

RBC Morphology: Moderate polychromasia, 3+ target cells, few schistocytes

Which of the following additional laboratory tests would yield informative diagnostic information for this patient?
A. Osmotic fragility
B. Hgb electrophoresis
C. Sugar water test
D. Bone marrow examination

Hematology/Correlate laboratory data with other laboratory data to assess test results/3

Answers to Questions 17–18

17. **D** β-Thalassemia minor can easily be detected by noting an abnormally elevated RBC count, a Hct that does not correlate with the elevated RBC count, in conjunction with a decreased MCV. Although thalassemia and IDA are both microcytic, hypochromic processes, thalassemia can be differentiated from IDA because the RBC count, Hgb, and Hct values are usually decreased along with the MCV in IDA. Although the RBC count is increased in PV, the Hct must also be greater than 50% to consider a diagnosis of PV.

18. **B** The findings of a moderate anemia, numerous target cells seen on a peripheral blood smear, as well as the presence of NRBCs are often associated with hemoglobinopathies. Hemoglobin electrophoresis at alkaline pH is a commonly performed test to correctly diagnose the type of hemoglobinopathy

BIBLIOGRAPHY

1. Harmening, D: Clinical Hematology and Fundamentals of Hemostasis, ed 3. FA Davis, Philadelphia, 1996.
2. Handin, RI, Lux SE, and Stossel, TP: Principles and Practice of Hematology. JB Lippincott, Philadelphia, 1995.
3. Jandl, JH: Blood Pathophysiology. Blackwell Scientific, Cambridge, England, 1991.
4. Koepke, JA: Practical Laboratory Hematology. Churchill Livingstone, New York, 1991.
5. Lotspeich-Steininger, CA, Stein-Martin, EA, and Koepke, JA (eds): Clinical Hematology: Principles, Procedures, Correlations. JB Lippincott, Philadelphia, 1992.
6. McKenzie, SB: Textbook of Hematology. Lea & Febiger, Philadelphia, 1988.
7. Turgeon, ML: Clinical Hematology: Theory and Procedures, ed 2. Little, Brown & Company, Boston 1993.
8. Williams, W (ed): Hematology. McGraw-Hill, New York, 1990.

CHAPTER TWO

Immunology

Basic Principles of Immunology

1. From the following, identify a specific component of the adaptive immune system that is formed in response to antigenic stimulation.
   A. Lysozyme
   B. Complement
   C. Commensal organisms
   D. Immunoglobulin

   Immunology/Apply knowledge of fundamental biological characteristics/Immune system/ Complement/1

2. Which two organs are considered the primary lymphoid organs where immunocompetent cells originate and mature?
   A. Thyroid and Peyer's patches
   B. Thymus and bone marrow
   C. Spleen and mucosal-associated lymphoid tissue (MALT)
   D. Lymph nodes and thoracic duct

   Immunology/Apply knowledge of fundamental biological characteristics/Immune system/ Organs/1

3. What type of B cells are formed after antigen stimulation?
   A. Plasma cells and memory B cells
   B. Mature B cells
   C. Antigen-dependent B cells
   D. Receptor-activated B cells

   Immunology/Apply knowledge of fundamental biological characteristics/Immune system/Cells/1

Answers to Questions 1–3

1. **D** Immunoglobulin is a specific part of the adaptive immune system and is formed only in response to a specific antigenic stimulation. Complement, lysozyme, and commensal organisms all act nonspecifically as a part of the adaptive immune system. These three components do not require any type of specific antigenic stimulation.

2. **B** The bone marrow and thymus are considered primary lymphoid organs because immunocompetent cells either originate or mature in them. Some immunocompetent cells mature or reside in the bone marrow (the source of all hematopoietic cells) until transported to the thymus, spleen, or Peyer's patches where they process antigen or manufacture antibody. T lymphocytes, after origination in the bone marrow, travel to the thymus to mature and differentiate.

3. **A** Mature B cells exhibit surface immunoglobulin that may cross-link a foreign antigen, thus forming the activated B cell and leading to capping and internalization of antigen. The activated B cell gives rise to plasma cells that produce and secrete immunoglobulins and memory cells that reside in lymphoid organs.

4. T cells travel from the bone marrow to the thymus for maturation. What is the correct order of the maturation sequence for T cells in the thymus?
   A. Bone marrow to the cortex; after thymic education, released back to peripheral circulation.
   B. Maturation and selection occur in the cortex; migration to the medulla; release of mature T cells to secondary lymphoid organs.
   C. Storage in either the cortex or medulla; release of T cells into the peripheral circulation.
   D. Activation and selection occur in the medulla; mature T cells stored in the cortex until activated by antigen.

   Immunology/Apply knowledge of fundamental biological characteristics/Immune system/Cells/1

5. Which CD marker appears during the first stage of T-cell development and remains present as an identifying marker for T cells?
   A. CD1
   B. CD2
   C. CD3
   D. CD4 or CD8

   Immunology/Apply principles of basic laboratory procedures/T Cells/Markers/1

6. Which markers are found on mature, peripheral helper T cells?
   A. CD1, CD2, CD4
   B. CD2, CD3, CD8
   C. CD1, CD3, CD4
   D. CD2, CD3, CD4

   Immunology/Apply knowledge of fundamental biological characteristics/T Cells/Markers/1

7. Which T cell expresses the CD8 marker and acts specifically to kill tumor or virally infected cells?
   A. Helper T
   B. T suppressor
   C. T cytotoxic
   D. T inducer/suppressor

   Immunology/Apply knowledge of fundamental biological characteristics/T cells/Cytokines/1

8. How are cytotoxic T cells (T_C cells) and natural killer (NK) cells similar?
   A. Require antibody to be present
   B. Effective against virally infected cells
   C. Recognize antigen in association with HLA class II markers
   D. Do not bind to infected cells

   Immunology/Apply knowledge of fundamental biological characteristics/Lymphocytes/Function/1

9. What is the name of the process by which phagocytic cells are attracted toward a substance such as a bacterial peptide?
   A. Diapedesis
   B. Degranulation
   C. Chemotaxis
   D. Phagosomasis

   Immunology/Apply knowledge of fundamental biological characteristics/Immune system/Cells/1

10. All of the following are immunologic functions of complement *except:*
    A. Induction of an antiviral state
    B. Opsonization
    C. Chemotaxis
    D. Anaphylatoxin formation

    Immunology/Apply knowledge of fundamental biological characteristics/Complement/Function/1

Answers to Questions 4–10

4. **B** Immature T cells travel from the bone marrow to the thymus to mature. Once in the thymus, T cells undergo a selection and maturation sequence that begins in the cortex and moves to the medulla of the thymus. Thymic factors such as thymosin and thymopoietin and cells within the thymus such as macrophages and dendritic cells assist in this sequence. After completion of the maturation cycle, T cells are released to secondary lymphoid organs to await antigen recognition and activation.

5. **B** The CD2 marker appears during the first stage of T-cell development and can be used to differentiate T cells from other lymphocytes. This T-lymphocyte receptor binds sheep red blood cells (RBCs). This peculiar characteristic was the basis for the classic E rosette test once used to enumerate T cells in peripheral blood.

6. **D** Mature, peripheral helper T cells have the CD2 (E rosette), CD3 (mature T cell), and CD4 (helper) markers.

7. **C** T cytotoxic cells recognize antigen in association with major histocompatibility complex (MHC) class I complexes and act against target cells that express foreign antigens. These include viral antigens and the human leukocyte antigens (HLA) that are the target of graft rejection.

8. **B** Both T_C and NK cells are effective against virally infected cells, and neither requires antibody to be present to bind to infected cells. NK cells do not exhibit MHC class restriction, whereas activation of T_C cells requires the presence of MHC class I molecules in association with the viral antigen.

9. **C** Chemotaxis is the process by which phagocytic cells are attracted toward an area where they detect a disturbance in the normal functions of body tissues. Products from bacteria and viruses, complement components, coagulation proteins, and cytokines from other immune cells may all act as chemotactic factors.

10. **A** Complement components are serum proteins that function in opsonization, chemotaxis, and anaphylatoxin formation but do not induce an antiviral state in target cells. This function is performed by interferons.

11. Which complement component is found in both the classic and alternative pathways?
A. C1
B. C4
C. Factor D
D. C3

Immunology/Apply knowledge of fundamental biological characteristics/Complement/Components/1

12. Which immunoglobulin(s) help(s) initiate the classic complement pathway?
A. IgA and IgD
B. IgM only
C. IgG and IgM
D. IgG only

Immunology/Apply of knowledge of fundamental biological characteristics/Complement/Activation/1

13. How is complement activity destroyed *in vitro*?
A. Heating serum at 56°C for 30 minutes
B. Keeping serum at room temperature of 22°C for 1 hour
C. Heating serum at 37°C for 45 minutes
D. Freezing serum at 0°C for 24 hours

Immunology/Apply knowledge of fundamental biological characteristics/Complement/Activation/1

14. What is the purpose of C3a, C4a, and C5a, the split-products of the complement cascade?
A. To bind with specific membrane receptors of lymphocytes and cause release of cytotoxic substances
B. To cause increased vascular permeability, contraction of smooth muscle, and release of histamine from basophils
C. To bind with membrane receptors of macrophages to facilitate phagocytosis and the removal of debris and foreign substances
D. To regulate and degrade membrane cofactor protein after activation by C3 convertase

Immunology/Apply knowledge of fundamental biological characteristics/Complement/Anaphylatoxins/1

15. Which region of the immunoglobulin molecule can bind antigen?
A. Fab (fragment antigen binding)
B. Fc (fragment crystallizable)
C. C_L
D. C_H

Immunology/Apply knowledge of fundamental biological characteristics/Immunoglobulin/Structure/1

16. What region determines the immunoglobulin class?
A. V_H
B. C_H
C. V_L
D. C_L

Immunology/Apply knowledge of fundamental biological characteristics/Immunoglobulin/Structure/1

17. Which immunoglobulin class(es) has/have a J chain?
A. IgM
B. IgE and IgD
C. IgM and sIgA
D. IgG3 and IgA

Immunology/Apply knowledge of fundamental biological characteristics/Immunoglobulin/Structure/1

Answers to Questions 11–17

11. **D** C3 is found in both the classic and alternative (alternate) pathways of the complement system. In the classic pathway, C3b forms a complex on the cell with C4b2a that enzymatically cleaves C5. In the alternative pathway, C3b binds to an activator on the cell surface. It forms a complex with factor B called C3bBb which, like C4b2a3b, can split C5.

12. **C** Both IgG and IgM are the immunoglobulins that help to initiate the activation of the classic complement pathway.

13. **A** Complement activity in serum *in vitro* is destroyed by heating the serum at 56°C for 30 minutes. In test procedures where complement may interfere with the test system, it may be necessary to destroy complement activity in the test sample by heat inactivation.

14. **B** C3a, C4a, and C5a are split-products of the complement cascade that participate in various biological functions such as vasodilation and smooth muscle contraction. These small peptides act as effector molecules that participate in the inflammatory response to assist in the destruction and clearance of foreign antigens.

15. **A** The Fab is the region of the immunoglobulin molecule that can bind antigen. Two Fab fragments are formed from hydrolysis of the immunoglobulin molecule by papain. Each consists of a light chain and the V_H and C_{H1} regions of the heavy chain. The variable regions of the light and heavy chains interact, forming a specific antigen-combining site.

16. **B** The composition and structure of the constant region of the heavy chain determines the immunoglobulin class of the molecule. The Fc fragment of an immunoglobulin molecule is formed by partial digestion with papain. The Fc fragment contains the C_{H2} and C_{H3} domains of the heavy chain, which are recognized by the antisera that define immunoglobulin class.

17. **C** Both IgM and secretory IgA have a J chain joining individual molecules together; the J chain in IgM joins five molecules and the J chain in sIgA joins two molecules.

18. Which immunoglobulin appears first in the primary immune response?
A. IgG
B. IgM
C. IgA
D. IgE

Immunology/Apply knowledge of fundamental biological characteristics/Immunoglobulin/Function/1

19. Which immunoglobulin appears in highest titer in the secondary response?
A. IgG
B. IgM
C. IgA
D. IgE

Immunology/Apply knowledge of fundamental biological characteristics/Immunoglobulin/Function/1

20. Which immunoglobulin(s) can cross the placenta?
A. IgG
B. IgM
C. IgA
D. IgE

Immunology/Apply knowledge of fundamental biological characteristics/Immunoglobulin/Function/1

21. Which immunoglobulin cross-links mast cells to release histamine?
A. IgG
B. IgM
C. IgA
D. IgE

Immunology/Apply knowledge of fundamental biological characteristics/Immunoglobulin/Function/1

22. All of the following are functions of immunoglobulins *except:*
A. Neutralize toxic substances
B. Facilitate phagocytosis through opsonization
C. Interact with T_C cells to lyse viruses
D. Combine with complement to destroy cellular antigens

Immunology/Apply knowledge of fundamental biological characteristics/Immunoglobulin/Function/1

23. Which of the following antigens is classified as an MHC class II antigen?
A. HLA-A
B. HLA-B
C. HLA-C
D. HLA-DR

Immunology/Apply knowledge of fundamental biological characteristics/MHC/HLA antigens/1

24. Which MHC class of antigens is necessary for antigen recognition by CD4-positive T cells?

A. Class I
B. Class II
C. Class III
D. No MHC molecule is necessary for antigen recognition.

Immunology/Apply knowledge of fundamental biological characteristics/MHC/Function/1

Answers to Questions 18–24

18. **B** The first antibody to appear in the primary immune response to an antigen is IgM. The titer of antiviral IgM (e.g., IgM antibody to cytomegalovirus [anti-CMV]) is more specific for acute or active viral infection than IgG, and may be measured to help differentiate active from prior infection.

19. **A** A high titer of IgG characterizes the secondary immune response. Consequently, IgG antibodies make up about 80% of the total immunoglobulin concentration in normal serum.

20. **A** IgG is the only immunoglobulin class that can cross the placenta. All subclasses of IgG can cross the placenta, but IgG2 crosses more slowly. This process requires recognition of the Fc region of the IgG by placental cells. These cells take up the IgG from the maternal blood and secrete it into the fetal blood, providing humoral immunity to the neonate for the first few months after delivery.

21. **D** IgE is the immunoglobulin that cross-links with basophils and mast cells. IgE causes the release of such immune response modifiers as histamine and mediates an allergic immune response.

22. **C** Cytotoxic T cells lyse virally infected cells directly, without requirement for specific antibody. The T_C cell is activated by viral antigen that is associated with MHC class I molecules on the surface of the infected cell. The activated T_C cell secretes several toxins, such as tumor necrosis factor, which destroy the infected cell and virions.

23. **D** The MHC region is located on the short arm of chromosome 6 and codes for antigens expressed on the surface of leukocytes and tissues. The MHC region genes control immune recognition; their products include the antigens that determine transplantation rejection. HLA-DR antigens are expressed on B cells. HLA-DR2, DR3, DR4, and DR5 antigens show linkage with a wide range of autoimmune diseases.

24. **B** Helper T lymphocytes (CD4-positive T cells) recognize antigens only in the context of a class II molecule. Because class II antigens are expressed on macrophages, monocytes, and B cells, the helper T-cell response is mediated by interaction with processed antigen on the surface of these cells.

25. Which of the following are products of HLA class III genes?
  A. T-cell immune receptors
  B. HLA-D antigens on immune cells
  C. Complement proteins C2, C4, and Factor B
  D. Immunoglobulin V_L regions

Immunology/Apply knowledge of fundamental biological characteristics/MHC/Function/1

Answer to Question 25

25. **C** Complement components C2 and C4 of the classic pathway and Factor B of the alternative pathway are class III molecules. HLA-A, HLA-B, and HLA-C antigens are classified as class I antigens, and HLA-D, HLA-DR, HLA-DQ, and HLA-DP antigens as class II antigens.

UNIT 2

Immunologic Procedures

1. Affinity between individual antigen and antibody molecules depends upon several types of bonds, such as ionic bonds, hydrophobic bonds, hydrogen bonds, and van der Waals forces. How is the strength of this attraction characterized?
   A. Avidity
   B. Specificity
   C. Reactivity
   D. Multivalency

   Immunology/Apply principles of basic laboratory procedures/1

2. A new test system to detect rheumatoid arthritis (RA) also reacts positively with the serum of up to 20% of patients with septic arthritis. What term describes the low specificity of this test system as an assay for RA?
   A. Cross-reactivity
   B. Cross-specificity
   C. Minimal equivalency
   D. Low bound equilibrium

   Immunology/Apply principles of basic laboratory procedures/RID/1

3. The detection of precipitation reactions depends upon the presence of maximal proportions of antigen and antibody. A patient's sample contains a large amount of antibody, but the reaction in a test system containing antigen is negative. What has happened?
   A. Performance error
   B. Low specificity
   C. A shift in the zone of equivalence
   D. Prozone phenomenon

   Immunology/Apply principles of basic laboratory procedures/2

4. Which part of the radial immunodiffusion (RID) test system contains the antisera?
   A. Center well
   B. Outer wells
   C. Gel
   D. Antisera may be added to any well.

Immunology/Apply principles of basic laboratory procedures/RID/Principle/1

Answers to Questions 1–4

1. **B** The antibody binding site may fit any number of epitopes of an antigen. The greater the specificity, however, the greater is the strength of the bond between the antigen and antibody. Specificity is considered a measure of the effectiveness of an immunologic test system.

2. **A** Cross-reactivity is the term that describes antibodies capable of reacting with two or more similar antigens. Antibodies formed in both conditions may recognize the antigen used in the test system. Such a test demonstrates a low specificity for RA and is a poor choice for a confirmatory test. However, if the assay demonstrates high sensitivity (a low percentage of false-negatives), it can be used as a screening test for RA.

3. **D** Although performance error and low specificity should be considered, if a test system fails to yield the expected reaction, excessive antibody preventing a precipitation reaction is usually the cause. Prozone occurs when antibody molecules saturate the antigen sites preventing cross-linking of the antigen-antibody complexes by other antibody molecules. Because the antigen and antibody do not react at equivalence, a visible product is not formed, leading to a false-negative result.

4. **C** In an RID test system, for example, one measuring hemopexin concentration, the gel would contain the anti-hemopexin. A standardized volume of serum containing the antigen is added to each well. Antigen diffuses from the well into the gel and forms a precipitin ring by reaction with antibody. At equivalence, the area of the ring is proportional to antigen concentration.

5. What corrective action should be taken if a patient's sample tested by RID exceeds the highest standard?
A. Dilute the sample.
B. Concentrate the standard.
C. Run a different standard.
D. Obtain a new sample.

Immunology/Evaluate laboratory data to recognize problems/RID/Testing/3

6. What is the most likely cause of a double precipitin ring in an RID test?
A. Presence of too much antibody
B. Presence of too much antigen
C. Defective gel
D. Presence of two antibodies

Immunology/Evaluate laboratory data to recognize problems/RID/Testing/3

7. What may happen if the gel is cut while filling the wells of an RID plate?
A. No problem
B. Irregular shaped ring; difficult to measure
C. Falsely high test result
D. Falsely low test result

Immunology/Apply knowledge to identify sources of error/RID/Testing/3

8. What is the interpretation when an Ouchterlony plate shows crossed lines between wells 1 and 2 (antigen is placed in the center well and antisera in wells 1 and 2)?
A. No reaction between wells 1 and 2
B. Partial identity between wells 1 and 2
C. Nonidentity between wells 1 and 2
D. Identity between wells 1 and 2

Immunology/Apply principles of basic laboratory procedures/Ouchterlony techniques/Interpretation/2

9. Why is radioimmunoassay (RIA) or enzyme immunoassay (EIA) the method of choice for detection of certain analytes, such as hormones, normally found in low concentrations?
A. Because of low cross-reactivity
B. Because of high specificity
C. Because of high sensitivity
D. Because test systems may be designed as both competitive and noncompetitive assays

Immunology/Apply principles of basic laboratory procedures/RIA/1

10. What comprises the reaction system in an enzyme-linked immunosorbent assay (ELISA)?
A. Enzyme-conjugate + substrate + chromogen
B. Enzyme + substrate
C. Enzyme + chromogen
D. Substrate + chromogen

Immunology/Apply principles of basic laboratory procedures/ELISA/1

11. What outcome results from improper washing of a tube or well after adding the enzyme-antibody conjugate in an ELISA system?
A. Result will be falsely decreased.
B. Result will be falsely increased.
C. Result will be unaffected.
D. Result is impossible to determine.

Immunology/Apply knowledge to identify sources of error/ELISA/3

Answers to Questions 5–11

5. **A** A sample exceeding the highest standard would indicate a large amount of antigen. The sample should be diluted and the result multiplied by the dilution factor.

6. **D** Two antibodies (or a single antibody that cross-reacts with two antigens) may be present in the gel. This will produce two rings provided the concentration of the two antigens is different.

7. **B** If the gel is nicked or cut, the diffusion pattern may be irregularly shaped and difficult or impossible to measure.

8. **C** Crossed lines indicate nonidentity between wells 1 and 2. The antibody from well 1 recognizes a different antigenic determinant than the antibody from well 2.

9. **C** RIA is extremely sensitive, but because of strict regulations for handling radioactive materials and safety concerns, it is used only when an alternative method is unavailable. The sensitivity of EIA methods producing fluorescent and chemiluminescent products can be equivalent to that of RIA. These detection systems have greatly diminished the number of analytes that must be measured by RIA.

10. **A** The ELISA test measures antibody using immobilized reagent antigen. The antigen is fixed to the walls of a tube or bottom of a microtiter well. Serum is added (and incubated) and the antibody binds, if present. After washing, the antigen-antibody complexes are detected by adding an enzyme labeled anti-immunoglobulin. Unbound enzyme label is removed by washing, and the bound enzyme label is detected by adding chromogenic substrate. The enzyme catalyzes the conversion of substrate to colored product.

11. **B** If unbound enzyme-conjugated anti-imunoglobulin is not washed away, it will catalyze conversion of substrate to colored product, yielding a falsely elevated result.

12. What would happen if the color reaction phase is prolonged in one tube or well of an ELISA test?
    A. Result will be falsely decreased
    B. Result will be falsely increased
    C. Result will be unaffected
    D. Impossible to determine

    Immunology/Apply knowledge to identify sources of error/ELISA/3

13. The absorbance of a sample measured by ELISA is greater than the highest standard. What corrective action should be taken?
    A. Extrapolate an estimated value from the highest reading.
    B. Repeat the test using a standard of higher concentration.
    C. Report the result as elevated greater than value of highest standard.
    D. Dilute the test sample.

    Immunology/Evaluate laboratory data to take corrective action according to predetermined criteria/ELISA/3

14. A patient was suspected of having a lymphoproliferative disorder. After several laboratory tests were completed, the patient was found to have an IgMκ paraprotein. In what sequence should the laboratory tests leading to this diagnosis have been performed?
    A. Serum and urine protein electrophoresis followed by immunoelectrophoresis (IEP) or immunofixation electrophoresis (IFE) on the positives.
    B. IEP of serum followed by IFE of serum if positive.
    C. IEP of serum followed by protein electrophoresis of serum if positive.
    D. Either serum protein electrophoresis or IEP could have led to the final conclusion. Only a single test should have been performed.

    Immunology/Evaluate laboratory data to reach conclusions/IEP/3

15. An IFE performed on a serum sample showed a narrow dark band in the lane containing anti-γ. How should this result be interpreted?
    A. Abnormally decreased IgG concentration
    B. Abnormal test result demonstrating monoclonal IgG
    C. Normal test result
    D. Impossible to determine without densitometric quantitation

    Immunology/Evaluate laboratory data to make identifications/IEP/2

16. What procedural step distinguishes immunoelectrophoresis from immunofixation electrophoresis?
    A. Electrophoresis of test sample.
    B. Reaction of test sample with antisera.
    C. Antisera are placed over the electrophoresed sample.
    D. No real difference in procedures.

    Immunology/Apply principles of basic laboratory procedures/IEP/1

Answers to Questions 12–16

12. **B** If the color reaction is not stopped within the time limits specified by the procedure, the enzyme will continue to act on the substrate, producing a falsely elevated test result.

13. **D** Any test sample that reads at a value above the highest standard in an ELISA test should be diluted and measured again.

14. **A** Serum and urine protein electrophoresis should be performed initially to detect the presence of an abnormal immunoglobulin which demonstrates restricted electrophoretic mobility. A patient producing only monoclonal light chains may not show any abnormal serum finding because the light chains may be excreted in the urine. A positive finding for either serum or urine should be followed by IEP or IFE on the positive specimen. This is required to confirm the presence of monoclonal immunoglobulin, to identify the heavy and light chain type, and to determine whether free monoclonal light chains are being produced.

15. **B** A *narrow* dark band formed in both the total immunoglobulin lane and lane containing anti-γ indicates the presence of a monoclonal IgG. A diffuse dark band would indicate a polyclonal increase in IgG that often accompanies chronic inflammatory disorders such as systemic lupus erythematosus (SLE).

16. **C** In immunofixation, the antiserum is placed over the electrophoresed sample and allowed to react. The antibodies are transferred to the gel by capillary action where they react with the antigens (if present), forming insoluble immune complexes that are visible within 1 hour of incubation. In immunoelectrophoresis, the antisera is added to a trough following electrophoretic separation of the sample proteins. The antibodies and antigens must diffuse through the gel before they meet. Incubation overnight is required in order to form insoluble immune complexes that are visible.

17. Which type of nephelometry is used to measure immune complex formation almost immediately after reagent has been added?
A. Rate
B. Endpoint
C. Continuous
D. One-dimensional

Immunology/Apply principles of basic laboratory procedures/Nephelometry/1

18. An immunofluorescence microscopy assay (IMA) was performed, and a significant antibody titer was reported. Positive and negative controls performed as expected. However, the clinical evaluation of the patient was not consistent with a positive finding. What is the most likely explanation of this situation?
A. The clinical condition of the patient changed since the sample was tested.
B. The pattern of fluorescence was misinterpreted.
C. The control results were misinterpreted.
D. The wrong cell line was used for the test.

Immunology/Apply principles of basic laboratory procedures/IMA/3

19. What corrective action should be taken when an indeterminate pattern occurs in an indirect IMA?
A. Repeat the test with a new sample.
B. Call the physician.
C. Have another person read the slide.
D. Dilute the sample and retest.

Immunology/Evaluate laboratory data to take corrective action according to predetermined criteria/IMA/3

20. All of the statements below regarding agglutination reactions used for serodiagnosis are true *except:*
A. Agglutination reactions are usually two-step processes involving sensitization and lattice formation.
B. Reactions can usually be observed visually.
C. Most agglutination reactions are direct reactions.
D. Carrier particles for antigen may be latex, RBCs, or yeast.

Immunology/Apply principles of basic laboratory procedures/Agglutination/1

21. What has happened in a titer, if tube Nos. 5–7 show a stronger reaction than tube Nos.1–4?
A. Prozone reaction
B. Postzone reaction
C. Equivalence reaction
D. Poor technique

Immunology/Evaluate data to determine possible inconsistent results/Serological titration/3

22. What is the titer in tube No. 8 if tube No. 1 is undiluted and dilutions are doubled?

A. 64
B. 128
C. 256
D. 512

Immunology/Calculate/Serological titration/2

Answers to Questions 17–22

17. **A** Rate nephelometry is used to measure formation of small immune complexes as they are formed under conditions of antibody excess. The rate of increase in photodetector output is measured within seconds or minutes and increases with increasing antigen concentration. Antigen concentration is determined by comparing the rate for the sample to that for standards using an algorithm that compensates for nonlinearity. In endpoint nephelometry, reactions are read after equivalence. Immune complexes will be of maximal size but may have a tendency to settle out of solution, thereby decreasing the amount of scatter.

18. **B** In an IMA, for example, an antinuclear antibody (ANA) test, the fluorescence pattern must be correlated correctly with the specificity of the antibodies. Both pathological and nonpathological antibodies can occur, and antibodies may be detected at a significant titer in a patient whose disease is inactive. Failure to correctly identify subcellular structures may result in misinterpretation of the antibody specificity, or a false-positive caused by nonspecific fluorescence.

19. **D** An unexpected pattern may indicate the presence of more than one antibody. Diluting the sample may help to clearly show the antibody specificities, if they are found in different titers.

20. **C** Most agglutination reactions represent passive or indirect agglutination where the carrier particles do not have naturally occurring antigens on their surfaces. Antigens are absorbed onto the surface of carrier particles to make the reactions more visible.

21. **A** In tube Nos.1–4, insufficient antigen is present to give a visible reaction because excess antibody has saturated all available antigen sites. After dilution of antibody, tube Nos.1–4 have the equivalent concentrations of antigen and antibody to allow formation of visible complexes.

22. **B** The antibody titer is reciprocal of the highest dilution of serum giving a positive reaction. For doubling dilutions, each tube has ½ the amount of serum as the previous tube. Because the first tube was undiluted (neat), the dilution in tube No. 8 is $(\frac{1}{2})^7$ and the titer equals 2^7 or 128.

23. The directions for a slide agglutination test instruct that after mixing the patient's serum and latex particles, the slide must be rotated for 2 minutes. What would happen if the slide were rotated for 10 minutes?
A. Possible false-positive
B. Possible false-negative
C. No effect
D. Depends on the amount of antibody present in the sample

Immunology/Apply principles of basic laboratory procedures/Agglutination/3

24. Which outcome indicates a negative result in a complement fixation test?
A. Hemagglutination
B. Absence of hemagglutination
C. Hemolysis
D. Absence of hemolysis

Immunology/Apply principles of basic laboratory procedures/Complement fixation/1

25. Lymphocytes have been improperly isolated from a sample for flow cytometric analysis. What control(s) would detect this problem?
A. Isotype(negative) control
B. Positive control
C. Both positive and negative control
D. Either positive or negative control

Immunology/Apply principles of basic laboratory procedures/Flow cytometry/controls/1

26. What control in flow cytometry establishes background fluorescence?
A. Isotype control
B. Positive control
C. Either isotype or positive control
D. Not necessary to establish background fluorescence

Immunology/Apply principles of basic laboratory procedures/Flow cytometry/Controls/1

27. If gating is not properly performed in flow cytometry, what happens to the test result?

A. No effect
B. Failure to isolate desired cell population
C. Falsely elevated results
D. Impossible to determine

Immunology/Apply principles of basic laboratory procedures/Flow cytometry/Controls/3

Answers to Questions 23–27

23. **A** Failure to follow directions, as in this case where the reaction was allowed to proceed beyond the recommended time, may result in a false-positive reading. Drying on the slide may lead to a possible erroneous reading of positive.

24. **C** In complement fixation, hemolysis indicates a negative test result. The absence of hemolysis indicates that complement was fixed in an antigen-antibody reaction and, therefore, that the specific complement binding antibody was present in the patient's serum. Consequently it was not available to react in the indicator system.

25. **B** The positive control is made by treating the sample lymphocytes with ficoll, which makes them fluorescent. If the lymphocyte population is contaminated by other cells, the fluorescence of nonlymphocytes extends the size of the gate. The positive control is used to establish the performance of the reagents, sample preparation method, and staining procedure, and to compare new reagent lots to currently used lots.

26. **A** The isotype or negative control is used to establish background fluorescence.

27. **B** Gating is the step performed to select the proper cell population for testing. Failure to properly perform this procedure will result in problems in isolating and counting the desired cell population. It is impossible to determine if the final result would be falsely elevated or falsely lowered by problems with gating.

UNIT 3

Infectious Diseases

1. Which serum antibody response usually characterizes the primary (early) stage of syphilis?
   A. Antibodies against syphilis are undetectable.
   B. Detected 1–3 weeks after appearance of the primary chancre.
   C. Detected in 50% of cases before the primary chancre disappears.
   D. Detected within 2 weeks after infection.

   Immunology/Correlate laboratory data with physiological processes/Syphilis/Testing/1

2. What substance is detected by the rapid plasma reagin (RPR) and Venereal Disease Research Laboratory (VDRL) tests for syphilis?
   A. Cardiolipin
   B. Reagin
   C. Specific antibody
   D. *Treponema pallidum*

   Immunology/Apply knowledge of fundamental biological characteristics/Syphilis/Testing/1

3. What type of antigen is used in the RPR card test?
   A. Live treponemal organisms
   B. Killed suspension of treponemal organisms
   C. Cardiolipin
   D. Tanned sheep cells

   Immunology/Apply principles of basic laboratory procedures/Syphilis/Testing/1

4. Which of the following is the most sensitive test to detect congenital syphilis?
   A. VDRL
   B. RPR
   C. Microhemagglutinin test for *T. pallidum* (MHA-TP)
   D. Polymerase chain reaction (PCR)

   Immunology/Apply principles of basic laboratory procedures/Syphilis/Testing/1

5. A biological false-positive reaction is *least* likely with which test for syphilis?
   A. VDRL
   B. Flourescent *T. pallidum* antibody absorption test (FTA-ABS)

C. RPR
D. All are equally likely to detect a false-positive

Immunology/Apply principles of basic laboratory procedures/Syphilis/Testing/1

Answers to Questions 1–5

1. **B** During the primary stage of syphilis, about 90% of patients develop antibodies between 1 and 3 weeks after appearance of the primary chancre.

2. **B** Reagin is the name for a nontreponemal antibody that appears in the serum of syphilis-infected persons. Reagin reacts with cardiolipin, a lipid-rich extract of beef heart and other animal tissues.

3. **C** Cardiolipin is extracted from animal tissues, such as beef hearts, and attached to carbon particles. In the presence of reagin, the particles will agglutinate.

4. **D** The PCR will amplify a very small amount of DNA from *T. pallidum* and allow for detection of the organism in the infant. Antibody tests such as VDRL and RPR may detect maternal antibody only, not indicating if the infant has been infected.

5. **B** The FTA-ABS test is more specific for *T. pallidum* than nontreponemal tests such as the VDRL and RPR and would be least likely to detect a biological false-positive. The FTA-ABS test uses heat inactivated serum that has been absorbed with the Reiter strain of *T. pallidum* to remove non-specific antibodies. Nontreponemal tests have a biological false-positive rate of 1%–10% depending upon the patient population tested. False-positives are caused commonly by infectious mononucleosis (IM), SLE, viral hepatitis, and human immunodeficiency virus (HIV) infection.

6. A 12-year-old girl has symptoms of fatigue and presents with a localized lymphadenopathy. Laboratory tests reveal a peripheral blood lymphocytosis, a positive RPR, and a positive spot test for IM. What test should be performed next?
A. HIV test by ELISA
B. VDRL
C. Epstein-Barr virus (EBV) specific antigen test
D. MHA-TP

Immunology/Correlate laboratory data with physiological processes/Syphilis/Testing/3

7. Which test is most likely to be positive in the tertiary stage of syphilis?
A. FTA-ABS
B. RPR
C. VDRL
D. Reagin screen test (RST)

Immunology/Correlate laboratory data with physiological processes/Syphilis/Testing/3

8. What is the most likely interpretation of the following syphilis serology results?
RPR: reactive; VDRL: reactive; MHA-TP: nonreactive
A. Neurosyphilis
B. Secondary syphilis
C. Syphilis that has been successfully treated
D. Biological false-positive

Immunology/Correlate laboratory data with physiological processes/Syphilis/Testing/2

9. Which specimen is the sample of choice to evaluate latent or tertiary syphilis?
A. Serum sample
B. Chancre fluid
C. CSF
D. Joint fluid

Immunology/Correlate laboratory data with physiological processes/Syphilis/Testing/1

10. Interpret the following quantitative RPR test results.
RPR titer: weakly reactive 1:8; reactive 1:8–1:64
A. Excess antibody, prozone effect
B. Excess antigen, postzone effect
C. Equivalence of antigen and antibody
D. Impossible to interpret; testing error

Immunology/Correlate laboratory data with physiological processes/Syphilis/Testing/2

11. Tests to identify infection with HIV fall into which three general classification types of tests?
A. Tissue culture, antigen, and antibody tests
B. Tests for antigens, antibodies, and genes
C. DNA probe, DNA amplification, and Western blot tests
D. ELISA, Western blot, and Southern blot

Immunology/Apply principles of basic laboratory procedures/HIV/Testing/1

Answers to Questions 6–11

6. **D** The patient's symptoms are nonspecific and could be attributed to many potential causes. However, the patient's age, lymphocytosis, and serology results point to infectious mononucleosis. The rapid spot test for antibodies seen in infectious mononucleosis is highly specific. The EBV specific antigen test is more sensitive, but is unnecessary when the spot test is positive. HIV infection is uncommon at this age and is often associated with generalized lymphadenopathy and a normal or reduced total lymphocyte count. IM antibodies are commonly implicated as a cause of biological false-positive nontreponemal tests for syphilis. Therefore, a treponemal test for syphilis should be performed to document this phenomenon in this case.

7. **A** The FTA-ABS or one of the treponemal tests is more likely to be positive than a nontreponemal test in the tertiary stage of syphilis. In some cases, systemic lesions have subsided by the tertiary stage and the nontreponemal tests become seronegative. Although the FTA-ABS is the most sensitive test for tertiary syphilis, it will be positive in both treated and untreated cases.

8. **D** A positive reaction with nontreponemal antigen and a negative reaction with a treponemal antigen is most likely caused by a biological false-positive nontreponemal test.

9. **C** Latent syphilis usually begins after the second year of untreated infection. In some cases the serological tests become negative. However, if neurosyphilis is present, cerebrospinal fluid serology will be positive and the CSF will display increased protein and pleocytosis characteristic of central nervous system infection.

10. **A** This patient may be in the secondary stage of syphilis and is producing excess antibody to *T. pallidum*. The test became strongly reactive only after the antibody was diluted.

11. **B** Two common methods for detecting antibodies to HIV are ELISA and Western blot. Two common methods for detecting HIV antigens are ELISA and immunofluorescence. Two common methods for detecting HIV genes are the Southern blot and DNA amplification using the polymerase chain reaction to detect viral nucleic acid in infected lymphocytes.

12. Which tests are considered screening tests for HIV?
    A. ELISA and rapid antibody tests
    B. Immunofluorescence, Western blot, radioim-munoprecipitation assay
    C. Culture, antigen capture assay, DNA amplification
    D. Reverse transcriptase and messenger RNA (mRNA) assay

    Immunology/Apply principles of basic laboratory procedures/HIV/Testing/1

13. Which tests are considered confirmatory tests for HIV?
    A. ELISA and rapid antibody tests
    B. Immunofluorescence assay (IFA), Western blot, and radioimmunoprecipitation assays (RIPA)
    C. Culture, antigen capture assay, polymerase chain reaction
    D. Reverse transcriptase and mRNA assay

    Immunology/Apply principles of basic laboratory procedures/HIV/Testing/1

14. Which is most likely a positive Western blot result for infection with HIV?
    A. Band at p24
    B. Band at gp60
    C. Bands at p24 and p31
    D. Bands at p24 and gp120

    Immunology/Evaluate laboratory data to recognize health and disease states/HIV/Western blot/2

15. A woman who has had five pregnancies tests positive for HIV by Western blot. What is the most likely reason for this result?
    A. Possible cross-reaction with herpes or EBV antibodies
    B. Interference from medication
    C. Cross reaction with HLA antigens in the Western blot
    D. Possible technical error

    Immunology/Evaluate laboratory data to recognize health and disease states/HIV/Western blot/3

16. Interpret the following results for HIV infection.
    ELISA: positive; repeat ELISA: negative; Western blot: no bands
    A. Positive for HIV
    B. Negative for HIV
    C. Indeterminate
    D. Further testing needed

    Immunology/Evaluate laboratory data to recognize health and disease states/HIV/Testing/2

17. Interpret the following results for HIV infection.
    ELISA: positive; Western blot: indeterminate; RIPA: negative
    A. Positive for human immunodeficiency virus, HIV-1

B. Positive for human immunodeficiency virus, HIV-2
C. Cross-reaction; biological false-positive
D. Impossible to determine

Immunology/Evaluate laboratory data to recognize health and disease states/HIV/Testing/2

Answers to Questions 12–17

12. **A** ELISA and rapid antibody tests (usually agglutination tests) are screening tests for HIV. The latter use polystyrene beads coated with HIV antigens to give visible agglutination following incubation with serum containing anti-HIV.

13. **B** IFAs, Western blot, and RIPAs are generally used as confirmatory tests for HIV. Currently, DNA or RNA amplification tests based upon the polymerase chain reaction are used for early detection of HIV infection and for initiating and following antiviral therapy.

14. **D** To be considered positive by Western blot, bands must be found for at least two of the following three HIV proteins: gp41, p24, and gp120 or 160. The p24 band denotes antibody to a *gag* protein. The gp160 is the precursor protein from which gp120 and gp41 are made; these are *env* proteins.

15. **C** Multiparous women often have HLA antibodies. The Western blot antigens are derived from HIV grown in human cell lines having HLA antigens. A cross-reaction with HLA antigen(s) in the Western blot could have occurred.

16. **B** These results are not indicative of an HIV infection and may be due to a testing error in the first ELISA assay. Known false-positive ELISA reactions occur in autoimmune diseases, syphilis, alcoholism, and lymphoproliferative diseases. A sample is considered positive for HIV if repeatedly positive by ELISA or other screening method and positive by a confirmatory method.

17. **C** Because the Western blot did not show a definite positive pattern, the RIPA assay was conducted to rule out cross-reactivity. The RIPA, highly specific for HIV, was negative. Therefore, the antibody detected in the other two assays is considered to be a biological false-positive.

18. What is the most likely explanation when antibody tests for HIV are negative, but a polymerase chain reaction test performed 1 week later is positive?
    A. Probably not HIV infection.
    B. Patient is in the "window phase" before antibody production.
    C. Tests were performed incorrectly.
    D. Clinical signs may be misinterpreted.

    Immunology/Correlate laboratory data with physiological processes/HIV/Testing/2

19. What criteria constitute the classification system for HIV infection?
    A. CD4-positive T-cell count and clinical symptoms
    B. Clinical symptoms, condition, and duration, and number of positive bands on Western blot
    C. Presence or absence of lymphadenopathy
    D. Positive bands on Western blot and CD8-positive T-cell count

    Immunology/Apply knowledge of fundamental biological characteristics/HIV/Helper T/1

20. What is the main difficulty associated with the development of an HIV vaccine?
    A. The virus has been difficult to culture; antigen extraction and concentration are extremely laborious.
    B. Human trials cannot be performed.
    C. Different strains of the virus are genetically diverse.
    D. Anti-idiotype antibodies cannot be developed.

    Immunology/Apply principles of basic immunology/ HIV/Vaccines/2

21. Which T helper to T suppressor ratio ($T_h:T_s$) is most likely in a patient with acquired immunodeficiency syndrome (AIDS)?
    A. 2:1
    B. 3:1
    C. 2:3
    D. 1:2

    Immunology/Correlate laboratory data with physiological processes/HIV/Testing/2

22. What is a disadvantage of using a culture technique for diagnosis of HIV infection?
    A. Time consuming
    B. Large amounts of sample required
    C. Difficult to grow
    D. Difficult to measure growth

    Immunology/Apply principles of basic laboratory procedures/HIV/Culture/1

23. Which method is used to test for HIV infection in infants who are born to HIV-positive mothers?
    A. ELISA
    B. Western blot
    C. Polymerase chain reaction
    D. Viral culture

    Immunology/Apply principles of special procedures/HIV/1

Answers to Questions 18–23

18. **B** In early seroconversion, patients may not be making enough antibodies to be detected by antibody tests. The period between infection with HIV and the appearance of detectable antibodies is called the *window phase*. Although this period has been reduced to a few weeks by sensitive enzyme immunoassays, patients at high risk or displaying clinical conditions associated with HIV disease should be tested again after waiting several more weeks.

19. **A** The classification system for HIV infection is based upon a combination of CD4-positive T-cell count (helper T cells) and various categories of clinical symptoms. Classification is important in determining treatment options and the progression of the disease.

20. **C** Vaccine development has been difficult primarily because of the genetic diversity among different strains of the virus, and new strains are constantly emerging. HIV-1 can be divided into two groups designated M (for main) and O (for outlier). The M group is further divided into 10 subtypes, designated A–J, based upon differences in the nucleotide sequence of the *gag* gene. A vaccine has yet to be developed that is effective for all of the subgroups of HIV-1.

21. **D** An inverted $T_h:T_s$ (less than 1.0) is a common finding in an AIDS patient. The Centers for Disease Control and Prevention requires a CD4-positive (helper T) cell count of less than 200/μL or 14% in the absence of an AIDS-defining illness (e.g., *Pneumocystis carinii* pneumonia) in the case surveillance definition of AIDS.

22. **A** The major disadvantage of culture techniques is that growth is very slow and then requires performance of a gene or antigen assay (e.g., immunofluorescence) to identify the virus.

23. **C** ELISA and Western blot will reflect primarily the presence of maternal antibody. The PCR uses small amounts of blood and does not rely on the antibody response. PCR amplifies small amounts of viral nucleic acid and can detect less than 200 copies of viral RNA per milliliter plasma. These qualities make PCR ideal for the testing of infants. PCR methods for HIV RNA include the Roche Amplicor reverse-transcriptase assay, the branched DNA (bDNA) signal amplification method, and the nucleic acid sequence-based amplification (NASBA) method.

24. What is the most likely cause when a Western blot or ELISA is positive for all controls and samples?
A. Improper pipetting
B. Improper washing
C. Improper addition of sample
D. Improper reading

Immunology/Evaluate laboratory data to recognize problems/HIV/Testing/3

25. What constitutes a diagnosis of viral hepatitis?
A. Abnormal test results for liver enzymes
B. Clinical signs and symptoms
C. Positive results for hepatitis markers
D. All of the above

Immunology/Evaluate laboratory data to recognize health and disease states/Hepatitis/Testing/2

26. Which of the following statements regarding infection with hepatitis D virus is true?
A. Occurs in patients with HIV infection
B. Does not progress to chronic hepatitis
C. Occurs in patients with hepatitis B
D. Is not spread through blood or sexual contact

Immunology/Apply knowledge of fundamental biological characteristics/Hepatitis/1

27. All of the following hepatitis viruses are spread through blood or blood products *except:*
A. Hepatitis A
B. Hepatitis B
C. Hepatitis C
D. Hepatitis D

Immunology/Apply knowledge of fundamental biological characteristics/Hepatitis/1

28. Which hepatitis B marker is the best indicator of early acute infection?
A. HBsAg
B. HBeAg
C. Anti-HBc
D. Anti-HBs

Immunology/Correlate laboratory data with physiological processes/Hepatitis/Testing/2

29. Which is the first antibody detected in serum after infection with hepatitis B virus (HBV)?
A. Anti-HBs
B. Anti-HBc
C. Anti-HBe
D. All are detectable at the same time.

Immunology/Correlate laboratory data with physiological processes/Hepatitis/Testing/2

30. Which antibody persists in low-level carriers of hepatitis B virus?
A. IgM anti-HBc
B. IgG anti-HBc
C. IgM anti-HBe
D. IgG anti-HBs

Immunology/Correlate laboratory data with physiological processes/Hepatitis/Testing/2

Answers to Questions 24–30

24. **B** Improper washing may not remove unbound enzyme conjugated anti-human globulin, and every sample may appear positive.

25. **D** To diagnose a case of hepatitis, the physician must consider clinical signs, as well as laboratory tests that measure liver enzymes and hepatitis markers.

26. **C** Hepatitis D virus is an RNA virus that requires the surface antigen or envelope of the hepatitis B virus for entry into the hepatocyte. Consequently, hepatitis D virus can only infect patients who are coinfected with hepatitis B.

27. **A** Hepatitis A is spread through the fecal-oral route and is the cause of infectious hepatitis. Hepatitis A virus has a shorter incubation period (2–7 weeks) than hepatitis B virus (1–6 months). Epidemics of hepatitis A virus can occur especially when food and water become contaminated with raw sewage. Hepatitis E virus is also spread via the oral-fecal route and, like hepatitis A virus, has a short incubation phase.

28. **A** Hepatitis B surface antigen (HBsAg) is the first marker to appear in hepatitis B virus infection. It is usually detected within 4 weeks of exposure (prior to the rise in transaminases) and persists for about 3 months after serum enzyme levels return to normal.

29. **B** Antibody to the hepatitis B core antigen (anti-HBc) is the first detectable hepatitis B antibody. It persists in the serum for 1–2 years postinfection, and is found in the serum of asymptomatic carriers of HBV. Because levels of total anti-HBc are high after recovery, IgM anti-HBc is a more useful marker for acute infection. Both anti-HBc and anti-HBs can persist for life, but only anti-HBs is considered protective.

30. **B** IgG antibodies to the hepatitis B core antigen (anti-HBc) can be detected in carriers who are HBsAg and anti-HBs negative. These persons are presumed infective even though the level of HBsAg is too low to detect.

31. What is the most likely explanation when a patient has clinical signs of viral hepatitis but tests negative for hepatitis markers?
A. Tests were performed improperly.
B. The patient does not have hepatitis.
C. The patient may be in the "core window."
D. Clinical evaluation was performed improperly.

Immunology/Correlate laboratory data with physiological processes/Hepatitis/Testing/3

32. Which hepatitis B markers should be performed on blood products?
A. HBsAg and anti-HBc
B. Anti-HBs and anti-HBc
C. HBeAg and HBcAg
D. Anti-HBs and HBeAg

Immunology/Apply principles of laboratory operations/Hepatitis/Testing/1

33. Which hepatitis antibody confers immunity against reinfection with hepatitis B virus?
A. Anti-HBc IgM
B. Anti-HBc IgG
C. Anti-HBe
D. Anti-HBs

Immunology/Correlate laboratory data with physiological processes/Hepatitis/Testing/1

34. Which test, other than serological markers, is most consistently elevated in viral hepatitis?
A. Antinuclear antibodies
B. Alanine aminotransferase (ALT)
C. Absolute lymphocyte count
D. Lactate dehydrogenase

Immunology/Correlate laboratory data with physiological processes/Hepatitis/Testing/1

35. If only anti-HBs is positive, which of the following can be ruled out?
A. Hepatitis B virus vaccination
B. Distant past infection with hepatitis B virus
C. Hepatitis B immune globulin (HBIG) injection
D. Chronic hepatitis B virus infection

Immunology/Correlate laboratory data with physiological processes/Hepatitis/Testing/2

36. Interpret the following results for EBV infection: IgG and IgM antibodies to viral capsid antigen (VCA) are positive.
A. Infection in the past
B. Infection with a mutual enhancer virus such as HIV
C. Current infection
D. Impossible to interpret; need more information

Immunology/Correlate laboratory data with physiological processes/EBV/Testing/2

37. Which statement concerning non-Forssman antibody is true?
A. Is not absorbed by guinea pig antigen
B. Is absorbed by guinea pig antigen
C. Does not agglutinate horse RBCs
D. Does not agglutinate sheep RBCs

Immunology/Apply principles of basic laboratory procedures/IM/Testing/1

Answers to Questions 31–37

31. **C** The patient may be in the "core window," the period when antigen is at low levels and IgG antibody has not yet reached detectable levels. IgM anti-HBc would be the only detectable marker in the serum of a patient in the core window phase of hepatitis B infection.

32. **A** Blood products are tested for HBsAg, an early indicator of infection, and anti-HBc, a marker that may persist for life. Following recovery from HBV infection, some patients demonstrate negative serology for HBsAg and anti-HBs, but are positive for anti-HBc. Such patients are considered infective.

33. **D** Anti-HBs appears later in infection than anti-HBc and is used as a marker for immunity following infection or vaccination, rather than for diagnosis of current infection.

34. **B** ALT is a liver enzyme and may be increased in hepatic disease. Highest levels occur in acute viral hepatitis, reaching 20–50 times the upper limit of normal.

35. **D** Persons with chronic HBV infection show a positive test result for anti-HBc (IgG or total) and HBsAg, but not anti-HBs. Patients with active chronic hepatitis have not become immune to the virus.

36. **C** Antibodies to both IgG and IgM VCA are found in a current infection with EBV. The IgG antibody may persist for life, but the IgM anti-VCA disappears within 4 months after the infection resolves.

37. **A** Non-Forssman antibody is not absorbed by guinea pig antigen. This is one of the principles of the Davidsohn differential test for antibodies to IM. These antibodies are non-Forssman; they are absorbed by sheep, horse, or beef RBCs but not by guinea pig kidney. Therefore, a heterophile titer remaining higher after absorption with guinea pig kidney than with beef RBCs indicates IM.

38. Given a heterophile antibody titer of 224, which of the results below indicate IM?

Absorption with guinea pig kidney	Absorption with beef cells
A. Two-tube titer reduction	Five-tube titer reduction
B. No titer reduction	No titer reduction
C. Five-tube titer reduction	Five-tube titer reduction
D. Five-tube titer reduction	No titer reduction

Immunology/Evaluate laboratory data to recognize health and disease states/IM/Testing/2

39. Given a heterophile antibody titer of 224, which of the results below indicate serum sickness?

Absorption with guinea pig kidney	Absorption with beef cells
A. Two-tube titer reduction	Five-tube titer reduction
B. No titer reduction	No titer reduction
C. Five-tube titer reduction	Five-tube titer reduction
D. Five-tube titer reduction	No titer reduction

Immunology/Evaluate laboratory data to recognize health and disease states/Serum sickness/Testing/2

40. Given a heterophile antibody titer of 224, which of the results below indicate an error in testing?

Absorption with guinea pig kidney	Absorption with beef cells
A. Two-tube titer reduction	Five-tube titer reduction
B. No titer reduction	No titer reduction
C. Five-tube titer reduction	Five-tube titer reduction
D. Five-tube titer reduction	No titer reduction

Immunology/Evaluate laboratory data to determine possible inconsistent results/IM/Testing/2

41. Blood products are tested for which virus before being transfused to newborns?
A. EBV
B. Human T-lymphotropic virus II (HTLV-II)
C. Cytomegalovirus (CMV)
D. Hepatitis D virus

Immunology/Apply principles of laboratory operations/CMV/Testing/1

42. What is the endpoint for the antistreptolysin O (ASO) test?
A. Highest-serum dilution that shows no hemolysis
B. Highest-serum dilution that shows hemolysis
C. Lowest-serum dilution that shows hemolysis
D. Lowest-serum dilution that shows no hemolysis

Immunology/Apply principles of basic laboratory procedures/ASO/Interpretation/1

43. Interpret the following antistreptolysin O (ASO) results.

Tube Nos. 1–4 (Todd unit 125): no hemolysis; Tube No. 5 (Todd unit 166): hemolysis
A. Positive Todd unit 125
B. Positive Todd unit 166
C. Negative
D. Impossible to interpret

Immunology/Evaluate laboratory data to make identifications/ASO/Interpretation/2

Answers to Questions 38–43

38. **A** Antibodies to infectious mononucleosis (non-Forssman antibodies) are not neutralized or absorbed by guinea pig antigen (but are absorbed by beef cell antigen). A positive test is indicated by at least a four-tube reduction in the heterophile titer after absorption with beef cells and no more than a three-tube reduction in titer after absorption with guinea pig kidney.

39. **C** In serum sickness, antibodies are neutralized by both guinea pig kidney and beef cell antigens, and at least a three-tube (eightfold) reduction in titer should occur after absorption with both.

40. **B** An individual with a 56 or higher titer in the presumptive test (significant heterophile antibodies) has either Forssman antibodies, non-Forssman antibodies, or both. A testing error has occurred if no reduction in the titer of antibody against sheep RBCs is observed after absorption because absorption should remove one or both types of sheep RBC agglutinins.

41. **C** CMV can be life-threatening if transmitted to a newborn through a blood product. HTLV-II is a rare virus, which like HIV, is a T-cell tropic RNA retrovirus. The virus has been associated with hairy cell leukemia, but this is not a consistent finding.

42. **A** SLO is an oxygen labile protein exotoxin produced by group A β-hemolytic *Streptococcus* (*S. pyrogenes*). If a patient has antibodies to streptolysin O, the antibodies will neutralize the exotoxin preventing hemolysis of RBCs. The highest serum dilution that shows no hemolysis is the endpoint titer for ASO.

43. **A** An ASO titer is expressed in Todd units as the last tube that neutralizes (*no* visible hemolysis) the streptolysin O (SLO). Most laboratories consider an ASO titer significant if it is 166 Todd units or higher. However, people with a recent history of streptococcal infection may demonstrate an ASO titer of 166 or higher; demonstration of a rise in titer from acute to convalescent serum is required to confirm a current streptococcal infection. ASO is commonly measured using a rapid latex agglutination assay. These tests show agglutination when the ASO concentration is 200 IU/mL or higher.

44. Which control shows the correct result for a valid ASO test?
  A. SLO control, no hemolysis
  B. Red cell control, no hemolysis
  C. Positive control, hemolysis in all tubes
  D. Hemolysis in both SLO and red cell control

Immunology/Apply principles of basic laboratory procedures/ASO/Controls/1

45. A streptozyme test was performed, but the result was negative, even though the patient showed clinical signs of a streptococcal throat infection. What should be done next?
  A. Either ASO or anti-deoxyribonuclease B (anti-DNase B) testing
  B. Another streptozyme test using diluted serum
  C. Antihyaluronidase testing
  D. Wait for 3–5 days and repeat streptozyme test

Immunology/Evaluate laboratory data to recognize health and disease states/ASO/Testing/3

46. Which test shows an increased titer due to *Mycoplasma pneumoniae* infection?
  A. ASO
  B. Cold agglutinins
  C. Heterophile antibodies
  D. Nonspecific warm autoantibodies

Immunology/Evaluate laboratory data to recognize health and disease states/2

47. How can interfering cold agglutinins be removed from a test sample?
  A. Centrifuge the serum and remove the top layer.
  B. Incubate the clot at 1°–4°C for several hours, then remove serum.
  C. Incubate the serum at 56°C in a water bath for 30 minutes.
  D. Use an anticoagulated sample.

Immunology/Apply principles of special procedures/Cold agglutinins/Testing/2

48. All tubes (dilutions) except the negative control are positive for cold agglutinins. This indicates:
  A. Contaminated red cells.
  B. A rare antibody against red cell antigens.
  C. The sample was stored at 4°C prior to separating serum and cells.
  D. Further serial dilution is necessary.

Immunology/Select course of action/Cold agglutinins/Testing/3

49. All positive cold agglutinin tubes remain positive after 37°C incubation except the positive control. What is the most likely explanation for this situation?
  A. High titer cold agglutinins
  B. Contamination of the test system
  C. Antibody other than cold agglutinins
  D. Faulty water bath

Immunology/Evaluate laboratory data to determine possible inconsistent results/Cold agglutinins/Testing/3

Answers to Questions 44–49

44. B The red cell control contains no SLO and should show no hemolysis. The SLO control contains no serum and should show complete hemolysis. An ASO titer cannot be determined unless both the RBC and SLO controls demonstrate the expected results.

45. A A streptozyme test is used for screening and contains several of the antigens associated with streptococcal products. Because some patients produce an antibody response to a limited number of streptococcal products, no single test is sufficiently sensitive to rule out infection. Clinical sensitivity is increased by performing additional tests when initial results are negative. The streptozyme test generally shows more false-positives and false-negatives than ASO and anti-DNase. A positive test for antihyaluronidase occurs in a smaller number of patients with recent streptococcal infections than ASO and anti-DNase.

46. B Cold agglutinin titers are increased in more than half of cases of primary atypical pneumonia caused by *M. pneumoniae*. Titers rise after the first week of acute illness and a fourfold rise in titer is considered evidence of infection. The antibody has I specificity, and is produced in many diseases other than mycoplasmal pneumonia. The cold agglutinin assay is nonspecific and may be negative in *Mycoplasma* infection. A more sensitive and specific alternative test is the measurement of IgM antibodies to *M. pneumoniae* by enzyme immunoassay.

47. B Cold agglutinins will attach to autologous red cells if incubated at 1°–4°C. The absorbed serum will be free of cold agglutinins.

48. D Cold agglutinins may be measured in patients who have cold agglutinin disease, a cold autoimmune hemolytic anemia. In such cases, titers can be as high as 10^6. If all tubes (dilutions) for cold agglutinins are positive, except the negative control, then a high titer of cold agglutinins is present in the sample. Further serial dilutions should be performed.

49. C Cold agglutinins do not remain reactive above 30°C, and agglutination must disperse following incubation at 37°C. The most likely explanation when agglutination remains after 37°C incubation is that a warm alloantibody or autoantibody is present.

50. Which increase in antibody titer (dilution) best indicates an acute infection?
A. From 1:2 to 1:8
B. From 1:4 to 1:16
C. From 1:16 to 1:256
D. From 1:64 to 1:128

Immunology/Correlate laboratory data with physiological processes/Antibody titers/1

51. Which of the following positive antibody tests may be an indication of recent vaccination or early primary infection for rubella in a patient with no clinical symptoms?
A. Only IgG antibodies positive
B. Only IgM antibodies positive
C. Both IgG and IgM antibodies positive
D. Fourfold rise in titer for IgG antibodies

Immunology/Apply principles of basic laboratory procedures/Rubella/Testing/2

52. Why is laboratory diagnosis difficult in cases of Lyme disease?
A. Clinical response may not be apparent upon initial infection; IgM antibody may not be detected until 3–6 weeks after the infection.
B. Laboratory tests may be designed to detect whole *Borrelia burgdorferi,* not flagellar antigen found early in infection.
C. Most laboratory tests are technically demanding and lack specificity.
D. Antibodies formed initially to *B. burgdorferi* may cross-react in antigen tests for autoimmune diseases.

Immunology/Correlate clinical signs with laboratory procedures/Lyme disease/Testing/2

53. Serological tests for which disease may give a false-positive result if the patient has Lyme disease?
A. AIDS
B. Syphilis
C. Cold agglutinins
D. Hepatitis C

Immunology/Evaluate laboratory data to determine possible inconsistent results/Lyme disease/Testing/3

Answers to Questions 50–53

50. **C** A fourfold or greater increase in antibody titer is usually indicative of an acute infection. In most serological tests a single high titer is insufficient evidence of acute infection unless specific IgM antibodies are measured because age, individual variation, immunologic status, and history of previous exposure (or vaccination) cause a wide variation in normal serum antibody titers.

51. **B** If only IgM antibodies are positive, then this result indicates a recent vaccination or an early primary infection.

52. **A** Lyme disease is caused by *B. burgdorferi,* a spirochete, and typical clinical symptoms such as rash or erythema chronicum migrans may be lacking in some infected individuals. Additionally, IgM antibody is not detectable by laboratory tests until 3–6 weeks after a tick bite, and IgG antibody develops later.

53. **B** Lyme disease is caused by a spirochete and may give positive results with some specific treponemal antibody tests for syphilis.

Autoimmune Diseases

1. What is a general definition for autoimmunity?
   A. Increase of tolerance to self-antigens
   B. Loss of tolerance to self-antigens
   C. Increase in clonal deletion of mutant cells
   D. Manifestation of immunosuppression

   Immunology/Apply knowledge of fundamental biological characteristics/Autoimmunity/ Definition/1

2. Which of the following is *not* an explanation for the development of autoimmune diseases?
   A. Loss/abnormality in T suppressor cells
   B. Abnormal expression of MHC class II molecules
   C. Suppression of anti-idiotypic antibodies
   D. Influence of hormones and environmental factors

   Immunology/Apply knowledge of fundamental biological characteristics/Autoimmunity/ Definition/1

3. Which disease is likely to show a rim (peripheral) pattern in an immunofluorescence (IF) microscopy test for ANA?
   A. Mixed connective tissue disease (MCTD)
   B. RA
   C. SLE
   D. Scleroderma

   Immunology/Correlate laboratory data with physiological processes/IF/2

4. What type of antibodies are represented by the peripheral or rim pattern of immunofluorescence in tests for antinuclear antibodies?
   A. Anti-histone antibodies
   B. Anti-dsDNA antibodies
   C. Anti–extractable nuclear antigen (anti-ENA) including anti-Sm (anti-Smith) and anti-RNP (antiribonucleoprotein) antibodies
   D. Anti-RNA antibodies

   Immunology/Correlate laboratory data with physiological processes/IF/1

5. What type of antibodies are represented by the solid or homogenous pattern in the immunofluorescence test for antinuclear antibodies?
   A. Antihistone antibodies
   B. Anticentromere antibodies
   C. Anti-ENA (anti-Sm and anti-RNP) antibodies
   D. Anti-RNA antibodies

   Immunology/Correlate laboratory data with physiological processes/IF/1

Answers to Questions 1–5

1. **B** Autoimmunity is a loss of tolerance to self-antigens and the subsequent formation of autoantibodies.

2. **C** The increase in reactivity of the anti-idiotypic antibodies may result in autoimmunity, where the antibodies react against self-antigens. Suppression would represent a normal reaction.

3. **C** The rim or peripheral pattern seen in indirect immunofluorescence techniques is most commonly found in cases of active SLE. The responsible autoantibody is highly correlated to anti-double-stranded DNA (anti-dsDNA).

4. **B** Anti-dsDNA antibodies are the primary antibodies represented by the peripheral or rim pattern. Some reactivity also occurs against single-stranded DNA and deoxyribonucleoproteins.

5. **A** Antihistone antibodies (and also anti-DNA antibodies) cause the solid or homogenous pattern, which is commonly found in patients with SLE, RA, mixed connective tissue disease, and Sjögren's syndrome. Antibodies to the centromere of chromosomes is a marker for the CREST (calcinosis, Raynaud's phenomenon, esophageal dysfunction, sclerodactyly, and telangiectasia) form of systemic sclerosis.

6. What disease is indicated by a high titer of anti-Sm (anti-Smith) antibody?
   A. Mixed connective tissue disease (MCTD)
   B. RA
   C. SLE
   D. Scleroderma

   Immunology/Correlate laboratory data with physiological processes/IF/2

7. Which disease is *least* likely when a nucleolar pattern occurs in an immunofluorescence test for antinuclear antibodies?
   A. MCTD
   B. Sjögren's syndrome
   C. SLE
   D. Scleroderma

   Immunology/Correlate laboratory data with physiological processes/IF/2

8. What antibodies are represented by the nucleolar pattern in the immunofluorescence test for antinuclear antibodies?
   A. Antihistone antibodies
   B. Anti-dsDNA antibodies
   C. Anti-ENA (anti-Sm and anti-RNP) antibodies
   D. Anti-RNA antibodies

   Immunology/Correlate laboratory data with physiological processes/IF/1

9. Which test would best distinguish between SLE and MCTD?
   A. Ouchterlony testing for anti-Sm and RNP antibodies.
   B. Immunofluorescence testing using *Crithidia* as substrate.
   C. Slide agglutination testing.
   D. Laboratory tests cannot distinguish between these disorders.

   Immunology/Evaluate laboratory data to recognize and report the need for additional testing/Autoimmune/Testing/3

10. When an antinuclear antibody test result does not fit a definite pattern, what should be done next?
    A. Report as inconclusive; retest in 6 weeks.
    B. Dilute sample and retest.
    C. Report as negative.
    D. Repeat the test.

    Immunology/Evaluate laboratory data to recognize and report the need for additional testing/Autoimmune/Testing/3

11. Which immunofluorescence pattern indicates the need for further testing by Ouchterlony immunodiffusion?
    A. Homogenous or solid
    B. Peripheral or rim
    C. Speckled
    D. Nucleolar

    Immunology/Evaluate laboratory data to recognize and report the need for additional testing/Autoimmune/Testing/3

Answers to Questions 6–11

6. **C** High titer anti-Sm is indicative of SLE. Anti-Sm is one of two antibodies against saline extractable nuclear antigens, the other being anti-RNP. These antibodies cause a speckled pattern of immunofluorescence.

7. **A** All of the diseases except MCTD may cause a nucleolar pattern of immunofluorescence. Nucleolar fluorescence is caused by anti-RNA antibodies and is seen in about 50% of patients with scleroderma.

8. **D** Anti-RNA antibodies are represented by the nucleolar pattern. This pattern may be seen in most systemic autoimmune diseases and is especially common in patients with scleroderma. Anti-RNA and anti-Sm are not usually found in patients with mixed connective tissue disease. This is a syndrome involving aspects of SLE, RA, scleroderma, and polymyoitis. The immunofluorescence pattern most often seen in MCTD is the speckled pattern caused by anti-RNP.

9. **A** The Ouchterlony (double) immunodiffusion method for detecting anti-Sm and anti-RNP antibodies should be positive for anti-RNP and negative for anti-Sm in MCTD. The test should be positive for anti-Sm antibodies and may be either positive or negative for anti-RNP antibodies in SLE.

10. **B** The sample should be diluted and retested because more than one antibody may be present. Dilution may reveal multiple antibodies at different titers and enable interpretation of the pattern of each.

11. **C** The speckled pattern can indicate a variety of autoimmune diseases that can be further distinguished by immunodiffusion using the Ouchterlony method or enzyme immunoassay for specific nuclear antigens. Those contributing to a positive speckled pattern include anti-Sm, anti-RNP, anti-SS-A (anti-Sjögren's syndrome antigen A), anti-SS-B (anti-Sjögren's syndrome antigen B), and anti-Scl-70 (antiscleroderma-70). Anti-SS-A and anti-SS-B react with small nuclear proteins and are associated with Sjögren's syndrome. Anti-Scl-70 is commonly seen in scleroderma and reacts with DNA topoisomerase.

12. Which of the following is used in rapid slide tests for detection of rheumatoid factors?
A. Whole IgM molecules
B. Fc portion of the IgG molecule
C. Fab portion of the IgG molecule
D. Fc portion of the IgM molecule

Immunology/Apply knowledge of fundamental biological characteristics/RA/Testing/1

13. Which of the following methods is *least* likely to give a definitive result for the diagnosis of RA?
A. Nephelometric measurement of anti-IgG
B. Agglutination testing for rheumatoid factor
C. ELISA of anti-IgG
D. Immunofluorescence testing for antinuclear antibodies

Immunology/Select routine laboratory procedures/Autoimmune/RA/Testing/1

14. Which disease might be indicated by antibodies to smooth muscle?
A. Atrophic gastritis
B. Active chronic hepatitis
C. Myasthenia gravis
D. Sjögren's syndrome

Immunology/Apply knowledge of fundamental biological characteristics/Autoimmune/Testing/1

15. Antibodies to thyroid peroxidase can be detected by using agglutination assays. Which of the following diseases may show positive results with this type of assay?
A. Graves' disease and Hashimoto's thyroiditis
B. Myasthenia gravis
C. Granulomatous thyroid disease
D. Addison's disease

Immunology/Select routine laboratory procedures/Autoimmune/Testing/1

16. What is the main use of laboratory tests to detect antibodies to islet cells and insulin in cases of insulin-dependent diabetes mellitus (IDDM)?
A. To regulate levels of injected insulin
B. To diagnose IDDM

C. To rule out the presence of other autoimmune diseases
D. To screen susceptible individuals prior to destruction of β cells

Immunology/Select routine laboratory procedures/Autoimmune/IDDM/Testing/1

Answers to Questions 12–16

12. **B** Rheumatoid factors react with the Fc portion of the IgG molecule and are usually IgM. This is the basis of rapid agglutination tests for RA. Particles of latex or cells are coated with IgG. Addition of serum containing rheumatoid factor results in visible agglutination.

13. **D** Patients with RA often show a homogenous pattern of fluorescence in tests for antinuclear antibodies. However, this pattern is seen in a wide range of systemic autoimmune diseases and in many normal persons at a titer below 10. The other three methods may be used to identify anti-IgG, which is required to establish a diagnosis of RA.

14. **B** Antibodies to smooth muscle are found in the serum of up to 70% of patients with active chronic hepatitis and up to 50% of patients with primary biliary cirrhosis.

15. **A** Antibodies to thyroid peroxidase may be detected in both Graves' disease (hyperthyroidism) and Hashimoto's thyroiditis (hypothyroidism). If a positive result is found to thyroid peroxidase, thyroxine levels can be measured to distinguish between the two diseases.

16. **D** Fasting hyperglycemia is the primary finding used to diagnose IDDM. For individuals with an inherited susceptibility to the development of IDDM, laboratory tests for the detection of antibodies to islet cells and insulin may help to initiate early treatment before complete destruction of β cells.

Hypersensitivity

1. Which of the following is a description of a type I hypersensitivity reaction?
   A. Ragweed antigen cross-links with IgE on the surface of mast cells causing release of preformed mediators and resulting in symptoms of an allergic reaction.
   B. Anti-Fy^a from a pregnant woman crosses the placenta and attaches to the Fy^a antigen-positive red cells of the fetus, destroying the red cells.
   C. Immune complex deposition occurs on the glomerular basement membrane of the kidney, leading to renal failure.
   D. Exposure to poison ivy causes sensitized T cells to release lymphokines that cause a localized inflammatory reaction.

   Immunology/Apply knowledge of fundamental biological characteristics/Hypersensitivity/IgE/2

2. Why is skin testing the most widely used method to test for a type I hypersensitivity reaction?
   A. It causes less trauma and is more cost-effective than other methods.
   B. It has greater sensitivity than *in vitro* measurements.
   C. It is more likely to be positive for IgE-specific allergens than other methods.
   D. It may be used to predict the development of further allergen sensitivity.

   Immunology/Apply principles of basic laboratory procedures/Hypersensitivity/Testing/1

3. Which *in vitro* test measures IgE levels against a specific allergen?
   A. Histamine release assay
   B. Radioimmunosorbent test (RIST)
   C. Radioallergosorbent test (RAST)
   D. Precipitin radioimmunosorbent test (PRIST)

   Immunology/Apply principles of basic laboratory procedures/Hypersensitivity/IgE testing/1

4. A patient who is blood group O is accidently transfused with group A blood. What antibody is involved in this type II reaction?

   A. IgM
   B. IgE
   C. IgG and IgE
   D. IgG

   Immunology/Apply principles of basic laboratory procedures/Hypersensitivity/Testing/1

Answers to Questions 1–4

1. **A** Type I immediate hypersensitivity (anaphylactic) responses are characterized by IgE molecules binding to mast cells via the Fc receptor. Cross-linking of surface IgE caused by binding of allergens causes the mast cell to degranulate, releasing histamine and other chemical mediators of allergy. Answer B describes a type II reaction; C describes a type III reaction; and D describes a type IV reaction.

2. **B** Skin testing is considered much more sensitive than *in vitro* tests that measure either total or antigen-specific IgE.

3. **C** The RAST measures specific IgE; the RIST and PRIST tests are radioimmunoassays that measure total IgE. The histamine release assay measures the amount of histamine. Allergen-specific IgE assays are available based upon solid-phase enzyme immunoassay. The allergen is covalently bound to a cellulose solid phase and reacts with specific IgE in the serum. After washing, enzyme (β-galactosidase) labeled monoclonal anti-IgE is added. The unbound antibody-conjugate is washed away and fluorogenic substrate (4-methylumbelliferyl-β-D-galactose) is added. Fluorescence is directly proportional to specific IgE.

4. **A** IgG and IgM are the antibodies involved in a type II cytotoxic reaction. Naturally occurring anti-A in the form of IgM is present in the blood of a group O individual and would cause an immediate transfusion reaction. Cell destruction occurs when antibodies bind to cells causing destruction via complement activation, thereby triggering intravascular hemolysis.

5. Which test would measure the coating of red cells by antibody as occurs in hemolytic transfusion reactions?
A. Indirect antiglobulin test (IAT)
B. Direct antiglobulin test (DAT)
C. ELISA
D. Hemagglutination

Immunology/Apply principles of basic laboratory procedures/Hemolytic reaction/1

6. Which test detects antibodies that have attached to tissues, resulting in a type II cytotoxic reaction?
A. Migration inhibition factor assay (MIF)
B. Direct IF
C. IEP
D. Hemagglutination

Immunology/Apply principles of basic laboratory procedures/Hemolytic reaction/1

7. Which of the following conditions will most likely result in a false-negative DAT test?
A. Insufficient washing of RBCs
B. Use of the wrong antiglobulin reagent
C. Use of excessive centrifugal force
D. Use of a sample obtained by finger puncture

Immunology/Apply knowledge to identify sources of error/Hemolytic reaction/3

8. Which of the following tests is used to detect circulating immune complexes in the serum of some patients with systemic autoimmune diseases such as rheumatoid arthritis?
A. Direct immunofluorescence
B. Enzyme immunoassay
C. Assay of cryoglobulins
D. Indirect antiglobulin test

Immunology/Apply knowledge of fundamental biological characteristics/Hypersensitivity/1

9. All of the following tests may be positive in a type III immune complex reaction *except:*
A. C1q-binding assay by RIA
B. Raji cell assay
C. CH$_{50}$ level
D. Mitogen response

Immunology/Apply principles of special laboratory procedures/Hypersensitivity/Testing/1

10. What immune elements are involved in a positive skin test for tuberculosis?
A. IgE antibodies
B. T cells and macrophages
C. NK cells and IgG antibody
D. B cells and IgM antibody

Immunology/Apply knowledge of fundamental biological characteristics/Hypersensitivity/1

Answers to Questions 5–10

5. **B** The DAT test measures antibody that has already coated RBCs *in vivo.* Direct antiglobulin and direct immunofluorescence tests use anti-immunoglobulin to detect antibody sensitized cells.

6. **B** The direct IF test detects the presence of antibody that may cause a type II cytotoxic reaction. For example, renal biopsies from patients with Goodpasture's syndrome exhibit a smooth pattern of fluorescence along the basement membrane after reaction with fluorescein isothiocyanate (FITC) conjugated anti-immunoglobulin. The reaction detects antibodies against the basement membrane of the glomeruli.

7. **A** Insufficient washing can cause incomplete removal of excess or unbound immunoglobulins and other proteins, which may neutralize the antiglobulin reagent.

8. **C** Most autoimmune diseases involve the formation of antigen-antibody complexes that deposit in the tissues, causing local inflammation and necrosis induced by complement activation, phagocytosis, WBC infiltration, and lysosomal damage. Some patients make monoclonal or polyclonal antibodies with rheumatoid factor activity that bind to serum immunoglobulins, forming aggregates that are insoluble at 4°C. These circulating immune complexes are detected by allowing a blood sample to clot at 37°C, transferring the serum to a sedimentation rate tube, and then incubating the serum at 4°C for 3 days.

9. **D** Mitogen stimulation is used to measure T-cell, B-cell, and null cell responsiveness, which is important in patients displaying anergy and other signs of immunodeficiency. The Raji cell assay identifies immune complexes. Raji cells are derived from a malignant B-cell line that demonstrates C3 receptors, but no surface membrane immunoglobulin. Immune complexes that have fixed complement will bind to Raji cells and can be identified using radiolabeled anti-immunoglobulin.

10. **B** T cells and macrophages are the immune elements primarily responsible for the clinical manifestations of a positive tuberculosis test. Reactions usually take 72 hours to reach peak development and are characteristic of localized type IV cell-mediated hypersensitivity. The skin reaction is characterized by a lesion containing a mononuclear cell infiltrate.

Immunoglobulins, Complement, and Cellular Testing

1. Which of the following symptoms in a young child may indicate an immunodeficiency syndrome?
   A. Anaphylactic reactions
   B. Severe rashes and myalgia
   C. Recurrent bacterial, fungal, and viral infections
   D. Weight loss, rapid heartbeat, breathlessness

   Immunology/Apply knowledge of fundamental biological characteristics/T cell/Testing/1

2. What screening test should be performed first in a young patient suspected of having an immune dysfunction disorder?
   A. Complete blood count (CBC) and white cell differential
   B. Chemotaxis assay
   C. Complement levels
   D. Bone marrow biopsy

   Immunology/Apply knowledge of fundamental biological characteristics/Testing/2

3. Which test should be performed when a patient has a reaction to transfused plasma products?
   A. Immunoglobulin levels
   B. T-cell count
   C. Hemoglobin levels
   D. Red cell enzymes

   Immunology/Evaluate laboratory and clinical data to specify additional tests/Testing/3

4. What is the "M" component in monoclonal gammopathies?
   A. IgM produced in excess
   B. μ Heavy chain produced in excess
   C. Malignant proliferation of B cells
   D. Monoclonal antibody or cell line

   Immunology/Apply knowledge of fundamental biological characteristics/Immunoglobulin/Testing/1

Answers to Questions 1–4

1. **C** An immunodeficiency syndrome should be considered in a young child who has a history of recurrent bacterial, fungal, and viral infections manifested after the disappearance of maternal IgG. Immunodeficiency disorders may involve deficiencies in production and/or function of lymphocytes and phagocytic cells or a deficiency in production of a complement factor. Choice of laboratory tests is based upon the patient's clinical presentation, age, and history.

2. **A** The first screening test performed in the initial evaluation of a young patient who is suspected of having an immune dysfunction is the CBC and differential. White cells that are decreased in number or abnormal in appearance may indicate further testing.

3. **A** A reaction to plasma products may be found in an IgA-deficient person who has formed anti-IgA antibodies. Immunoglobulin levels would aid in this determination. Selective IgA deficiency is the most common immunodeficiency disease and is characterized by serum IgA levels below 5 mg/dL. IgA is usually absent from secretions, but the B-cell count is usually normal.

4. **D** The "M" component refers to any monoclonal protein or cell line produced in a monoclonal gammopathy such as multiple myeloma.

5. A child suspected of having an inherited humoral immunodeficiency disease is given diphtheria/tetanus vaccine. Two weeks after the immunization his level of antibody to the specific antigens is measured. Which result is expected for this patient?
  A. Increased levels of specific antibody
  B. No change in the level of specific antibody
  C. An increase in IgG-specific antibody but not IgM-specific antibody
  D. Increased levels of nonspecific antibody

Immunology/Evaluate laboratory data/Immunoglobulins/Testing/2

6. Which disease may be expected to show an IgM spike on an electrophoretic pattern?
  A. Hypogammaglobulinemia
  B. Multicystic kidney disease
  C. Waldenström's macroglobulinemia
  D. Wiskott-Aldrich syndrome

Immunology/Evaluate laboratory data to make identifications/Immunoglobulins/Testing/2

7. In testing for DiGeorge's syndrome, what type of laboratory analysis would be most helpful in determining the number of mature T cells?
  A. Complete blood count
  B. Nitroblue tetrazolium (NBT) test
  C. T-cell enzyme assays
  D. Flow cytometry

Immunology/Evaluate laboratory data to make identifications/T cells/Testing/2

8. Interpret the following description of an immuno-electrophoresis assay of urine: heavy bowed arcs with anti-κ and anti-λ antisera when compared to the normal control.
  A. Normal
  B. Light chain disease
  C. Increased polyclonal Fab fragments
  D. Multiple myeloma

Immunology/Evaluate laboratory data to make identifications/Immunoglobulins/Testing/2

9. What laboratory test would help in the diagnosis of a case of multiple myeloma in which only free monoclonal κ chains are produced?
  A. Serum protein electrophoresis
  B. IFE on serum
  C. Histology of lymphoid tissues
  D. Immunofixation electrophoresis on urine

Immunology/Evaluate laboratory data to make identifications/Immunoglobulins/Testing/2

10. What is measured in the CH_{50} assay?
  A. RBC quantity needed to agglutinate 50% of antibody
  B. Complement needed to lyse 50% of RBCs

  C. Complement needed to lyse 50% of antibody-sensitized RBCs
  D. Antibody and complement needed to sensitize 50% of RBCs

Immunology/Apply principles of basic laboratory procedures/Complement/Testing/1

Answers to Questions 5–10

5. **B** In an immunodeficient patient, the expected levels of specific antibody to the antigens in the vaccine would be decreased or not present. This response provides evidence of deficient antibody production.

6. **C** Waldenström's macroglobulinemia is a malignancy of plasmacytoid lymphocytes involving both the bone marrow and lymph nodes. The malignant cells secrete monoclonal IgM and are in transition from B cells to plasma cells. In contrast to multiple myeloma, osteolytic bone lesions are not found.

7. **D** DiGeorge's syndrome is caused by a developmental failure or hypoplasia of the thymus, and results in a deficiency of T lymphocytes and cell-mediated immune function. The T-cell count is low, but the level of immunoglobulins is usually normal. Flow cytometry is most helpful in determining numbers and subpopulations of T cells.

8. **C** Heavy bowed arcs seen with both anti-κ and anti-λ antisera indicate excessive light-chain excretion. Light-chain disease would show a heavy restricted arc for one of the light chain reactions, but not both. The finding of excess λ and κ chains indicates a polyclonal gammopathy with increased immunoglobulin turnover, and excretion of the light chains as Fab fragments.

9. **D** The monoclonal κ chains may be cleared completely in the urine and not detected in a serum sample. A 24-hour urine sample may be needed to reveal the presence of the κ chains.

10. **C** The CH_{50} is the amount of complement needed to lyse 50% of standardized hemolysin-sensitized sheep RBCs. It is expressed as the reciprocal of the serum dilution resulting in 50% hemolysis. Low levels are associated with deficiency of some complement components and active systemic autoimmune diseases in which complement is being consumed.

11. What type of disorders would show a decrease in C3, C4, and CH_{50}?
   A. Autoimmune disorders such as SLE and RA
   B. Immunodeficiency disorders such as common variable immunodeficiency
   C. Tumors
   D. Bacterial, viral, fungal, or parasitic infections

Immunology/Evaluate laboratory data to make identifications/Complement/Testing/2

12. All of the following tests measure phagocyte function *except:*
   A. Leukocyte adhesion molecule analysis
   B. Hydrogen peroxide production
   C. NBT test
   D. IL-2 (interleukin-2) assay

Immunology/Apply principles of basic laboratory procedures/Phagocyte/Testing/1

Answers to Questions 11–12

11. **A** The pattern of decreased C3, C4, and CH_{50} indicates classic pathway activation. This results in consumption of complement and is associated with SLE, serum sickness, subacute bacterial endocarditis, and other immune complex diseases. The inflammatory response seen in malignancy and acute infections gives rise to an increase in complement components. Immunodeficiency caused by an inherited deficiency in complement comprises only about 1% of immunodeficiency diseases. Such disorders reduce the CH_{50} but involve a deficient serum level of only one complement factor.

12. **D** Hydrogen peroxide and NBT tests are used to diagnose chronic granulomatous disease, an inherited disorder in which phagocytic cells fail to kill microorganisms due to a defect in peroxide production (respiratory burst). Leukocyte adhesion deficiency is associated with a defect in the production of integrin molecules on the surface of WBCs and their granules. IL-2 is a cytokine produced by activated T_h and B cells. It causes B-cell proliferation and increased production of antibody, interferon, and other cytokines. IL-2 can be measured by EIA and is used to detect transplant rejection, which is associated with an increase in the serum and urine level.

Tumor Testing and Transplantation

1. A patient had surgery for colorectal cancer. After surgery, the patient received chemotherapy for 6 months. The test for carcinoembryonic antigen (CEA) was normal at this time. One year later, the bimonthly CEA was elevated (above 10 ng/mL). An examination and biopsy revealed the recurrence of a small tumor. What was the value of the results provided by the CEA test in this clinical situation?
   A. Diagnostic information
   B. Information for further treatment
   C. Information on the immunologic response of the patient
   D. No useful clinical information in this case

   Immunology/Apply principles of basic laboratory procedures/Tumor/Testing/1

2. A carbohydrate antigen 125 assay (CA 125) was performed on a woman with ovarian cancer. After treatment the levels fell significantly. An examination performed later revealed the recurrence of the tumor, but the CA 125 levels remained low. How can this finding be explained?
   A. Test error.
   B. CA 125 was the wrong laboratory test; α fetoprotein (AFP) is a better test to monitor ovarian cancer.
   C. CA 125 may not be sensitive enough when used alone to monitor tumor development.
   D. CA 125 is not specific enough to detect only one type of tumor.

   Immunology/Apply principles of basic laboratory procedures/Tumor/Testing/3

3. What is the correct procedure upon receipt of a test request for human chorionic gonadotropin (HCG) on the serum from a 60-year-old man?
   A. Return the request; HCG is not performed on men.
   B. Perform a qualitative HCG test to see if HCG is present.

C. Perform the test; HCG may be increased in testicular tumors.
D. Perform the test but use different standards and controls.

Immunology/Correlate laboratory data with physiological processes/Tumor/HCG/3

Answers to Questions 1–3

1. **B** CEA is a glycoprotein that is elevated in about 60% of patients with colorectal cancer and one-third or more patients with pulmonary, gastric, and pancreatic cancers. CEA may be positive in smokers, patients with cirrhosis, Crohn's disease, and other nonmalignant conditions. Because sensitivity for malignant disease is low, CEA is not recommended for use as a diagnostic test. However, an elevated CEA after treatment is evidence of tumor recurrence and the need for second-look surgery.

2. **C** CA 125 is a tumor associated carbohydrate antigen that is elevated in 70%–80% of patients with ovarian cancer and about 20% of patients with pancreatic cancer. While an increase in CA 125 may indicate recurrent or progressive disease, a decrease in CA 125 does not necessarily indicate the absence of tumor growth.

3. **C** HCG is normally tested for in pregnancy; it is increased in approximately 60% of patients with testicular tumors and a lesser percentage of those with ovarian, GI, breast, and pulmonary tumors. Malignant cells secreting HCG may produce only the β subunit; therefore, qualitative and quantitative tests that detect only intact hormone may not be appropriate.

4. Would an HCG test using a monoclonal antibody against the β subunit of HCG likely be affected by an increased level of follicle-stimulating hormone (FSH)?
A. Yes, the β subunit of FSH is identical to HCG.
B. No, the test would be specific for the β subunit of HCG.
C. Yes, a cross-reaction would occur because of structural similarities.
D. No, the structure of FSH and HCG are not at all similar.

Immunology/Evaluate laboratory data to check for sources of error/HCG/Testing/3

5. Which of the following substances, sometimes used as a tumor marker, is increased two- or threefold in a normal pregnancy?
A. Alkaline phosphatase (ALP)
B. Calcitonin
C. Adrenocortocotropic hormone (ACTH)
D. Neuron-specific enolase

Immunology/Tumor markers/Testing/1

6. What is an advantage of performing a prostate-specific antigen (PSA) test for prostate cancer?
A. PSA is stable in serum and not affected by digital-rectal exam.
B. PSA is increased only in prostatic malignancy.
C. A normal serum level rules out malignant prostatic disease.
D. The percentage of free PSA is elevated in persons with malignant disease.

Immunology/Correlate laboratory data with physiological processes/Tumor/PSA/1

7. Which method is the most sensitive for quantitation of AFP?
A. Double immunodiffusion
B. Electrophoresis
C. Enzyme immunoassay
D. Particle agglutination

Immunology/Select appropriate method/AFP/1

Answers to Questions 4–8

4. **B** Luteinizing hormone, FSH and HCG share a common α subunit but have different β subunits. A test for HCG using a monoclonal antibody would be specific for HCG provided the antibody was directed against an antigenic determinant on the carboxy terminal end of the β subunit.

5. **A** Isoenzymes of ALP are sometimes used as tumor markers but have a low specificity because they are also increased in nonmalignant diseases. These include the placental-like (heat-stable) ALP isoenzymes, which are found (infrequently) in some malignancies such as cancer of the lung; bone-derived ALP, which is a marker for metastatic bone cancer; and the fast-migrating liver isoenzyme, which is a marker for metastatic liver cancer. ACTH is secreted as an ectopic hormone in some patients with cancer of the lung. Calcitonin is a hormone produced by the medulla of the thyroid and is increased in the serum of patients with medullary thyroid carcinoma. Neuron-specific enolase is an enzyme that is used as a tumor marker primarily for neuroblastoma.

6. **A** PSA is a glycoprotein with protease activity that is specific for the prostate gland. High levels may be caused by prostate malignancy, benign prostatic hypertrophy, or prostatitis, but PSA is not increased by physical examination of the prostate. PSA has a sensitivity of 80% and a specificity of about 75% for prostate cancer. The sensitivity is sufficiently high to warrant its use as a screening test, but sensitivity for stage A cancer is below 60%. Most of the serum PSA is bound to protease inhibitors such as α-1 antitrypsin. Early studies indicate that patients with borderline PSA levels (4–10 ng/mL) and a low percentage of free PSA are more likely to have cancer of the prostate than patients with a normal percentage of free PSA.

7. **C** AFP is a glycoprotein that is produced in about 80%–90% of patients with hepatoma and in a lower percentage of patients with other tumors, including retinoblastoma, breast, uterine, and pancreatic cancer. The upper reference limit for serum is only 10 ng/mL, which requires a sensitive method of assay such as EIA. The high analytical sensitivity of immunoassays permits detection of reduced AFP levels in maternal serum associated with Down syndrome, as well as elevated levels associated with spina bifida.

8. How is HLA typing used in the investigation of genetic diseases?
A. For prediction of the severity of the disease
B. For genetic linkage studies
C. For direct diagnosis of disease
D. Is not useful in this situation

Immunology/Correlate clinical and laboratory data/HLA typing/1

9. Select the best donor for a man, blood type AB, in need of a kidney transplant.
A. His brother, type AB, HLA matched for class II antigens
B. His mother, type B, HLA matched for class I antigens
C. His cousin, type O, HLA matched for major class II antigens
D. Cadaver donor, type O, HLA matched for some class I and II antigens

Immunology/Correlate data with other laboratory data to assess test results/Transplantation/Testing/3

10. Interpret the following microcytotoxicity result: A9 and B12 cells damaged; A1 and Aw19 cells intact.
A. Positive for A1 and Aw19; negative for A9 and B12
B. Negative for A1 and Aw19; positive for A9 and B12
C. Error in test system; retest
D. Impossible to determine

Immunology/Evaluate laboratory data to make identifications/Transplantation/Testing/2

11. Which method can be used to crossmatch recipients and organ donors for HLA-D compatibility?
A. Flow cytometry
B. Mixed lymphocyte culture (MLC)
C. Primed lymphocyte test (PLT)
D. Restriction fragment length polymorphism (RFLP)

Immunology/Apply principles of special procedures/Transplantation/HLA typing/1

12. SITUATION: Cells type negative for all HLA antigens. What is the most likely cause?
A. Too much supravital dye was added.
B. Rabbit complement is inactivated.
C. All leukocytes are dead.
D. Antisera is too concentrated.

Immunology/Evaluate laboratory data to check for sources of error/HLA typing/3

13. What method may be used for tissue typing instead of serologic HLA typing?
A. PCR
B. Southern blotting
C. RFLP
D. All of the above

Immunology/Apply principles of special procedures/Transplantation/HLA typing/1

Answers to Questions 9–13

8. **B** HLA typing is useful in predicting some genetic diseases and for genetic counseling because certain HLA types show strong linkage to some diseases. HLA typing is not specifically used to diagnose a disease or assess its severity. In linkage studies a disease gene can be predicted because it is located next to the locus of a normal gene with which it segregates. For example, the relative risk of developing ankylosing spondylitis is 87% in persons who are positive for HLA-B27. Analysis of family pedigrees for the linkage marker and disease can be used to determine the probability that a family member will inherit the disease gene.

9. **A** A twin or sibling donor of the same blood type, and HLA matched for class II antigens, is the best donor in this situation. Class II antigens (HLA-D, HLA-DR, DQ, and DP) determine the ability of the transplant recipient to recognize the graft. The HLA genes are located close together on chromosome 6, and crossover between HLA genes is rare. Siblings with closely matched class II antigens most likely inherited the same class I genes. The probability of siblings inheriting the same HLA haplotypes from both parents is 1:4.

10. **B** The microcytotoxicity test is based upon the reaction of specific antisera and HLA antigens on test cells. Cells damaged by the binding of antibody and complement are detected with a supravital dye such as eosin.

11. **B** Flow cytometry can be used in transplantation to type serologically defined HLA antigens. The one-way mixed lymphocyte reaction is used to identify HLA-D antigens on the donor's lymphocytes. HLA-D incompatibility is associated with the recognition phase of allograft rejection. The primed lymphocyte test is used to identify HLA-DP antigens.

12. **B** Inactive rabbit complement may not become fixed to antibodies that have bound test leukocytes; therefore, no lysis of cells will occur. When the supravital dye is added, all cells will appear negative (exclude the dye) for all HLAs.

13. **D** PCR, Southern blotting, and testing for RFLPs may all be used to identify HLA genes. Many laboratories use PCR technology for the routine determination of HLA type.

Immunology Problem Solving

1. Which of the following serial dilutions contains an incorrect factor?
   A. 1:4, 1:8, 1:16
   B. 1:1, 1:2, 1:4
   C. 1:5, 1:15, 1:45
   D. 1:2, 1:6, 1:12

   Immunology/Apply knowledge to recognize sources of error/Serological titration/3

2. A patient was tested for syphilis by the RPR method and was reactive. An FTA-ABS test was performed and the result was negative. Subsequent testing showed the patient to have a high titer of anticardiolipin antibodies (ACAs) by the ELISA method. Which routine laboratory test is most likely to be abnormal for this patient?
   A. Activated partial thromboplastin time (APTT)
   B. Anti–smooth muscle antibodies
   C. Aspartate aminotransferase (AST)
   D. C3 assay by immunonephelometry

   Immunology/Apply knowledge to recognize sources of error/Anticardiolipin/3

3. Inflammation involves a variety of biochemical and cellular mediators. Which of the following may be increased within 72 hours after an initial infection?
   A. Neutrophils, macrophages, antibody, complement, α_1-antitrypsin
   B. Macrophages, T cells, antibody, haptoglobin, fibrinogen
   C. Neutrophils, macrophages, complement, fibrinogen, C-reactive protein
   D. Macrophages, T cells, B cells, ceruloplasmin, complement

   Immunology/Apply principles of basic immunologic response/Inflammation/2

Answers to Questions 1–3

1. **D** All the dilutions are multiplied by the same factor in a progression except the last one. 1:2 to 1:6 is × 3, whereas 1:6 to 1:12 is × 2. Threefold dilutions of a 1:2 dilution would result in a 1:6 followed by a 1:18.

2. **A** Approximately 50%–70% of patients with ACA also have the lupus anticoagulant (LAC) in their serum. The LAC is an immunoglobulin that interferes with *in vitro* coagulation tests: prothrombin time (PT), APTT, and dilute viper venom time (dRVVT). These tests require phospholipid for the activation of factor X. About 30% of patients with antibodies to cardiolipin or phospholipids will have a biological false-positive RPR result. Anti-smooth muscle is most commonly associated with chronic active hepatitis, and increased AST with necrotic liver diseases. Although ACA and LAC may be associated with SLE, the majority of patients with these antibodies do not have lupus and would have a normal C3 level.

3. **C** The correct list, in which *all* mediators are involved in an inflammatory response within 72 hours after initial infection, is neutrophils, macrophages, complement, fibrinogen, and C-reactive protein. Phagocytic cells, acute phase reactants, and fibrinolytic factors enter the site of inflammation. Antibody and lymphocytes do not enter until later.

4. An 18-month-old boy has recurrent sinopulmonary infections and septicemia. Bruton's X-linked immunodeficiency syndrome is suspected. Which test result would be markedly decreased?
   A. Serum IgG, IgA, and IgM
   B. Total T-cell count
   C. Both B- and T-cell counts
   D. Lymphocyte proliferation with phytohemagglutinin stimulation

   Immunology/Correlate laboratory data with physiological processes/Immunodeficiency/Testing/2

5. A patient received five units of fresh frozen plasma (FFP) and developed a severe anaphylactic reaction. He has a history of respiratory and gastrointestinal infections. Posttransfusion studies showed all five units to be ABO-compatible. What immunologic test would help to determine the cause of this transfusion reaction?
   A. Complement levels, particularly C3 and C4
   B. Flow cytometry for T-cell counts
   C. Measurement of immunoglobulins
   D. NBT test for phagocytic function

   Immunology/Determine laboratory tests/Immunodeficiency/Testing/3

6. An IEP and IFE both revealed excessive amounts of polyclonal IgM and low concentrations of IgG and IgA. What is the most likely explanation of these findings and best course of action?
   A. Proper amounts of antisera were not added; repeat both tests.
   B. Test specimen was not added properly; repeat both procedures.
   C. Patient has common variable immunodeficiency; perform B-cell count.
   D. Patient has immunodeficiency with hyper-M; perform immunoglobulin levels.

   Immunology/Correlate laboratory data with physiological processes/Immunodeficiency/Testing/3

7. **SITUATION:** A 54-year-old man was admitted to the hospital after having a seizure. Many laboratory tests were performed, including an RPR, but none of the results were positive. The physician suspects a case of late (tertiary) syphilis. Which test should be performed next?
   A. Repeat RPR, then perform VDRL.
   B. Treponemal test such as MHA-TP on serum.
   C. VDRL on CSF.
   D. No laboratory test is positive for late (tertiary) syphilis.

   Immunology/Correlate laboratory data with physiological processes/Syphilis/Testing/3

8. A patient came to his physician complaining of a rash, severe headaches, stiff neck, and sleep problems. Laboratory tests of significance were an elevated sedimentation rate (ESR) and slightly increased liver enzymes. Further questioning of the patient revealed that he had returned from a hunting trip in upstate New York 4 weeks ago. His physician ordered a serological test for Lyme disease, and the assay was negative. What is the most likely explanation of these results?
   A. The antibody response is not sufficient to be detected at this stage.
   B. The clinical symptoms and laboratory results are not characteristic of Lyme disease.
   C. The patient likely has an early infection with hepatitis B virus.
   D. Laboratory error has caused a false-negative result.

   Immunology/Correlate laboratory data with physiological processes/Lyme testing/Testing/3

Answers to Questions 4–8

4. **A** A patient with Bruton's X-linked agammaglobulinemia presents with clinical symptoms related to recurrent infections, demonstrated in the laboratory by decreased or absent immunoglobulins. Peripheral blood B cells are absent or markedly reduced, but T cells are normal in number and function. Because phytohemagglutinin is a T-cell mitogen, the lymphocyte proliferation test using PHA would be normal for this patient.

5. **C** The patient had an anaphylactic reaction to a plasma product. This, combined with the history of respiratory and gastrointestinal infections, suggests a selective IgA deficiency. Measurement of immunoglobulins would be helpful in this case. A low serum IgA and normal IgG substantiates the diagnosis of selective IgA deficiency. Such patients frequently produce anti-IgA, which is often responsible for a severe transfusion reaction when ABO-compatible plasma is administered.

6. **D** The same finding on two different procedures decreases the possibility of a technical error. This finding is consistent with an immunodeficiency of IgG and IgA and an abundance of IgM. Patients with common variable immunodeficiency have low serum IgG, IgA, and IgM, but a normal number of B cells that exhibit a maturation defect.

7. **B** Serum antibody tests such as RPR and VDRL are often negative in cases of late syphilis. However, treponemal tests remain positive in over 95% of cases. The VDRL test on CSF is the most specific test for diagnosis of neurosyphilis. It should be used as the confirmatory test when the serum treponemal test is positive. However, the CSF VDRL is limited in sensitivity and would not be positive if the serum MHA-TP or FTA-ABS was negative.

8. **A** The antibody response to *B. burgdorferi* may not develop until several weeks after initial infection. The antibody test should be followed by a test such as PCR to detect the DNA of the organism. Regardless of the test outcome, if the physician suspects Lyme disease, treatment should begin immediately.

9. A 19-year-old girl came to her physician complaining of a sore throat and fatigue. Upon physical examination, lymphadenopathy was noted. Reactive lymphocytes were noted on the differential, but a rapid test for IM antibodies was negative. Liver enzymes were only slightly elevated. What test(s) should be ordered next?
A. Hepatitis testing
B. EBV serological panel
C. HIV confirmatory testing
D. Bone marrow biopsy

Immunology/Correlate laboratory data with physiological processes/EBV/Testing/3

10. A patient received two units of RBCs following surgery. Two weeks after the surgery, the patient was seen by his physician and exhibited mild jaundice and slightly elevated liver enzymes. Hepatitis testing, however, was negative. What should be done next?
A. Nothing until more severe or definitive clinical signs develop.
B. Repeat hepatitis testing immediately.
C. Repeat hepatitis testing in a few weeks.
D. Check blood bank donor records and contact donor(s) of transfused units.

Immunology/Correlate laboratory data with physiological processes/Hepatitis/Testing/3

11. A hospital employee has just received the third dose of hepatitis vaccine. She wants to donate blood next week. Which of the following results are expected from the hepatitis screen, and will she be allowed to donate blood?
A. HBsAg, positive; anti-HBc, negative. She may donate.
B. HBsAg, negative; anti-HBc, positive. She may not donate.
C. HBsAg, positive; anti-HBc, positive. She may not donate.
D. HBsAg, negative; anti-HBc, negative. She may donate.

Immunology/Correlate laboratory data with physiological processes/Hepatitis/Testing/3

12. A pregnant woman came to her physician with a maculopapular rash on her face and neck. Her temperature was 37.7°C (100°F). Rubella tests for both IgG and IgM antibody were positive. What positive test(s) would reveal a diagnosis of congenital rubella syndrome in her baby after birth?
A. Positive rubella tests for both IgG and IgM antibody.
B. Positive rubella test for IgM.
C. Positive rubella test for IgG.
D. No positive test is revealed in congenital rubella syndrome.

Immunology/Correlate laboratory data with physiological processes/Rubella/Testing/3

13. SITUATION: A patient with RA has acute pneumonia but a negative throat culture. The physician suspects an infection with *M. pneumoniae* and requests an IgM-specific antibody test. The test is performed directly on serial dilutions of serum less than 4 hours old. The result is positive, giving a titer of 1:32. However, the test is repeated 3 weeks later, and the titer remains at 1:32. What best explains these results?
A. IgM-specific antibodies do not increase fourfold between acute and convalescent serum.
B. The results are not significant because the initial titer was not accompanied by a positive test for cold agglutinins.
C. Rheumatoid factor caused a false-positive test result.
D. Insufficient time had elapsed between measurement of acute and convalescent samples.

Immunology/Apply knowledge to recognize sources of error/IgM testing/3

Answers to Questions 9–13

9. **B** An EBV serological panel would give a more accurate assessment than a rapid slide IM test. The time of appearance of the various antibodies to the viral antigens differ according to the clinical course of the infection.

10. **C** The level of HBsAg may not have reached detectable levels, and antibodies to HBc and HCV would not have yet developed. Waiting 1 or 2 weeks and repeating the tests may reveal evidence of hepatitis virus infection.

11. **D** She may donate if she is symptom-free. The response to hepatitis B vaccine would include a positive result for anti-HBs, a test not normally a part of routine donor testing. She will be negative for HBsAg and anti-HBc.

12. **B** A finding of IgG is not definitive for congenital rubella syndrome because IgG crosses the placenta from the mother; however, demonstration of IgM, even in a single neonatal sample, is diagnostic.

13. **C** The IgM-specific antibody test for *M. pneumoniae* detects antibodies to mycoplasmal membrane antigens and, unlike cold agglutinins, is specific for *M. pneumoniae*. A positive result (titer of 1:32 or higher) occurs during the acute phase in about 87% of *M. pneumoniae* infections and does not need to be confirmed by assay of convalescent serum. However, patients with RA may show a false-positive reaction because rheumatoid factor in their serum can react with the conjugated anti-IgM used in the test. For this reason, serum from patients known or suspected to have rheumatoid factor (RF) must be pretreated. The serum is heated to 56°C to aggregate the RF, and the aggregated immunoglobulin is removed by a chromatography minicolumn.

14. A patient has a prostatic-specific antigen level of 60 ng/mL the day before surgery to remove a localized prostate tumor. One week following surgery the serum PSA was determined to be 8 ng/mL by the same method. What is the most likely cause of these results?
A. Incomplete removal of the malignancy
B. Cross-reactivity of the antibody with another tumor antigen
C. Testing too soon after surgery
D. Hook effect with the PSA assay

Immunology/Apply knowledge to recognize inconsistent results/Tumor markers/3

15. A patient with symptoms associated with SLE and scleroderma was evaluated by immunofluorescence microscopy for ANAs using the HEp-2 cell line as substrate. The cell line displayed a mixed pattern of fluorescence that could not be separated by serial dilutions of the serum. Which procedure would be most helpful in determining the antibody profile of this patient?
A. Use of a different tissue substrate
B. Absorption of the serum using the appropriate tissue extract
C. Ouchterlony technique
D. ELISA tests for nuclear antigens

Immunology/Apply knowledge to identify laboratory tests/ANA/Testing/3

16. A patient with joint swelling and pain tested negative for serum RF by both latex agglutination and ELISA methods. What other test would help establish a diagnosis of RA in this patient?
A. Analysis of synovial fluid
B. ANA testing
C. Flow cytometry
D. Complement levels

Immunology/Correlate laboratory data with physiological processes/RA/Testing/3

17. What is the main advantage of the recovery and re-infusion of autologous stem cells?
A. It slows the rate of rejection of transplanted cells.
B. It prevents graft-versus-host disease.
C. No HLA testing is required.
D. Engraftment occurs in a more efficient sequence.

Immunology/Apply knowledge of fundamental biological characteristics/Transplantation/2

18. A transplant patient began to show signs of rejection 8 days after receipt of the transplanted organ, and the organ was removed. What immune elements might be found in the rejected organ?
A. Antibody and complement
B. Primarily antibody
C. Macrophages
D. T cells

Immunology/Correlate laboratory data and basic immune response/Transplantation/Rejection/3

Answers to Questions 14–18

14. C When monitoring the level of a tumor marker for treatment efficacy or recurrence, the half-life of the protein must be considered when determining the testing interval. PSA has a half-life of almost 4 days and would not reach normal levels after surgery for approximately 3–4 weeks. The hook effect is the result of very high antigen levels giving a lower than expected result in a double antibody sandwich assay.

15. D Many patients with multiorgan autoimmune disease display symptoms that overlap two or more diseases and have complex mixtures of serum autoantibodies. The HEp-2 substrate is the most sensitive cell line for immunofluorescent microscopy because it contains cells in various mitotic stages, which exposes the serum to more antigens. Use of a nonhuman substrate such as *Crithidia* may help to identify dsDNA antibodies but would not aid in differentiating all of the antibodies in a complex mixture. Ouchterlony immunodiffusion helps to identify specific ANAs but has limited sensitivity. The best method is ELISA because it is more sensitive than immunofluorescence microscopy and can quantitate antibodies to specific antigens. ELISA is often used to measure antibodies to extractable nuclear antigens, which may be partially or completely lost during fixation of cells used for immunofluorescent microscopy. These antibodies cause a speckled pattern and are seen in a wide range of autoimmune diseases. Identification of the ENA specificities is helpful in differentiating these diseases.

16. A Analysis of synovial fluid would help to distinguish RA from other causes of arthritis such as gout and septic arthritis. The absence of rheumatoid factors from serum does not rule out a diagnosis of RA, and more than half of patients who are diagnosed with RA present initially with a negative serum result. The serum RF test will eventually be positive in 80%–90% of patients who meet the clinical criteria for RA. Conversely, a positive test for RF (and ANA) is nonspecific and is not by itself sufficient evidence of RA. Because RF may be present in the fluid from an affected joint before it appears in serum, the evaluation of joint fluid should include this test.

17. B The main advantage to the patient for the reinfusion of autologous stem cells is that the procedure prevents graft-versus-host disease, especially in the immunocompromised patient. Although HLA testing is not required, this is not the primary advantage for patient care.

18. D Acute rejection occurs within 3 weeks of transplantation. The immune elements most likely to be involved in an acute rejection are T cells in a type IV, delayed hypersensitivity (cell-mediated) reaction. Preformed antibody, and possibly complement, is usually involved in hyperacute (immediate) rejection and chronic rejection.

19. A patient with ovarian cancer who has been treated with chemotherapy is being monitored for recurrence using serum CA 125, CA 50, and CA 15–3. Six months after treatment the CA 15–3 is elevated, but the CA 125 and CA 50 remained low. What is the most likely explanation of these findings?
A. Ovarian malignancy has recurred.
B. CA 15–3 is specific for breast and indicates metastatic breast cancer.
C. Testing error occurred in the measurement of CA 15–3 caused by poor analytical specificity.
D. The CA 15–3 elevation is spurious and probably benign.

Immunology/Correlate laboratory data with physiological processes/Tumor markers/Testing/3

20. An initial and repeat ELISA test for antibodies to HIV-1 are both positive. A Western blot shows a single band at gp160. The patient shows no clinical signs of HIV infection, and the patient's helper T-cell count is normal. Based upon these results which conclusion is correct?
A. Patient is diagnosed as HIV-1-positive.
B. Patient is diagnosed as HIV-2-positive.
C. Results are inconclusive.
D. Patient is diagnosed as HIV-1-negative.

Immunology/Apply knowledge to recognize inconsistent results/HIV/3

Answers to Questions 19–20

19. **A** Although CA 125 is the most commonly used tumor marker for ovarian cancer, not all ovarian tumors produce CA 125. Greatest sensitivity in monitoring for recurrence is achieved when several markers known to be increased in the malignant tissue type are measured simultaneously, and when the markers are elevated (by malignancy) prior to treatment. In addition to limited sensitivity, no single tumor maker is entirely specific. Carbohydrate and other oncofetal antigens are produced by several malignant and benign conditions. Although testing errors may occur in any situation, measurements of carbohydrate antigens use purified monoclonal antibodies with very low cross-reactivities.

20. **C** The Western blot is used as a confirmatory test for HIV, but it is not as sensitive as enzyme immunoassay tests using polyvalent HIV antigens derived from cloned HIV genes. The Western blot test is considered positive only if antibodies to two of three viral antigens—p24, gp41, and gp160/120—are detected. The presence of a single band is indeterminate. Over the course of the next 3 months, two or more antibodies will be detected if the patient is HIV-positive; however, antibodies to a single viral protein may be caused by a cross-reaction, and this patient may fail to seroconvert. This result should be reported as indeterminate, and the patient should be retested in 3 months. Alternatively, a more sensitive confirmatory test such as PCR or immunofluorescence may be performed.

BIBLIOGRAPHY

1. Bryant, NJ: Laboratory Immunology and Serology. WB Saunders, Philadelphia, 1992.
2. Kuby, J: Immunology, ed 2. WH Freeman, 1994.
3. Leffell, MS, Donnenberg, AD, Rose, NR, (eds): Handbook of Human Immunology. CRC Press, Boca Raton, FL, 1997.
4. Roitt, I: Essential Immunology. Blackwell Scientific, Boston, 1996.
5. Roitt, I, Brostoff, J, Male, D: Immunology, ed 4. CV Mosby, London, 1996.
6. Rose, NR: Manual of Clinical Laboratory Immunology. American Society for Microbiology, Washington, DC, 1997.
7. Stephens, CD: Clinical Immunology and Serology: A Laboratory Perspective. FA Davis, Philadelphia, 1996.
8. Stites, DP, Terr, AI, Parslow, TG: Medical Immunology, Appleton and Lange, East Norwalk, CT, 1997.
9. Turgeon, ML: Immunology and Serology in Laboratory Medicine, ed 2. CV Mosby, Philadelphia, 1996.

Immunohematology

Genetics and Immunology of Blood Groups

1. What type of routine testing does the blood bank technologist perform when determining the blood group of a patient?
   A. Genotyping
   B. Phenotyping
   C. Both genotyping and phenotyping
   D. Depends on the type of test request

   Blood bank/Apply knowledge of laboratory operations/Genetics/1

2. Which genetic events most commonly affect the expression of genes within the ABO blood group system?
   A. Mutations that cause aberrant expressions of group A and group B
   B. Cis and trans effects that cause unequal expressions of group A and group O
   C. Crossovers that produce exchange of genetic material, especially in subgroups of A
   D. Amorphs that cause expression of an undetectable group such as group O

   Blood bank/Apply knowledge of fundamental biological characteristics/Genetics/ABO/2

3. Carla has the blood group antigens Fy^a, Fy^b, and Xg^a. Fred shows expression of none of these antigens. What factor(s) may account for the absence of these antigens in Fred?
   A. Gender
   B. Race
   C. Gender and race
   D. Medication or pathological condition

   Blood bank/Apply knowledge of fundamental biological characteristics/Genetics/ABO/2

4. Which of the following statements is true?
   A. An individual with the *BO* genotype is homozygous for B.
   B. An individual with the *BB* genotype is homozygous for B.
   C. An individual with the *OO* genotype is heterozygous for O.
   D. An individual with the *AB* genotype is homozygous for A and B.

   Blood bank/Apply knowledge of fundamental biological characteristics/Genetics/ABO/1

5. Which genotype is heterozygous for C?
   A. *DCe/dce*
   B. *DCE/DCE*
   C. *Dce/dce*
   D. None of the above

   Blood bank/Apply knowledge of fundamental biological characteristics/Genetics/Rh/2

Answers to Questions 1–5

1. **B** Phenotyping, or the physical expression of a genotype, is the type of testing routinely performed in the blood bank. An individual, for example, may have the *AO* genotype but phenotypes as group A.

2. **D** One of the primary genetic effects seen in the ABO group is the nonexpression of the blood group O. A genetic expression with no detectable product is considered an amorph.

3. **C** The frequency of Duffy antigens Fy^a and Fy^b varies with race. The Fy(a-b-) phenotype occurs in almost 70% of blacks and is very rare in whites. The Xg^a antigen is X-linked and, therefore, expressed more frequently in women (who may inherit the antigen from either parent) than men.

4. **B** An individual having the *BB* genotype has inherited the B gene from both parents and, therefore, is homozygous for B.

5. **A** The genotype *DCe/dce* contains one C and one c gene and is heterozygous for C (and c).

6. Which genotype(s) will give rise to the Bombay phenotype?
   A. *HH* only
   B. *HH* and *Hh*
   C. *Hh* and *hh*
   D. *hh* only

   Blood bank/Apply knowledge of fundamental biological characteristics/ABO grouping/Bombay/1

7. Adults who have the *Le, Se,* and *H* genes will exhibit which Lewis antigen(s) on their red cells?
   A. Le^a
   B. Le^b
   C. Both Le^a and Le^b
   D. Neither Le^a nor Le^b

   Blood bank/Apply knowledge of fundamental biological characteristics/Lewis system/2

8. Which list represents three pairs of antithetical antigens for the Kell system?
   A. K/K, Kb^p/Ka^p, Jx^a/Jx^b
   B. k/k, Ko^x/Kp^x, Jp^a/Jp^b
   C. K/k, Kp^a/Kp^b, Js^a/Js^b
   D. K^x/K^o, Ks^a/Ks^b, Jp^a/Jp^b

   Blood bank/Apply knowledge of fundamental biological characteristics/Genetics/Kell system/1

9. Why is the study of genetics important to blood banking?
   A. For use in population studies in order to provide proper blood products
   B. For use in paternity studies to identify the father of a child
   C. For use in antibody or antigen studies to assist in the identification of unknown antibodies or antigens
   D. All of the above

   Blood bank/Apply knowledge of fundamental biological characteristics/Genetics/1

10. What blood type is *not* possible for an offspring of AO and BO persons?
   A. AB
   B. A or B
   C. O
   D. All are possible

   Blood bank/Apply knowledge of fundamental biological characteristics/Genetics/ABO/2

11. The alleged father of a child in a disputed case of paternity is blood group AB. The mother is group O and the child is group O. What type of exclusion is this?
   A. Direct/primary/first order
   B. Probability
   C. Random
   D. Indirect/secondary/second order

   Blood bank/Evaluate laboratory data to verify test results/Genotype/Paternity testing/2

12. The results of DNA typing are summarized as follows: the child demonstrates some markers in common with the mother but also has a few markers that are missing from both the mother and the alleged father. What type of exclusion is this?
   A. Direct/primary/first order.
   B. Indirect/secondary/second order.
   C. Random.
   D. He is not excluded; he should be the father.

   Blood bank/Evaluate laboratory data to verify test results/Genotype/Paternity testing/2

Answers to Questions 6–12

6. **D** The Bombay phenotype will be expressed only when no H substance is present. The O$_h$ type is expressed by the genotype *hh.*

7. **B** An individual with the *Le* gene who also inherits the *Se* (secretor) and *H* genes will have Le^b adsorbed onto the red cells.

8. **C** K(Kell)/k(Cellano), Kp^a(Penny)/Kp^b(Rautenberg), and Js^a(Sutter)/Js^b (Matthews) are the antithetical antigens for the Kell system.

9. **D** Blood bankers need a basic knowledge of genetics because of the application in population studies to provide blood products, paternity testing, and identification of unknown antibodies or antigens. Knowledge of the frequency of expression of certain antigens helps in testing for blood products and in detecting antigens. Blood cell and protein antigens are expressions of specific alleles that an offspring inherits from both parents. Parentage may sometimes be excluded or confirmed based upon the pattern of inheritance.

10. **D** A mating between AO and BO persons can result in an offspring with a blood type of A, B, AB, or O.

11. **D** An indirect/secondary/second order exclusion occurs when a genetic marker is absent in the child but should have been transmitted by the alleged father. In this case either A or B should be present in the child.

12. **A** A direct/primary/first order exclusion occurs when a genetic marker is present in the child that is absent from the mother and the alleged father.

13. ABO and human leukocyte antigen (HLA) testing give a W value of 80%. Is further testing indicated?
A. No, this W value is over 50% and indicates paternity.
B. Yes, a W value must be at least 95% to suggest paternity.
C. No, this W value indicates nonpaternity.
D. Yes, the W value must be 100% to indicate paternity.

Blood bank/Select course of action/Paternity testing/W value/2

14. What is the *first* criterion in paternity testing?
A. Positive identification of individuals being tested
B. Age of the child (at least 1 year old)
C. Ethnic group or race of the individuals
D. Credentials of the testing agency

Blood bank/Apply knowledge of laboratory operations/Paternity testing/1

15. Why do IgM antibodies, such as those formed against the ABO antigens, have the ability to directly agglutinate red blood cells (RBCs) and cause visible reactions?
A. IgM antibodies are larger molecules and have the ability to bind more antigen.
B. IgM antibodies tend to clump together more readily to bind more types of antigens.
C. IgM antibodies are found in greater concentrations than IgG molecules.
D. IgM antibodies are not limited by subclass specificity.

Blood bank/Apply knowledge of fundamental biological characteristics/Antibodies/1

16. What factors influence the physical attachment of antibodies to RBC antigens?
A. Concentration of antibodies and antigens
B. Temperature
C. Presence of potentiators
D. All of the above

Blood bank/Apply knowledge of fundamental biological characteristics/Antibodies and antigens/1

17. What type of antibody response usually causes problems for transfusion patients?
A. Primary
B. Secondary
C. Both primary and secondary
D. Tolerance

Blood bank/Apply knowledge of fundamental biological characteristics/Antibody response/1

18. How may a technologist distinguish between a reaction caused by immune agglutination and nonimmune agglutination?
A. Check patient factors, appearance of reaction, and circumstances and factors of testing.
B. Check physical factors involved in sensitization first; then check for instrument and reagent failure.
C. Check patient factors first because nonimmune agglutination is most often related to problems with the patient sample.
D. It is impossible to distinguish immune from nonimmune agglutination.

Blood bank/Evaluate laboratory data to verify test results/Antibodies/2

Answers to Questions 13–18

13. **B** Other tests, such as red cell enzymes or other blood groups must be performed to bring the W value to at least 95% to suggest paternity.

14. **A** Positive identification of the alleged father must be made by using at least two forms of identification, such as driver's license or social security card, and a photograph. A heel print of the baby may also be required as positive identification of the baby.

15. **A** An IgM molecule has the potential to bind up to 10 antigens, as compared to a molecule of IgG, which can bind only two.

16. **D** Concentration of antibodies and antigens, temperature, and the presence of potentiators are all factors that affect the physical attachment of antibodies and RBC antigens.

17. **B** The secondary response, with rapid IgG production, can cause life-threatening transfusion reactions.

18. **A** Always check, *in order,* patient factors, appearance of reaction, and circumstances and factors of testing; any of these may cause nonimmune agglutination.

ABO Blood Group System

1. Which of the following distinguishes between the blood groups A_1 and A_2?
   A. A_2 antigen will not react with anti-A; A_1 will react strongly (4+).
   B. An A_2 person may form anti-A_1; an A_1 person will not form anti-A.
   C. An A_1 person may form anti-A_2; an A_2 person will not form anti-A_1.
   D. A_2 antigen will not react with anti-A from a nonimmunized donor; A_1 will react with any anti-A.

   Blood bank/Apply knowledge of fundamental biological characteristics/ABO blood group/1

2. A patient's serum is incompatible with O cells. The patient's RBCs give a negative reaction to anti-H lectin. What is the most likely cause of these results?
   A. The patient may be a subgroup of A.
   B. The patient may have an immunodeficiency.
   C. The patient may be a Bombay.
   D. The patient may have developed alloantibodies.

   Blood bank/Apply principles of special procedures/ABO blood group/3

3. What antibodies are formed by a Bombay individual?
   A. Anti-A and anti-B
   B. Anti-H
   C. Anti-A,B
   D. Anti-A, anti-B, and anti-H

   Blood bank/Apply knowledge of fundamental biological characteristics/ABO blood group/ Bombay/1

4. Interpret the following typing results:
   Anti-A, 1+; anti-B, neg; A1 cells, 1+; B cells, 4+

   A. The patient is group A with autoantibodies.
   B. The patient is group O with acquired A antigen.
   C. The patient is group AB with excessive A_1.
   D. The patient may be A_2 with anti-A_1.

   Blood bank/Evaluate laboratory data to recognize problems/ABO discrepancy/2

Answers to Questions 1–4

1. **B** The group A_1 comprises both A_1 and A antigens. Anti-A will react with both A_1- and A_2-positive RBCs. A person who is group A_2 may form anti-A_1, but an A_1 person will not form anti-A (which would cause autoagglutination).

2. **C** Bombay cells are the only group incompatibile with O cells, and the red cells of a Bombay show a negative reaction to anti-H because the cells contain no H substance.

3. **D** A Bombay individual has no expressed A, B, or H antigens; therefore, anti-A, anti-B, and anti-H are formed. Because a Bombay individual has these antibodies, the only compatible blood must be from a Bombay donor.

4. **D** A group O person will show reactions of equal strength with A_1 and B cells. The weak reaction in the forward grouping with anti-A indicates group A, not O. The weak reaction in the reverse grouping, with A_1 cells, indicates the presence of anti-A.

5. Which typing results characterize a secretor who is group O?
A. Anti-A + saliva + A cells = positive; anti-B + saliva + B cells = negative; anti-H + saliva + O cells = negative
B. Anti-A + saliva + A cells = positive; anti-B + saliva + B cells = positive; anti-H + saliva + O cells = positive
C. Anti-A + saliva + A cells = positive; anti-B + saliva + B cells = positive; anti-H + saliva + O cells = negative
D. Anti-A + saliva + A cells = negative; anti-B + saliva + B cells = negative; anti-H + saliva + O cells = negative

Blood bank/Evaluate laboratory data to make identifications/Saliva neutralization/2

6. Which of the following results is characteristic of an ABO nonsecretor?
A. All negative indicator cells for anti-A, anti-B, and anti-H
B. All positive indicator cells for anti-A, anti-B, and anti-H
C. Positive indicator cells for anti-A and anti-B; negative for anti-H
D. Positive indicator cells for anti-H; negative for anti-A and anti-B

Blood bank/Evaluate laboratory data to make identifications/Saliva neutralization/2

7. What reagents should be used to resolve an A subgroup with anti-A_1?
A. Anti-B from a nonimmunized donor; O cells; autocontrol
B. A different lot of A_1 cells; new bottle of anti-A; new sample
C. A_2 cells; anti-A_1 lectin; anti-H; anti-A,B; O cells
D. Anti-H; anti-A,B; A_2 cells; Bombay cells

Blood bank/Apply principles of special procedures/RBC/ABO discrepancy/3

8. Which typing results are most likely to occur when a patient has an "acquired B" antigen?
A. Anti-A, 4+ anti-B, 3+ A_1 cells, neg B cells, neg
B. Anti-A, 3+ anti-B, neg A_1 cells, neg B cells, neg
C. Anti-A, 4+ anti-B, 1+ A_1 cells, neg B cells, 4+
D. Anti-A, 4+ anti-B, 4+ A_1 cells, 2+   B cells, neg

Blood bank/Evaluate laboratory data to recognize problems/ABO discrepancy/2

9. Given the following typing reactions, what is the most appropriate first course of action?

Anti-A, 4+; anti-B, 4+; A1 cells, neg; B cells, 4+

A. Perform an autocontrol and, if negative, interpret as group AB.
B. Wash the red cells before retyping; interpret the same results as group O.
C. Perform an antibody identification panel to determine presence of alloantibodies.

D. Wash the red cells and dilute the serum before retyping.

Blood bank/Evaluate laboratory data to recognize problems/ABO discrepancy/3

Answers to Questions 5–9

5. **C** The result is consistent for a secretor group O, in which soluble H antigens from saliva have neutralized anti-H typing reagent. No antigen is left to react with reagent O cells. No A or B antigens are present in a group O individual, so no A or B antigen is available to bind with the anti-A or anti-B antiserum. When A and B cells are added, a positive result is obtained.

6. **B** If no soluble antigens are found in secretions, then antibodies in the reagents are free to bind to the corresponding antigens on reagent red cells. This results in agglutination when anti-A, anti-B, and anti-H are mixed with saliva and the respective antigen-positive RBCs.

7. **C** The most complete and correct list of reagents to resolve an A subgroup with anti-A_1 includes A_2 cells, anti-A_1 lectin, anti-H, anti-A,B, and O cells. Confirmation of the subgroup and the presence of anti-A_1 must be tested before a conclusion may be drawn by the investigator. Anti-A,B would determine if the test sample was a group O or A. A negative result with A_2 cells would indicate anti-A_1 and not an alloantibody. Anti-A_1 lectin agglutinates only A_1-positive RBCs. Anti-H detects A subgroups, and O cells rule out alloantibodies.

8. **C** In forward typing a 1+ reaction with anti-B is suspicious because of the weak reaction and the "normal" reverse grouping that appears to be group A. This may be indicative of an acquired antigen. In cases of acquired B antigen, the reverse grouping is the same as for a group A person. Choice A is indicative of group AB; B is indicative of a group A who may be immunocompromised; D may be caused by a mistyping or an antibody against antigens on reverse cells.

9. **D** This situation could be a problem with either forward typing (anti-B should not have been positive) or reverse typing (B cells should not have been positive). The result cannot be interpreted as AB because of the positive reaction with B cells in the reverse grouping. The patient cannot be group O given the positive reactions with anti-A and anti-B and negative reaction with group A_1 cells. The patient may have an alloantibody reacting with the B cells; an antibody screen should be performed to confirm or rule this out. The first action should be to wash the cells and dilute the serum before retesting. This will resolve a discrepancy caused by excessive protein coating the RBCs.

10. What should be done if all forward and reverse ABO results and the autocontrol are positive?
    A. Wash the cells with warm saline; autoadsorb the serum at 4°C.
    B. Retype the sample using a different lot number of reagents.
    C. Use polyclonal typing reagents.
    D. Report the sample as group AB.

    Blood bank/Evaluate laboratory and clinical data to specify additional tests/RBC/ABO discrepancy/3

11. What should be done if all forward and reverse ABO results are negative?
    A. Perform additional testing such as typing with anti-A$_1$ lectin, and anti-A,B.
    B. Incubate at 22°C or 4°C to enhance weak expression.
    C. Repeat the tests with new reagents.
    D. Run an antibody identification panel.

    Blood bank/Evaluate laboratory and clinical data to specify additional tests/RBC/ABO discrepancy/3

12. Interpret the following results:

    | Unknown cells: | Anti-A, neg | Anti-B, 4+ |
    | Unknown serum: | A$_1$ cells, 4+ | B cells, 4+ |

    A. A$_1$ with acquired B
    B. Room temperature reactive alloantibody
    C. Bombay
    D. Cold autoantibody

    Blood bank/Evaluate laboratory data to recognize problems/ABO discrepancy/2

13. A transplant patient was retyped when she was transferred from another hospital. What is the most likely cause of the following results?

    | Patient's cells: | Anti-A, neg | Anti-B, 4+ |
    | Patient's serum: | A$_1$ cells, neg | B cells, neg |

    A. Viral infection
    B. Alloantibodies
    C. Immunodeficiency
    D. Autoimmune hemolytic anemia

    Blood bank/Evaluate laboratory data to recognize health and disease states/ABO discrepancy/3

14. What reaction would be the same for an A$_1$ and an A$_2$ individual?
    A. Positive reaction with anti-A$_1$ lectin
    B. Positive reaction with A$_1$ cells
    C. Equal reaction with anti-H
    D. Positive reaction with anti-A,B

    Blood bank/Evaluate laboratory data to make identifications/ABO discrepancy/2

15. Which of the following results would be indicative of polyagglutination (using monoclonal typing reagents)?

	Anti-A	Anti-B	A$_1$ cells	B cells
A.	Anti-A 2+mf	Anti-B neg	A$_1$ cells 4+	B cells 4+
B.	Anti-A neg	Anti-B neg	A$_1$ cells 4+	B cells 4+
C.	Anti-A 2+	Anti-B 2+	A$_1$ cells 4+	B cells 4+
D.	Anti-A 4+	Anti-B 4+	A$_1$ cells 2+	B cells neg

Blood bank/Evaluate laboratory data to make identification/ABO discrepancy/3

Answers to Questions 10–15

10. **A** These results point to a cold autoantibody. Washing the cells with warm saline may elute the autoantibody allowing a valid forward type to be performed. The serum should be adsorbed using washed cells until the autocontrol is negative. Then the adsorbed serum should be used for the reverse grouping.

11. **B** All negative results may be due to weakened antigens or antibodies. Room temperature or lower incubation temperature may enhance expression of weakened antigens or antibodies.

12. **D** A cold reactive autoantibody might be reacting with reverse grouping cells to give a positive reaction. Perform an autocontrol. If positive, dilute the serum and perform a secretor study, or wash the red cells and repeat the forward typing.

13. **C** A transplant patient is probably taking immunosuppressive medication. Immunosuppression can contribute to the loss of normal blood group antibodies as well as other types of antibodies.

14. **D** Anti-A,B should react positively with group A or B and any subgroup of A or B (with the exception of A$_m$). An A$_1$ (not A$_2$) would react with anti-A$_1$ lectin; only an A$_2$ individual with anti-A$_1$ would give a positive reaction with A$_1$ cells; an A$_2$ would react more strongly with anti-H than an A$_1$.

15. **A** A mixed field positive reaction in the forward type in an individual who normally appears to be group O would be indicative of polyagglutination caused by bacterial infection.

16. Which condition would most likely be responsible for the following typing results?

Patient's cells: Anti-A, neg   Anti-B, neg

Patient's serum: A₁ cells, neg   B cells, 4+

A. Immunodeficiency
B. Masking of antigens by the presence of massive amounts of antibody
C. Weak or excessive antigen(s)
D. Impossible to determine

Blood bank/Apply principles of basic laboratory procedures/ABO discrepancy/3

17. Which of the following results is discrepant?

Anti-A, neg; anti-B, 4+; A₁ cells, neg; B cells, neg

A. Negative B cells
B. Positive reaction with anti-B
C. Negative A₁ cells
D. No problem with this typing

Blood bank/Evaluate laboratory data to recognize problems/ABO discrepancy/3

Answers to Questions 16–17

16. **C** Excessive A substance, such as may be found in some types of tumors, may be neutralizing the anti-A. Weak A subgroups may fail to react with anti-A and require additional testing techniques (e.g., room temperature incubation) before their expression is apparent.

17. **C** The reverse typing should agree with the forward typing in this result. The 4+ reaction with anti-B indicates group B. A positive reaction is expected with A₁ cells in the reverse group.

Rh Blood Group System

1. A complete Rh typing for antigens C, c, D, E, and e revealed negative results for C, D, and E. How is this individual designated?
   A. Rh-positive
   B. Rh-negative
   C. Rh-positive for c and e
   D. Impossible to determine

   Blood bank/Apply knowledge of fundamental biological characteristics/Rh typing/1

2. How is an individual classified with genotype *DCe/dce*?
   A. Rh-positive
   B. Rh-negative
   C. Rh$_{null}$
   D. Rh-enhanced

   Blood bank/Apply knowledge of fundamental biological characteristics/Rh typing/2

3. An Rh typing revealed all Rh antigens as negative. What could be the problem with this typing?
   A. Test performance error.
   B. Problem with reagents.
   C. Patient Rh$_{null}$.
   D. Any of the above may be true.

   Blood bank/Apply knowledge of fundamental biological characteristics/Rh typing/2

4. Which donor unit is selected for a recipient with anti-c?
   A. *r'r*
   B. *R⁰R¹*
   C. *R²r″*
   D. *r'rʸ*

   Blood bank/Apply knowledge of fundamental biological characteristics/Rh typing/3

5. Which genotype usually shows the strongest reaction with anti-D?
   A. *DCE/DCE*

B. *Dce/dCe*
C. *D—/D—*
D. *-CE/-ce*

Blood bank/Apply knowledge of fundamental biological characteristics/Rh typing/1

Answers to Questions 1–5

1. **B** *Rh-positive* refers to the presence of D antigen; *Rh-negative* refers to the absence of the D antigen. These designations are for D antigen only and do not involve other Rh antigens.

2. **A** This individual has the D antigen and is classified as Rh-positive. Any genotype containing the D antigen will be considered Rh-positive.

3. **D** Testing problems, such as performance errors and faulty reagents, may account for an Rh typing that appeared negative for all the Rh antigens. The test should be repeated. The problem, however, may be the patient, who may be Rh$_{null}$ and have no Rh antigens.

4. **D** The designation *r'* is *dCe* and *rʸ* is *dCE*, neither of which contains the c antigen. The other three Rh types contain the c antigen and could not be used for a person with anti-c.

5. **C** The phenotype that results from *D—/D—* is classified as enhanced D because it shows a stronger reaction than expected with anti-D. Such cells have a greater amount of D antigen than normal. This is thought to result from a larger quantity of precursor being available to the D genes because there is no competition from other Rh genes.

6. Why is testing for Rh antigens and antibodies different from ABO testing?
   A. ABO reactions are primarily due to IgM antibodies and usually occur at room temperature; Rh antibodies are IgG, and agglutination usually requires incubation and enhancement media.
   B. ABO antigens are attached to receptors on the outside of the red cell and do not require any special enhancement for testing; Rh antigens are loosely attached to the red cell membrane and require enhancement for detection.
   C. Both ABO and Rh antigens and antibodies have similar structures, but Rh antibodies are configured so that special techniques are needed to facilitate binding to Rh antigen.
   D. There is no difference in ABO and Rh testing; both may be conducted at room temperature with no special enhancement needed for reaction.

   Blood bank/Apply knowledge of fundamental biological characteristics/Rh system/1

7. Testing reveals a weak D (D^u) that reacts 1+ after indirect antiglobulin testing (IAT). How is this result classified?
   A. Rh-positive
   B. Rh-negative; D^u-positive
   C. Rh-negative
   D. Rh-positive; D^u-positive

   Blood bank/Apply knowledge of standard operating procedures/Components/Rh label/2

8. What is one possible genotype for a patient who develops anti-C antibody?
   A. R^1r
   B. R^1R^1
   C. $r'r$
   D. rr

   Blood bank/Apply knowledge of fundamental biological characteristics/Rh typing/2

9. A patient developed a combination of Rh antibodies: anti-C, anti-E, and anti-D. Can compatible blood be found for this patient?
   A. Almost impossible to find blood lacking the C, E, and D antigens
   B. rr blood could be used without causing a problem.
   C. R^0R^0 may be used because it lacks all three of these antigens.
   D. Although rare, r^yr may be obtained from close relatives of the patient.

   Blood bank/Apply knowledge of fundamental biological characteristics/Rh antibodies/1

10. A patient tests positive for weak D, but also appears to have anti-D in his serum. What may be the problem?

   A. Mixup of samples or testing error.
   B. Most weak D individuals make anti-D.
   C. The problem could be due to a disease state.
   D. A D mosaic may make antibodies to missing antigen parts.

   Blood bank/Apply knowledge to identify sources of error/Rh antibodies/2

11. Which offspring is *not* possible from a mother who is R^1R^2 and a father who is R^1r?
   A. DcE/DcE
   B. DCe/DCe
   C. DcE/DCe
   D. DCe/dce

   Blood bank/Evaluate laboratory data to verify test results/Rh system/Paternity testing/2

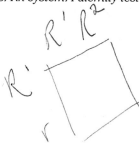

Answers to Questions 6–11

6. **A** Detection of ABO and Rh antigens and antibodies requires different reaction conditions. ABO antibodies are naturally occurring IgM molecules and react best at room temperature. Rh antibodies are generally immune IgG molecules that result from transfusion or pregnancy. Detection usually requires incubation and enhancement techniques.

7. **A** Blood tested for D^u that shows a 1+ reaction after IAT is classified as Rh-positive. The weak D designation is not noted in the reporting of the result.

8. **D** Only rr (*dce/dce*) does not contain the C antigen. Normally, people will not develop antibodies to their own antigens.

9. **B** The genotype rr (*dce/dce*) lacks D, C, and E antigens and would be suitable for an individual who has developed antibodies to all three antigens. This is the most common Rh-negative genotype and is found in nearly 14% of white blood donors.

10. **D** The D antigen is made up of different parts designated as a mosaic. If an individual lacks parts of the antigen, he or she may make antibodies to the missing parts if exposed to the whole D antigen.

11. **A** *DcE/DcE* (R^2R^2) is not possible because R^2 can be inherited only from the mother and is not present in the father.

12. Which genotype would most likely show dosage effect for both C and e antigens?
  A. *dce/dce*
  B. *dCE/dCE*
  C. *DCE/DcE*
  D. *DCe/DcE*

  Blood bank/Evaluate laboratory data to verify test results/Rh system/Rh testing/2

13. What antibodies could an R^1R^1 individual make if exposed to R^2R^2 blood?
  A. Anti-e and anti-C
  B. Anti-E and anti-c
  C. Anti-E and anti-C
  D. Anti-e and anti-c

  Blood bank/Apply knowledge of fundamental biological characteristics/Rh antibodies/2

14. Interpret this Rh phenotype: —/—
  A. No problem, Rh-negative
  B. D mosaic
  C. Rh$_{null}$
  D. Loss of Rh antigens through disease

  Blood bank/Evaluate laboratory data to make identifications/Rh system/Rh antigens/2

15. What techniques are necessary for D^u testing?
  A. Saline + 22°C incubation
  B. Albumin or LISS + 37°C incubation
  C. Saline + 37°C incubation
  D. 37°C incubation + IAT

  Blood bank/Apply knowledge of basic laboratory procedure/Rh system/D^u testing/2

16. A patient types as AB and appears to be Rh-positive on slide typing. What additional test should be performed for tube typing?
  A. Rh-negative control
  B. Direct antiglobulin test (DAT)
  C. Low-protein Rh antisera
  D. No additional testing is needed

  Blood bank/Evaluate laboratory data to verify test results/Rh system/D^u testing/2

17. Which of the following will *not* facilitate detection of D^u antigen?
  A. Incubation at 37°C
  B. Anti-C3d monospecific antihuman globulin (AHG) reagent
  C. Monoclonal antisera
  D. IAT

  Blood bank/Apply knowledge of basic laboratory procedure/Rh system/D^u testing/2

18. What might happen if an Rh viewbox temperature were 60°C?
  A. False-positive typing results due to excessively high temperature

  B. False-negative typing results due to excessively low temperature
  C. No adverse consequence to this action
  D. False-positive typing results due to activation of fibrin

  Blood bank/Apply knowledge to identify sources of error/Rh system/Rh slide testing/3

Answers to Questions 12–18

12. **D** In the genotype *DCe/DcE,* both C and e (and C and E) are heterozygous, which may result in dosage effect. The agglutination reaction between these antigens and the respective antisera will be weaker than for cells from a homozygote.

13. **B** The R^1R^1 (DCe/DCe) individual does not have the E or c antigen and could make anti-E and anti-c antibodies when exposed to R^2R^2 (DcE/DcE) cells.

14. **C** A person who is Rh$_{null}$ shows no Rh antigens on his/her RBCs. Loss of Rh antigens is very unlikely to happen because Rh antigens are integral parts of the RBC membrane. The Rh$_{null}$ phenotype can result from either genetic suppression of the Rh genes or inheritance of amorphic genes at the Rh locus.

15. **D** D^u testing requires both 37°C incubation and the IAT procedure.

16. **A** An Rh-negative control (patient cells in saline or 6% albumin) should be run if a sample appears to be AB in the forward typing. The ABO test serves as the Rh control for other ABO types.

17. **B** Anti-C3d AHG will detect complement-coated cells and will not detect anti-D (IgG) attached to D^u-positive cells.

18. **A** Rh viewbox temperatures should be 40°–50°C. An excessive temperature will most likely cause a false-positive test for the D antigen because drying may cause the slide to appear as if agglutination has occurred.

19. Given the following results, what course of action should be followed in order to determine the patient's Rh type?

Anti-A	Anti-B	A cells	B cells	Autocontrol	Anti-D	DAT
4+	Neg	Neg	4+	1+	4+	Neg

  A. Rh typing is probably correct; no further action is needed.

  B. Wash the patient's cells and retype.

  C. Wash the patient's cells in warm saline and repeat the Rh typing.

  D. Obtain a new sample and repeat all tests.

Blood bank/Evaluate sources of error/Rh system/3

20. What is the purpose of adding antibody-coated red cells to all negative AHG tubes?

  A. To ensure proper tube reading

  B. To ensure proper cell washing and addition of AHG reagent

  C. To check for hemolysis or reaction of complement

  D. To check for attachment of additional antibody

Blood bank/Apply principles of basic laboratory procedures/AHG testing/1

Answers to Questions 19–20

19. **C** There appears to be no problem with ABO typing, and no antibody is coating the patient's red cells (negative DAT). The patient's serum may contain a cold-reacting antibody directed only against the patient's own RBCs. Check the patient's records for a previous diagnosis and repeat the Rh typing.

20. **B** The addition of red cells coated with antibody (available commercially) ensures proper cell washing and addition of AHG reagent. If the cells agglutinate, then the test was performed properly.

Testing for Antibodies

1. A patient has the Lewis phenotype Le(a-b-). An antibody panel reveals the presence of anti-Le^a. Another patient with the phenotype Le(a-b+) has a positive antibody screen, but a panel reveals no conclusive antibody. Should anti-Le^a be considered as a possibility for the patient with the Le(a-b+) phenotype?
   A. Anti-Le^a should be considered as a possible antibody for this patient.
   B. Anti-Le^a may be a possible antibody, but further studies are needed.
   C. Anti-Le^a is not a likely antibody because even Le^b individuals secrete some Le^a.
   D. Anti-Le^a may be found in saliva, but is not detectable in serum.

   Blood bank/Apply knowledge of fundamental biological characteristics/Blood groups/2

2. A technologist is having great difficulty resolving an antibody mixture. One of the antibodies is anti-Le^a. This antibody is not clinically significant in this situation, but it needs to be removed to reveal the possible presence of an underlying antibody of clinical significance. What can be done?
   A. Perform an enzyme panel.
   B. Neutralize the serum with saliva.
   C. Neutralize the serum with hydatid cyst fluid.
   D. Use 2-aminoethylisothiouronium (AET) to treat the panel cells.

   Blood bank/Apply knowledge of fundamental biological characteristics/Blood groups/3

3. What type of blood should be given an individual who has an anti-Le^b that reacts 1+ at the IAT phase?
   A. Blood that is negative for the Le^b antigen.
   B. Blood that is negative for both the Le^a and the Le^b antigen.
   C. Blood that is positive for the Le^b antigen.
   D. Lewis antibodies are not clinically significant, so any type of blood may be given.

   Blood bank/Apply knowledge of fundamental biological characteristics/Blood group antibodies/3

4. Which of the following statements is true concerning the MN phenotype?
   A. Antigen typing is enhanced for both antigens.
   B. Dosage effect may be seen for both M and N antigens.
   C. Both M or N antigens are impossible to detect due to cross-interference.
   D. MN is a rare phenotype seldom found in routine antigen typing.

   Blood bank/Apply knowledge of fundamental biological characteristics/Blood groups/2

Answers to Questions 1–4

1. **C** Anti-Le^a is produced primarily by persons with the Le(a-b-) phenotype because Le(a-b+) persons will still have some Le^a antigen present in saliva. Although Le^a is not present on their red cells, Le(a-b+) persons will not form anti-Le^a.

2. **B** Saliva from an individual with the Le gene will contain the Le^a antigen. This will combine with anti-Le^a, neutralizing the antibody. Panel cells treated with AET lose reactivity with anti-K, not anti-Le^a. Hydatid cyst fluid neutralizes anti-P$_1$.

3. **A** Lewis antibodies are generally not considered clinically significant unless they react near 37°C or at the IAT phase; for example, 1+ at IAT.

4. **B** Dosage effect is the term used to describe the phenomenon of weak agglutination when an antibody reacts with a cell that is heterozygous for the corresponding antigen. Dosage effect is a characteristic of the genotype *MN* because the M and N antigens are heterozygous on the same cell. This causes a weaker reaction than seen with RBCs of either the *MM* or *NN* genotype which carry a greater amount of the corresponding antigen.

5. Anti-M is sometimes found with reactivity detected at the immediate spin (IS) phase that persists in strength to the IAT phase. What is the main testing problem with a strong anti-M?
  A. Anti-M may not allow detection of a clinically significant antibody.
  B. Compatible blood may not be found for the patient with a strongly reacting anti-M.
  C. The anti-M cannot be removed from the serum.
  D. The anti-M may react with the patient's own cells, causing a positive autocontrol.

Blood bank/Apply knowledge of fundamental biological characteristics/Blood groups/2

6. A patient is suspected of having paroxysmal cold hemoglobinuria. Which pattern of reactivity is characteristic of the Donath-Landsteiner antibody, which causes this condition?
  A. The antibody attaches to RBCs at 4°C and causes hemolysis at 37°C.
  B. The antibody attaches to RBCs at 37°C and causes agglutination at the IAT phase.
  C. The antibody attaches to RBCs at 22°C and causes hemolysis at 37°C.
  D. The antibody attaches to RBCs and causes agglutination at the IAT phase.

Blood bank/Apply knowledge of fundamental biological characteristics/Blood group antibodies/1

7. How can interfering anti-P_1 antibody be removed from a mixture of antibodies?
  A. Neutralization with saliva
  B. Agglutination with human milk
  C. Combination with urine
  D. Neutralization with hydatid cyst fluid

Blood bank/Apply principles of special procedures/Blood group antibodies/1

8. A patient is scheduled to undergo open heart surgery. He has anti-P_1 antibody. How should blood be selected?
  A. Negative for the P_1 antigen.
  B. Positive for the P_1 antigen.
  C. Either positive or negative for the P_1 antigen.
  D. Compatible blood cannot be easily selected; suggest that surgery be postponed.

Blood bank/Correlate clinical and laboratory data/Blood group antibodies/2

9. An antibody shows high titered reactions in all test phases. All screen and panel cells are positive. The serum is then tested with a cord cell and the reaction is negative. What antibody is suspected?
  A. Anti-i
  B. Anti-I
  C. Anti-H
  D. Anti-p

Blood bank/Apply principles of special procedures/Antibody ID/2

10. Which group of antibodies are commonly found as cold agglutinins?
  A. Anti-K, Anti-k, Anti-Js^b
  B. Anti-D, Anti-e, Anti-C
  C. Anti-M, Anti-N
  D. Anti-Fy^a, Anti-Fy^b

Blood bank/Apply knowledge of fundamental biological characteristics/Blood group antibodies/1

11. Which antibody does *not* usually give a mixed-field reaction?
  A. Anti-Lu^a
  B. Anti-Di^a
  C. Anti-Sd^a
  D. A_3 cells with anti-A

Blood bank/Apply knowledge of fundamental biological characteristics/Blood group antibodies/1

Answers to Questions 5–11

5. **A** While anti-M may not be clinically significant, a strong reacting anti-M that persists through to the IAT phase may interfere with detection of a clinically significant antibody that reacts only at IAT.

6. **A** The Donath-Landsteiner antibody has anti-P specificity with biphasic activity. The antibody attaches to RBCs at 4°C and then causes the red cells to hemolyze when warmed to 37°C.

7. **D** Hydatid cyst fluid contains P_1 substance, which can neutralize anti-P_1 antibody.

8. **A** Anti-P_1 antibodies are IgM and are usually not clinically significant. In cases of cold surgery, such as open heart surgery, however, P antibodies may cause problems and must be identified and titered.

9. **B** Adult cells contain mostly I antigen, and anti-I would react with all adult cells found on screen or panel cells. Cord cells, however, contain mostly i antigen and would react negatively or only weakly positive with anti-I.

10. **C** Antibodies to the M and N antigens are IgM antibodies commonly found as cold agglutinins.

11. **B** Anti-Di^a does not give a mixed-field reaction. Anti-Lu^a and anti-Sd^a give a mixed-field pattern of reactivity.

12. What is true concerning the acquisition of K-negative donor units?
  A. Blood must be provided by rare donor files.
  B. Close relatives must be screened as potential donors.
  C. Ninety percent of donor units will be K-negative.
  D. It depends upon the racial composition of the blood donors.

Blood bank/Calculate/Hemotherapy/1

13. The k (Cellano) antigen is a high-frequency antigen and is found on most red cells. How often would one expect to find the corresponding antibody, anti-k?
  A. Often, because it is a high-frequency antibody.
  B. Rarely, because most individuals have the antigen and therefore would not develop the antibody.
  C. Depends upon the population because certain racial and ethnic groups show a higher frequency of anti-k.
  D. Impossible to determine without consulting regional blood group antigen charts.

Blood bank/Calculate/Hemotherapy/1

14. Which procedure would help to distinguish between an anti-e and anti-Fyᵃ in an antibody mixture?
  A. Lower pH of test serum.
  B. Run an enzyme panel.
  C. Use a thiol reagent.
  D. Run a regular panel.

Blood bank/Apply principles of special procedures/Antibody ID/2

15. Which characteristics are true of *all three* of the following antibodies: anti-Fyᵃ, anti-Jkᵃ, and anti-K?
  A. Detected at the IAT phase; may cause hemolytic disease of the newborn (HDN) and transfusion reactions
  B. Not detected with enzyme-treated cells; may cause delayed transfusion reactions
  C. Requires the IAT technique for detection; usually not responsible for causing HDN
  D. May show dosage effect; may cause severe hemolytic transfusion reactions

Blood bank/Apply principles of special procedures/Antibody ID/2

16. What reagent or procedure is used to distinguish Kidd and Kell antibodies?
  A. Ficin enzyme panel
  B. Chloroquine
  C. LISS media
  D. AET

Blood bank/Apply principles of special procedures/Antibody ID/3

17. A technologist performs an antibody study and finds 1+ and weak positive reactions for several of the panel cells. The reactions do not fit a pattern. An enzyme panel, several selected cell panels, and antigen typing of the patient's red cells do not reveal any additional information. The serum is diluted and retested, but the same reactions persist. What type of antibody may be causing these results?
  A. High incidence
  B. Low incidence
  C. High-titer low-avidity (HTLA)
  D. HLA

Blood bank/Evaluate laboratory data to make identifications/Antibody ID/2

Answers to Questions 12–17

12. **C** The K antigen is found in approximately 9%–10% of the population. Ninety percent of donor units, therefore, should be negative for the K antigen.

13. **B** The k antigen is found with a frequency of 99.8%; therefore, the k-negative person is rare. Because k-negative individuals are very rare, the occurrence of anti-k is also rare.

14. **B** Enzyme-treated cells will not react with Duffy antibodies. Rh antibodies react more strongly with enzyme-treated panel cells. An enzyme panel, therefore, would enhance reactivity of anti-e and destroy reactivity to anti-Fyᵃ.

15. **A** Anti-Fyᵃ, anti-Jkᵃ, and anti-K are usually detected at IAT and all may cause HDN and transfusion reactions that may be hemolytic. Although anti-Fyᵃ demonstrates dosage effect and anti-Jkᵃ may react weakly with antigen-positive cells, anti-K usually reacts well with either homozygous or heterozygous K antigen-positive cells.

16. **D** Red cells treated with AET lose reactivity to Kell antibodies; therefore, Kell antibodies, if present, would fail to react with AET-treated red cells. Chloroquine is used to remove autoantibodies from RBCs, allowing the cells to be typed. Chloroquine can also be used to prepare RBCs that will adsorb the autoantibodies.

17. **C** HTLA antibodies may persist in reaction strength, even when diluted. These antibodies are directed against high-frequency antigens (such as Chᵃ) that are also present in soluble form in plasma. They are not clinically significant but, when present, are responsible for a high incidence of incompatible crossmatches.

Cell

No.	D	C	E	c	e	f	Cw	V	K	k	Kpa	Kpb	Jsa	Jsb	Fya	Fyb	Jka	Jkb	Xga	Lea	Leb	S	s	M	N	P1	Lua	Lub
1	+	+	0	0	+	0	+	0	0	+	0	+	0	+	0	+	0	+	+	+	0	0	+	0	+	0	0	+
2	+	+	0	0	+	0	0	0	+	+	0	+	0	+	+	+	+	+	+	0	+	+	0	+	+	0	0	+
3	+	0	+	+	0	0	0	0	0	+	0	+	0	+	+	0	+	+	0	0	+	+	+	+	+	+s	0	+
4	0	+	0	+	+	+	0	0	0	+	0	+	0	+	+	+	+	+	+	0	+	0	+	+	+	0	0	+
5	0	0	+	+	+	+	0	0	+	+	0	+	0	+	+	+	+	0	0	0	+	0	+	+	+	+s	0	+
6	0	0	0	0	+	+	0	0	0	+	0	+	0	+	+	+	+	+	+	+	0	+	+	+	0	+	0	+
7	0	0	0	+	+	+	0	+	+	0	+	0	+	0	0	+	0	+	0	+	0	+	0	+	0	+s	0	+
8	0	0	0	+	+	+	0	0	0	+	0	+	0	+	0	+	0	+	+	0	0	+	+	+	0	+	+	+
9	+	+	0	0	+	0	0	0	0	+	0	+	0	+	+	+	+	+	+	+	0	0	+	+	+	+	0	+
10	+	0	0	+	+	+	0	0	0	+	0	+	0	+	0	0	+	+	+	0	0	0	+	0	0	+s	0	+

18. An antibody is detected in a pregnant woman and is suspected of being the cause of fetal distress. The antibody reacts at the IAT phase and causes *in-vitro* hemolysis. What is the most likely antibody specificity?
A. Anti-Le^a
B. Anti-Lu^a
C. Anti-Lu^b
D. Anti-Xg^a

Blood bank/Evaluate laboratory data to make identifications/Antibody ID/2

19. What sample is best for detecting complement-dependent antibodies?
A. Plasma stored at 4°C for no longer than 24 hours
B. Serum stored at 4°C for no longer than 48 hours
C. Either serum or plasma stored at 20°–24°C no longer than 6 hours
D. Serum heated at 56°C for 30 minutes

Blood bank/Apply principles of basic laboratory procedures/Antibody ID/3

20. Which antibody would *not* be detected by group O screen cells?
A. Anti-N
B. Anti-A$_1$
C. Anti-Di^a
D. Anti-k

Blood bank/Apply principles of special procedures/Antibody ID/3

Using the antigen profile chart, answer questions 21 and 22.

21. Given the following pattern of reactivity at the IAT phase, select the most likely antibody specificity.

Cell number	1	2	3	4	5	6	7	8	9	10
Reaction	2+	1+	1+	±	0	±	0	2+	1+	1+

A. Anti-Fy^b
B. Anti-Jk^b
C. Anti-e
D. Anti-c and anti-K

Blood bank/Apply principles of special procedures/Antibody ID/2

22. Given the following pattern of reactivity, select the most likely antibodies in the serum.

Cell number	1	2	3	4	5	6	7	8	9	10
Reaction 37° C	1+	1+	0	±	0	0	0	0	1+	0
IAT	2+	2+	0	±	2+0	2+	0		1+	0

A. Anti-S and anti-E
B. Anti-E and anti-K
C. Anti-Le^a and anti-Fy^b
D. Anti-C and anti-K

Blood bank/Apply principles of special procedures/Antibody ID/3

Answers to Questions 18–22

18. **C** Of the antibodies above only Lu^b is detected in the IAT phase, causes *in-vitro* hemolysis, and may cause HDN.

19. **B** Serum stored at 4°C for no longer than 48 hours preserves complement activity. Plasma is inappropriate because most anticoagulants chelate Ca^{2+} needed for activation of complement. Heating the serum to 56°C will destroy complement.

20. **B** ABO antibodies are not detected by group O screen cells.

21. **B** The pattern clearly fits that of anti-Jk^b, an antibody that usually reacts best at IAT. The weaker reactions are due to dosage effect found on cells with both Jk^a and Jk^b antigens.

22. **D** The pattern fits anti-C at 37°C, which becomes stronger at the IAT phase. The additional antibody is anti-K, which appears only at the IAT phase.

Compatibility Testing

1. **SITUATION**: An emergency trauma patient requires transfusion. Six units of blood are ordered stat. There is no time to draw a patient sample. O-negative blood is released. When will compatibility testing be performed?
   A. Compatibility testing must be performed before blood is issued.
   B. Compatibility testing will be performed when a patient sample is available.
   C. Compatibility testing may be performed immediately using donor serum.
   D. Compatibility testing is not necessary when blood is released in emergency situations.

   Blood bank/Apply knowledge of laboratory operations/Crossmatch/1

2. How would autoantibodies or abnormal proteins affect compatibility testing?
   A. No effect.
   B. Screen cells would be positive.
   C. All tests (ABO, Rh, screen cells, A/C, cross-match) may show abnormal results.
   D. Results would depend on the specificity of the abnormal proteins or autoantibodies.

   Blood bank/Evaluate laboratory data to make identifications/Antibody ID/3

3. What is the most likely explanation when screen cells and panel cells are positive and the autocontrol is negative?
   A. Nonspecific alloantibodies
   B. High-frequency alloantibodies or mixture of alloantibodies
   C. Specific IgG and IgM antibodies
   D. Autoantibodies or abnormal proteins

   Blood bank/Evaluate laboratory data to make identifications/Antibody identification/3

4. What is the most common cause of transfusion reactions?
   A. Donor units with low-incidence antigens
   B. Disease states of recipients
   C. Clerical errors
   D. Patient alloantibodies

   Blood bank/Apply knowledge to identify sources of error/Transfusion reaction/1

5. Can crossmatching be performed on October 14, using a patient sample drawn on October 12?
   A. Yes, a new sample would not be needed.
   B. Yes, but only if the previous sample has no alloantibodies.
   C. No, a new sample is needed because the 2-day limit has expired.
   D. No, a new sample is needed for each testing.

   Blood bank/Apply knowledge of standard operating procedures/Crossmatch/2

Answers to Questions 1–5

1. **B** When patient serum is available, it will be crossmatched with donor cells. Patient serum might contain antibodies against antigens on donor cells that may destroy donor cells. If an incompatibility is discovered, the problem will be reported immediately to the patient's physician.

2. **C** Autoantibodies or abnormal protein(s) may cause positive reactions with screen cells, panel cells, donor cells, and patient cells. The positive autocontrol may be indicative of this problem.

3. **B** High-frequency alloantibodies or a mixture of alloantibodies may cause screen cells and panel cells to be positive. A negative autocontrol would rule out autoantibodies or an abnormal protein.

4. **C** Clerical errors account for more transfusion reactions than testing or patient problems.

5. **A** Compatibility testing may be performed on a patient sample within 3 days of the scheduled transfusion.

6. A type and screen was performed on a 32-year-old woman, and the patient was typed as AB-negative. There are no AB-negative units in the blood bank. What should be done?
A. Order AB-negative units from a blood supplier.
B. Check inventory of A-, B-, and O-negative units.
C. Ask the patient to make a preoperative autologous donation.
D. Nothing, the blood will probably not be used.

Blood bank/Apply principles of basic laboratory procedures/Crossmatch/2

7. What ABO type(s) may donate to any other ABO type?
A. A-negative, B-negative, AB-negative, or O-negative
B. O-negative
C. AB-negative
D. AB-negative, A-negative, B-negative

Blood bank/Apply knowledge of fundamental biological characteristics/Crossmatch/2

8. What type(s) of red cells is (are) acceptable to transfuse to an O-negative patient?
A. A-negative, B-negative, AB-negative, or O-negative
B. O-negative
C. AB-negative
D. AB-negative, A-negative, B-negative

Blood bank/Apply knowledge of fundamental biological characteristics/Crossmatch/2

9. A technologist removed four units of blood from the blood bank refrigerator and placed them on the counter. A clerk was waiting to take the units for transfusion. As she checked the paperwork, she noticed that one of the units was leaking onto the counter. What should she do?
A. Issue the unit if red cells appear normal.
B. Reseal the unit.
C. Discard the unit.
D. Call the medical director and ask for an opinion.

Blood bank/Apply knowledge of standard operating procedures/Crossmatch/1

10. A 46-year-old woman came into the hospital for a hysterectomy. What testing will *most likely* be performed on her?
A. Only a three-cell screen IS
B. Cell panel to quickly identify alloantibodies
C. No testing needed
D. Type and screen

Blood bank/Apply knowledge of standard operating procedures/Crossmatch/1

11. A patient received 15 units of blood in 4 hours due to a gunshot wound. Six hours later he received

another four units. Ten hours later he got another two units. What testing was required on these two units?
A. IS crossmatch or forward typing ABO
B. ABO, Rh, crossmatch
C. ABO, forward and reverse typing
D. Antibody screen and ABO typing

Blood bank/Apply knowledge of standard operating procedures/Crossmatch/1

12. A patient showed positive results with screen cells and four donor units. The patient autocontrol was negative. What was the most likely antibody?
A. Anti-H
B. Anti-S
C. Anti-Kp^a
D. Anti-k

Blood bank/Evaluate laboratory data to make identifications/Incompatible crossmatch/3

Answers to Questions 6–12

6. **B** An AB person is the universal recipient and may receive any type blood; because only a type and screen was ordered and blood may not be used, check inventory for A-, B-, and O-negative units.

7. **B** An O-negative individual has no A or B antigen and may donate red cells to any other ABO type.

8. **B** An O-negative individual has both anti-A and anti-B and may receive only O-negative red cells.

9. **C** Leaking may indicate a broken seal or a puncture, which indicates possible contamination of the unit, even if the red cells appear normal. The unit should be discarded.

10. **D** Most hysterectomies do not require blood except in unusual circumstances; a type and screen would be performed in the blood bank.

11. **A** This patient meets the criteria for a massively transfused patient. Confirmation of ABO type is the most important testing criterion for a massively transfused patient, who often loses blood almost as quickly as the blood is transfused. The patient is not exposed to the red cells long enough to mount an immune response and form antibodies. ABO typing, therefore, may be accomplished through either an IS crossmatch or forward typing.

12. **D** Anti-k (Cellano) is a high-frequency alloantibody that would react with screen cells and most donor units. The negative autocontrol rules out autoantibodies. Anti-H and anti-S are cold antibodies and anti-Kp^a is a-low frequency alloantibody.

13. Screen cells and crossmatch are positive on IS only, and the autocontrol is negative. Identify the problem.
A. Cold alloantibody
B. Cold autoantibody
C. Abnormal protein
D. Antibody mixture

Blood bank/Evaluate laboratory data to make identifications/Incompatible crossmatch/3

14. Six units are crossmatched. Five units are compatible, one unit is incompatible, and the recipient's antibody screen is negative. Identify the problem.
A. Patient may have a high-frequency alloantibody.
B. Patient may have an abnormal protein.
C. Donor unit may have a positive DAT.
D. Donor may have high-frequency antigens.

Blood bank/Evaluate laboratory data to make identifications/Incompatible crossmatch/3

15. What should be done with a donor unit with a positive DAT?
A. Discard the unit.
B. Antigen type the unit for high-frequency antigens.
C. Wash the donor cells and use the washed cells for testing.
D. Perform a panel on the incompatible unit.

Blood bank/Apply principles of special procedures/Incompatible crossmatch/3

16. Screen cells, crossmatch, and patient autocontrol are positive in all phases of the crossmatch. Identify the problem.
A. Specific cold alloantibody
B. Specific cold autoantibody
C. Abnormal protein or nonspecific autoantibody
D. Cold and warm alloantibody mixture

Blood bank/Evaluate laboratory data to make identifications/Incompatible crossmatch/3

17. What is the first step in a crossmatch after identification of patient antibodies?
A. Perform a DAT on patient cells and donor units.
B. Antigen type patient cells and any donor cells to be crossmatched.
C. Adsorb any antibodies from the patient serum.
D. Obtain a different enhancement medium for testing.

Blood bank/Apply principles of special procedures/Incompatible crossmatch/1

18. What is the disposition of a donor unit that contains an antibody?
A. The unit must be discarded.
B. Only the plasma may be used to make components.
C. The antibody must be adsorbed from the unit.
D. The unit may be labeled indicating that it contains antibody and released into inventory.

Blood bank/Apply knowledge of laboratory operations/Hemotherapy/Blood components/1

19. Given a situation where screen cells, crossmatch, autocontrol, and DAT (anti-IgG) are all positive, what procedure should be performed next?
A. Adsorption using rabbit stroma
B. Antigen typing of the patient's cells
C. Elution followed by a cell panel on the eluate
D. Selected cell panel

Blood bank/Apply principles of special procedures/Incompatible crossmatch/3

20. A crossmatch and screen cells are 2+ at IS, 1+ at 37°C, and negative at the IAT phase. Identify the most likely problem.
A. Combination of antibodies
B. Cold antibody(s)
C. Rouleaux
D. Test error

Blood bank/Evaluate laboratory data to make identifications/Incompatible crossmatch/3

Answers to Questions 13–20

13. A A cold alloantibody would show a reaction with screen cells and donor units only at IS phase. The negative autocontrol rules out autoantibodies and abnormal protein.

14. C The incompatible donor unit may have an antibody coating the red cells, or the patient may have a low-frequency alloantibody. High-frequency antibodies or antigens would agglutinate all units and screen cells.

15. A The incompatible unit may have red cells coated with antibody or complement. If red cells are sensitized, then some problem exists with the donor. Discard the unit.

16. C An abnormal protein or nonspecific autoantibody would cause antibody screen, crossmatch, and patient autocontrol to be positive. Alloantibodies would not cause a positive patient autocontrol.

17. B Antigen typing of the patient's cells confirms the antibody identification; antigen typing of donor cells helps ensure the crossmatch of compatible donor units.

18. D The unit may be used in the general blood inventory if it is properly labeled and only cellular elements are used.

19. C A positive DAT using anti-IgG indicates that antibodies are coating the patient cells. An eluate would be helpful to remove the antibody, followed by a cell panel in order to identify it.

20. B The reaction pattern fits that of a cold antibody reacting at IS phase and of sufficient titer to persist at 37°C incubation. The reactions disappear after IAT testing.

21. What corrective action should be taken when rouleaux causes positive test results?
A. Wash cells and dilute serum.
B. Perform an autoadsorption.
C. Run a panel.
D. Perform an elution.

Blood bank/Apply principles of special procedures/Testing problem/3

22. All of the following are reasons for performing an adsorption *except:*
A. Separation of mixtures of antibodies
B. Removal of interfering antibodies
C. Confirmation of weak antigens on red cells
D. Identification of antibodies causing a positive DAT

Blood bank/Apply principles of special procedures/Antibody identifications/2

23. A patient's sample showed positive results for all testing at IS. What procedure would help prepare this sample for testing?
A. Elution
B. Adsorption and prewarmed technique
C. ZZAP reagent
D. pH alteration of serum

Blood bank/Apply principles of special procedures/Antibody identification/2

24. What is needed for detection of some drug-induced antibodies?
A. Panel cells
B. Polyspecific antihuman globulin (AHG) sera
C. Enzyme-treated cells
D. Drug-coated cells

Blood bank/Apply principles of special procedures/Antibody identification/1

25. A warm, nonspecific autoantibody was causing a positive DAT. How can these antibodies be removed from red cells?
A. ZZAP
B. Cold elution
C. Thiol reagents
D. AET

Blood bank/Apply principles of special procedures/Antibody identification/2

26. How can IgM antibodies be separated from IgG antibodies?
A. Warm elution
B. Thiol reagents
C. Adsorption with antigen-specific red cells
D. Impossible to separate

Blood bank/Apply principles of special procedures/Antibody identification/1

27. A patient had a transfusion reaction. His red cells revealed a positive DAT; however, his antibody screen was negative. What procedure would remove the antibody from his red cells to allow identification of the probable cause of the transfusion reaction?
A. Elution
B. Adsorption
C. AET
D. Washing cells and diluting serum

Blood bank/Apply principles of special procedures/Antibody identification/3

28. In the IAT phase, what action should be taken if tubes are negative after addition of check cells (reagent-sensitized cells)?
A. Repeat the test; replace AHG reagent and check the cell washer.
B. Add additional check cells.
C. Add additional AHG reagent.
D. Record all results as negative.

Blood bank/Apply knowledge to identify sources of error/Reagent QC/3

Answers to Questions 21–28

21. **A** Rouleaux may be dispersed or lessened by washing the patient's red cells and replacing the serum with saline. Testing may be performed using the washed cells.

22. **D** Antibodies causing a positive DAT would be coating red cells and would require an elution, not an adsorption, to identify them.

23. **B** This sample probably contains cold antibodies. Adsorption or the prewarmed technique can help to remove cold antibodies from patient serum or to prevent them from interfering with other testing.

24. **D** Only drug-coated cells, specific for the drug, can detect drug-induced antibodies. These antibodies may be found in patients with drug-induced hemolytic anemia.

25. **A** ZZAP reagent causes IgG antibodies to lose their integrity and dissociate from the surface of red cells.

26. **B** Thiol abolishes the activity of IgM antibodies and permits detection of IgG antibodies.

27. **A** A positive DAT indicates that antibody is coating red cells; a negative antibody screen indicates that all of the antibody is on the cells; an elution would remove the antibody and allow for identification of the antibody.

28. **A** Negative check cells may be due to a problem with the AHG reagent or to inadequate cell washing.

UNIT 6

Transfusion Reactions

1. A patient had a transfusion reaction. The technologist began the laboratory investigation of the transfusion reaction by assembling pre- and posttransfusion specimens and all paperwork and computer printouts. He checked the patient's records and talked to the nurse in charge of the patient. What should he do first?
   A. Perform a DAT on the posttransfusion sample.
   B. Check for a clerical error.
   C. Repeat ABO and Rh typing of patient and donor unit.
   D. Perform antibody screen on the posttransfusion sample.

   Blood bank/Apply knowledge of standard operating procedures/Transfusion reaction/2

2. A trauma patient had a severe hemolytic reaction just minutes after receiving a blood transfusion. What is the most likely cause?
   A. Immediate, nonimmunologic; probably due to volume overload
   B. Delayed immunologic; probably due to an antibody such as anti-Jk^a
   C. Delayed nonimmunologic; probably due to iron overload
   D. Immediate, immunologic; probably due to clerical error, ABO incompatibility

   Blood bank/Apply knowledge of fundamental biological characteristics/Transfusion reaction/2

3. A patient has a hemolytic reaction to blood transfused 8 days ago. What is the most likely cause?
   A. Immediate, nonimmunologic; probably due to volume overload
   B. Delayed immunologic; probably due to an antibody such as anti-Jk^a
   C. Delayed nonimmunologic; probably due to iron overload
   D. Immediate, immunologic; probably due to clerical error, ABO incompatibility

Blood bank/Apply knowledge of fundamental biological characteristics/Transfusion reaction/2

4. What would be the result of group A blood given to a group O patient?
   A. Nonimmune transfusion reaction
   B. Immediate hemolytic transfusion reaction
   C. Delayed hemolytic transfusion reaction
   D. No problem

Blood bank/Apply knowledge of fundamental biological characteristics/Transfusion reaction/2

Answers to Questions 1–4

1. **B** Over 90% of transfusion reactions are due to some type of clerical error. The most time-saving approach would be to check all paperwork before any laboratory testing.

2. **D** A trauma patient probably received blood on emergency release. An immediate, hemolytic reaction may be due to an immunological cause, for example, a preformed antibody. The most likely problem for this scenario is an immediate, immunologic reaction due to clerical error or ABO mix-up.

3. **B** A transfusion reaction that occurs several days after a transfusion of blood products is probably a delayed immunologic reaction due to an antibody formed against donor antigens. This is a classic example of a reaction caused by an antibody such as anti-Jk^a.

4. **B** Group A blood given to a group O patient would cause an immediate hemolytic transfusion reaction because a group O patient has anti-A and anti-B antibodies and would destroy A cells.

5. All of the following are part of the preliminary evaluation of a transfusion reaction *except:*
   A. Check pre- and posttransfusion samples for color of serum.
   B. Perform ABO and Rh recheck.
   C. DAT on the posttransfusion sample.
   D. Panel on pre- and posttransfusion sample.

Blood bank/Apply knowledge of standard operating procedures/Transfusion reaction/1

6. All of the following tests should be done if a hemolytic transfusion reaction has taken place *except:*
   A. Recrossmatch and repetition of the antibody screen
   B. Adsorption using pre- and posttransfusion samples
   C. Gram stain and culture of the unit
   D. Chemistry, coagulation, and urine tests

Blood bank/Apply principles of special procedures/Transfusion reaction/1

7. An alloantibody has caused an immediate hemolytic transfusion reaction. What is the most likely result for the DAT?
   A. 4+ positive.
   B. Mixed field.
   C. Result is dependent upon the amount of red cell destruction by attached antibody; positive, negative, or mixed field.
   D. If transfused incompatible red cells are destroyed, then result may be negative.

Blood bank/Apply knowledge of standard operating procedures/Transfusion reaction/1

8. Is hematuria a sign of transfusion reaction in a recently transfused patient?
   A. Hematuria is indicative of a severe hemolytic reaction.
   B. Hematuria may indicate a delayed hemolytic reaction.
   C. Not significant; intact RBCs indicate bleeding and not hemolysis.
   D. Significant only if hematuria is accompanied by an increase in bilirubin.

Blood bank/Apply knowledge of fundamental biological characteristics/Transfusion reaction/3

Answers to Questions 5–8

5. **D** The preliminary evaluation of a transfusion reaction includes checking the color of serum, performing ABO and Rh checks, and a DAT on the posttransfusion sample. A panel would not be a part of the preliminary evaluation.

6. **B** Performing an adsorption would not add any information to the investigation and would probably be useless and unproductive. A Gram stain and culture of the unit may indicate if a contaminated unit could have caused the transfusion reaction. Chemistry, coagulation, and urine tests may indicate the extent of the transfusion reaction.

7. **D** Although a positive DAT is the usual finding in an acute extravascular transfusion reaction, the DAT may be negative in an immediate hemolytic reaction because the red cells are destroyed by antibody and complement.

8. **C** Hematuria is not caused by a transfusion reaction and indicates bleeding within the urinary tract system. However, intravascular hemolysis causes shock, fever, and hemoglobinuria and frequently results in renal failure and disseminated intravascular coagulation.

Components

1. A male cancer patient with a hemoglobin of 6 g/dL was admitted to the hospital with acute abdominal pain. Small bowel resection was indicated, but the attending physician wanted to raise the patient's hemoglobin to 12 g/dL before surgery. How many units of RBCs would most likely be required to accomplish this?
   A. Two
   B. Three
   C. Six
   D. Eight

   Blood bank/Apply knowledge of fundamental biological characteristics/Blood components/RBCs/2

2. A shipment of packed RBCs, platelets, and leukocyte-reduced RBCs arrived in the same container, at 1°–6°C. What should be done?
   A. Place all units in the 1°–6°C blood bank refrigerator.
   B. Reject the shipment.
   C. Prepare the RBC units for freezing.
   D. Accept red cell products; return or discard the platelets.

   Blood bank/Select course of action/Blood components/RBCs/3

3. Four units of packed RBCs were brought to the nurses' station at 10:20 AM. Two units were transfused immediately, and one unit was transfused at 10:40 AM. The remaining unit was returned to the blood bank at 11:00 AM. The units were not refrigerated after leaving the blood bank. What problem(s) is (are) present in this situation?
   A. The only problem is with the returned unit; the 30-minute limit has expired and the unit cannot be used.
   B. The unit should not have been transfused at 10:40 AM because the time limit has expired; this unit and the remaining unit should have been returned to the blood bank.

C. The returned unit may be held for this patient for 48 hours but cannot be used for another patient.
D. No problems; all actions were performed within the allowable time limits.

Blood bank/Select course of action/Blood components/RBCs/3

Answers to Questions 1–3

1. **C** One unit of RBCs will raise the hemoglobin level by approximately 1 to 1.5 g/dL, and the hematocrit by 3%–4%. Results will vary depending upon the age of the blood, and the blood volume and hydration status of the patient. Six units will raise the hemoglobin to at least 12 g/dL.

2. **D** The transport and storage temperature for RBC products is 1°–6°C. Platelets should be shipped at 20°–24°C in an insulated container to protect them from extreme heat or cold.

3. **A** There is a 30-minute time limit for a unit of RBCs that is not kept under proper storage conditions (1°–6°C).

4. Five years ago a patient made an autologous donation for a surgical procedure. The two units were not used, and 3 days later, the patient requested that the two units be frozen. This patient is having cosmetic surgery next week that may require transfusion. Which statement is consistent with acceptable blood banking policy?
A. The units cannot be used because too much time had elapsed between donation and freezing.
B. The cells may be transfused if proper freezing, thawing, washing, and transfusion procedures are followed.
C. The units should be discarded because too much time elapsed between freezing and the date of surgery.
D. Autologous units are donated only for one specific transfusion purpose and should not be used for an unrelated incident.

Blood bank/Apply knowledge of standard operating procedures/Blood components/Autologous donation/2

5. Which of the following is acceptable according to American Association of Blood Banks (AABB) standards?
A. Rejuvenated RBCs may be made within 3 days of outdate and transfused or frozen within 24 hours of rejuvenation.
B. Frozen RBCs must be prepared within 30 minutes of collection and may be used within 10 years.
C. Irradiated RBCs must be treated within 8 hours of collection and transfused within 6 hours.
D. Leukocyte-reduced RBCs must be prepared within 6 hours of collection and transfused within 6 hours of preparation.

Blood bank/Apply knowledge of laboratory operations/Blood components/RBCs/2

6. Which condition requires administration of red cells through a 37°C blood warmer?
A. Exchange transfusion
B. Urticaria
C. Chronic lymphocytic leukemia
D. Graft-versus-host disease

Blood bank/Apply knowledge of laboratory operations/Blood components/RBCs/2

7. All of the following are advantages of using packed RBCs instead of whole blood *except:*
A. Minimizes circulatory overload
B. Minimizes exposure to large volumes of electrolytes
C. Decreases transfusion time
D. Minimizes exposure to large volumes of anticoagulants

Blood bank/Apply knowledge of fundamental biological characteristics/Blood components/RBCs/1

8. All of the following statements are true *except:*
A. Centrifugation is an acceptable method for preparing leukocyte-reduced RBCs.
B. Graft-versus-host disease may be prevented by visual inspection of units before transfusion.
C. Circulatory overload may be prevented by the administration of packed RBCs.
D. Leukodepletion filters may prevent febrile transfusion reactions.

Blood bank/Apply principles of special procedures/Blood components/Preparation of Components/1

Answers to Questions 4–8

4. **B** Red cells may be frozen within 6 days of collection and remain viable for 10 years. Frozen cells may be shipped and used for any purpose within the 10-year time limit.

5. **A** Rejuvenated RBCs may be prepared within 3 days of the outdate of the unit and washed and transfused or frozen within 24 hours. A unit of RBCs may be frozen within 6 days of collection. An RBC unit can be irradiated anytime prior to the expiration date; once irradiated the unit must be transfused within 28 days. Leukocyte-reduced RBCs should be prepared within 6 hours of collection, but must be given within 24 hours if prepared using an open system. Leukocyte-reduced RBCs prepared using a closed system may be kept until the original expiration date.

6. **A** The transfusion of cold blood may cause hypothermia in the patient. This situation must be avoided, especially during exchange transfusion. A blood warmer may be used in any condition, but its use becomes particularly critical during the demanding process of exchange transfusion.

7. **C** Packed RBCs actually have increased transfusion time because of greater viscosity than whole blood.

8. **B** Although visual inspection is important in evaluating possible bacterial contamination of units, graft-versus-host disease may be prevented by irradiation. Irradiation prevents blast transformation of leukocytes.

9. All of the following statements regarding fresh frozen plasma (FFP) are true *except:*
  A. FFP must be prepared within 24 hours of collection.
  B. After thawing, FFP must be transfused within 24 hours.
  C. Storage temperature for FFP is −18°C or lower.
  D. When thawed, FFP must be stored between 1°–6°C.

Blood bank/Apply knowledge of standard operating procedures/Blood components/RBCs/1

10. What may be done to RBCs before transfusion to a patient with cold agglutinin disease in order to reduce the possibility of a transfusion reaction?
  A. Irradiate to prevent graft-versus-host disease.
  B. Wash with 0.9% saline.
  C. Warm to 37°C with a blood warmer.
  D. Transport so that temperature is maintained at 20°–24°C.

Blood bank/Apply knowledge of standard operating procedures/Hemotherapy/RBCs/2

11. A unit of packed RBCs is split using the open system. One of the half units is used. What may be done with the second half unit?
  A. Must be issued within 24 hours
  B. Must be issued within 48 hours
  C. Must be discarded
  D. Retains the original expiration date

Blood bank/Apply knowledge of laboratory operations/Blood components/RBCs/2

12. What should be done if a noticeable clot is found in an RBC unit?
  A. Issue the unit; the blood will be filtered.
  B. Issue the unit; note the presence of a clot on the release form.
  C. Filter the unit in the blood bank before issue.
  D. Do not issue the unit.

Blood bank/Select course of action/Hemotherapy/RBCs/3

13. Which of the following units may be used to prepare platelets?
  A. A unit placed at 1°–6°C immediately after collection
  B. A unit centrifuged at 1°–6°C 30 minutes after collection
  C. A unit placed at 20°–24°C for 3 hours
  D. A unit placed at 20°–24°C for 10 hours

Blood bank/Apply knowledge of basic laboratory procedures/Blood components/RBCs/1

14. A patient has hypofibrinogenemia. What component is the *best* choice for transfusion?
  A. Granulocytes
  B. Cryoprecipitate
  C. FFP
  D. Platelet concentrate

Blood bank/Apply knowledge of standard operating procedures/Blood components/RBCs/1

15. What component(s) is/are indicated for patients who have anti-IgA antibodies?
  A. Whole blood
  B. Packed RBCs
  C. Washed, leukocyte-reduced, or frozen deglycerolized RBCs
  D. Granulocyte preparations

Blood bank/Select course of action/Hemotherapy/RBCs/2

16. Which statement applies when preparing FFP or cryoprecipitate for transfusion?
  A. FFP and cryoprecipitate do not need to be the same Rh type as the patient.
  B. No antigen typing is required for transfusion of plasma products.
  C. Antibody screening of plasma products is not required.
  D. All blood components must be matched for both ABO group and Rh type.

Blood bank/Apply knowledge of standard operating procedures/Blood components/RBCs/1

Answers to Questions 9–16

9. **A** FFP must be prepared 8 hours after collection if the anticoagulant is citrate phosphate dextrose (CPD), citrate phosphate double dextrose (CP2D), or citrate phosphate dextrose adenine (CPDA-1); or within 6 hours if the anticoagulant is acid citrate dextrose (ACD).

10. **C** A patient having cold agglutinins might have a reaction to a cold blood product. The product should be warmed to body temperature, 37°C, before transfusion.

11. **A** The other half unit must be issued within 24 hours if an open system is used to split the unit.

12. **D** A unit having a noticeable clot should not be issued for transfusion to a patient. The clot may be an indication of contamination or bacterial growth.

13. **C** A unit used for making platelets may be kept at 20°–24°C for up to 8 hours.

14. **B** Although FFP and cryoprecipitate both contain fibrinogen, cryoprecipitate is a more concentrated source of fibrinogen.

15. **C** Patients with anti-IgA antibodies should not receive components containing plasma. Washed, leukocyte-reduced, or frozen deglycerolized RBCs contain very little plasma.

16. **A** No Rh antigens are found on plasma products because no cellular elements should be present in the products. Plasma products must be compatible with the patient's RBCs. Therefore, plasma products must be ABO-compatible because antibodies in the plasma would bind to the corresponding antigen on the patient's RBCs.

17. What component may *not* be prepared if whole blood is spun at 1°–6°C?
   A. Packed red cells
   B. Platelets
   C. Leukocyte-reduced red blood cells
   D. FFP

   Blood bank/Apply knowledge of standard operating procedures/Blood components/Processing/1

18. What is a special condition for the storage of platelets?
   A. Room temperature, 20°–24°C.
   B. No other components may be stored with platelets.
   C. Platelets must be stored upright in separate containers.
   D. Platelets require constant agitation at 20°–24°C.

   Blood bank/Apply knowledge of standard operating procedures/Blood components/Processing/1

19. Transfusion of an irradiated blood product is indicated in all of the following conditions *except:*
   A. Exchange transfusion
   B. Bone marrow transplant
   C. Human immunodeficiency virus (HIV) patient
   D. Warm autoimmune hemolytic anemia (WAIHA)

   Blood bank/Select course of action/Hemotherapy/Irradiation/2

20. A rare type RBC unit has expired on Tuesday. What can be done with this unit on Thursday?
   A. The unit may be frozen.
   B. The unit may be rejuvenated, then used or frozen.
   C. The unit must be discarded.
   D. The unit may be washed.

   Blood bank/Apply principles of special procedures/Blood components/RBCs/2

21. Four units of pooled platelets show visible signs of red cell contamination. Under which condition can this product be transfused?
   A. The product must be ABO- and Rh-compatible and crossmatched, if patient has alloantibodies.
   B. The product can be transfused only if the red cells are filtered and removed.
   C. The product should be irradiated prior to transfusion.
   D. The product may be transfused regardless of the patient's ABO and Rh type.

   Blood bank/Apply knowledge of standard operating procedures/Blood components/Platelets/2

22. All of the statements below regarding granulocyte transfusion are true *except:*
   A. Granulocytes are stored at room temperature, 20°–24°C.
   B. Granulocytes may be used for the short-term control of severe infection.

C. Granulocytes are administered with a microaggregate filter.
D. Because of 24-hour expiration, granulocytes may be administered before all serological testing is completed.

Blood bank/Apply knowledge of standard operating procedures/Blood components/Granulocytes/1

23. What component(s) may be shipped together with FFP?
   A. Frozen RBCs and cryoprecipitate.
   B. Platelets.
   C. Packed RBCs and granulocytes.
   D. No other component may be shipped with FFP.

   Blood bank/Apply knowledge of standard operating procedures/Blood components/FFP/1

24. What procedure should be followed in order to prevent contamination of FFP during thawing?
   A. Place the unit directly into a clean water bath.
   B. Seal the unit in an outer, separate bag prior to placing in the water bath.
   C. Thaw at 1°–6°C.
   D. When half-thawed, transfer the FFP to another bag.

   Blood bank/Apply knowledge of standard operating procedures/Blood components/FFP/1

Answers to Questions 17–24

17. **B** Whole blood must be spun at 20°–24°C in order to prepare platelets.

18. **D** Platelets are stored at 20°–24°C and require agitation during storage to prevent platelet aggregation. Granulocytes are also stored at 20°–24°C but do not require agitation.

19. **D** WAIHA would not normally require an irradiated product. Irradiated products are given to immunocompromised patients to prevent graft-versus-host disease.

20. **B** Rejuvenation of red cells may be performed up to 3 days after the red cells expire.

21. **A** Platelet products sometimes contain red cells; any product that contains greater than 5 mL of RBCs must be ABO- and Rh-compatible and crossmatched, particularly if a patient has alloantibodies to red cell antigens.

22. **C** A microaggregate filter will trap the granulocytes and not permit passage through the IV line.

23. **A** FFP requires dry ice for shipment. Frozen RBCs and cryoprecipitate also require dry ice.

24. **B** To prevent contamination of FFP during thawing in a water bath, seal the bag of FFP in a separate bag prior to placing it in the water bath.

25. What laboratory testing is required for stem cell preparations?
A. The same testing is required as for any red cell product.
B. Only ABO and Rh typing are required; a cross-match is not needed because progenitor cells have not acquired expression of the red cell antigens.
C. Only antigen testing is required.
D. No testing is required.

Blood bank/Apply knowledge of standard operating procedures/Blood components/Stem cells/1

26. Which component has the longest expiration date?
A. Cryoprecipitate
B. FFP
C. Frozen RBCs
D. Platelet concentrate

Blood bank/Apply knowledge of standard operating procedures/Blood components/Expiration date/1

27. All of the following are advantages of using single donor rather than random donor platelets *except:*
A. Less preparation time
B. Less antigen exposure for patients
C. May be HLA matched
D. No pooling is required

Blood bank/Apply principles of special procedures/Blood components/Platelets/1

28. Select the patients below for which transfusion of buffy coats are *best* indicated.
A. Immunocompromised leukemia patients
B. Patients with low WBC counts
C. Patients with bone marrow failure
D. Newborns with severe infections

Blood bank/Select course of action/Blood components/Buffy coats/1

29. Which preparation may be made from autologous leukapheresis lymphocytes?
A. Leukocytes
B. Buffy coats
C. Lymphocyte-activated killer (LAK) cells
D. Transfer factor

Blood bank/Apply principles of special procedures/LAK cells/1

30. **SITUATION:** A cancer patient recently developed a severe infection. The patient's hemoglobin is 8 g/dL owing to chemotherapy with a drug known to cause bone marrow depression and immunodeficiency. Which blood products are indicated for this patient?
A. Liquid plasma and cryoprecipitate
B. Crossmatched platelets and washed RBCs
C. Factor IX concentrate and FFP
D. Irradiated RBCs, platelets, and granulocytes

Blood bank/Correlate clinical and laboratory data/Blood components/3

Answers to Questions 25–30

25. **A** Stem cells contain antigens; therefore, ABO, Rh, and crossmatching are required.

26. **C** Frozen RBCs may be kept for up to 10 years. FFP and cryoprecipitate expire in 1 year. Platelet concentrates expire in 5 days.

27. **A** Single donor platelets require more preparation time than random donor platelets because they are prepared by plateletpheresis on a single donor, a procedure that may require 1–3 hours. Pooling random donor platelets in equivalent amounts (usually 5–6 units) may require only a few minutes.

28. **D** Buffy coats are low-volume white cell concentrates prepared from random donor units and are indicated primarily to control severe infections in newborns. Because of the low volume of the component, leukocytes, not buffy coats, would be indicated for adults with conditions that may make them susceptible to infections.

29. **C** LAK cells are collected by apheresis from the patient and treated with interleukin-2 (IL-2) to enhance activities such as tumor killing. Because LAK cells are the patient's own cells, there are no problems with graft-versus-host disease, antibody response, or any other adverse transfusion reactions.

30. **D** This cancer patient may be immunocompromised from the medication but needs to receive RBCs for anemia; therefore, irradiated RBCs are indicated. Platelets may be needed to control bleeding, and granulocytes may be indicated for short-term control of severe infection.

UNIT 8

Donors

1. Which of the following individuals is acceptable as a blood donor?
A. A 29-year-old man who received the hepatitis B vaccine last week.
B. A 21-year-old woman who had her nose pierced last week.
C. A 30-year-old man who lived in Zambia for 3 years and returned last month.
D. A 54-year-old man who tested positive for hepatitis C virus (HCV) last year, but has no active symptoms of the disease.

Blood bank/Apply knowledge of standard operating procedures/Donor requirements/2

2. **SITUATION:** A 17-year-old girl comes to the blood center to donate blood. She weighs 90 pounds and has a hemoglobin of 13 g/dL. She tells the interviewer that she helped to care for her HIV-positive cousin for a week last month. Which condition is cause for rejecting her as a donor?
A. Age; she is too young.
B. Her weight is too low.
C. Hemoglobin is too low.
D. Living with an HIV-positive individual.

Blood bank/Apply knowledge of standard operating procedures/Donor requirements/1

3. Which immunization has the longest deferral period?
A. HBIG (hepatitis B immune globulin) injection
B. Rubella vaccine
C. Flu vaccine
D. Yellow fever vaccine

Blood bank/Apply knowledge of standard operating procedures/Donor requirements/1

4. The following blood donors regularly give blood. Which donor may donate on September 10?
A. A 40-year-old woman who last donated on July 23.
B. A 28-year-old man who had plateletpheresis on August 24.

C. A 52-year-old man who made an autologous donation 2 days ago.
D. A 23-year-old woman who donated blood for her aunt on August 14.

Blood bank/Apply knowledge of standard operating procedures/Donor requirements/2

Answers to Questions 1–4

1. **A** If the donor is symptom-free, there is no deferral period for the hepatitis B vaccine. Individuals who have had body piercing or been institutionalized are given a 12-month deferral. Individuals who lived in a malarial area or who received antimalarial drugs are deferred for 3 years. A positive test for hepatitis C is cause for permanent deferral.

2. **D** Her age and hemoglobin meet donor criteria. Her weight, although low, does not disqualify her as a donor; she may donate, but not a 450-mL unit. Because she cared for her HIV-positive cousin for a week, she lived in close contact with this individual. This would disqualify her as a donor.

3. **A** Deferral for HBIG injection is 12 months. Deferral for rubella vaccine is 4 weeks. The deferral period for the flu vaccine lasts until the donor is symptom-free. Deferral for the yellow fever vaccine is 2 weeks.

4. **B** A plateletpheresis donor must wait at least 48 hours between donations. The waiting period following an autologous donation is at least 3 days. An 8-week interval must pass between all other types of donations.

5. Which of the following contraindicates accepting a donor for plateletpheresis?
   A. Platelet count of 75×10^9/L
   B. Plasma loss of 800 mL from plasmapheresis 1 week ago
   C. Plateletpheresis performed 3 days ago
   D. Aspirin ingestion 7 days ago

Blood bank/Apply knowledge of standard operating procedures/Donor requirements/1

6. Which of the following donors could be accepted for blood donation?
   A. A former drug addict who has been drug-free for the past 3 years
   B. A triathelete with a pulse of 45
   C. A man who is in remission from lymphoma
   D. A woman treated for gonorrhea 8 months ago

Blood bank/Apply knowledge of standard operating procedures/Donor requirements/1

7. Which physical examination result is cause for rejecting a blood donor?
   A. Weight of 105 lb
   B. Pulse of 75
   C. Temperature of 99.3°F
   D. Diastolic pressure of 110 mm Hg

Blood bank/Apply knowledge of standard operating procedures/Donor requirements/1

8. Which situation is *not* a cause for indefinite deferral of a donor?
   A. History of contact with prostitutes.
   B. Donation of a unit of blood that transmitted hepatitis B virus (HBV) to a recipient.
   C. Receipt of human growth hormone 30 years ago.
   D. Accidental needle stick 1 year ago; negative for infectious diseases.

Blood bank/Apply knowledge of standard operating procedures/Donor requirements/1

9. The tubing on a donor blood collection set begins to leak halfway through a donation. What should be done?
   A. Repair the leak by placing tape over the tubing.
   B. Continue the donation but be careful to use a sterile container to contain the leaking blood.
   C. Discontinue the donation.
   D. Remove the damaged set and begin collection of another unit from the donor's other arm.

Blood bank/Select course of action/Donor processing/Unacceptable donor set/3

10. A blood donor appears to be very nervous and anxious about donation. He has never donated before but passes all physical criteria and gives acceptable responses to the interview. Choose the correct course of action.
   A. Reject him as a donor.
   B. Make him lie down and breathe deeply prior to donation.
   C. Accept him; there is no obvious reason to reject him.
   D. Call the medical director and ask his opinion.

Blood bank/Select course of action/Donor requirements/3

Answers to Questions 5–10

5. **A** To be eligible for plateletpheresis the platelet count should be at least 150×10^9/L. Plasma loss exceeding 1000 mL, less than 48 hours since the last pheresis, and aspirin ingestion within 3 days of donation are all contraindications for plateletpheresis.

6. **B** Atheletes may have a pulse below 50 and may still be acceptable as blood donors. Drug addiction is cause for permanent deferral, as is a major illness such as cancer. The deferral period following treatment for syphilis or gonorrhea is 12 months.

7. **D** Diastolic pressure must not be higher than 100 mm Hg. Donors weighing less than 110 pounds may donate up to 12% of their blood volume (volume = weight in kg/50 × 450 mL). Oral temperature must not be greater than 99.5°F. Blood pressure limits for donation are 180 mm Hg for systolic and 100 mm Hg for diastolic pressure. The limit for hemoglobin is 12.5 g/dL and for hematocrit 38%.

8. **D** An accidental needle stick would not be a cause for indefinite deferral of a donor. The deferral time would be 1 year.

9. **C** If the set is leaking, then the sterility of the system has been compromised. The collection set and the blood collected must be discarded. The donor should not be subjected to a second venipuncture.

10. **A** A potential donor who appears anxious about donation may have problems during the donation, such as fainting, nausea, or hyperventilation. He should be rejected as a donor in order to avoid potential problems.

11. A woman begins to breathe rapidly while donating blood. Choose the correct course of action.
  - A. Continue the donation; rapid breathing is not a reason to discontinue a donation.
  - B. Withdraw the needle, raise her feet, and administer ammonia.
  - C. Discontinue the donation and provide a paper bag.
  - D. Tell her to sit upright and apply cold compresses to her forehead.

Blood bank/Select course of action/Donor processing/Donor adverse reaction/3

12. A donor bag is half-filled during donation when the blood flow stops. Select the correct course of action.
  - A. Closely observe the bag for at least 3 minutes; if blood flow does not resume, withdraw the needle.
  - B. Remove the needle immediately and discontinue the donation.
  - C. Check and reposition needle if necessary; if blood flow does not resume, withdraw the needle.
  - D. Withdraw the needle and perform a second venipuncture in the other arm.

Blood bank/Select course of action/Donor processing/3

13. Who is the best candidate for a predeposit autologous donation?
  - A. A 45-year-old man who is having elective surgery in 2 weeks; he has anti-k.
  - B. A 23-year-old female leukemia patient with a hemoglobin of 10 g/dL.
  - C. A 12-year-old boy who has hemophilia.
  - D. A 53-year-old woman who has a severe skin infection.

Blood bank/Select course of action/Donor processing/Autologous donation/2

14. Can an autologous donor donate blood on Monday, if he is having surgery on Friday?
  - A. Yes, he can donate up to 72 hours before surgery.
  - B. No, he cannot donate within 7 days of surgery.
  - C. Yes, he can donate, but only half a unit.
  - D. No, he cannot donate within 4 days of surgery.

Blood bank/Apply knowledge of standard operating procedures/Autologous donation/2

15. Which of the conditions below is acceptable for an autologous blood donation?
  - A. The donation is scheduled to take place 2 days before surgery is to be performed.
  - B. The final donation is scheduled for 2 days after the current donation.
  - C. Type and screen results reveal the donor to have an anti-Fy^a.
  - D. The donor's hematocrit is 30%.

Blood bank/Apply knowledge of standard operating procedures/Autologous donation/1

16. Which of the following is true concerning blood salvage?
  - A. Requires ABO, Rh, and IS crossmatch before re-infusion
  - B. May be released for use by other recipients if patient meets all donor criteria
  - C. Eliminates the risk of dilutional coagulopathy
  - D. Must be returned to patient within 6 hours of collection or stored up to 24 hours at 1°–6°C

Blood bank/Apply knowledge of standard operating procedures/Blood salvage/2

Answers to Questions 11–16

11. C This woman is hyperventilating; therefore, the donation should be discontinued. A paper bag should be provided for the donor to breathe into in order to increase the CO_2 in the donor's air.

12. C If blood flow has stopped, check needle first. If the blood flow does not resume after repositioning, then withdraw needle and discontinue the donation. Do not perform a second venipuncture on the donor.

13. A The 45-year-old man with anti-k is the best candidate for predeposit autologous donation because compatible blood will be hard to find if he needs blood after surgery. The other candidates may not be good choices for donation because the process may prove harmful to them.

14. A An autologous donor can donate up to 72 hours before the expected surgery.

15. C Many individuals make an autologous donation because they have alloantibodies that may pose problems in compatibility testing and acquisition of compatible blood. Their autologous blood would always be compatible. An autologous donation must be made at least 72 hours prior to surgery, and no less than 3 days following the previous donation. The hematocrit must be 33% or higher.

16. D Recovered blood must be returned to the patient within 6 hours if stored at 20°–24°C or up to 24 hours if stored at 1°–6°C. If blood is not immediately reinfused, it must be ABO- and Rh-typed. Salvaged blood is never used for another recipient and has the disadvantage of possible dilutional coagulopathy due to the removal of platelets and plasma.

17. What is the term for intraoperative withdrawal of autologous blood with the immediate replacement of compatible fluids and replacement of autologous units after surgery and major bleeding has stopped?
A. Therapeutic bleeding
B. Normovolemic hemodilution
C. Intraoperative autologous intervention
D. Hemodiluted blood salvage

Blood bank/Apply knowledge of standard operating procedures/Normovolemic hemodilution/1

18. Which of the following may be transfused to another person provided that it meets all donor criteria?
A. Therapeutic bleeding and intraoperative autologous blood salvage
B. Intraoperative blood salvage and postraumatic blood salvage
C. Preoperative autologous donation
D. Therapeutic donation

Blood bank/Apply knowledge of standard operating procedures/Hemotherapy/1

Answers to Questions 17–18

17. **B** Normovolemic hemodilution is useful mainly for those patients who do not have time to donate before surgery. The withdrawal of one or two units just prior to surgery is replaced by crystalloid or colloid solutions. The patient's own autologous blood is reinfused after surgery after most bleeding has stopped.

18. **C** Preoperative autologous donations may be released into the general blood inventory if the patient or donor meets all homologous donor criteria.

Hemolytic Disease of the Newborn

1. All of the following may be reasons for a positive DAT on cord cells of a newborn infant *except:*
   A. High concentrations of Wharton's jelly on cord cells
   B. Immune anti-A from an O mother on the cells of an A baby
   C. Immune anti-D from an Rh-negative mother on the cells of an Rh-positive baby
   D. Immune anti-K from a K-negative mother on the cells of a K-negative baby

   Blood bank/Correlate clinical and laboratory data/Hemolytic disease of the newborn/ DAT/2

2. A group O mother gives birth to a normal, healthy infant. The direct antiglobulin test on cord cells, however, is weakly positive. The DAT-negative control is negative. No antibodies are detected in the mother's serum. What is the most likely cause of the positive DAT?
   A. Cord cells were not properly washed.
   B. Immune anti-A or anti-B from the mother has coated cord cells.
   C. A low-titer antibody was below the detection level of screen and panel cells.
   D. A technical error has occurred.

   Blood bank/Correlate clinical and laboratory data/Hemolytic disease of the newborn/ DAT/2

3. What should be done when a woman who is 24 weeks pregnant has a positive antibody screen?
   A. Perform an antibody identification panel; titer if necessary.
   B. No need to do anything until 30 weeks of pregnancy.
   C. Administer Rh immune globulin (RhIg) prophy-lactically.
   D. Adsorb the antibody onto antigen-positive cells.

   Blood bank/Apply knowledge of standard operating procedures/Hemolytic disease of the newborn/Antibody testing/2

4. All of the following are interventions for fetal distress caused by maternal antibodies attacking fetal cells *except:*
   A. Intrauterine transfusion
   B. Plasmapheresis on the mother
   C. Transfusion of antigen-positive cells to the mother
   D. Early induction of labor

   Blood bank/Apply knowledge of standard operating procedures/Hemolytic disease of the newborn/Clinical intervention/2

Answers to Questions 1–4

1. **D** Immune anti-K from the mother would not coat the baby's red cells if the red cells did not contain the K antigen; therefore, the DAT would be negative.

2. **B** Immune anti-A or anti-B from a mother may coat the cord cells of the infant, if the infant is group A or B. This results in either mild HDN or no disease, as in the case here. Although a technical error could have occurred, the negative control for the DAT was negative, making the possibility of technical error unlikely.

3. **A** The identification of the antibody is very important at this stage of the pregnancy. If the antibody is determined to be clinically significant, then a titer may determine the level of antibody and the need for clinical intervention.

4. **C** Transfusion of antigen-positive cells to the mother who already has an antibody might cause a transfusion reaction and/or evoke an even stronger antibody response, possibly causing more harm to the fetus.

5. Cord cells are washed six times and the DAT and negative control are still positive. What should be done next?
A. Obtain a heelstick sample.
B. Record the DAT as positive.
C. Obtain another cord sample.
D. Perform an elution on the cord cells.

Blood bank/Select course of action/Hemolytic disease of the newborn/DAT/2

6. What may be done if HDN is caused by maternal anti-K?
A. Give Kell immune globulin.
B. Monitor the mother's antibody level.
C. Prevent formation of K-positive cells in the fetus.
D. Not a problem; anti-K will not cause HDN.

Blood bank/Apply principles of special procedures/Hemolytic disease of the newborn/Antibody formation/2

7. Should an O-negative mother receive Rh immune globulin (RhIg) if a positive direct antiglobulin test on the newborn is caused by immune anti-A?
A. No, the mother is not a candidate for RhIg because of the positive DAT.
B. Yes, but only if the baby's type is Rh-negative.
C. Yes, but only if the baby's type is Rh-positive.
D. No, the baby's problem is unrelated to Rh blood group antibodies.

Blood bank/Correlate clinical and laboratory data/Hemolytic disease of the newborn/RhIg/3

8. Should an A-negative woman who has just had a miscarriage receive RhIg?
A. Yes, but only if she does not already have anti-D from a previous pregnancy.
B. No, the type of the baby is unknown.
C. Yes, but only a minidose regardless of trimester.
D. No, RhIg is given for term pregnancies only.

Blood bank/Apply knowledge of standard operating procedures/Hemotherapy/RhIg/2

9. A group O mother has given birth to an infant who appears, upon initial testing, to be group AB. What should be done next?
A. Nothing, report the result.
B. Retype both using a different lot number of anti-A and anti-B antisera.
C. Question the phlebotomist about the identity of the samples.
D. Check all labels; repeat the tests; obtain new samples if results are the same.

Blood bank/Correlate clinical and laboratory data/Hemolytic disease of the newborn/Genetics/3

10. Which of the following patients would be a candidate for RhIg?
A. B-positive mother; B-negative baby; first pregnancy; no anti-D in mother

B. O-negative mother; A-positive baby; second pregnancy; no anti-D in mother
C. A-negative mother; O-negative baby; fourth pregnancy; anti-D in mother
D. AB-negative mother; B-positive baby; second pregnancy; anti-D in mother

Blood bank/Correlate clinical and laboratory data/Hemolytic disease of the newborn/RhIg/2

11. How many doses of RhIg are administered for a fetal cell bleed of 25 mL?
A. None are required for 25 mL or less.
B. 2.
C. 3.
D. 4.

Blood bank/Calculate/Hemolytic disease of the newborn/RhIg/2

Answers to Questions 5–11

5. **A** If the cord cells contain excessive Wharton's jelly, then further washing or obtaining another cord sample will not solve the problem. A heelstick sample will not contain Wharton's jelly and should give a true DAT result.

6. **B** Anti-D is the only antibody for which prevention of HDN is possible. If a pregnant woman develops anti-K, she will be monitored to determine if the antibody level and signs of fetal distress necessitate clinical intervention.

7. **C** RhIg is immune anti-D and is given to Rh-negative mothers who give birth to Rh-positive babies, and who do not have anti-D already formed from previous pregnancies or transfusion.

8. **A** When the fetus is Rh-positive or the Rh status of the fetus is unknown, termination of the pregnancy from any cause presents a situation in which the patient should receive RhIg.

9. **D** A clerical, sampling, or testing error may have occurred because an O mother cannot have a group AB infant. Repeating the tests will determine whether a testing error has occurred. If not, new samples should be collected after making a positive identification of both the mother and infant.

10. **B** An O-negative mother who gives birth to an A-positive baby and has no anti-D formed from a previous pregnancy would be a candidate for RhIg. A mother who already has anti-D or a mother who gives birth to an Rh-negative baby is not a candidate for RhIg.

11. **B** A 300-μg dose of RhIg protects for 30 mL fetal cells. The volume of fetal blood is divided by 30 mL. The result is rounded up if the remainder is 0.5 or higher, and one additional dose is added.

12. How many doses of RhIg are indicated for a Kleinhauer-Betke result of 2.0%?
A. 1
B. 2
C. 3
D. 4

Blood bank/Calculate/Hemolytic disease of the newborn/RhIg/2

13. Anti-E is detected in the serum of a woman in the first trimester of pregnancy. The first titer for anti-E is 32. Two weeks later, the antibody titer is 64 and then 128 after another 2 weeks. Clinically, there are beginning signs of fetal distress. What may be done?
A. Induce labor for early delivery.
B. Perform plasmapheresis to remove anti-E from the mother.
C. Administer RhIg to the mother.
D. Perform intrauterine transfusion using E-negative cells.

Blood bank/Correlate clinical and laboratory data/Hemolytic disease of the newborn/2

14. What testing is done for exchange transfusion when the mother's serum contains an alloantibody?
A. Complete crossmatch and antibody screen
B. ABO, Rh, antibody screen, and crossmatch
C. ABO, Rh, and antibody screen
D. ABO and Rh only

Blood bank/Apply knowledge of standard operating procedures/Hemolytic disease of the newborn/Hemotherapy/1

15. Which blood type may be transfused to an AB-positive baby who has HDN caused by anti-D?
A. AB-negative or O-negative
B. AB-positive or O-positive
C. AB-negative only
D. O-negative only

Blood bank/Select course of action/Hemolytic disease of the newborn/Hemotherapy/2

16. All of the following tests are routinely performed on a cord blood sample *except:*
A. Forward typing ABO
B. Antibody screen
C. Rh typing
D. DAT

Blood bank/Apply knowledge of laboratory operations/Hemolytic disease of the newborn/Cord blood/1

17. What test should be performed on blood that will be transfused to an acidotic or hypoxic infant?
A. Cytomegalovirus (CMV)
B. Hemoglobin S (Hgb S)
C. Epstein-Barr virus (EBV)
D. HLA

Answers to Questions 12–17

12. **D** The Kleinhauer-Betke acid elution test is used to estimate the volume of fetal RBCs in the maternal circulation. The percentage of fetal RBCs is multiplied by 50 (the factor for maternal blood volume). The result is divided by 30 (the volume of fetal blood requiring one dose of RhIg) and the result is rounded up if the remainder is 0.5 or higher. Since this is an estimate of the fetal bleed, one additional dose is added. In this case, 2.0×50 mL = 100 mL fetal blood; 100 mL ÷ 30 mL per dose = 3.3 + 1 = 4 doses.

13. **B** Plasmaphresis will remove excess anti-E from the mother and provide a temporary solution to the problem until the fetus is mature enough to be delivered. The procedure may need to be performed several times, depending upon how quickly and how high the levels of anti-E are formed by the mother. Administration of RhIg (anti-D) would not contribute to solving this problem caused by anti-E. Intrauterine transfusion would not be performed before week 20, and would be considered only if there is evidence of severe hemolytic disease.

14. **B** ABO (forward) and Rh are required. An antibody screen using either the neonatal serum or maternal serum is required. A crossmatch is necessary as long as maternal antibody persists in the infant's blood.

15. **A** Either AB-negative or O-negative RBCs may be given to an AB-positive baby because both types are ABO-compatible and lack the D antigen.

16. **B** An antibody screen is not performed on a cord blood sample because a baby does not make antibodies until approximately 6 months of age. Any antibodies detected in a cord blood sample would have come from the mother.

17. **B** Hgb S testing should be performed on blood to be given in an exchange transfusion to an acidotic or hypoxic infant. If the blood is positive for Hgb S, the cells may sickle under conditions of low oxygen.

18. An exchange transfusion is indicated for an infant weighing 1000 g at birth. The donor blood must meet all of the following criteria *except:*

A. HLA-matched
B. CMV-negative
C. O-negative units, less than 5 days old
D. Irradiated

Blood bank/Correlate clinical and laboratory data/Hemolytic disease of the newborn/Selection of blood products/2

Answer to Question 18

18. **A** Blood selected for exchange transfusion should be CMV-negative (to prevent transmission of CMV that may be fatal to an infant), O-negative, less than 5 days old (fresh units with no A or B antigens) and irradiated (to prevent graft-versus-host disease). HLA matching is not a consideration for selecting blood for exchange transfusion.

Serological Testing of Blood Products

1. Why is serological testing important for blood products?
   A. Some carriers of disease may appear asymptomatic.
   B. Diseases may have long incubation periods between initial infection and manifestation of disease symptoms.
   C. To protect the health of the recipient.
   D. All of the above.

   Blood bank/Correlate clinical and laboratory data/Processing/1

2. Which tests to detect HIV are required for blood products?
   A. Anti-HIV-1 and anti-HIV-2
   B. HIV-1 Ag and HIV-2 Ag
   C. Anti-HIV-1, anti-HIV-2, and HIV-1 Ag
   D. Anti-HIV-1, anti-HIV-2, HIV-1 Ag, and HIV-2 Ag

   Blood bank/Apply knowledge of standard operating procedures/Processing/1

3. Which test results for HIV would necessitate discarding the donated blood?
   A. Two positive ELISAs; Western blot bands at p24 and gp160
   B. One positive ELISA; Western blot band at p41
   C. Two positive ELISAs; Western blot band at gp120
   D. Two negative ELISAs; Western blot bands at gp 120 and 160

   Blood bank/Apply knowledge of standard operating procedures/Processing/2

4. **SITUATION:** A man comes to the donor center to donate blood. He appears to be in good health and passes the physical exam. His answers on the donor questionnaire reveal no high-risk behaviors. He has recently recovered from an upper respiratory tract infection that he attributed to the flu. He says that his girlfriend has not been feeling well for about 3 months. He is not aware that he has contracted HIV from her. What will be the most likely outcome of serological testing on his blood?
   A. He will test positive for anti-HIV-1.
   B. He will test negative for anti-HIV-1 and HIV-1 Ag.
   C. He may be in the "window phase" of infection and test negative for all HIV tests.
   D. He may test positive for anti-HIV-1, but negative for HIV-1 Ag.

   Blood bank/Correlate clinical and laboratory data/Processing/2

Answers to Questions 1–4

1. **D** Serological testing is performed to protect the health of the recipient. Serological testing will identify most carriers of disease who are asymptomatic at the time of donation, and donors with infectious diseases that have a long incubation period, such as hepatitis B.

2. **C** The antibody tests for HIV-1 and HIV-2 and the antigen test for HIV-1 are all required for blood products.

3. **A** Samples initially reactive on screening by ELISA should be retested by ELISA in duplicate. A sample reactive in one or both tests should be tested using a confirmatory method such as Western blot. The presence of antibody to two of the following—gp41, p24, gp160 or 120— is indicative of HIV infection.

4. **C** The *window phase* represents a period between infection and the development of serologically detectable markers. If this donor is in the early stages of infection, both his antigen and antibody tests may be negative. Highly sensitive new immunoassays for HIV-1 antibodies have reduced the window phase to a few weeks. Nucleic acid tests on pooled donor samples are being evaluated as a means to reduce the window phase further.

5. A new hospital employee comes to donate blood and tells the blood center nurse that she received the hepatitis B vaccine 4 weeks ago as part of her employee physical exam. If she is accepted as a blood donor, what results will be revealed by serological testing on her unit?
  A. She will not be accepted as a blood donor; deferral period for hepatitis B vaccine is 1 year.
  B. Her blood will be positive for hepatitis B surface antigen (HBsAg).
  C. Her blood will be positive for HbsAg and anti-hepatitis B core antigen (anti-HBc).
  D. Her blood will be negative for all hepatitis markers tested for in donor blood.

Blood bank/Apply knowledge of standard operating procedures/Processing/3

6. What happens to a donor unit that tests positive for anti-hepatitis C virus (anti-HCV)?
  A. The plasma may be used to prepare FFP or cryoprecipitate; cellular elements are discarded.
  B. Cellular elements are used to prepare red cells and platelets; plasma must be discarded.
  C. The unit may not be discarded based upon the results of one test; other hepatitis markers should be examined.
  D. The unit must be discarded.

Blood bank/Apply knowledge of standard operating procedures/Processing/1

7. A unit tests positive for syphilis using the rapid plasma reagin test (RPR). The microhemagglutination assay–*Treponema pallidum* (MHA-TP) on the same unit is negative. What is the disposition of the unit?
  A. The unit may be used to prepare components.
  B. The donor must be contacted and questioned further. If the RPR result is most likely a false-positive, then the unit may be used.
  C. The unit must be discarded.
  D. Cellular components may be prepared but must be irradiated before issue.

Blood bank/Apply knowledge of standard operating procedures/Processing/2

8. What is the *best* method to prevent virus transfer from blood products?
  A. Donor screening
  B. Virucidal processes for plasma products
  C. Microwaving of the blood products
  D. Washing red cells

Blood bank/Apply principles of special procedures/Processing/1

9. Which of the following is routinely tested for in all blood products?
  A. *T. pallidum*
  B. *Borrelia burgdorferi*
  C. *Yersinia enterocolitica*
  D. *Plasmodium falciparum*

Blood bank/Apply principles of basic laboratory procedures/Processing/1

10. What disease is tested on the donor unit before transfusing it to an immunocompromised patient or a newborn?
  A. Syphilis
  B. Sickle cell trait or disease
  C. Lyme disease
  D. CMV

Blood bank/Apply knowledge of laboratory operations/Processing/1

Answers to Questions 5–10

5. **D** She will produce anti-HbsAg as a result of receiving the vaccine; this marker is not normally tested for in donor blood.

6. **D** The whole unit must be discarded even if only one serological test, for example, anti-HCV, is positive.

7. **C** Even a biological false-positive result may be indicative of some type of disease process, and the unit should be discarded.

8. **A** Careful donor screening, especially during the interview process, may uncover high-risk behaviors that may place the donor in a high-risk category for a disease that could possibly be passed to others through blood products.

9. **A** Of the four organisms above, only *T. pallidum* is tested for in donor blood.

10. **D** Blood products are tested for CMV before they are given to immunocompromised patients or newborns. CMV infection may prove life threatening to these individuals.

UNIT 11

Immunohematology Problem Solving

1. Is there a discrepancy between the following blood typing and secretor study results?

   Blood typing results:

Anti-A	Anti-B	A_1 cell	B cell
4+	0	0	4+

   Secretor results:
   Anti-A + saliva + A_1 cells: 0
   Anti-B + saliva + B cells: 4+
   Anti-H + saliva + O cells: 0

   A. No problem, the sample is from a group A secretor.
   B. Blood types as A and saliva types as B.
   C. Blood types as A, but secretor study is inconclusive.
   D. No problem, the sample is from a group A nonsecretor.

   Blood bank/Evaluate laboratory data to make identifications/Saliva neutralization/2

2. What is the best course of action given the following test result? (Assume that the patient has not been recently transfused.)

Anti-A	Anti-B	A_1 Cells	B Cells
Mixed field	0	1+	4+

   A. Nothing, typing is normal.
   B. Type patient cells with anti-A_1 lectin and type serum with A_2 cells.
   C. Retype patient cells; type with anti-H and anti-A,B; use screen cells on patient serum; run patient autocontrol.
   D. Both B and C are correct.

   Blood bank/Apply principles of special procedures/RBC/ABO discrepancy/3

Answers to Questions 1–2

1. **A** The blood typing result demonstrates A antigen on the red cells and anti-B in the serum. The secretor result reveals the A antigen in the saliva. The A antigen neutralized the anti-A, preventing agglutination when A_1 cells were added. Each blood type (except a Bombay) contains some H antigen; therefore, the H antigen in the saliva would be bound by the anti-H reagent. No agglutination would occur when the O cells are added.

2. **D** The patient may be a subgroup of A, possibly an A_3, as indicated by the mixed field result in forward grouping. The reverse grouping shows weak agglutination with A_1 cells, possibly indicating anti-A_1 (sometimes present in the serum of subgroups of A). A positive reaction with anti-A,B would help to differentiate an A subgroup from group O. Anti-A_1 lectin would help to determine if the forward typing represents an A subgroup or A_1. The degree of agglutination with anti-H may also help to determine if an A subgroup is present. If A_2 cells are not agglutinated by the patient's serum, the result would indicate the presence of anti-A_1. If the patient's serum agglutinates A_2 cells, then an autoantibody (patient autocontrol) or alloantibody (screen cells) must be considered.

3. SITUATION: Five consecutive patient samples give the same blood typing results as shown below:

Anti-A	Anti-B	A_1 Cells	B Cells
0	4+	4+	4+

What action should be taken first?
A. Report all results as group B.
B. Wash the RBCs of all five samples and retype using anti-A,B.
C. Retype the patient samples using anti-B from a nonimmunized donor.
D. Check all labels and then retype all five samples.

Blood bank/Evaluate laboratory data to recognize problems/ABO discrepancy/3

4. When a patient's sample shows a discrepancy between forward and reverse grouping with missing or weak reactions, what can be done to enhance these reactions?
A. Nothing can be done to enhance weak ABO reactions.
B. Incubate 15–30 minutes at room temperature or 4°C.
C. Test with new reagents.
D. Centrifuge the patient's serum to concentrate antibodies, and use a heavier suspension of the patient's cells.

Blood bank/Apply knowledge of fundamental biological characteristics/ABO discrepancy/2

5. A patient initially types as group AB with a positive Rh. What should be done next?
A. The patient's sample must be retyped to confirm group AB.
B. The Rh typing should be repeated.
C. An autocontrol should be performed.
D. Report patient as group AB, Rh-positive.

Blood bank/Apply knowledge of routine laboratory procedures/Rh typing/2

6. Which of the following typings would be unlikely to show expression of D^u?
A. *DcE/dce*
B. *Dce/dCe*
C. *DCe/dce*
D. All would require testing for D^u.

Blood bank/Apply knowledge of fundamental biological characteristics/Rh typing/3

7. An obstetric patient, 34 weeks pregnant, shows a positive antibody screen at the indirect antiglobulin phase of testing. She is group B, Rh-negative. This is her first pregnancy. She has no prior history of transfusion. What is the most likely explanation for the positive antibody screen?
A. She has developed an antibody to fetal red cells.

B. She probably does not have antibodies because this is her first pregnancy, and she has not been transfused. Check for technical error.
C. She received RhIg at 28 weeks' gestation.
D. Impossible to determine without further testing.

Blood bank/Correlate clinical and laboratory data/HDN/3

Answers to Questions 3–7

3. **D** Five consecutive samples having a forward grouping of B and reverse grouping of O would not occur by chance. A mix-up of samples and/or reagents most likely occurred while typing the five samples. If the error persists after repeating the tests, then new samples should be obtained and tested with new typing reagents.

4. **B** Sometimes weak or missing reactions may be enhanced by incubation at room temperature or 4°C.

5. **C** In the situation of an A, B, or O patient, the ABO typing serves as a control for Rh typing because at least one forward reaction will be negative for agglutination. When the patient types as AB and Rh-positive, an autocontrol using the patient's cells in saline or 6%–8% albumin is performed. A negative control confirms that the positive typing results were not caused by autoagglutination or rouleaux.

6. **A** D antigen in *trans* position to C (*Dce/dCe*) and D antigen in *cis* position to C (*DCe/dce*) may show weakened expression of D. E antigen in *cis* position to D (*DcE/dce*) may show enhanced D, and would not require incubation and AHG testing.

7. **C** Because the patient has never been transfused or pregnant, she probably has not formed any atypical antibodies. Because she is Rh-negative, she would have received a dose of RhIg at 28 weeks if her prenatal antibody screen had been negative. Although technical error cannot be ruled out, it is far less likely than RhIg administration.

8. A patient's serum contains a mixture of antibodies. One of the antibodies is identified as anti-D. Anti-Jk^a or anti-Fy^a and possibly another antibody are present. What technique(s) may be helpful to identify the other antibody(s)?
A. Enzyme panel; select cell panel
B. Thiol reagents
C. Lowering the pH and increasing the incubation time
D. Using albumin as an enhancement media in combination with selective adsorption

Blood bank/Apply principles of special procedures/Antibody ID/3

9. An anti-M reacts strongly through all phases of testing. Which of the following techniques would *not* contribute to removing this reactivity so that more clinically significant antibodies may be revealed?
A. Acidifying the serum
B. Prewarmed technique
C. Adsorption with homozygous cells
D. Testing with enzyme-treated red cells

Blood bank/Apply principles of special procedures/Antibody ID/3

10. The reactivity of an unknown antibody could be anti-Jk^a, but the antibody identification panel does not fit this pattern conclusively. Which of the following would *not* be effective in determining if the specificity is anti-Jk^a?
A. Testing with enzyme-treated red cells
B. Select panel of homozygous cells
C. Testing with AET-treated cells
D. Increased incubation time

Blood bank/Apply principles of special procedures/Antibody ID/3

11. A cold-reacting antibody is found in the serum of a recently transfused patient and is suspected to be anti-I. The antibody identification panel shows reactions with all cells at room temperature including the autocontrol. The reaction strength varies from 2 to 4+. What procedure would help to distinguish this antibody from other cold-reacting antibodies?
A. Autoadsorption technique
B. Neutralization using saliva
C. Autocontrol using ZZAP reagent–treated cells
D. Reaction with cord cells

Blood bank/Apply principles of special procedures/Antibody ID/3

Answers to Questions 8–11

8. **A** An enzyme panel would help to distinguish between anti-Jk^a (reaction enhanced) and anti-Fy^a (destroyed). Anti-D, however, would also be enhanced and may mask reactions that may distinguish another antibody. A select panel of cells negative for anti-D may help to reveal an additional antibody or antibodies.

9. **A** Lowering the pH will actually enhance reactivity of anti-M. Prewarming (anti-M is a cold-reacting antibody), cold adsorption with homozygous M cells, and testing the serum with enzyme-treated red cells (destroys M antigens) are all techniques to remove reactivity of anti-M.

10. **C** AET denatures Kell antigens and prevents the interference of Kell antibodies during testing for the presence of other antibodies. Because the detection of Kidd antibodies is subject to dosage effect, selection of cells homozygous for the Jk^a antigen (and longer incubation) would help to detect the presence of the corresponding antibody. Enzyme-treated red cells would also react more strongly in the presence of Kidd antibodies.

11. **D** Because RBCs contain variable amounts of I antigen, reactions with anti-I often vary in agglutination strength. However, because this patient was recently transfused, the variation in reaction strength may be the result of an antibody mixture. Although autoadsorption would remove the anti-I, this procedure does not confirm the antibody specificity and can result in removal of other antibodies as well. Cord cells express primarily i antigen with very little I antigen. Anti-I would react weakly or negatively with cord RBCs. ZZAP removes IgG antibodies from red cells. Because anti-I is usually IgM and always has an IgM component, the use of the ZZAP reagent would not be of value.

12. An antibody identification panel reveals the presence of anti-Le^b and a possible second specificity. Saliva from which person would be best to neutralize this Le^b antibody?

	Lewis	ABO	Secretor
A.	Le	H	sese
B.	Le	hh	Se
C.	Le	H	Se
D.	lele	hh	sese

Blood bank/Apply principles of special procedures/Antibody ID/3

13. Which two blood group systems are similar in that the red-cell antigens are highly antigenic and may lead to the formation of clinically significant antibodies; the lack of normal antigens leads to damaged red cells and resultant anemic conditions; and there is usually no problem finding antigen-negative blood for patients with antibodies to the most common antigens of the systems?
A. Rh and Kell
B. P and I
C. MNSs and Lewis
D. Duffy and Kidd

Blood bank/Correlate clinical and laboratory data/Blood group antigens/2

14. A sample from a patient who appeared to have had a delayed transfusion reaction was tested at night in the blood bank. A weak-reacting antibody was detected at the indirect antiglobulin phase. The following morning the antibody panel was repeated, but no antibody was found. Which is the most likely explanation of these findings?
A. The wrong patient sample was tested the previous night.
B. The antibody was an anti-Kidd and deteriorated rapidly.
C. Panel cells were contaminated.
D. The incubator may not have been at the proper temperature.

Blood bank/Evaluate laboratory data to determine possible inconsistent results/Transfusion reaction/3

15. Red cells from a recently transfused patient were DAT-positive when tested with anti-IgG. Screen cells and a panel performed on the patient's serum showed very weak reactions with inconclusive results. What procedure could help to identify the antibody?
A. Elution followed by a panel on the eluate
B. Adsorption followed by a panel on the adsorbed serum
C. Enzyme panel
D. Antigen typing the patient's red cells

Blood bank/Apply principles of special procedures/Antibody identification/3

16. A patient types as O-positive. All three screen cells and red cells from two O-positive donor units show agglutination after incubation at 37°C and increase in reactivity at the IAT phase of testing. What action should be taken next?

A. Perform an autocontrol and direct antiglobulin test on the patient.
B. Perform an enzyme panel.
C. Perform an elution.
D. Choose another two units and repeat the crossmatch.

Blood bank/Select course of action/Incompatible crossmatch/3

Answers to Questions 12–16

12. **C** Lewis antibodies are usually not clinically significant but may interfere with the testing for clinically significant antibodies. Lewis antibodies are most easily removed by neutralizing them with soluble Lewis substance. The Lewis antigens are secreted into saliva and plasma and are adsorbed onto the red cells. Le^b substance is made by adding an L-fucose to both the terminal and next-to-last sugar residue on the type 1 precursor chain. This requires the *Le, H,* and *Se* genes. Since some examples of anti-Le^b react only with group O or A$_2$ RBCs, neutralization is best achieved if the saliva comes from a person who is group O.

13. **A** Rh and Kell systems are among the most antigenic of all blood group systems. Exposure to a small amount of antigen-positive cells in a negative recipient may invoke antibody production. K$_{null}$ and Rh$_{null}$ do not produce Kell and Rh red-cell antigens and the absence of these antigens leads to damaged cells. Damaged cells are removed by the spleen and anemic conditions may result from this action. K-negative and D-negative blood are easy to locate.

14. **B** Kidd antibodies easily deteriorate and may fall to undetectable levels in a very short time. Although technical errors and performance errors may occur in any testing system or situation, the clue to this problem is that the patient had symptoms of a delayed transfusion reaction. Kidd antibodies may be responsible for this type of transfusion reaction.

15. **A** If the red cells show a positive DAT, then IgG antibody has coated incompatible, antigen-positive cells. If screen cells and panel cells show missing or weak reactions, most of the antibody is on the red cells and would need to be eluted before it can be detected. An elution procedure followed by a panel performed on the eluate would help to identify the antibody.

16. **A** All screen cells and all units are positive at both 37°C and the IAT phase. This indicates the possibility of a high-frequency alloantibody or a warm autoantibody. An autocontrol would help to make this distinction. A positive autocontrol indicates an autoantibody; a negative autocontrol indicates an alloantibody. A DAT would be performed to determine if an antibody has coated the patient's red cells and is directed against screen cells and donor cells.

17. Four units of blood are ordered for a patient. Blood bank records are checked and indicate that 5 years ago this patient had an anti-Jk^b. Units are typed for the Jk^b antigen, and those units negative for Jk^b are selected for crossmatch. After initial testing is completed, the patient types as A-positive with a negative antibody screen, and units appear to be compatible. What should be the next course of action?
   A. Run an enzyme panel to detect weak anti-Jk^b.
   B. Issue the units.
   C. Increase the incubation time in order to detect weak anti-Jk^b.
   D. Get another patient sample, check all labels, and retest.

Blood bank/Apply principles of laboratory operations/Compatibility testing/3

18. An antibody screen and crossmatch for six units of red blood cells was performed. All units were incompatible at the indirect antiglobulin phase, but the antibody screen was negative. The patient's autocontrol was negative, and there was no ABO problem. What should be done next?
   A. Repeat the antibody screen using new screen cells.
   B. Antigen type patient cells for low-frequency antigens.
   C. Perform a DAT on samples from all of the donor units.
   D. Crossmatch with samples from six other donor units.

Blood bank/Evaluate laboratory data to determine possible inconsistent results/Incompatible crossmatch/3

19. A cord cell typing appears to be AB-positive with a 2+ DAT. The baby was born normal and healthy to an O-negative mother. Is there a problem here?
   A. No problem, the mother probably received an antenatal dose of RhIg that coated the baby's cells before birth.
   B. No problem, the positive DAT is due to an ABO incompatibility; the baby was not affected.
   C. A technical problem exists because the DAT should not have been positive; repeat the DAT with a negative control.
   D. A problem exists because an AB baby is not possible with an O mother; wash the cells and retype. Perform a negative control for the DAT.

Blood bank/Evaluate laboratory data to determine possible inconsistent results/ABO/3

20. An O-negative mother with no record of any previous pregnancies gives birth to her first child, a B-positive baby. The DAT is weakly positive (+/−). The DAT negative control is negative. The antibody screen is negative. The baby appears healthy but develops mild jaundice after two days, which is treated with phototherapy. The baby goes home after 4 days in the hospital without complications. What is the most likely explanation for the weakly positive DAT?
   A. A technical error

   B. A low titer anti-D
   C. Immune anti-B from the mother
   D. A maternal antibody against a low-incidence antigen

Blood bank/Correlate clinical and laboratory data/HDN/2

Answers to Questions 17–20

17. **B** The amount of anti-Jk^b in patient's serum may have fallen to undetectable levels. The antibody may not be demonstrable in the present sample. Regardless of the presence of detectable antibody, if records indicate the presence of a previous antibody, units should be selected that are antigen-negative for the respective antibody. If antigen-negative units appear compatible, then the units may be issued.

18. **A** If all units are incompatible, then the problem is most likely with the patient's sample. If only one or two units are incompatible, then the problem may be a positive DAT on the unit(s), or an antibody in the patient's serum against an antigen of low frequency that is absent from the screen cells. An antibody should have been detected by the screen cells. A set of new screen cells and possibly a panel should be performed in order to detect the antibody or antibodies.

19. **D** An O mother cannot have an AB baby. Since the baby appears normal and healthy, the positive DAT is probably not due to an alloantibody. The cord cells may be washed and typed again, making certain to perform a negative control for the DAT. If the problem is not resolved, clerical and sample checks should be performed, and if no problem is found, testing should be repeated using a heelstick sample.

20. **C** The history of the baby and mother are consistent with a mild case of ABO-induced HDN. Since this is a first pregnancy, anti-D or other antibodies are unlikely. The O-negative mother may, however, have an immune anti-B that crossed the placenta and attached to the offspring's group B RBCs. The baby was only mildly affected and was treated briefly with phototherapy.

BIBLIOGRAPHY

1. American Association of Blood Banks Standards, ed 18. Arlington, VA, 1997.
2. Harmening, D: Modern Blood Banking and Transfusion Practices. FA Davis, Philadelphia, 1994.
3. Issitt, PD: Applied Blood Group Serology. Montgomery Scientific Publications, Miami, 1985.
4. Quinley, E: Immunohematology: Principles and Practice. JB Lippincott, Philadelphia, 1993.
5. Rudmann, SV: Textbook of Blood Banking and Transfusion Medicine. WB Saunders, Philadelphia, 1995.
6. Turgeon, ML: Fundamentals of Immunohematology. Lea and Febiger, Philadelphia, 1995.
7. Venegelen-Tyler, V: American Association of Blood Banks Technical Manual, ed 12. Arlington, VA, 1996.

CHAPTER FOUR

Clinical Chemistry

Instrumentation

1. Which formula correctly describes the relationship between absorbance and %T?
   A. $A = 2 - \log \%T$
   B. $A = \log 1/T$
   C. $A = -\log T$
   D. All of the above

   Chemistry/Identify basic principle(s)/
   Instrumentation/2

2. A solution that has a transmittance of 1.0 %T would have an absorbance of:
   A. 1.0
   B. 2.0
   C. 1%
   D. 99%

   Chemistry/Calculate/Beer's law/2

3. In absorption spectrophotometry:
   A. Absorbance is directly proportional to transmittance.
   B. Percent transmittance is directly proportional to concentration.
   C. Percent transmittance is directly proportional to the light path length.
   D. Absorbance is directly proportional to concentration.

   Chemistry/Define fundamental
   characteristics/Beer's law/1

4. Which wavelength would be absorbed strongly by a red-colored solution?
   A. 450 nm
   B. 585 nm
   C. 600 nm
   D. 650 nm

   Chemistry/Define fundamental characteristics/
   Spectrophotometry/2

Answers to Questions 1–4

1. **D** Absorbance is proportional to the inverse log of transmittance.
   $$A = -\log T = \log 1/T$$
   Multiplying the numerator and denominator by 100 gives:
   $$A = \log (100/100 \times T)$$
   $100 \times T = \%T$, substituting %T for $100 \times T$ gives:
   $$A = \log 100/\%T$$
   $$A = \log 100 - \log \%T$$
   $$A = 2 - \log \%T$$

   For example, if %$T = 10.0$, then
   $$A = 2 - \log 10.0$$
   $$\log 10.0 = 1.0$$
   $$A = 2-1 = 1.0$$

2. **B** $A = 2 - \log \%T$
   $$A = 2 - \log 1.0$$
   The log of $1.0 = 0$
   $$A = 2.0$$

3. **D** Beer's law states that $A = a \times b \times c$, where a is the absorbtivity coefficient (a constant), b is the path length, and c is concentration. Absorbance is directly proportional to both b and c. Doubling the path length results in incident light contacting twice the number of molecules in solution. This causes absorbance to double, the same effect as doubling the concentration of molecules.

4. **A** A solution transmits light corresponding in wavelength to its color, and usually absorbs light of wavelengths complementary to its color. A red solution transmits light of 600–650 nm and strongly absorbs 400–500 nm light.

5. A green-colored solution would show highest transmittance at:
A. 475 nm
B. 525 nm
C. 585 nm
D. 620 nm

Chemistry/Define fundamental characteristics/ Spectrophotometry/2

6. SITUATION: A technologist is performing an enzyme assay at 340 nm using a visible range spectrophotometer. After setting the wavelength and adjusting the readout to zero %T with the light path blocked, a cuvet with deionized water is inserted. With the light path fully open and the 100%T control at maximum, the instrument readout will not rise above 90%T. What is the most appropriate first course of action?
A. Replace the source lamp.
B. Insert a wider cuvet into the light path.
C. Measure the voltage across the lamp terminals.
D. Replace the instrument fuse.

Chemistry/Select course of action/Spectrophotometry/3

7. Which type of monochromator produces the purest monochromatic light in the UV range?
A. A diffraction grating and a fixed exit slit
B. A sharp cutoff filter and a variable exit slit
C. Interference filters and a variable exit slit
D. A prism and a variable exit slit

Chemistry/Select component/Spectrophotometry/2

8. Which monochromator specification is required in order to measure the true absorbance of a compound having a natural absorption bandwidth of 30 nm?
A. 50-nm bandpass
B. 25-nm bandpass
C. 15-nm bandpass
D. 5-nm bandpass

Chemistry/Select component/Spectrophotometry/2

9. Which photodetector is most sensitive to low levels of light?
A. Barrier layer cell
B. Photodiode
C. Diode array
D. Photomultiplier tube

Chemistry/Define fundamental characteristics/ Instrumentation/1

10. Which condition is a common cause of stray light?
A. Unstable source lamp voltage
B. Improper wavelength calibration
C. Dispersion from second order spectra
D. Misaligned source lamp

Chemistry/Identify source of error/Spectrophotometry/2

Answers to Questions 5–10

5. **B** Green light consists of wavelengths from 500–550 nm. A green-colored solution with a transmittance maximum of 525 nm and a 50-nm bandpass transmits light of 525 nm and absorbs light below 475 nm and above 575 nm. A solution that is green would be quantitated using a wavelength that it absorbs strongly, such as 450 nm.

6. **A** Visible spectrophotometers are usually supplied with a tungsten source lamp. Tungsten lamps produce a continuous range of wavelengths from about 320–1200 nm. Output increases as wavelength becomes longer and is poor below 400 nm. As the lamp envelope darkens with age, the amount of light reaching the photodetector at 340 nm becomes insufficient to set the blank reading to 100%T. Deuterium or hydrogen lamps produce ultraviolet-rich spectra optimal for ultraviolet (UV) work. Halogen, mercury vapor, and xenon give moderate visible and ultraviolet output.

7. **D** Diffraction gratings and prisms both produce a continuous range of wavelengths. A diffraction grating produces a uniform separation of wavelengths. A prism produces much better separation of high-frequency light because refraction is greater for higher energy wavelengths. Instruments using a prism and a variable exit slit can produce UV light of a very narrow bandpass. The adjustable slit is required in order to allow sufficient light to reach the detector to set 100%T.

8. **D** *Bandpass* refers to the range of wavelengths passing through the sample. The narrower the bandpass, the greater is the photometric resolution. Bandpass can be made smaller by reducing the width of the exit slit. Accurate absorbance measurements require a bandpass less than one-fifth the natural bandpass of the chromophore.

9. **D** The photomultiplier tube uses dynodes of increasing voltage to amplify the current produced by the photosensitive cathode. It is 10,000 times as sensitive as a barrier layer cell, which has no amplification. A photomultiplier tube requires a DC regulated lamp because it responds to light fluctuations caused by the AC cycle.

10. **C** Stray light is caused by the presence of any light other than the wavelength of measurement reaching the detector. It is most often caused by second order spectra, deteriorated optics, light dispersed by a darkened lamp envelope, and extraneous room light.

11. A linearity study is performed on a visible spectrophotometer at 650 nm and the following absorbance readings are obtained:

Concentration of Standard	Absorbance
10.0 mg/dL	0.20
20.0 mg/dL	0.41
30.0 mg/dL	0.62
40.0 mg/dL	0.79
50.0 mg/dL	0.92

The study was repeated using freshly prepared standards and reagents, but results were identical to those above. What is the most likely cause of these results?
A. Wrong wavelength used
B. Insufficient chromophore concentration
C. Matrix interference
D. Stray light

Chemistry/Evaluate source of error/Spectro-photometry/3

12. Which type of filter is best for measuring stray light?
A. Wratten
B. Didymium
C. Sharp cutoff
D. Neutral density

Chemistry/Evaluate source of error/Spectro-photometry/2

13. Which of the following materials is best suited for verifying the wavelength calibration of a spectrophotometer?
A. Neutral density filters
B. Potassium dichromate solutions traceable to the National Bureau of Standards reference
C. Wratten filters
D. Holmium oxide glass

Chemistry/Identify standard operating procedure/Spectrophotometry/2

14. A chopper is used in a dual-beam spectrophotometer in order to:
A. Reduce the number of moving parts
B. Facilitate wavelength scanning
C. Obviate the need for matched detectors
D. Reduce stray light

Chemistry/Define fundamental characteristics/Spectrophotometry/1

15. The half-band width of a monochromator is defined by:
A. The range of wavelengths passed at 50% maximum transmittance
B. One-half the lowest wavelength of optical purity
C. The wavelength of peak transmittance
D. One-half the wavelength of peak absorbance

Chemistry/Define fundamental characteristics/Spectrophotometry/1

Answers to Questions 11–15

11. **D** Stray light is the most common cause of loss of linearity at high-analyte concentrations. Transmitted incident light is lowest when absorption is highest. Therefore, stray light is a greater percentage of the detector response when sample concentration is high. Stray light is usually most significant when measurements are made at the extremes of the visible spectrum because lamp output and detector response are low.

12. **C** Sharp cutoff filters transmit almost all incident light until the cutoff wavelength is reached. At that point, they cease to transmit light. Because they give an "all or none effect" only stray light reaches the detector when the selected wavelength is beyond the cutoff.

13. **D** Wavelength accuracy is verified by determining the wavelength reading that gives the highest absorbance (or transmittance) when a substance with a narrow natural bandpass (sharp absorbance or transmittance peak) is scanned. For example, didymium glass has a sharp absorbance peak at 585 nm. Therefore, an instrument should give its highest absorbance reading when the wavelength dial is set at 585 nm. Holmium oxide produces a very narrow absorbance peak at 361 nm; likewise, the hydrogen lamp of a UV spectrophotometer produces a 656-nm emission line that can be used to verify wavelength. Neutral density filters and dichromate solutions are used to verify absorbance accuracy or linearity. A Wratten filter is a wide-bandpass filter made by placing a thin layer of colored gelatin between two glass plates and is unsuitable for spectrophotometric calibration.

14. **C** An optical chopper consists of a rotating sector mirror that alternately passes incident light through sample and reference cuvets. The chopper is synchronized with mirrors that recombine the light beam before striking the detector. The detector produces a square wave representing the ratio of sample and reference signals.

15. **A** Half-band width is a measure of bandpass made using a solution or filter having a narrow natural bandpass (transmittance peak). The wavelength giving maximum transmittance is set to $100\%T$ (or $0\,A$). Then, the wavelength dial is adjusted downward, until a readout of $50\%T$ ($0.301\,A$) is obtained. Next, the wavelength is adjusted upward until $50\%T$ is obtained. The wavelength difference is the half-band width. The narrower the half-band width, the better the photometric resolution of the instrument.

16. The term *dark current* as used in spectrophotometry refers to:
   A. Drift in the $100\%T$ reading of a spectrophotometer
   B. The $\%T$ reading when the reagent blank is measured
   C. Flow of current from a phototube caused by high gain on its anode
   D. Electron flow through the readout circuit induced by the magnetic field of the power supply transformer

Chemistry/Define fundamental characteristics/ Spectrophotometry/1

17. The reagent blank corrects for absorbance caused by:
   A. The color of reagents
   B. Sample turbidity
   C. Bilirubin and hemolysis
   D. All of the above

Chemistry/Identify basic principle(s)/Reaction/2

18. Which instrument requires a highly regulated DC power supply?
   A. A spectrophotometer with a barrier layer cell
   B. A colorimeter with multilayer interference filters
   C. A spectrophotometer with a photomultiplier tube
   D. A densitometer with a photodiode detector

Chemistry/Select component/ Spectrophotometry/2

19. Which of the following is an advantage of a spectrophotometer with a diode array detector over a spectrophotometer with a photomultiplier tube?
   A. Measurement at multiple wavelengths simultaneously
   B. Correction for fluctuation in source lamp intensity
   C. Greater optical resolution
   D. Greater optical sensitivity

Chemistry/Define fundamental characteristics/ Spectrophotometry/2

20. Which statement regarding reflectometry is true?
   A. The relation between reflectance density and concentration is linear.
   B. Single point calibration can be used to determine concentration.
   C. 100% reflectance is set with an opaque film called a white reference.
   D. The diode array is the photodetector of choice.

Chemistry/Apply principles of special procedures/ Instrumentation/2

Answers to Questions 16–20

16. C Dark current is the current generated by a detector when the light path is blocked to prevent incident light from striking it. Phototubes and photomultiplier tubes will leak a small amount of current because electrons are drawn through the circuit by the high positive voltage applied to the anode or dynodes.

17. A When a spectrophotometer is set to $100\%T$ with the reagent blank instead of water, the absorbance of reagents is automatically subtracted from each unknown reading. The reagent blank does not correct for absorbance caused by interfering chromogens in the sample such as bilirubin, hemolysis, or turbidity.

18. C When AC voltage regulators are used to isolate source lamp power, light output fluctuates as the voltage changes. Because this occurs at 60 Hz, it is not detected by eyesight or slow-responding detectors. Photomultiplier tubes are sensitive enough to respond to the AC frequency and require a DC regulated power supply.

19. A A diode array detector contains hundreds of photo diodes in a fixed alignment with the monochromator. Each diode gives a linear increase in current with increasing transmitted light, allowing the instrument microprocessor to construct a spectral absorbance curve for the solution being measured. However, diode spacing restricts optical resolution, which is usually in the range of 1–5 nm. Unlike a photomultiplier tube, signal amplification does not take place at the detector and each diode is stimulated by only a small fraction of the light leaving the exit slit. This results in less optical sensitivity than is available with a photomultiplier tube. Photodiode array detectors have largely replaced dual beam scanning spectrophotometers because they are much faster.

20. C Reflectometry does not follow Beer's law, but the relationship between concentration and reflectance can be described by a logistic formula or algorithm that can be solved for concentration. For example, $K/S = (1 - R)^2/2R$, where K = Kubelka-Munk absorptivity constant, S = scattering coefficient, R = reflectance density. K/S is proportional to concentration. The white reference is analogous to the $100\%T$ setting in spectrophotometry and serves as a reference signal. $D_r = \log R_0/R_1$, where D_r is the reflectance density, R_0 is the white reference signal, and R_1 is the photodetector signal for the test sample.

21. Bichromatic filter photometers can correct for interfering substances if:
A. The energy outputs from both filters are equal.
B. Both wavelengths pass through the sample simultaneously.
C. The side band is a harmonic of the primary wavelength.
D. The chromogen has the same absorbance at both wavelengths.

Chemistry/Apply principles of special procedures/ Instrumentation/2

22. Which instrument requires a primary and secondary monochromator?
A. Flame photometer
B. Atomic absorption spectrophotometer
C. Fluorometer
D. Nephelometer

Chemistry/Apply principles of special procedures/ Instrumentation/1

23. Which of the statements below about fluorometry is accurate?
A. Fluorometry is less sensitive than spectrophotometry.
B. Fluorometry is less specific than spectrophotometry.
C. Unsaturated cyclic molecules are often fluorescent.
D. Fluorescence is directly proportional to temperature.

Chemistry/Apply principles of special procedures/ Instrumentation/2

24. Which statement about fluorescence polarization immunoassay (FPIA) is true?
A. Rotation of free antigen conjugate is faster than antibody-bound conjugate.
B. Fluorescence by free antigen conjugate is unpolarized.
C. Analyte concentration is related inversely to polarized fluorescence.
D. All of the above.

Chemistry/Apply principles of special procedures/ Instrumentation/2

25. Light scattering when wavelength is greater than ten times particle diameter is described by:
A. Rayleigh's law
B. The Beer-Lambert law
C. Mie's law
D. The Rayleigh-Debye law

Chemistry/Apply principles of special procedures/ Instrumentation/2

26. Which statement regarding nephelometry is true?
A. Nephelometry is less sensitive than absorption spectrophotometry.
B. Nephelometry follows Beer's law.
C. The optical design is identical to a turbidimeter except that a HeNe laser light source is used.

D. The detector response is directly proportional to concentration.

Chemistry/Apply principles of special procedures/ Instrumentation/2

Answers to Questions 21–26

21. **A** In bichromatic photometry the absorbance of sample is measured at two different wavelengths. The primary wavelength is at or near the absorbance maximum. An interfering substance having the same absorbance at both primary and secondary (side band) wavelengths does not affect the absorbance difference (*Ad*).

22. **C** A fluorometer uses a primary monochromator to isolate the wavelength for excitation, and a secondary monochromator to isolate the wavelength emitted by the fluorochrome.

23. **C** Increasing temperature results in more random collision between molecules by increasing their motion. This causes energy to be dissipated as heat instead of fluorescence. Temperature is inversely proportional to fluorescence. Fluorescence is more sensitive than spectrophotometry because the detector signal can be amplified when dilute solutions are measured. It is also more specific than spectrophotometry because both the excitation and emission wavelengths are characteristics of the compound being measured.

24. **D** In FPIA, antigen in patient's sample competes with antigen conjugated to a fluorochrome (tracer) for a limited number of antibodies. When antibody binds to the tracer, it slows its rotation. This increases the emission of plane polarized fluorescence. Polarized fluorescence is inversely related to concentration and can be measured without the need to separate free and antibody-bound tracer.

25. **A** Rayleigh's law states that when the incident wavelength is much longer than the particle diameter there is maximum backscatter and minimum right-angle scatter. The Rayleigh-Debye law predicts maximum right-angle scatter when wavelength and particle diameter approach equality. In nephelometry, the relationship between wavelength and diameter determines the angle at which the detector is located.

26. **D** In nephelometry the detector output is proportional to concentration (as opposed to turbidimetry where the detector is behind the cuvet). The detector(s) is/are usually placed at an angle between 25° and 90° to the incident light depending upon the application. Nephelometers, like fluorometers, are calibrated to read zero with the light path blocked, and sensitivity can be increased up to 1000 times by amplification of the detector output or photomultiplier tube gain.

27. The purpose of the nebulizer and atomizer in an atomic absorption spectrophotometer that uses a flame is to:
A. Convert ions to atoms
B. Cause ejection of an outer shell electron
C. Reduce evaporation of the sample
D. Burn off organic impurities

Chemistry/Apply principles of basic procedures/ Instrumentation/2

28. Internal standards are *not* needed in atomic absorption spectrophotometry because:
A. Changes in aspiration have little effect on the number of ground state atoms.
B. Atomic absorption instruments have a stable light path.
C. The instrument measures only one atom at a time.
D. The instrument source lamp is used for a reference voltage.

Chemistry/Apply principles of special procedures/ Instrumentation/2

29. A flameless atomic absorption spectrophotometer dehydrates and atomizes a sample using:
A. A graphite capillary furnace
B. An electron gun
C. A thermoelectric semiconductor
D. A thermospray platform

Chemistry/Apply principles of special procedures/ Instrumentation/1

30. Interference in atomic absorption spectrophotometry caused by differences in viscosity is called:
A. Absorption interference
B. Matrix effect
C. Ionization interference
D. Quenching

Chemistry/Evaluate sources of error/ Instrumentation/2

31. All of the following are required when measuring magnesium by atomic absorption spectrophotometry *except:*
A. A hollow cathode lamp with a magnesium cathode
B. A chopper to prevent optical interference from magnesium emission
C. A monochromator to isolate the magnesium emission line at 285 nm
D. A 285-nm reference beam to correct for background absorption

Chemistry/Select methods/Reagents/Media/ Electrolytes/2

32. When measuring calcium by atomic absorption spectrophotometry, which is required?
A. An organic extraction reagent to deconjugate calcium from protein
B. An internal standard
C. A magnesium chelator
D. Lanthanum oxide to chelate phosphates

Chemistry/Select methods/Reagents/Media/ Electrolytes/2

Answers to Questions 27–32

27. **A** The atomizer of the atomic absorption spectrophotometer consists of either a nebulizer and flame or graphite furnace. The nebulizer disperses the sample evenly into the flame. Heat is used to evaporate water and break the ionic bonds of salts, forming atoms. The flame also excites a small percentage of the atoms, which release a characteristic emission line.

28. **A** The steady state between ground state and excited atoms in a flame or graphite furnace favors the ground state by more than 10,000:1. Small fluctuations in aspiration rate or flame temperature have an insignificant effect on the number of ground state atoms, but have a pronounced effect on the number excited.

29. **A** Flameless atomic absorption uses a hollow tube of graphite with quartz ends. The tube is heated by current in order to char the sample, and argon is injected into the capillary to distribute the atoms. The furnace is more sensitive than a flame atomizer and more efficient in atomizing thermostable salts. However, it is prone to greater matrix interference and is slower than the flame atomizer because it must cool down before injection of the next sample.

30. **B** Significant differences in aspiration and atomization result when the matrix of sample and unknowns differ. Differences in viscosity and protein content are major causes of matrix error. Matrix effects can be reduced by using protein-based calibrators and diluting both standards and samples prior to assay.

31. **D** Atomic absorption requires a lamp with a cathode made from the metal to be assayed. The lamp emits the line spectrum of the metal providing the wavelength that the atoms can absorb. The chopper pulses the source light, allowing it to be discriminated from light emitted by excited atoms. A monochromator eliminates light emitted by the ideal gas in the lamp. Wide bandpass light or Zeeman correction (splitting the incident light into side bands by a magnetic field) may be used to correct for background absorption.

32. **D** An acidic diluent such as hydrochloric acid (HCl) will displace calcium bound to albumin. However, calcium forms a thermostable bond with phosphate that causes chemical interference in atomic absorption. Lanthanum displaces calcium, forming lanthanum phosphate, and eliminates interference from phosphates. Unlike colorimetric methods for calcium (e.g., *o*-cresolphthalein complexone) magnesium does not interfere since it does not absorb the 422.7-nm emission line from the calcium hollow cathode lamp.

33. Ion-selective analyzers using *undiluted* samples have an advantage over a flame photometer because they:
A. Can measure whole blood
B. Are not subject to pseudohyponatremia caused by high lipids
C. Do not require an internal standard or flammable gas
D. All of the above

Chemistry/Apply knowledge to identify sources of error/Electrolytes/2

34. Select the equation describing the potential that develops at the surface of an ion-selective electrode.
A. Van Deemter equation
B. Van Slyke equation
C. Nernst equation
D. Henderson-Hasselbalch equation

Chemistry/Define fundamental characteristics/ Instrumentation/1

35. The reference potential of a silver-silver chloride electrode is determined by the:
A. Concentration of the potassium chloride filling solution
B. Surface area of the electrode
C. Activity of total anion in the paste covering the electrode
D. The concentration of silver in the paste covering the electrode

Chemistry/Define fundamental characteristics/ Instrumentation/1

36. The term RT/nF in the Nernst equation defines the:
A. Potential at the ion-selective membrane
B. Slope of the electrode
C. Decomposition potential
D. Isopotential point of the electrode

Chemistry/Define fundamental characteristics/ Instrumentation/1

37. The ion-selective membrane used to measure potassium is made of:
A. High-borosilicate glass membrane
B. Polyvinyl chloride dioctylphenyl phosphonate ion exchanger
C. Valinomycin gel
D. Calomel

Chemistry/Apply principles of basic laboratory procedures/Electrolytes/1

38. The response of a sodium electrode to a tenfold increase in sodium concentration should be:
A. A tenfold drop in potential
B. An increase in potential of approximately 60 mV
C. An increase in potential of approximately 10 mV
D. A decrease in potential of approximaely 10 mV

Chemistry/Calculate/Electrolytes/2

Answers to Questions 33–38

33. D Ion-selective analyzers measure the electrolyte dissolved in the fluid phase of the sample in millimoles per liter of plasma water. When undiluted blood is assayed, the measurement is independent of colloids such as protein and lipid. Hyperlipemic samples cause falsely low sodium measurements when assayed by flame photometry and ion-selective analyzers requiring dilution because lipids displace plasma water containing the electrolytes.

34. C The Van Deemter equation describes the relation between the velocity of mobile phase to column efficiency in gas chromatography. The Henderson-Hasselbalch equation is used to determine the pH of a solution containing a weak acid and its salt. Van Slyke developed an apparatus to measure CO_2 and O_2 content using a manometer.

35. A The activity of any solid or ion in a saturated solution is unity. For a silver electrode covered with silver chloride paste, the Nernst equation is $E = E^o - RT/nF \times 2.3 \log_{10} [Ag^o \times Cl^-]/[AgCl]$. Because silver and silver chloride have an activity of 1.0, and all components except chloride are constants, the potential of the reference electrode is determined by the chloride concentration of the filling solution.
$$E = E^o - RT/nF \times 2.3 \log_{10}[Cl^-] = E^o - 59.2\ mV \times \log[Cl^-]\ \text{(at room temperature)}.$$

36. B In the term RT/nF, R = the molar gas constant, T = temperature in degrees Kelvin, F = Faraday's constant, and n = the number of electrons donated per atom of reductant. The slope depends upon the temperature of the solution and the valence of the reductant. At room temperature, the slope is 59.2 mV for a univalent ion and 29.6 mV for a divalent ion.

37. C Valinomycin is an antibiotic with a highly selective reversible binding affinity for potassium ions. Sodium electrodes are usually composed of a glass membrane with a high content of aluminum silicate. Calcium and lithium ion-selective electrodes are made from organic liquid ion exchangers called neutral carrier ionophores. Calomel is made of mercury covered with a paste of mercurous chloride (Hg^o/Hg_2Cl_2) and is used as a reference electrode for pH.

38. B The Nernst equation predicts an increase of approximately 60 mV per tenfold increase in sodium activity. For sodium, $E = E^o + RT/nF \times 2.3 \log_{10}[Na^+]$. $RT/nF \times 2.3 = 60$ mV at 37°C. Therefore, $E = E^o + 60\ mV \times \log_{10}[Na^+]$. If sodium concentration is 10 mmol/L, then $E = E^o + 60\ mV \times \log_{10}[10] = E^o + 60$ mV. If sodium concentration increases from 10 mmol/L to 100 mmol/L, then $E = E^o + 60\ mV \times \log_{10}[100] = E^o + 60\ mV \times 2 = E^o + 120$ mV.

39. Which of the electrodes below is a current-producing (amperometric) rather than a voltage-producing (potentiometric) electrode?
A. Clark electrode
B. Severinghaus electrode
C. pH electrode
D. Ionized calcium electrode

Chemistry/Define fundamental characteristics/ Instrumentation/1

40. Which of the following would cause a "response" error from an ion-selective electrode for sodium when measuring serum but *not* calibrator?
A. Interference from other electrolytes
B. Protein coating the ion-selective membrane
C. An overrange in sodium concentration
D. Protein binding to sodium ions

Chemistry/Identify source of error/Electrolytes/2

41. In polarography, the voltage needed to cause depolarization of the cathode is called the:
A. Half-wave potential
B. Isopotential point
C. Decomposition potential
D. Polarization potential

Chemistry/Define fundamental characteristics/ Instrumentation/1

42. Persistent noise from an ion-selective electrode is most often caused by:
A. Contamination of sample
B. Blocked junction at the salt bridge
C. Overrange from high concentration
D. Improper calibration

Chemistry/Identify source of error/Electrolytes/2

43. Which element is reduced at the cathode of a Clark polarographic electrode?
A. Silver
B. Oxygen
C. Chloride
D. Potassium

Chemistry/Define fundamental characteristics/ Instrumentation/1

44. Which of the following statements accurately characterizes the coulometric titration of chloride?
A. The indicator electrodes generate voltage.
B. Constant current must be present across the generator electrodes.
C. Silver ions are formed at the generator cathode.
D. Chloride concentration is inversely proportional to titration time.

Chemistry/Define fundamental characteristics/ Instrumentation/2

Answers to Questions 39–44

39. **A** The Clark electrode is composed of two half cells that generate current, not voltage. It is used to measure partial pressure of oxygen (PO_2), and is based upon an amperometric method called polarography. When -0.8 V is applied to the cathode, O_2 is reduced causing current to flow. Current is proportional to the PO_2 of the sample.

40. **B** Response is the time required for an electrode to reach maximum potential. Ion-selective analyzers use a microprocessor to monitor electrode response, slope, drift, and noise. When an electrode gives an acceptable response time when measuring aqueous calibrator, but not when measuring serum, the cause is often protein build-up on the membrane.

41. **C** In polarography, a minimum negative voltage must be applied to the cathode to cause reduction of metal ions (or O_2) in solution. This is called the decomposition potential. It is concentration-dependent (dilute solutions require greater negative voltage), and can be determined using the Nernst equation.

42. **B** Electrode noise most often results from an unstable junction potential. Most reference electrodes contain a high concentration of KCl internal solution used to produce the reference potential. This forms a salt bridge with the measuring half-cell by contacting sample, but is kept from equilibrating via a barrier called a *junction*. When this junction becomes blocked by salt crystals, the reference potential will be unstable, resulting in fluctuation in the analyzer readout.

43. **B** The Clark electrode is designed to measure oxygen. O_2 diffuses through a gas-permeable membrane covering the electrode. It is reduced at the cathode, which is usually made of platinum wire. Electrons are supplied by the anode, which is made of silver. The net reaction is $4\,KCl + 2\,H_2O + O_2 + 4\,Ag° \rightarrow 4\,AgCl + 4\,KOH$.

44. **B** The Cotlove chloridometer is based upon the principle of coulometric titration with amperometric detection. Charge in the form of silver ions is generated by oxidation of silver wire at the generator anode. Silver ions react with chloride ions, forming insoluble silver chloride (AgCl). When all of the chloride is titrated, free silver ions are detected by reduction back to elemental silver, which causes an increase in current across the indicator electrodes (a pair of silver electrodes with a voltage difference of about 1.0 V DC). Charge or titration time is directly proportional to chloride concentration as long as the rate of oxidation remains constant at the generator anode.

45. In the coulometric chloride titration:
  A. Acetic acid in the titrating solution furnishes the counter ion for reduction.
  B. The endpoint is detected by amperometry.
  C. The titrating reagent contains a phosphate buffer to keep pH constant.
  D. Nitric acid (HNO_3) is used to lower the solubility of AgCl.

Chemistry/Apply principles of special procedures/ Electrolytes/2

46. Which of the following compounds can interfere with the coulometric chloride assay?
  A. Bromide
  B. Cyanide
  C. Cysteine
  D. All the above

Chemistry/Apply knowledge to identify sources of error/Electrolytes/2

47. All of the following compounds contribute to the osmolality of plasma *except:*
  A. Lipids
  B. Creatinine
  C. Drug metabolites
  D. Glucose

Chemistry/Apply knowledge of fundamental biological characteristics/Osmolality/2

48. One mole per kilogram H_2O of any solute will cause all of the following *except:*
  A. Lower the freezing point by 1.86°C
  B. Raise vapor pressure by 0.3 mm Hg
  C. Raise the boiling point by 0.52°C
  D. Raise osmotic pressure by 22.4 atm

Chemistry/Apply knowledge of fundamental biological characteristics/Osmolality/2

49. What component of a freezing point osmometer measures the sample temperature?
  A. Thermistor
  B. Thermocouple
  C. Capacitor
  D. Electrode

Chemistry/Apply principles of special procedures/ Osmometry/1

50. What type of measuring circuit is used in a freezing point osmometer?
  A. Electrometer
  B. Potentiometer
  C. Wheatstone bridge
  D. Thermal conductivity bridge

Chemistry/Apply principles of special procedures/Osmometry/1

51. Which measurement principle is employed in a vapor pressure osmometer?
  A. Seebeck
  B. Peltier
  C. Hayden
  D. Darlington

Chemistry/Apply principles of special procedures/ Osmometry/1

Answers to Questions 45–51

45. **B** Reduction of Ag^+ back to Ag^o generates the current, which signals the endpoint. The titrating reagent contains HNO_3, acetic acid, H_2O, and either gelatin or polyvinyl alcohol. The HNO_3 furnishes nitrate, which is reduced at the generator cathode, forming ammonium ions. The ammonium becomes oxidized back to nitrate at the indicator anode. Gelatin or polyvinyl alcohol is needed to prevent pitting of the generator anode. Acetic acid lowers the solubility of AgCl preventing dissociation back to Ag^+.

46. **D** Chloride assays based upon either coulometric or chemical titration are subject to positive interference from other anions and electronegative radicals that may be titrated instead of chloride ions.

47. **A** Osmolality is the concentration (in moles) of dissolved solute per kilogram solvent. Proteins and lipids are not in solution, and do not contribute to osmolality. The nonionized solutes such as glucose and urea contribute one osmole per mole per kilogram water, whereas dissociated salts contribute one osmole per mole of each dissociated ion or radical.

48. **B** Both freezing point and vapor pressure are lowered by increasing solute concentration. Boiling point and osmotic pressure are raised. Increasing solute concentration of a solution opposes a change in its physical state and lowers the concentration of H_2O molecules.

49. **A** A thermistor is a temperature-sensitive resistor. The resistance to current flow increases as temperature falls. The temperature at which a solution freezes can be determined by measuring the resistance of the thermistor. Resistance is directly proportional to the osmolality of the sample.

50. **C** The resistance of the thermistor is measured using a network of resistors called a Wheatstone bridge. When the sample is frozen, the bridge is balanced using a calibrated variable resistor, so that no current flows to the readout. The resistance required to balance the meter is equal to the resistance of the thermistor.

51. **A** The Seebeck effect refers to the increase in voltage across the opposite ends of a thermocouple caused by decreasing temperature. Increasing osmolality lowers the dew point of a sample. When sample is cooled to its dew point, the voltage change across the thermocouple is directly proportional to osmolality.

52. The freezing point osmometer differs from the vapor pressure osmometer in that only the freezing point osmometer:
A. Cools the sample
B. Is sensitive to ethanol
C. Requires a thermoelectric module
D. Requires calibration with aqueous standards

Chemistry/Apply principles of special procedures/ Osmometry/2

53. The method for measuring iron by plating the metal and then oxidizing it is called
A. Polarography
B. Coulometry
C. Anodic stripping voltometry
D. Amperometry

Chemistry/Apply principles of special procedures/ Instrumentation/1

54. The term *isocratic* is used in high-performance liquid chromatography (HPLC) to mean the:
A. Mobile phase is at constant temperature.
B. Stationary phase is equilibrated with the mobile phase.
C. Mobile phase consists of a constant solvent composition.
D. Flow rate of the mobile phase is regulated.

Chemistry/Apply principles of special procedures/ High-performance liquid chromatography/1

55. The term *reverse phase* is used in HPLC to indicate that the mobile phase is:
A. More polar than the stationary phase
B. Liquid and the stationary phase is solid
C. Organic and the stationary phase is aqueous
D. A stronger solvent than the stationary phase

Chemistry/Apply principles of special procedures/ High-performance liquid chromatography/1

56. What is the primary means of solute separation in HPLC using a C18 column?
A. Anion exchange
B. Size exclusion
C. Partitioning
D. Cation exchange

Chemistry/Apply principles of special procedures/ High-performance liquid chromatography/1

57. The most commonly used detector for clinical gas-liquid chromatography (GLC) is based upon:
A. Ultraviolet light absorbance at 254 nm
B. Flame ionization
C. Refractive index
D. Thermal conductance

Chemistry/Apply principles of special procedures/Gas chromatography/1

58. What type of detector is used in high-performance liquid chromatography with electrochemical detection (HPLC-ECD)?
A. Calomel electrode
B. Conductivity electrode
C. Glassy carbon electrode
D. Polarographic electrode

Chemistry/Apply principles of special procedures/ High-performance liquid chromatography/1

Answers to Questions 52–58

52. B Alcohol enters the vapor phase so rapidly that it evaporates before the dew point of the sample is reached. Therefore, ethanol does not contribute to osmolality as measured using the vapor pressure osmometer. Freezing point osmometers measure alcohol and can be used in emergency room settings to estimate ethanol toxicity.

53. C Anodic stripping voltometry is used to measure lead and iron. The cation of the metal is plated onto a mercury cathode by applying a negative charge. The voltage of this electrode is reversed until the plated metal is oxidized back to a cation. Current produced by oxidation of the metal is proportional to concentration.

54. C An isocratic separation uses a single mobile phase of constant composition, pH, and polarity, and requires a single pump. Some HPLC separations use a gradient mobile phase to increase distance between peaks. Gradients are made by mixing two or more solvents using a controller to change the proportions of solvent components.

55. A In reverse phase HPLC the separation takes place using a nonpolar sorbent (stationary phase) such as octadecylsilane (C18). Solutes that are nonpolar are retained longer than polar solutes. Most clinical separations of drugs, hormones, and metabolites use reverse phase because aqueous mobile phases are far less toxic and flammable.

56. C Stationary phases (column packings) used in HPLC separate solutes by multiple means, but in reverse phase HPLC the relative solubility between the mobile phase and stationary phase is most important and depends upon solvent polarity, pH, and ionic strength.

57. B Volatile solutes can be detected in GLC using flame ionization, thermal conductivity, electron capture, and mass spectroscopy. In flame ionization, energy from a flame is used to excite the analytes as they elute from the column. The flame is made by igniting a mixture of hydrogen, carrier gas, and air. Current is produced when an outer shell electron is ejected from the excited analyte.

58. C HPLC-ECD uses a glassy carbon measuring electrode and a silver-silver chloride reference. The analyte is oxidized or reduced by holding the glassy carbon electrode at a positive voltage (oxidization) or negative voltage (reduction). The resulting current flow is directly proportional to concentration. Phenolic groups such as catecholamines can be measured by HPLC-ECD.

59. In gas chromatography the elution order of volatiles is usually based upon the:
A. Boiling point
B. Molecular size
C. Carbon content
D. Polarity

Chemistry/Apply principle of special procedures/Gas chromatography/2

60. Select the chemical that is used in most HPLC procedures to decrease solvent polarity.
A. Hexane
B. Nonane
C. Chloroform
D. Acetonitrile

Chemistry/Apply principles of special procedures/Biochemical/2

61. In thin-layer chromatography (TLC), the distance the solute migrates divided by the distance the solvent migrates is the:
A. t_R
B. K_d
C. R_f
D. pK

Chemistry/Apply principles of special procedures/High-performance liquid chromatography/1

62. Which reagent is used in TLC to extract cocaine metabolites from urine?
A. Acid and sodium chloride
B. Alkali and organic solvent
C. Chloroform and sodium acetate
D. Neutral solution of ethyl acetate

Chemistry/Apply principles of special procedures/Biochemical/2

63. What is the purpose of an internal standard in HPLC and GC methods?
A. Compensate for variation in extraction and injection
B. Correct for background absorbance
C. Compensate for changes in flow rate
D. Correct for coelution of solutes

Chemistry/Apply principles of special procedures/Chromatography/2

64. What is the confirmatory method for measuring drugs of abuse?
A. HPLC
B. Enzyme-multiplied immunoassay technique (EMIT)
C. Gas chromatography with mass spectroscopy (GC-MS)
D. TLC

Chemistry/Select instruments to perform test/Drugs of abuse/2

65. Which of the following isotopes has a half-life best suited to radioimmunoassay (RIA)?

A. Tritium
B. Iodine 131 (^{131}I)
C. Iodine 125 (^{125}I)
D. Carbon 14 (^{14}C)

Chemistry/Apply principles of special procedures/RIA/1

Answers to Questions 59–65

59. **A** The order of elution is dependent upon the velocity of the analyte. Usually the lower the boiling point of the compound, the greater its velocity or solubility in carrier gas.

60. **D** All of the compounds mentioned have nonpolar properties. Because most HPLC is reverse phase (a polar solvent is used), hexane and nonane are too nonpolar. Acetonitrile is more polar and less toxic than chloroform and along with methanol is a common polarity modifier for HPLC.

61. **C** R_f is the distance migrated by the solute divided by the distance migrated by the solvent. The t_R refers to the retention time of the solute in HPLC or gas chromatography (GC). The K_d is the partition coefficient, and is a measure of the relative affinity of solutes for the stationary phase. The solute with the greater K_d will be retained longer. The pK is the negative logarithm of K, the ionization constant, and is a measure of ionization.

62. **B** Alkaline drugs such as cocaine, amphetamine, and morphine are extracted at alkaline pH. Ideally, the pH of the extracting solution should be 2 pH units greater than the negative log of dissociation constant (pK_a) of the drug. More than 90% of the drug will be un-ionized and will extract in ethyl acetate or another organic solvent.

63. **A** Internal standards should have the same affinity as the analyte for the extraction reagents. Dividing peak height (or area) of all samples (standards and unknowns) by the peak height (or area) of the internal standard reduces error caused by variation in extraction recovery and injection volume.

64. **C** GC-MS determines the mass spectrum of the compounds eluting from the analytic column. Each substance has a unique and characteristic spectrum of mass fragments. This spectrum is compared to spectra in a library of standards to determine the percent match. A match of greater than 95% is considered confirmatory.

65. **C** The half-life of ^{131}I is 8 days, making it too short for application in RIA. The half-life of ^{125}I is 60 days and will give an acceptable dose-reponse curve in RIA for at least 90 days. Tritium and ^{14}C are β emitters and have very long half-lives (12.3 and 5730 years, respectively).

66. The process by which an isotope with a high neuron/proton (N/P) ratio stabilizes is called:
A. α Decay
B. β Decay
C. γ Emission
D. Negatron emission

Chemistry/Apply principles of special procedures/ RIA/1

67. Which functional group of protein antigens is commonly labeled using ^{125}I?
A. Carboxyl groups
B. Terminal amino groups
C. Tyrosine residues
D. Peptide bonds

Chemistry/Apply knowledge of fundamental biological characteristics/Antigen/2

68. The detector utilized in gamma (γ) counters is a solid crystal composed of:
A. Sodium iodide activated with thallium
B. Selenium
C. Gallium
D. Magnesium chloride and silicon

Chemistry/Apply principles of special procedures/ Instrumentation/1

69. Scintillation counters discriminate between different isotopes by using a:
A. Frequency counter
B. Pulse height analyzer
C. Photomultiplier tube
D. Polarizer

Chemistry/Apply principles of special procedures/ Instrumentation/1

70. Which of the following eliminates counting errors caused by high gain in liquid scintillation counters?
A. Internal standard
B. Dual isotope labeling
C. Primary and secondary scintillators
D. Matched photomultiplier tubes

Chemistry/Apply knowledge to identify sources of error/RIA/2

71. Which of the statements below regarding radioisotopes is true?
A. Half-life is directly related to mass.
B. Solid crystal counters are needed for β emitters.
C. Radiation is measured in mass units.
D. Lead shields are required around detectors to reduce background counts.

Chemistry/Apply knowledge of fundamental biological characteristics/RIA/2

Answers to Questions 66–71

66. **B** β Decay results in conversion of a neutron to a proton by emission of a β particle. For example, ^{14}C loses a β particle and becomes ^{14}N. The mass number does not change, but the atomic number is increased from 6 to 7.

67. **C** The ^{125}I tags tyrosine residues by halogenating the phenolic ring, forming iodotyrosine. The reaction is catalyzed by chloramine T. Free ^{125}I is removed by reduction to iodide followed by anion exchange chromatography.

68. **A** When a γ ray enters the sodium iodide crystal, it transfers some of its energy to an outer shell electron. The electron is ejected and strikes other atoms, which are in turn excited. When excited atoms return to the ground state, they release energy. When light at a wavelength of 400–500 nm is emitted, it causes a voltage pulse from the photomultiplier tube.

69. **B** Each isotope emits radiation of a characteristic energy measured in electron volts. This energy determines the amount of light energy emitted by the crystal, and thus the amplitude of the voltage pulse. The pulse height analyzer consists of upper and lower thresholds. Only voltage pulses of an amplitude between these limits are counted.

70. **D** Spontaneous firing of the photomultiplier tubes (PMTs) may occur leading to falsely high counts. This is especially true in liquid scintillation counters that use PMTs with dynodes at high positive voltages to increase sensitivity. Error is eliminated by use of two matched PMTs that must pulse simultaneously in order to generate a count.

71. **D** Half-life, not mass, is a measure of the quantity of radioactivity. The ratio of half-life to mass is called *specific activity*. This should be high to reduce the mass of tracer required for RIA. β particles cannot penetrate the enclosure around a solid crystal counter and must be measured by dissolving the tracer in a scintillation cocktail. γ Radiation penetrates matter easily, and detectors must be shielded to prevent interference from radiation sources such as radioactive reagents.

72. When working with radioisotopes, one safety requirement not applicable to general laboratory areas is:
A. All tests are performed under a fume hood.
B. All measuring is done using disposable labware.
C. A record is kept of the radioactivity of all discarded reagents.
D. Special radiation proof gowns must be worn.

Chemistry/Apply principles of basic laboratory procedures/Laboratory safety/1

Answer to Question 72

72. **C** The same general safety practices of other areas of the clinical laboratory; for example, universal precautions, proper barrier protection, no mouth pipeting, no eating or drinking, are applied to the RIA laboratory. Fume hoods are needed only if working with volatile materials, and no special radiation shielding of personnel is required when working with radioisotopes used in routine *in vitro* clinical diagnostic testing. Additional precautions include wearing of radiation exposure badges, performing tests only in designated areas, labeling all radioactive materials, storage only in approved areas, disposal in approved sinks and waste containers, measuring any spills for radioactivity before and following decontamination, and keeping a log of all radioactivity received and discarded.

Blood Gases, pH, and Electrolytes

1. Which of the following represents the Henderson-Hasselbalch equation as applied to blood pH?
   A. $pH = 6.1 + \log HCO_3^-/P_{CO_2}$
   B. $pH = 6.1 + \log HCO_3^-/(0.03 \times P_{CO_2})$
   C. $pH = 6.1 + \log dCO_2/HCO_3^-$
   D. $pH = 6.1 + \log (0.03 \times P_{CO_2})/HCO_3^-$

   Chemistry/Calculate/Acid-base/1

2. What is the P_{O_2} of calibration gas containing 20.0% O_2, when the barometric pressure is 30 in.?
   A. 60 mm Hg
   B. 86 mm Hg
   C. 143 mm Hg
   D. 152 mm Hg

   Chemistry/Calculate/Blood gas/2

3. What is the blood pH when the partial pressure of carbon dioxide (P_{CO_2}) is 60 mm Hg and the bicarbonate is 18 mmol/L?
   A. 6.89
   B. 7.00
   C. 7.10
   D. 7.30

   Chemistry/Calculate/Acid-base/2

4. Which of the following best represents the reference (normal) range for arterial pH?
   A. 7.35–7.45
   B. 7.42–7.52
   C. 7.38–7.68
   D. 6.85–7.56

   Chemistry/Apply knowledge of fundamental biological characteristics/Acid-base/1

5. What is the normal ratio of bicarbonate to dissolved carbon dioxide (HCO_3:dCO_2) in arterial blood?
   A. 1:10
   B. 10:1
   C. 20:1
   D. 30:1

Chemistry/Apply knowledge of fundamental biological characteristics/Acid-base/1

Answers to Questions 1–5

1. **B** The Henderson-Hasselbalch equation describes the pH of a buffer made up of a weak acid and its salt. $pH = pK_a + \log$ salt/acid, where pK_a is the negative logarithm of the dissociation constant of the acid.

2. **C** Convert barometric pressure in inches to mm Hg by multiplying by 25.4 (mm/in.). Next, subtract the vapor pressure of H_2O at 37°C, 47 mm Hg, to give dry gas pressure. Multiply dry gas pressure by the %O_2:

   25.4 mm/in. $\times$ 30 in. = 762 mm Hg
   762 mm Hg − 47 mm Hg (vapor pressure) = 715 mm Hg (dry gas pressure)
   0.20 $\times$ 715 mm Hg = 143 mm Hg P_{O_2}

3. **C** Solve using the Henderson-Hasselbalch equation. $pH = pK' + \log HCO_3^-/(0.03 \times P_{CO_2})$, where pK', the negative logarithm of the combined hydration and dissociation constants for dissolved CO_2 and carbonic acid, is 6.1 and 0.03 is the solubility coefficient for CO_2 gas.

   $pH = 6.1 + \log 18/(0.03 \times 60) = 6.1 + \log 18/1.8$
   $pH = 6.1 + \log 10$. Because $\log 10 = 1$, $pH = 7.10$

4. **A** The reference range for arterial blood pH is 7.35–7.45 and is only 0.03 pH units lower for venous blood owing to the buffering effects of hemoglobin (Hgb) known as the chloride-isohydric shift. Most laboratories consider less than 7.20 and greater than 7.60, the critical values for pH.

5. **C** When the ratio of HCO_3:dCO_2 is 20:1, the log of salt/acid becomes 1.3. Substituting this in the Henderson-Hasselbalch equation and solving for pH gives $pH = 6.1 + \log 20$; $pH = 6.1 + 1.3 = 7.4$. Acidosis results when this ratio is decreased, and alkalosis when it is increased.

6. What is the P_{CO_2} if the dCO_2 is 1.8 mmol/L?
   A. 24 mm Hg
   B. 35 mm Hg
   C. 60 mm Hg
   D. 72 mm Hg

   Chemistry/Calculate/Blood gas/2

7. In the Henderson-Hasselbalch expression pH = 6.1 + log HCO_3^-/dCO_2 the 6.1 represents:
   A. The combined hydration and dissociation constants for CO_2 in blood at 37°C
   B. The solubility constant for CO_2 gas
   C. The dissociation constant of H_2O
   D. The ionization constant of sodium bicarbonate ($NaHCO_3$)

   Chemistry/Apply knowledge of fundamental biological characteristics/Acid-base/1

8. Which of the following contributes the most to the serum total CO_2
   A. P_{CO_2}
   B. dCO_2
   C. HCO_3^-
   D. Carbonium ion

   Chemistry/Apply knowledge of fundamental biological characteristics/Acid-base/2

9. What other measurement in addition to bicarbonate is needed to calculate buffer base?
   A. Hgb concentration
   B. Dissolved O_2 concentration
   C. Inorganic phosphorus (P_i)
   D. All of the above

   Chemistry/Apply knowledge of fundamental biological characteristics/Acid-base/2

10. Which of the following effects results from exposure of a normal arterial blood sample to room air?
   A. P_{O_2} increased P_{CO_2} decreased   pH increased
   B. P_{O_2} decreased P_{CO_2} increased   pH decreased
   C. P_{O_2} increased P_{CO_2} decreased   pH decreased
   D. P_{O_2} decreased P_{CO_2} decreased   pH decreased

   Chemistry/Evaluate laboratory data to recognize problems/Blood gas/3

11. Which of the following formulas for O_2 content is correct?
   A. O_2 Content = %O_2 saturation/100 × Hgb g/dL × 1.34 mL/g + (0.003 × P_{O_2})
   B. O_2 Content = P_{O_2} × 0.0306 mmol/L/mm
   C. O_2 Content = O_2 saturation × Hgb g/dL × 0.003 mL/g
   D. O_2 Content = O_2 capacity × 0.003 mL/g

   Chemistry/Calculate/Blood gas/1

12. The normal difference between alveolar and arterial P_{O_2} ($PA_{O_2}-Pa_{O_2}$ difference) is:
   A. 3 mm Hg
   B. 10 mm Hg

C. 40 mm Hg
D. 50 mm Hg

Chemistry/Apply knowledge of fundamental biological characteristics/Blood gas/2

Answers to Questions 6–12

6. **C** Dissolved CO_2 is calculated from the measured P_{CO_2} × 0.0306, the solubility coefficient for CO_2 gas in blood at 37°C.

   $$dCO_2 = P_{CO_2} \times 0.03$$
   $$\text{Therefore, } P_{CO_2} = dCO_2/0.03$$
   $$P_{CO_2} = 1.8 \text{ mmol/L} \div 0.03 = 60 \text{ mm Hg}$$

7. **A** The equilibrium constant, K_h, for the hydration of CO_2 ($dCO_2 + H_2O \rightarrow H_2CO_3$) is only about $2.3 \times 10^{-3}M$, making dCO_2 far more prevalent than carbonic acid. The dissociation constant, K_d, for the reaction $H_2CO_3 \rightarrow H^+ + HCO_3^-$ is about $2 \times 10^{-4}M$. The product of these constants is the combined equilibrium constant, K'. The negative logarithm of K' is the pK', which is 6.103 in blood at 37°C.

8. **C** The total CO_2 is the sum of the dCO_2, H_2CO_3 (carbonic acid or hydrated CO_2), and bicarbonate (as mainly $NaHCO_3$). When serum is used to measure total CO_2, the dCO_2 is insignificant because all the CO_2 gas has escaped into the air. Therefore, serum total CO_2 is equivalent to the bicarbonate concentration.

9. **A** Buffer base refers to all forms of base that will titrate hydrogen ions. The major blood buffers contributing to buffer base (in order of concentration) are bicarbonate, Hgb, protein, and phosphate.

10. **A** The P_{O_2} of air at sea level (21% O_2) is about 150 mm Hg. The P_{CO_2} of air is only about 0.3 mm Hg. Consequently, blood releases CO_2 gas and gains O_2 when exposed to air. Loss of CO_2 shifts the equilibrium of the bicarbonate buffer system to the right, decreasing hydrogen ion concentration and blood becomes more alkaline.

11. **A** Oxygen content is the sum of O_2 bound to Hgb and O_2 dissolved in the plasma. It is dependent upon the Hgb concentration and the percentage of Hgb bound to O_2 (O_2 saturation). Each gram of Hgb binds 1.34 mL of O_2. The dissolved O_2 is determined from the solubility coefficient of O_2 (0.003 mL/mm Hg) and the P_{O_2}. O_2 Content = % Sat/100 × Hgb in g/dL × 1.34 + (0.003 × P_{O_2}).

12. **B** The $PA_{O_2}-Pa_{O_2}$ difference results from the low ratio of ventilation to perfusion in the base of the lungs. This blood has a low O_2 saturation, causing it to take up O_2 from blood leaving other well-ventilated areas of the lung.

13. A decreased $PAO_2 - PaO_2$ difference is found in:
  A. A/V (arteriovenous) shunting
  B. V/Q (ventilation/perfusion) inequality
  C. Ventilation defects
  D. All of the above

Chemistry/Evaluate laboratory data to recognize health and disease states/Blood gas/2

14. Bichromatic measurement of oxyhemoglobin concentration is performed at:
  A. 577/548 nm
  B. 450/410 nm
  C. 340/380 nm
  D. 400/600 nm

Chemistry/Apply principles of special procedures/Hemoglobin/1

15. Correction of pH for a patient with a body temperature of 38°C would require:
  A. Subtraction of 0.015
  B. Subtraction of 0.01%
  C. Addition of 0.020
  D. Subtraction of 0.020

Chemistry/Calculate/Acid-base/2

16. Select the anticoagulant of choice for blood gas studies.
  A. Sodium citrate 3.2%
  B. Lithium heparin 100 U/mL blood
  C. Sodium citrate 3.8%
  D. Ammonium oxalate 5.0%

Chemistry/Apply knowledge of standard operating procedures/Specimen collection and handling/1

17. A patient's blood gas results are as follows:

pH = 7.26; dCO_2 = 2.0 mmol/L; HCO_3^- = 29 mmol/L

These results would be classified as:
  A. Metabolic acidosis
  B. Metabolic alkalosis
  C. Respiratory acidosis
  D. Respiratory alkalosis

Chemistry/Evaluate laboratory data to recognize health and disease states/Acid-base/3

18. A patient's blood gas results are:

pH = 7.50; PCO_2 = 55 mm Hg; HCO_3^- = 40 mmol/L

These results indicate:
  A. Respiratory acidosis
  B. Metabolic alkalosis
  C. Respiratory alkalosis
  D. Metabolic acidosis

Chemistry/Evaluate laboratory data to recognize health and disease states/Acid-base/3

19. Which set of results is consistent with uncompensated metabolic acidosis?

A. pH 7.34	HCO_3 18 mmol/L	PCO_2 32 mm Hg
B. pH 7.25	HCO_3 15 mmol/L	PCO_2 35 mm Hg
C. pH 7.30	HCO_3 16 mmol/L	PCO_2 28 mm Hg
D. pH 7.45	HCO_3 22 mmol/L	PCO_2 40 mm Hg

Chemistry/Evaluate laboratory data to recognize health and disease states/Acid-base/3

Answers to Questions 13–19

13. **C** Patients with A/V shunts, V/Q inequalities, and cardiac failure will have an increased $PAO_2 - PaO_2$ difference. However, patients with ventilation problems have low alveolar PO_2 owing to retention of CO_2. This reduces the $PAO_2 - PaO_2$ difference.

14. **A** Oxyhemoglobin is measured as an absorbance ratio, where the numerator represents a wavelength of high absorbance for oxyhemoglobin and the denominator an isobestic wavelength (all Hgb pigments have the same absorbtivity coefficient). The absorbance ratio increases linearly with increasing oxyhemoglobin concentration.

15. **A** The pH decreases by 0.015 for each degree Celsius above the 37°C. Because the blood gas analyzer measures pH at 37°C, the *in vivo* pH would be 0.015 pH units below the measured pH.

16. **B** Heparin is the only anticoagulant that does not alter the pH of blood; heparin salts must be used for pH and blood gases. Solutions of heparin are air-equilibrated and must be used sparingly to prevent contamination of the sample by gas in the solution.

17. **C** Imbalances are classified as respiratory when the primary disturbance is with PCO_2 because PCO_2 is regulated by ventilation. PCO_2 = dCO_2/0.03 or 60 mm Hg (normal 35–45 mm Hg). Increased dCO_2 will increase hydrogen ion concentration, causing acidosis. Bicarbonate is moderately increased, but a primary increase in $NaHCO_3$ causes alkalosis. Thus, the cause of this acidosis is CO_2 retention (respiratory acidosis), and it is partially compensated by renal retention of bicarbonate.

18. **B** A pH above 7.45 corresponds with alkalosis. Both bicarbonate and PCO_2 are elevated. Bicarbonate is the conjugate base and is under metabolic (renal) control, while PCO_2 is an acid and is under respiratory control. Increased bicarbonate (but not increased CO_2) results in alkalosis; therefore, the classification is metabolic alkalosis, partially compensated by increased PCO_2.

19. **B** Metabolic acidosis is caused by bicarbonate deficit. If uncompensated, the respiratory system is not excreting CO_2 at an increased rate; pH and bicarbonate are low, but PCO_2 is normal.

20. Which of the following will shift the O_2 dissociation curve to the left?
A. Anemia
B. Hyperthermia
C. Hypercapnia
D. Alkalosis

Chemistry/Calculate clinical and laboratory data/ Blood gas/2

21. Which would be consistent with partially compensated respiratory acidosis?
A. pH increased PCO_2 increased Bicarbonate increased
B. pH increased PCO_2 decreased Bicarbonate decreased
C. pH decreased PCO_2 decreased Bicarbonate decreased
D. pH decreased PCO_2 increased Bicarbonate increased

Chemistry/Evaluate laboratory data to recognize health and disease states/3

22. Which condition results in metabolic acidosis with severe hypokalemia and chronic alkaline urine?
A. Diabetic ketoacidosis
B. Phenformin-induced acidosis
C. Renal tubular acidosis
D. Acidosis caused by starvation

Chemistry/Correlate clinical and laboratory data/ Acid-base and Electrolytes/2

23. Which of the following mechanisms is responsible for metabolic acidosis?
A. Bicarbonate deficiency
B. Excessive retention of dissolved CO_2
C. Accumulation of volatile acids
D. Hyperaldosteronism

Chemistry/Apply knowledge of fundamental biological characteristics/Acid-base/1

24. Which of the following disorders is associated with lactate acidosis?
A. Diarrhea
B. Renal tubular acidosis
C. Hypoaldosteronism
D. Alcoholism

Chemistry/Correlate clinical and laboratory data/ Acid-base/2

25. Which of the following is the primary mechanism of compensation for metabolic acidosis?
A. Hyperventilation
B. Release of epinephrine
C. Aldosterone release
D. Bicarbonate excretion

Chemistry/Apply knowledge of fundamental biological characteristics/Acid-base/2

Answers to Questions 20–25

20. D A left shift in the oxyhemoglobin dissociation curve signifies an increase in the affinity of Hgb for O_2. This occurs in alkalosis, hypothermia, and in those hemoglobinopathies such as Hgb Chesapeake that increase the binding of O_2 to heme. A right shift in the oxyhemoglobin dissociation curve lowers the affinity of Hgb for O_2. This occurs in anemia due to increased 2,3-diphosphoglycerate (2,3-DPG), with increased body temperature, increased hydrogen ion concentration, hypercapnia (increased PCO_2), and in some hemoglobinopathies, such as Hgb Kansas.

21. D Acidosis = low pH; respiratory = disturbance of PCO_2; a low pH is caused by increased PCO_2. In partially compensated respiratory acidosis, the metabolic component of the buffer system, bicarbonate, is retained. This helps to compensate for retention of PCO_2 by titrating hydrogen ions. The compensatory component always moves in the same direction as the cause of the acid-base disturbance.

22. C Metabolic acidosis can be caused by any condition which lowers bicarbonate. In nonrenal causes the kidneys will attempt to compensate by increased acid excretion. However, in renal tubular acidosis (RTA), an intrinsic defect in the tubules prevents bicarbonate reabsorption. This causes alkaline instead of acidic urine. Excretion of bicarbonate as potassium bicarbonate ($KHCO_3$) results in severe hypokalemia.

23. A Metabolic acidosis is caused by bicarbonate deficiency and metabolic alkalosis by bicarbonate excess. Respiratory acidosis is caused by PCO_2 retention (defective ventilation), and respiratory alkalosis is caused by PCO_2 loss (hyperventilation). Important causes of metabolic acidosis include renal failure, diabetic ketoacidosis, lactate acidosis, and diarrhea.

24. D Lactate acidosis often results from hypoxia, which causes a deficit of nicotinamide adenine dinucleotide, the oxidized form (NAD^+). This promotes the reduction of pyruvate to lactate regenerating NAD^+ needed for glycolysis. In alcoholic acidosis, oxidation of ethanol to acetaldehyde consumes the NAD^+. In diabetes, lactate acidosis can result from depletion of Krebs cycle intermediates. Diarrhea and renal tubular acidosis result in metabolic acidosis via bicarbonate loss. Hypoaldosteronism causes metabolic acidosis via hydrogen and potassium ion retention.

25. A In metabolic acidosis the respiratory center is stimulated by chemoreceptors in the carotid sinus causing hyperventilation. This results in increased release of CO_2. Respiratory compensation begins almost immediately unless blocked by pulmonary disease or respiratory therapy. Hyperventilation can bring the PCO_2 down to approximately 10–15 mm Hg.

26. The conditions below are all causes of alkalosis. Which condition is associated with *respiratory* (rather than metabolic) alkalosis?
A. Anxiety
B. Hypovolemia
C. Hyperaldosteronism
D. Hypoparathyroidism

Chemistry/Correlate clinical and laboratory data/ Acid-base/2

27. Which of the following conditions is associated with both metabolic and respiratory alkalosis?
A. Hyperchloremia
B. Hypernatremia
C. Hyperphosphatemia
D. Hypokalemia

Chemistry/Correlate clinical and laboratory data/ Acid-base/2

28. In uncompensated metabolic acidosis which of the following will be normal?
A. Plasma bicarbonate
B. PCO_2
C. p50
D. Total CO_2

Chemistry/Correlate clinical and laboratory data/Acid-base/2

29. Which of the following conditions is classified as normochloremic acidosis?
A. Diabetic ketoacidosis
B. Chronic pulmonary obstruction
C. Uremic acidosis
D. Diarrhea

Chemistry/Correlate clinical and laboratory data/ Acid-base/2

30. Which PCO_2 value would be seen in maximally compensated metabolic acidosis?
A. 15 mm Hg
B. 30 mm Hg
C. 40 mm Hg
D. 60 mm Hg

Chemistry/Evaluate laboratory data to recognize health and disease states/Blood gas/3

31. Why are three levels used for quality control of pH and blood gases?
A. Systematic errors can be detected earlier than with two controls.
B. Protein coating will first affect controls that differ from the calibration values.
C. Precision for gas measurements differs in the high and low ranges.
D. All of the above.

Chemistry/Select appropriate controls/Acid-base/2

32. A single-point calibration is performed between each blood gas sample in order to:
A. Correct the electrode slope

B. Correct electrode and instrument drift
C. Compensate for temperature variance
D. Prevent contamination by the previous sample

Chemistry/Apply knowledge of standard operating procedures/Blood gas/2

Answers to Questions 26–32

26. **A** Respiratory alkalosis is caused by hyperventilation, which leads to decreased PCO_2. Anxiety and drugs sush as epinephrine that stimulate the respiratory center are common causes of respiratory alkalosis. Excess aldosterone increases net acid excretion by the kidneys. Low parathyroid hormone causes increased bicarbonate reabsorption resulting in alkalosis. Hypovolemia increases the relative concentration of bicarbonate. This is common and is termed dehydrational alkalosis, chloride responsive alkalosis, or alkalosis of sodium deficit.

27. **D** Hypokalemia is both a cause and result of alkalosis. In alkalosis hydrogen ions may move from the cells into the extracellular fluid and potassium into the cells. In hypokalemia caused by overproduction of aldosterone, hydrogen ions are secreted by the renal tubules. This increase in net acid excretion results in metabolic alkalosis.

28. **B** The normal compensatory mechanism for metabolic acidosis is respiratory hyperventilation. In uncompensated cases, the PCO_2 is not reduced, indicating a concomitant problem in respiratory control.

29. **A** Bicarbonate deficit will lead to hyperchloremia unless the bicarbonate is replaced by an unmeasured anion. In diabetic ketoacidosis, acetoacetate and other ketoacids replace bicarbonate. The chloride remains normal or low and there is an increased anion gap.

30. **A** In metabolic acidosis hyperventilation increases the ratio of bicarbonate to dissolved CO_2. The extent of compensation is limited by the rate of both gas diffusion and diaphragm contraction. The lower limit is between 10 and 15 mm Hg PCO_2, which is the maximum compensatory effect.

31. **D** Error detection occurs sooner when more controls are used. Some errors, such as those resulting from temperature error and protein coating of electrodes, are not as pronounced near the calibration point, as in the acidosis and alkalosis range.

32. **B** Calibration using a single standard corrects the instrument for error at the labeled value of the calibrator but does not correct for analytic errors away from the set point. A two-point calibration adjusts the slope response of the electrode, eliminating proportional error caused by poor electrode performance.

33. In which condition would hypochloremia be expected?
A. Respiratory alkalosis
B. Metabolic acidosis
C. Metabolic alkalosis
D. All of the above

Chemistry/Correlate clinical and laboratory data/Blood gas electrolytes/2

34. Given the following serum electrolyte data, determine the anion gap.

Na = 132 mmol/L; Cl = 90 mmol/L; HCO_3^- = 22 mmol/L
A. 12 mmol/L
B. 20 mmol/L
C. 64 mmol/L
D. Cannot be determined from the information provided

Chemistry/Calculate/Electrolytes/2

35. Which of the following conditions will cause an increased anion gap?
A. Diarrhea
B. Hypoaldosteronism
C. Hyperkalemia
D. Renal failure

Chemistry/Correlate clinical and laboratory data/Electrolyte/2

36. Alcoholism, liver failure, and hypoxia induce acidosis by causing:
A. Depletion of cellular NAD^+
B. Increased excretion of bicarbonate
C. Increased retention of PCO_2
D. Loss of carbonic anhydrase

Chemistry/Apply knowledge of fundamental biological characteristics/Acid-base/2

37. Which of the following is the primary mechanism causing respiratory alkalosis?
A. Hyperventilation
B. Deficient alveolar diffusion
C. Deficient pulmonary perfusion
D. Parasympathetic inhibition

Chemistry/Apply knowledge of fundamental biological characteristics/Acid-base/2

38. Excessive administration of oxygen can cause which of the following conditions?
A. Acidosis
B. O_2 saturation of Hgb approaching 100%
C. Optic nerve damage
D. All of the above

Chemistry/Correlate clinical and laboratory data/Blood gas/2

Answers to Questions 33–38

33. **C** Chloride is the major extracellular anion and is retained or lost to preserve electroneutrality. Low chloride will occur in metabolic alkalosis because excess bicarbonate is retained. It also will occur in partially compensated respiratory acidosis because the kidneys compensate by increased retention of bicarbonate.

34. **B** The anion gap is defined as unmeasured anions minus unmeasured cations. It is calculated by subtracting the measured anions (bicarbonate and chloride) from the serum sodium (or sodium plus potassium). A normal anion gap is approximately 8–16 mmol/L.
Anion gap = Na − (HCO_3 + Cl)
Anion gap = 132 − (90 + 22) = 20 mmol/L

35. **D** An increased anion gap occurs when there is production or retention of anions other than bicarbonate or chloride (measured anions). For example, in renal failure retention of phosphates and sulfates (as sodium salts) increases the anion gap. Other common causes of metabolic acidosis with an increased anion gap are diabetic ketoacidosis and lactate acidosis. The anion gap may also be increased in the absence of an acid-base disorder. Common causes include hypocalcemia, drug overdose, and laboratory error when measuring electrolytes.

36. **A** Oxygen debt and liver failure block oxidative phosphorylation preventing nicotinamide adenine dinucleotide, the reduced form (NADH) from being oxidized back to NAD^+. Oxidation of ethanol to acetate results in accumulation of NADH. When NAD^+ is depleted, glycolysis cannot proceed. It is regenerated by reduction of pyruvate to lactate causing lactate acidosis.

37. **A** Hyperventilation via stimulation of the respiratory center (or induced by a respirator) is the mechanism of respiratory alkalosis. Causes include low PO_2, anxiety, fever, and drugs that stimulate the respiratory center. Acute respiratory alkalosis is often uncompensated because renal compensation is not rapid. Uncompensated respiratory alkalosis is characterized by an elevated pH and a low PCO_2 with normal bicarbonate.

38. **D** When O_2 saturation of venous blood is greatly elevated, Hgb cannot release O_2. Oxyhemoglobin cannot bind CO_2 or hydrogen ions and acidosis results. Pure O_2 may cause neurological damage leading to convulsion and blindness especially in infants. It can induce respiratory failure by causing pulmonary hemorrhage, edema, and hyalinization.

39. Which of the following conditions is associated with an increase in ionized calcium (Ca_I) in the blood?
A. Alkalosis
B. Hypoparathyroidism
C. Hyperalbuminemia
D. Malignancy

Chemistry/Correlate clinical and laboratory data/ Electrolytes/2

40. Which of the following laboratory results is consistent with primary hypoparathyroidism?
A. Low calcium; high (P_i)
B. Low calcium; low P_i
C. High calcium; high P_i
D. High calcium; low P_i

Chemistry/Correlate clinical and laboratory data/Electrolytes/2

41. Which of the following conditions is associated with hypophosphatemia?
A. Rickets
B. Multiple myeloma
C. Renal failure
D. Hypervitaminosis D

Chemistry/Correlate laboratory data with physiological processes/Electrolytes/2

42. Which of the following test results is a specific marker for osteoporosis?
A. High urinary calcium
B. High serum P_i
C. Low serum calcium
D. High urinary α-2N-telopeptide

Chemistry/Correlate laboratory data with physiological processes/Electrolytes/2

Answers to Questions 39–42

39. **D** Increased Ca_I occurs in hyperparathyroidism, malignancy, and acidosis. Ca_I is elevated in primary hyperparathyroidism due to resorption of calcium from bone. Many nonparathyroid malignancies create products called parathyroid hormone-related proteins that stimulate the parathyroid receptors of cells. Acidosis alters the equilibrium between bound and free calcium, favoring ionization. Hyperalbuminemia increases the total calcium by increasing the protein-bound fraction, but does not affect the Ca_I.

40. **A** Parathyroid deficiency causes reduced resorption of calcium from bone, increased renal excretion of calcium, and decreased renal excretion of phosphorus. It is distinguished from other causes of hypocalcemia by Ca_I, which is reduced only by primary hypoparathyroidism and alkalosis.

41. **A** Rickets can result from dietary phosphate deficiency, vitamin D deficiency, or an inherited disorder of either vitamin D or phosphorus metabolism. Vitamin D–dependent rickets (VDDR) can be reversed by megadoses of vitamin D. Type I is caused by a deficiency in renal cells of 1-α-hydroxylase, an enzyme which converts 25 hydroxyvitamin D to the active form, 1,25 hydroxyvitamin D. Type II is caused by a deficiency in the vitamin D receptor of bone tissue. Vitamin D–resistant rickets (VDRR) is caused by a deficiency in the renal reabsorption of phosphate. Consequently, affected persons (usually men because it is most commonly X-linked) have a normal serum calcium and a low P_i.

42. **D** Commonly used markers for other bone diseases such as serum or urinary calcium, P_i, alkaline phosphatase (ALP), and vitamin D are neither sensitive nor specific for osteoporosis. Calcium and phosphorus are usually within normal limits. Although estrogen deficiency reduces formation of 1,25 hydroxyvitamin D (1,25 hydroxycholecalciferol) promoting postmenopausal osteoporosis, the 1,25 hydroxy-vitamin D is low in only 30%–35% of cases, and low levels may be caused by other bone disorders. α-2N-telopeptide of type I collagen (Ntx) is a collagen fragment produced during bone resorption and is the most specific marker for osteoporosis.

43. The serum level of which of the following laboratory tests is decreased in both VDDR and VDRR?
A. Vitamin D
B. Calcium
C. P_i
D. Parathyroid hormone

Chemistry/Correlate laboratory data with physiological processes/Electrolytes/2

44. Which of the following is the most accurate measurement of P_i in serum?
A. Rate of unreduced phosphomolybdate formation at 340 nm
B. Measurement of phosphomolybdenum blue at 680 nm
C. Use of aminonaptholsulfonic acid to reduce phosphomolybdate
D. Formation of a complex with malachite green dye

Chemistry/Apply principles of basic laboratory procedures/Biochemical/2

45. What is the percentage of serum calcium that is ionized (Ca_I)?
A. 30%
B. 45%
C. 60%
D. 80%

Chemistry/Apply knowledge of fundamental biological characteristics/Electrolytes/1

46. Which of the following conditions will cause erroneous Ca_I results? Assume that the samples are collected and stored anaerobically, kept at 4°C until measurement, and stored for no longer than 1 hour.
A. Slight hemolysis during venipuncture
B. Assay of whole blood collected in sodium oxalate
C. Analysis of serum in a barrier gel tube stored at 4°C until the clot has formed
D. Analysis of whole blood collected in sodium heparin, 20 U/mL (low heparin tube)

Chemistry/Apply knowledge to recognize sources of error/Specimen collection and handling/3

47. Which of the following conditions is associated with a low serum magnesium?
A. Addison's disease
B. Hemolytic anemia
C. Hyperparathyroidism
D. Pancreatitis

Chemistry/Correlate clinical and laboratory data/Electrolytes/2

Answers to Questions 43–47

43. C Persons with VDDR and VDRR have a low P_i. However, persons with VDDR have a decreased calcium as well. Parathyroid hormone (PTH) is increased in persons with VDDR because calcium is the primary stimulus for PTH release, but not in persons with VDRR. Vitamin D levels vary depending upon the type of rickets and the vitamin D metabolite that is measured. 1,25-Hydroxyvitamin D (calcitriol) is the active form of vitamin D. It is low in type I but high in type II VDDR. It may be either normal or low in VDRR.

44. A The colorimetric method of Fiske and SubbaRow for P_i reacts ammonium molybdate with P_i, forming ammonium phosphomolybdate $(NH_4)_3[PMo_3O_{12}])$. A reducing agent, aminonaptholsulfonic acid (ANS), is added, forming phosphomolybdenum blue. The product is unstable and requires sulfuric acid, making precipitation of protein a potential source of error. These problems are avoided by measuring the rate of formation of unreduced phosphomolybdate at 340 nm.

45. B Calcium exists in serum in three forms: protein-bound, ionized, and complexed (as undissociated salts). Only Ca_I is physiologically active. Protein-bound and Ca_I each account for approximately 45% of total calcium, and the remaining 10% is complexed. The term "free" calcium refers to the sum of complexed and Ca_I.

46. B Unlike P_i, the intracellular calcium level is not significantly different from plasma calcium, and calcium is not greatly affected by diet. Whole blood collected with 5–20 U/mL heparin and stored on ice no longer than 2 hours is the sample of choice for Ca_I. Blood gas syringes prefilled with 100 U/mL heparin should not be used because the high heparin concentration will cause low results. Citrate, oxalate, and ethylenediaminetetraacetic acid (EDTA) must not be used because they chelate calcium. Serum may be used provided that the sample is iced, kept capped while clotting, and assayed within 2 hours (barrier gel tubes may be stored longer).

47. D Low magnesium can be caused by gastrointestinal loss as occurs in diarrhea and pancreatitis (loss of Mg and Ca as soaps). Hyperparathyroidism causes increased release of both calcium and magnesium from bone. Addison's disease (adrenocorticosteroid deficiency) may be associated with increased magnesium accompanying hyperkalemia. Hemolytic anemia causes increased release of magnesium as well as potassium from damaged red blood cells (RBCs).

48. When measuring calcium with a complexometric dye, magnesium is kept from interfering by
A. Using an alkaline pH
B. Adding 8-hydroxyquinoline
C. Measuring at 450 nm
D. Complexing to EDTA

Chemistry/Apply principles of basic laboratory procedures/Biochemical/1

49. Which electrolyte measurement is *least* affected by hemolysis?
A. Potassium
B. Calcium
C. P_i
D. Magnesium

Chemistry/Apply knowledge to recognize sources of error/Specimen collection and handling/2

50. Which of the following conditions is associated with hypokalemia?
A. Addison's disease
B. Hemolytic anemia
C. Digoxin intoxication
D. Alkalosis

Chemistry/Correlate clinical and laboratory data/Electrolytes/2

51. Which electrolyte is *least* likely to be elevated in renal failure?
A. Potassium
B. Magnesium
C. P_i
D. Sodium

Chemistry/Correlate clinical and laboratory data/Electrolytes/2

52. Which of the following is the primary mechanism for vasopressin (ADH) release?
A. Hypovolemia
B. Hyperosmolar plasma
C. Renin release
D. Reduced renal blood flow

Chemistry/Apply knowledge of fundamental biological characteristics/Osmolality/2

53. Which of the following conditions is associated with hypernatremia?
A. Diabetes insipidus
B. Hypoaldosteronism
C. Burns
D. Diarrhea

Chemistry/Correlate clinical and laboratory data/Electrolytes/2

Answers to Questions 48–53

48. **B** Complexometric methods can be used to measure either magnesium or calcium. Interference in calcium assays is prevented by addition of 8-hydroxyquinoline which chelates magnesium. When magnesium is measured, ethyleneglycol bistetraacetic acid (EGTA) or EDTA is used to chelate calcium. Dyes often used for both magnesium and calcium assay are calmagite and methylthymol blue.

49. **B** Potassium, phosphorus, and magnesium are the major intracellular ions, and even slight hemolysis will cause falsely elevated results. Serum samples with visible hemolysis (20 mg/dL free Hgb) should be redrawn.

50 **D** Addison's disease, adrenocortical insufficiency, results in low levels of adrenal corticosteroid hormones, including aldosterone and cortisol. Because these hormones promote reabsorption of sodium and secretion of potassium by the collecting tubules, patients with Addison's disease display hyperkalemia and hyponatremia. Hemolytic anemia and digoxin intoxication cause release of intracellular potassium. Alkalosis causes potassium to move from the extracellular fluid into the cells as hydrogen ions move from the cells into the extracellular fluid to compensate for alkalosis.

51. **D** Reduced glomerular filtration coupled with decreased tubular secretion causes accumulation of potassium, magnesium, and P_i. Poor tubular reabsorption of sodium offsets reduced glomerular filtration. Unfiltered sodium draws both chloride and water causing osmotic equilibration between filtrate, serum, and the tissues. Serum sodium is often normal even when total body sodium is elevated.

52. **B** ADH is released by the posterior pituitary in response to increased plasma osmolality. Normally, this is triggered by release of aldosterone caused by ineffective arterial pressure in the kidney. Aldosterone causes sodium reabsorption, which raises plasma osmolality; release of ADH causes reabsorption of water, which increases blood volume and restores normal osmolality. A deficiency of ADH, diabetes insipidus, results in dehydration and hypernatremia. An excess of ADH, syndrome of inappropriate ADH release (SIADH), results in dilutional hyponatremia. This may be caused by regional hypovolemia, hypothyroidism, central nervous system injury, drugs, and malignancy.

53. **A** Diabetes insipidus results from failure to produce ADH. Because the collecting tubules are impermeable to water in the absence of ADH, severe hypovolemia and dehydration result. Hypovolemia stimulates aldosterone release, causing sodium reabsorption, which worsens the hypernatremia. Burns, hypoaldosteronism, diarrhea, and diuretic therapy are common causes of hyponatremia.

54. Which of the following conditions is more often associated with total body sodium excess than hypernatremia?
A. Renal failure
B. Congestive heart failure
C. Hepatic cirrhosis
D. All of the above

Chemistry/Correlate clinical and laboratory data/Electrolytes/2

55. Which of the following conditions involving electrolytes is described correctly?
A. Pseudohyponatremia occurs only when sodium measurements are performed by flame photometry.
B. Potassium levels are slightly higher in heparinized plasma than in serum.
C. Hypoalbuminemia causes low total calcium but does not affect Ca_I.
D. Hypercalcemia may be induced by low serum magnesium.

Chemistry/Correlate clinical and laboratory data/ Electrolytes/2

56. Which of the following laboratory results is usually associated with cystic fibrosis?
A. Sweat chloride greater than 70 mmol/L
B. Low serum sodium and chloride
C. Deficiency of fecal trypsin
D. All of the above

Chemistry/Evaluate laboratory data to recognize health and disease states/Electrolytes/2

57. When performing a sweat chloride collection, which of the following steps will result in analytical error?
A. Using unweighed gauze soaked in pilocarpine nitrate on the inner surface of the forearm
B. Using unweighed gauze soaked in saline on the outside of the arm
C. Leaving the preweighed gauze on the inside of the arm exposed to air during collection
D. Rinsing the collected sweat from the gauze pad using chloride titrating solution

Chemistry/Apply knowledge to recognize sources of error/Specimen collection and handling/3

58. Which electrolyte level best correlates with plasma osmolality?
A. Sodium
B. Chloride
C. Bicarbonate
D. Calcium

Chemistry/Apply knowledge of fundamental biological characteristics/Electrolytes/2

Answers to Questions 54–58

54. D When water is retained along with sodium, total body sodium excess results rather than hypernatremia. Heart failure causes sodium and water retention by reducing blood flow to the kidneys. Cirrhosis causes obstruction of hepatic lymphatics and portal veins leading to local hypertension and accumulation of ascites fluid.

55. C When serum albumin is low, the equilibrium between bound and Ca_I is shifted, producing increased Ca_I. This inhibits release of PTH by negative feedback until the Ca_I level returns to normal. Potassium is released from platelets and leukocytes during coagulation causing serum levels to be higher than plasma. Pseudohyponatremia is caused by fat displacing plasma water and will occur whenever samples are diluted before measurement because the dilution is affected by the volume of fat in the sample. Only ion-selective electrodes that measure whole blood or undiluted serum are unaffected. Magnesium is needed for release of PTH; therefore, hypocalcemia can be associated with both magnesium deficiency and magnesium excess.

56. D Cystic fibrosis causes obstruction of the exocrine glands including the sweat glands, mucus glands, and pancreas. Newborns with pancreatic involvement may be detected by failure of stool to clear an x-ray emulsion, but this test requires confirmation. More than 98% of affected infants have elevated sweat sodium and chloride levels and low serum levels. A sweat chloride level exceeding 70 mmol/L confirms the clinical diagnosis.

57. C The sweat chloride procedure requires the application of pilocarpine to stimulate sweating, and the use of iontophoresis (application of 0.16-mA current for 5 minutes) to bring the sweat to the surface. The only gauze that needs to be preweighed is the pair of 2-in.^{2} pads that will be applied to the skin after iontophoresis. During the 30-minute collection of sweat, the gauze must be completely covered to prevent contamination and loss of sweat by evaporation. The Gibson-Cooke reference method for sweat chloride uses the Schales and Schales method (titration by $Hg[NO_3]_2$ with diphenylcarbazone indicator) to assay 1.0 mL of sweat eluted from the gauze with 5 mL of water. A Cotlove chloridometer is often used to measure sweat chloride. The sweat is eluted from the gauze with the titrating solution to facilitate measurement.

58. A Sodium and chloride are the major extracellular ions. Chloride passively follows sodium, making sodium the principal determinant of plasma osmolality.

59. Which formula is most accurate in predicting plasma osmolality?
A. Na + 2(Cl) + BUN + glucose
B. 2(Na) + 2(Cl) + glucose + urea
C. 2(Na) + (glucose ÷ 18) + (BUN ÷ 2.8)
D. Na + Cl + K + HCO₃

Chemistry/Calculate/Osmolality/2

60. Which of the following conditions will cause an increased osmolal gap?
A. Diabetic ketoacidosis
B. Drug overdose
C. Renal failure
D. All of the above

Chemistry/Correlate clinical and laboratory data/Osmolality/2

Answers to Questions 59–60

59. **C** Calculated plasma osmolality is based upon measurement of sodium, glucose, and urea. Because sodium associates with a counter ion, two times the sodium estimates the millimoles per liter of sodium and anions. Some laboratories multiply by 1.86 instead of 2 to correct for undissociated salts. Dividing glucose by 18 converts from milligrams per deciliter to millimole per liter. Dividing blood urea nitrogen (BUN) by 2.8 converts from milligram per deciliter BUN to millimole per liter urea.

60. **D** The osmolal gap is the difference between measured and calculated plasma osmolality. An osmolal gap exceeding 12 mOsm/kg is significant, and in emergency room settings is a sensitive indicator of alcohol or drug overdose.

UNIT 3

Glucose, Hemoglobin, Iron, and Bilirubin

1. Which of the biochemical processes below is promoted by insulin?
   A. Glycogenolysis
   B. Gluconeogenesis
   C. Lipolysis
   D. Uptake of glucose by cells

   Chemistry/Apply knowledge of fundamental biological characteristics/Carbohydrate/1

2. Which of the following hormones promotes hyperglycemia?
   A. Cortisol
   B. Growth hormone
   C. Epinephrine
   D. All of the above

   Chemistry/Apply knowledge of fundamental biological characteristics/Carbohydrate/1

3. Which of the following is characteristic of type 1 diabetes mellitus?
   A. Requires an oral glucose tolerance test for diagnosis
   B. Is the most common form of diabetes mellitus
   C. Usually occurs after age 40
   D. Requires insulin replacement to prevent ketosis

   Chemistry/Correlate clinical and laboratory data/Biological manifestation of disease/2

4. Which of the following is characteristic of type 2 diabetes mellitus?
   A. Insulin levels are consistently low.
   B. Most cases require a 3-hour oral glucose tolerance test to diagnose.
   C. Hyperglycemia is often controlled without insulin replacement.
   D. The condition is associated with unexplained weight loss.

Chemistry/Correlate clinical and laboratory data/Biological manifestation of disease/2

Answers to Questions 1–4

1. **D** Insulin reduces blood glucose levels by increasing glucose uptake by cells. It promotes lipid and glycogen production, induces synthesis of glycolytic enzymes, and inhibits formation of glucose from pyruvate and Krebs cycle intermediates.

2. **D** Cortisol and growth hormone promote gluconeogenesis, and epinephrine stimulates glycogenolysis. All three may cause abnormal glucose tolerance.

3. **D** Type 1, or juvenile diabetes, is also termed *insulin-dependent diabetes* because patients must be given insulin to prevent ketosis. Type 1 accounts for only about 10%–20% of cases of diabetes mellitus and is usually diagnosed by a fasting blood glucose (FBG). An FBG of 126 mg/dL or higher on more than one instance is diagnostic. Approximately 95% of patients produce autoantibodies against the β cells of the pancreatic islets. There is genetic association between type 1 diabetes and human leukocyte antigens (HLAs) DR3 and DR4.

4. **C** Type 2, or *late-onset diabetes,* is associated with a defect in the receptor site for insulin. Insulin levels may be low, normal, or high. Patients do not require insulin to prevent ketosis, and hyperglycemia can be controlled in most patients by diet and drugs that promote insulin release. Patients are usually obese and over 40 years of age. Type 2 accounts for 80%–90% of all diabetes mellitus.

5. Which of the following results is confirmatory for diabetes mellitus?
  A. FBG of 120 mg/dL
  B. Two-hour postprandial glucose of 160 mg/dL
  C. Two-hour oral glucose tolerance values of 255 and 205 mg/dL.
  D. Random urine glucose of 250 mg/dL

  Chemistry/Evaluate laboratory data to recognize health and disease states/Carbohydrate/2

6. Select the appropriate reference range for fasting blood glucose.
  A. 40–100 mg/dL   (2.22–5.55 mmol/L)
  B. 60–140 mg/dL   (3.33–7.77 mmol/L)
  C. 65–109 mg/dL   (3.61–6.10 mmol/L)
  D. 75–150 mg/dL   (4.16–8.32 mmol/L)

  Chemistry/Apply knowledge of fundamental biological characteristics/Carbohydrate/1

7. When preparing a patient for an oral glucose tolerance test (OGTT), which of the following conditions will lead to erroneous results?
  A. The patient remains ambulatory for 3 days prior to the test.
  B. Carbohydrate intake is restricted to below 150 g/day for 3 days prior to test.
  C. No food, coffee, tea, or smoking is allowed 8 hours before and during the test.
  D. Seventy-five grams of glucose is administered to an adult patient following a 10- to 12-hour fast.

  Chemistry/Apply knowledge to recognize sources of error/Glucose tolerance test/3

8. Which of the following results at 2 hours would be classified as impaired glucose tolerance?
  A. 105 mg/dL
  B. 130 mg/dL
  C 150 mg/dL
  D. 204 mg/dL

  Chemistry/Evaluate laboratory data to recognize health and disease states/Glucose tolerance/2

9. Which statement regarding gestational diabetes mellitus (GDM) is correct?
  A. Is diagnosed using the same oral glucose tolerance criteria as in nonpregnancy
  B. Converts to diabetes mellitus after pregnancy in 60%–75% of cases
  C. Presents no increased health risk to the fetus
  D. Is defined as glucose intolerance originating during pregnancy

  Chemistry/Evaluate laboratory data to recognize health and disease states/Glucose tolerance test/2

10. Which of the following findings is characteristic of all forms of clinical hypoglycemia?
  A. A fasting blood glucose value below 55 mg/dL
  B. High fasting insulin levels
  C. Neuroglycopenic symptoms at the time of low blood sugar

D. Decreased serum C peptide

Chemistry/Correlate clinical and laboratory data/Carbohydrate/2

Answers to Questions 5–10

5. **C** Urine glucose depends upon renal threshold, kidney function, and hydration status, and is useful only as a screening test for hyperglycemia. Diabetes is indicated by any of the following on more than a single occasion: a random glucose ≥200 mg/dL when overt symptoms are present; an FBG ≥126mg/dL; a glucose ≥200 mg/dL at 2 hours following a 75-g oral dose of glucose.

6. **C** Reference ranges vary slightly depending upon method and specimen type. Enzymatic methods specific for glucose have an upper limit of normal no greater than 109 mg/dL. Although 65 mg/dL is considered the 2.5 percentile, a fasting level below 50 mg/dL is often seen without associated clinical hypoglycemia.

7. **B** Standardized OGTTs require that patients receive at least 150 grams of carbohydrate per day for 3 days prior to the test in order to stabilize the synthesis of inducible glycolytic enzymes. The OGTT is to be used only for cases difficult to diagnose.

8. **C** With the exception of pregnant women, impaired glucose tolerance (IGT) is defined by the American Diabetes Association as a fasting glucose ≥ 110 mg/dL but <126 mg/dL (called impaired fasting glucose [IFG]), or a 2-hour OGTT ≥140 mg/dL but <200 mg/dL at 2 hours.

9. **D** Control of GDM reduces perinatal complications such as respiratory distress syndrome, high birth weight, and neonatal jaundice. Women at risk are screened between 24 and 28 weeks' gestation. A 3-hour OGTT is used to confirm gestational diabetes following a challenge with 100 g glucose. At least two of the following cutoffs must be exceeded: fasting, 105 mg/dL or higher; 1-hour, 190 mg/dL or higher; 2-hour 165 mg/dL or higher; 3-hour, 145 mg/dL or higher. GDM converts to diabetes mellitus within 10 years in 30%–40% of cases.

10. **C** Clinical hypoglycemia can be caused by insulinoma, drugs, or reactive hypoglycemia. Reactive hypoglycemia is characterized by delayed or excessive insulin output after eating and is very rare. Fasting insulin is normal but postprandial levels are increased. High fasting insulin levels (usually >6 μg/L) are seen in insulinoma, and patients with insulinoma almost always display fasting hypoglycemia. C peptide is a subunit of proinsulin that is hydrolyzed when insulin is released. In hypoglycemia, low levels indicate an exogenous insulin source, whereas high levels indicate overproduction of insulin.

11. Which statement regarding glycated (glycosylated) Hgb (G-Hgb) is true?
    A. Has a sugar attached to the C-terminal end of the β chain
    B. Is a highly reversible aminoglycan
    C. Reflects the extent of glucose regulation in the 8- to 12-week interval prior to sampling
    D. All of the above

    Chemistry/Correlate laboratory data with physiological processes/Carbohydrate/2

12. Which statement regarding measurement of G-Hgb is true?
    A. Levels do not need to be done fasting.
    B. Affinity chromatography is more temperature-dependent than cation exchange.
    C. Chromatography is the only technique that is clinically useful.
    D. All methods measure the same G-Hgb fraction.

    Chemistry/Apply knowledge to recognize sources of error/Carbohydrate/2

13. Which of the following is the reference method for measuring serum glucose?
    A. Somogyi-Nelson
    B. Hexokinase
    C. Glucose oxidase
    D. Glucose dehydrogenase

    Chemistry/Select method/Carbohydrate/2

14. Polarographic methods for glucose analysis are based upon which principle of measurement?
    A. Nonenzymatic oxidation of glucose
    B. The rate of O_2 depletion
    C. Chemiluminescence caused by formation of adenosine triphosphate (ATP)
    D. The change in electrical potential as glucose is oxidized

    Chemistry/Apply principles of basic laboratory procedures/Carbohydrate/2

15. Select the enzyme that is most specific for β-D-glucose.
    A. Hexokinase
    B. G-6-PD
    C. Phosphohexisomerase
    D. Glucose oxidase

    Chemistry/Apply knowledge of fundamental biological characteristics/Biochemical/1

Answers to Questions 11–15

11. **C** G-Hgb results from the nonenzymatic attachment of a sugar such as glucose to the N-terminal valine of the β chain. The reaction is nonreversible and is related to the time-averaged blood glucose concentration over the life span of the RBCs. There are three G-Hgb fractions designated A_{1a}, A_{1b}, and A_{1c}. Both total G-Hgb and A_{1c} are used to determine the adequacy of insulin therapy. The time-averaged blood glucose is approximated by the formula (G-Hgb $\times$ 33.3) − 86 mg/dL, and insulin adjustments can be made to bring this level to within reference limits. Also, glycated protein assay (called fructosamine) provides similar data for the period between 2 and 4 weeks before sampling.

12. **A** Because G-Hgb represents the average blood glucose 2–3 months prior to blood collection, the dietary status of the patient on the day of the test has no effect upon the results. G-Hgb can be assayed using cation exchange chromatography, weak affinity chromatography, ion-capture immunoassay, or electrophoresis. The affinity method has replaced cation exchange because the latter is subject to more temperature variation and interference from abnormal Hgbs. The affinity method uses boronyl groups, which form a diol bond with the G-Hgbs. The nonglycohemoglobins are washed from the column, and the total G-Hgb is eluted with sorbitol.

13. **B** The hexokinase method is considered more accurate than glucose oxidase methods because the coupling reaction using glucose-6-phosphate dehydrogenase (G-6-PD) is highly specific. The hexokinase method may be done on serum or plasma collected using heparin, EDTA, fluoride, oxalate, or citrate. The method can also be used for urine, cerebrospinal fluid, and serous fluids.

14. **B** Polarographic glucose analyzers measure the rate of oxygen consumption as glucose is oxidized. Glucose oxidase catalyzes the oxidation of glucose by O_2 under first-order conditions, forming hydrogen peroxide (H_2O_2), which must not breakdown reforming O_2. This is prevented by adding molybdate and iodide. Molybdate catalyzes the oxidation of iodide to iodine and H_2O by peroxide. In addition, catalase and ethanol may be used. Catalase catalyzes the formation of acetaldehyde and H_2O from peroxide and ethanol.

15. **D** Glucose oxidase is the most specific enzyme reacting with only β-D-glucose. However, the peroxidase coupling reaction used in the glucose oxidase method is subject to positive and negative interference. Therefore, hexokinase is used in the reference method although it will phosphorylate some other hexoses including mannose, fructose, and glucosamine.

16. Select the coupling enzyme used in the hexokinase method for glucose.
A. G-6-PD
B. Peroxidase
C. Glucose dehydrogenase
D. Glucose-6-phosphatase

Chemistry/Apply knowledge of basic laboratory procedures/Carbohydrate/1

17. Which glucose method is subject to falsely low results caused by ascorbate?
A. Hexokinase
B. Glucose dehydrogenase
C. Trinder glucose oxidase
D. Polarography

Chemistry/Apply knowledge to recognize sources of error/Carbohydrate/2

18. Which of the following is a potential source of error in the hexokinase method?
A. Galactosemia
B. Hemolysis
C. Sample collected in fluoride
D. Ascorbic acid

Chemistry/Apply knowledge to recognize sources of error/Carbohydrate/2

19. Which statement about glucose in cerebrospinal fluid (CSF) is correct?
A. Levels below 40 mg/dL occur in septic meningitis, cancer, and multiple sclerosis.
B. CSF glucose is usually 50%–65% of the plasma glucose level.
C. Hyperglycorrhachia is caused by hyperglycemia.
D. All of the above

Chemistry/Correlate laboratory data with physiological processes/Cerebrospinal fluid/2

20. In peroxidase coupled glucose methods, which reagent complexes with the chromogen?
A. Nitroprusside
B. Phenol
C. Tartrate
D. Hydroxide

Chemistry/Apply knowledge of basic laboratory procedures/Carbohydrate/1

21. Which of the following is classified as a mucopolysaccharide storage disease?
A. Pompe's disease
B. Von Gierke disease
C. Hers' disease
D. Hurler's syndrome

Chemistry/Correlate clinical and laboratory data/Carbohydrates/1

22. Identify the enzyme deficiency responsible for type I glycogen storage disease (von Gierke's disease).
A. Glucose-6-phosphatase
B. Glycogen phosphorylase
C. Glycogen synthetase
D. β-Glucosidase

Chemistry/Correlate clinical and laboratory data/Carbohydrates/2

Answers to Questions 16–22

16. **A** The hexokinase reference method uses a protein-free filtrate prepared with barium hydroxide (BaOH) and zinc sulfate ($ZnSO_4$). Hexokinase catalyzes the phosphorylation of glucose in the filtrate using ATP as the phosphate donor. Glucose-6-phosphate (glucose-6-PO_4) is oxidized to 6-phosphogluconate and NAD^+ is reduced to NADH using G-6-PD. The increase in absorbance at 340 nm is proportional to glucose concentration.

17. **C** Although glucose oxidase is specific for β-D-glucose, the coupling (indicator) reaction is prone to negative interference from ascorbate, uric acid, acetoacetic acid, and other reducing agents. These compete with dye (e.g., o-dianisidine) for peroxide, resulting in less dye being oxidized to chromophore.

18. **B** The hexokinase method can be performed on serum or plasma using heparin, EDTA, citrate, or oxalate. RBCs contain glucose-6-PO_4 and intracellular enzymes that generate NADH, causing positive interference. Therefore, hemolyzed samples require a serum blank correction (subtraction of the reaction rate with hexokinase omitted from the reagent).

19. **D** High glucose in CSF is a reflection of hyperglycemia and not central nervous system disease. Low levels are significant and are most often associated with bacterial or fungal meningitis, malignancy in the central nervous system, and some cases of subarachnoid hemorrhage, rheumatoid meningitis, and multiple sclerosis.

20. **B** The coupling step in the Trinder glucose oxidase method uses peroxidase to catalyze the oxidation of a dye by H_2O_2. Dyes such as 4-aminophenozone or 4-aminoantipyrine are coupled to phenol to form a quinoneimine dye that is red and is measured at about 500 nm.

21. **D** Hurler's syndrome is an autosomal recessive disease resulting from a deficiency of iduronidase. Glycosaminoglycans (mucopolysaccharides) accumulate in the lysosomes. Multiple organ failure and mental retardation occur, resulting in early mortality. Excess deramtan and heparin sulfate are excreted in urine. Other mucopolysaccharidoses (MPS storage diseases) are Hunter's, Scheie's, Sanfilippo's, and Morquio's syndromes.

22. **A** Type I glycogen storage disease, von Gierke's disease, is an autosomal recessive deficiency of glucose-6-phosphatase. Glycogen accumulates in tissues causing hypoglycemia, ketosis, and fatty liver. Pompe's disease (α-glucosidase deficiency) and Hers' disease (phosphorylase deficiency) are also forms of glycogenosis.

23. Which of the following abnormal laboratory results is found in von Gierke's disease?
A. Hyperglycemia
B. Increased glucose response to epinephrine administration
C. Metabolic alkalosis
D. Hyperlipidemia

Chemistry/Correlate clinical and laboratory data/Carbohydrate/2

24. The D-xylose absorption test is used for the differential diagnosis of which two diseases?
A. Pancreatic insufficiency from malabsorption
B. Primary from secondary disorders of glycogen synthesis
C. Type 1 and type 2 diabetes mellitus
D. Generalized from specific carbohydrate intolerance

Chemistry/Correlate clinical and laboratory data/D-xylose absorption/2

25. Which of the statements below about carbohydrate intolerance is true?
A. Galactosemia results from deficiency of galactose-1-phosphate (galactose-1-PO$_4$) uridyl transferase.
B. Galactosemia results in a positive test for reducing sugars in urine.
C. Lactase deficiency results in diarrhea after milk ingestion.
D. All of the above.

Chemistry/Correlate clinical and laboratory data/Carbohydrate/2

26. Which of the statements below regarding iron metabolism is correct?
A. The dietary requirement for adult men is about 1–2 mg/day.
B. Normally 40%–50% of ingested iron is absorbed.
C. The daily requirement is higher for pregnant and menstruating women.
D. Absorption increases with the amount of iron in the body stores.

Chemistry/Apply knowledge of fundamental biological characteristics/Iron/1

27. Which of the processes below occurs when iron is in the oxidized (Fe^{3+}) state?
A. Absorption by intestinal epithelium
B. Binding to transferrin and incorporation into ferritin
C. Incorporation into protoporphyrin IX to form functional heme
D. Reaction with chromogens in colorimetric assays

Chemistry/Apply knowledge of fundamental biological characteristics/Iron/1

Answers to Questions 23–27

23. **D** Von Gierke's disease (type I glycogen storage disease) results from a deficiency of glucose-6-phosphatase. This blocks the hydrolysis of glucose-6-PO$_4$ to glucose and P$_i$, preventing degradation of glycogen to glucose. The disease is associated with increased triglyceride levels because fats are mobilized for energy and lactate acidosis caused by increased glycolysis. A presumptive diagnosis is made when intravenous galactose administration fails to increase serum glucose, and can be confirmed by demonstrating glucose-6-phosphatase deficiency or decreased glucose production in response to epinephrine.

24. **A** Xylose is a pentose that is absorbed without the help of pancreatic enzymes and is not metabolized. In normal adults more than 25% of the dose is excreted into the urine after 5 hours. Low blood or urine levels are seen in malabsorption syndrome, sprue, Crohn's disease, and other intestinal disorders, but not pancreatitis.

25. **D** Galactose is metabolized to galactose-1-PO$_4$ by the action of galactokinase. Galactose-1-PO$_4$ uridine diphosphate (UDP) transferase converts galactose-1-PO$_4$ to glucose. Deficiency of either enzyme causes elevated blood and urine galactose. Tests for reducing sugars employing copper sulfate are used to screen for galactose, lactose, and fructose in urine. A positive test is followed by TLC to identify the sugar, and demonstration of the enzyme deficiency in RBCs.

26. **C** For adult men and nonmenstruating women approximately 1–2 mg/day of iron is needed to replace the small amount lost mainly by exfoliation of cells. Because 5%–10% of dietary iron is absorbed normally, the daily dietary requirement in this group is 10–20 mg/day. Menstruating women have an additional requirement of 1 mg/day and pregnant women 2 mg/day. Absorption efficiency will increase in iron deficiency and decrease in iron overload. Iron absorption is enhanced by low gastric pH and is increased by alcohol ingestion.

27. **B** Intestinal absorption occurs only if the iron is in the reduced (Fe^{2+}) state. After absorption, Fe^{2+} is oxidized to Fe^{3+} by gut mucosal cells. Transferrin and ferritin bind iron efficiently only when in the oxidized state. Iron within Hgb binds to O$_2$ by coordinate bonding, which occurs only if the iron is in the reduced state. Likewise, in colorimetric methods, Fe^{2+} forms coordinate bonds with carbon and nitrogen atoms of the chromogen.

28. Which of the following is associated with low serum iron and high total iron-binding capacity (TIBC)?
A. Anemia associated with pregnancy
B. Hepatitis
C. Nephrosis
D. Noniron deficiency anemias
Chemistry/Correlate clinical and laboratory data/Iron/2

29. Which condition is associated with the *lowest* percent saturation of transferrin?
A. Hemochromatosis
B. Anemia of chronic infection
C. Iron deficiency anemia
D. Noniron deficiency anemia
Chemistry/Correlate clinical and laboratory data/Iron/2

30. Which condition is most often associated with a high serum iron level?
A. Nephrosis
B. Chronic infection or inflammation
C. Polycythemia vera
D. Noniron deficiency anemias
Chemistry/Correlate clinical and laboratory data/Iron/2

31. Which of the following is likely to occur first in iron deficiency anemia?
A. Decreased serum iron
B. Increased TIBC
C. Decreased serum ferritin
D. Increased transferrin
Chemistry/Correlate clinical and laboratory data/Iron/2

32. Which formula provides the best estimate of serum transferrin?
A. Serum Fe/TIBC
B. TIBC (μg/dL) $\times$ 0.70 = Transferrin in mg/dL
C. Percent iron saturation $\times$ TIBC (μg/dL)/1.2 + 0.06 mg/dL
D. Serum Fe (μg/dL) $\times$ 1.25 = Transferrin (μg/dL)
Chemistry/Calculate/Iron/2

33. Which statement regarding the diagnosis of iron deficiency is correct?
A. Serum iron levels are always higher at night than during the day.
B. Serum iron levels begin to fall before the body stores become depleted.
C. A normal level of serum ferritin rules out iron deficiency.
D. A low serum ferritin is diagnostic of iron deficiency.
Chemistry/Correlate clinical and laboratory data/Iron/2

Answers to Questions 28–33

28. **A** Iron deficiency anemia is the principal cause of low serum iron and high TIBC because it promotes increased transferrin. Pregnancy without iron supplementation depletes maternal iron stores. Iron-supplemented pregnancy and use of contraceptives increase both iron and TIBC. Nephrosis causes low iron and TIBC due to loss of both iron and transferrin by the kidneys. Hepatitis causes increased release of storage iron, resulting in high levels of iron and transferrin. Noniron deficiency anemias may cause high iron and usually show low TIBC and normal or high ferritin.

29. **C** Percent saturation = Serum Fe $\times$ 100/TIBC. Normally, transferrin is one-third saturated with iron. In iron deficiency states, the serum iron falls but transferrin rises. This causes the numerator and denominator to move in opposite directions resulting in very low percent saturation (about 10%). The opposite occurs in hemochromatosis and sideroblastic anemia resulting in an increased percent saturation.

30. **D** Pernicious anemia and sideroblastic anemia produce high serum iron and low TIBC. Anemia associated with chronic infection causes a low serum iron but, unlike iron deficiency, causes a low (or normal) TIBC and does not cause low ferritin.

31. **C** Body stores must be depleted of iron before serum iron falls. Thus, serum ferritin falls in the early stages of iron deficiency, making it a more sensitive test than serum iron in uncomplicated cases. Ferritin levels are low only in iron deficiency. However, concurrent illness such as malignancy, infection, and inflammation may promote ferritin release from the tissues causing the serum ferritin to be normal in iron deficiency.

32. **B** Transferrin is the principal iron transport protein, and TIBC is directly related to serum transferrin concentration. Each mole of transferrin binds two moles of iron. Transferrin, a β-globulin, has a molecular size of about 77,000. The atomic weight of iron is about 55.8. The TIBC in micrograms per deciliter multiplied by 0.7 estimates transferrin concentration in milligrams per deciliter. This formula slightly overestimates transferrin because some of the iron added in the TIBC assay binds to other proteins.

33. **D** Serum iron levels are falsely elevated by hemolysis and subject to diurnal variation. Levels are highest in the morning and lowest at night, but this pattern is reversed in persons who work at night. A low ferritin is specific for iron deficiency. However, only about 1% of ferritin is in the vascular system. Any disease that increases ferritin release may mask iron deficiency.

34. Which statement about iron methods is true?
  A. Interference from Hgb can be corrected by a serum blank.
  B. Colorimetric methods measure binding of Fe^{2+} to a ligand such as ferrozine.
  C. Atomic absorption is the method of choice for measurement of serum iron.
  D. Serum iron can be measured by potentiometry.

Chemistry/Apply principles of special procedures/Iron/2

35. Which of the statements below regarding the TIBC assay is correct?
  A. All TIBC methods require addition of excess iron to saturate transferrin.
  B. All methods require the removal of unbound iron.
  C. Measurement of TIBC is specific for transferrin-bound iron.
  D. The chromogen used must be different from the one used for measuring serum iron.

Chemistry/Apply principles of special procedures/ Iron/2

36. Which of the statements below regarding the metabolism of bilirubin is true?
  A. It is formed by hydrolysis of the α methene bridge of biliverdin.
  B. It is reduced to biliverdin prior to excretion.
  C. It is a product of porphyrin metabolism.
  D. It is produced from the destruction of RBCs.

Chemistry/Apply knowledge of fundamental biological characteristics/Bilirubin/1

37. Bilirubin is transported from reticuloendothelial cells to the liver by:
  A. Albumin
  B. Bilirubin-binding globulin
  C. Haptoglobin
  D. Transferrin

Chemistry/Apply knowledge of fundamental biological characteristics/Bilirubin/1

38. In the liver bilirubin is conjugated by addition of:
  A. Vinyl groups
  B. Methyl groups
  C. Hydroxyl groups
  D. Glucuronyl groups

Chemistry/Apply knowledge of fundamental biological characteristics/Bilirubin/1

39. Which enzyme is responsible for the conjugation of bilirubin?
  A. β-Glucuronidase
  B. UDP-glucuronyl transferase
  C. Bilirubin oxidase
  D. Biliverdin reductase

Chemistry/Apply knowledge of fundamental biological characteristics/Bilirubin/1

Answers to Questions 34–39

34. **B** Atomic absorption is not the method of choice for serum iron because matrix error and variation of iron recovered by extraction cause bias and poor precision. Most methods use HCl to deconjugate Fe^{3+} from transferrin followed by reduction to Fe^{2+}. This reacts with a neutral ligand such as ferrozine, tripyridyltriazine (TPTZ), or bathophenanthroline to give a blue complex. Anodic stripping voltammetry can also be used to measure serum iron. Hemolysis must be avoided because RBCs contain a much higher concentration of iron than does plasma.

35. **A** Some of the iron added to serum for TIBC assay binds to proteins other than transferrin. When excess iron is removed by ion exchange or alumina gel columns, the TIBC can be determined by the same method as used for serum iron. Alternatively, the excess iron can be assayed after removing protein-bound iron by precipitation. In this case, iron added − unbound (excess) iron = unsaturated iron binding capacity (UIBC); UIBC + serum iron = TIBC. To avoid bias in calculating percent iron saturation, the chromogen used for TIBC should be the same as used for serum iron.

36. **D** Metabolism of porphyrins yields uroporphrins and coproporphyrins, not bilirubin. RBC destruction determines the rate of bilirubin production. Reticuloendothelial cells in the spleen digest Hgb and release the iron from heme. The tetrapyrrole ring is opened at the α methene bridge by heme oxygenase, forming biliverdin. Bilirubin is formed by reduction of biliverdin at the γ methene bridge. It is complexed to albumin and transported to the liver.

37. **A** Albumin transports bilirubin, haptoglobin transports free Hgb, and transferrin transports ferric iron. When albumin binding is exceeded, unbound bilirubin, called free bilirubin, increases. This may cross the blood-brain barrier resulting in kernicterus.

38. **D** The esterification of glucuronic acid to the propionyl side chains of the inner pyrrole rings (I and II) makes bilirubin water soluble. Conjugation is required before bilirubin can be excreted via the bile.

39. **B** β-Glucuronidase hydrolyzes glucuronide from bilirubin, hormones, or drugs. It is used prior to organic extraction to deconjugate urinary metabolites (e.g., total cortisol). Biliverdin reductase forms bilirubin from biliverdin (and heme oxygenase forms biliverdin from heme). Bilirubin oxidase is used in an enzymatic bilirubin assay in which bilirubin is oxidized back to biliverdin and the rate of bilirverdin formation is measured at 410 nm. Most conjugated bilirubin is diglucuronide. The liver makes a small amount of monoglucuronide and other glycosides.

40. The term δ-*bilirubin* refers to:
A. Water-soluble bilirubin
B. Free unconjugated bilirubin
C. Bilirubin tightly bound to albumin
D. Direct-reacting bilirubin

Chemistry/Apply knowledge of fundamental biological characteristics/Bilirubin/1

41. Which of the following processes is part of the normal metabolism of bilirubin?
A. Both conjugated and unconjugated bilirubin are excreted into the bile.
B. Methene bridges of bilirubin are reduced by intestinal bacteria forming urobilinogens.
C. Most of the bilirubin delivered into the intestine is reabsorbed.
D. Bilirubin and urobilinogen reabsorbed from the intestine are mainly excreted by the kidneys.

Chemistry/Apply knowledge of fundamental biological characteristics/Bilirubin/1

42. Which of the following is a characteristic of conjugated bilirubin?
A. It is water-soluble.
B. It reacts more slowly than unconjugated bilirubin.
C. It is more stable than unconjugated bilirubin.
D. All of the above.

Chemistry/Apply knowledge of fundamental biological characteristics/Bilirubin/1

43. Which of the following statements regarding urobilinogen is true?
A. It is formed in the intestines by bacterial reduction of bilirubin.
B. It consists of three distinct water-soluble pigments differing by extent of reduction.
C. It is measured by its reaction with *p*-dimethylaminobenzaldehyde.
D. All of the above.

Chemistry/Apply knowledge of fundamental biological characteristics/Bilirubin/1

44. Which statement regarding bilirubin metabolism is true?
A. Bilirubin undergoes rapid photo-oxidation when exposed to daylight.
B. Bilirubin excretion is inhibited by barbiturates.
C. Bilirubin excretion is increased by chlorpromazine.
D. Bilirubin is excreted only as the diglucuronide.

Chemistry/Evaluate laboratory data to recognize problems/Bilirubin/2

45. Which condition is caused by deficient secretion of bilirubin into the bile canaliculi?
A. Gilbert's disease
B. Neonatal hyperbilirubinemia
C. Dubin-Johnson syndrome
D. Crigler-Najjar syndrome

Chemistry/Correlate laboratory data with physiologic processes/Bilirubin/2

Answers to Questions 40–45

40. **C** HPLC separates bilirubin into four fractions: α = unconjugated, β = monoglucuronide, γ = diglucuronide, δ = irreversibly albumin bound. δ Bilirubin is a separate fraction from the unconjugated bilirubin, which is bound loosely to albumin. δ Bilirubin and conjugated bilirubin react with diazo reagent in the direct bilirubin assay.

41. **B** Most of the conjugated bilirubin delivered into the intestine is deconjugated by β-glucuronidase and then reduced by intestinal flora to form three different reduction products collectively called urobilinogens. The majority of bilirubin and urobilinogen in the intestine are not reabsorbed. Most of that which is reabsorbed is re-excreted by the liver. The portal vein delivers blood from the bowel to the sinusoids. Hepatocytes take up about 90% of the returned bile pigments and secrete them again into the bile. This process is termed the *enterohepatic circulation.*

42. **A** Conjugated bilirubin refers to bilirubin mono- and diglucuronides. Conjugated bilirubin reacts almost immediately with the aqueous diazo reagent without need for a nonpolar solvent. Historically, conjugated bilirubin has been used synonymously with direct-reacting bilirubin, although the latter includes the δ-bilirubin fraction when measured by the Jendrassik-Grof method. Conjugated bilirubin is excreted in both bile and urine. It is easily photo-oxidized and has very limited stability. For this reason, bilirubin standards are usually prepared from unconjugated bilirubin stabilized by the addition of alkali and albumin.

43. **D** Urobilinogen is a collective term given to the reduction products of bilirubin formed by the action of enteric bacteria. Urobilinogen excretion is increased in hemolytic anemia and decreased in obstructive jaundice (cholestatic disease).

44. **A** Samples for bilirubin analysis must be protected from direct sunlight. Drugs may have a significant *in vivo* effect on bilirubin levels. Barbiturates lower serum bilirubin by increasing excretion. Other drugs such as chlorpromazine cause cholestasis and increase the serum bilirubin. Although most conjugated bilirubin is in the form of diglucuronide, some monoglucuronide and other glycosides are excreted. In glucuronyl transferase deficiency some bilirubin is excreted as sulfatides.

45. **C** Dubin-Johnson syndrome (type 2 hyperbilirubinemia) is inherited as an autosomal recessive condition producing mild jaundice from accumulation of conjugated bilirubin. Total and direct bilirubin are elevated, but other liver function is normal.

46. In hepatitis the rise in serum conjugated bilirubin can be caused by:
A. Secondary renal insufficiency
B. Failure of the enterohepatic circulation
C. Enzymatic conversion of urobilinogen to bilirubin
D. Extrahepatic conjugation

Chemistry/Correlate laboratory data with physiologic processes/Bilirubin/2

47. Which of the following is a characteristic of obstructive jaundice?
A. The ratio of direct to total bilirubin is greater than 1:2.
B. Conjugated bilirubin is elevated, but unconjugated bilirubin is normal.
C. Urinary urobilinogen is increased.
D. Urinary bilirubin is normal.

Chemistry/Correlate clinical and laboratory data/ Bilirubin/2

48. Which of the following would cause an increase in only the unconjugated bilirubin?
A. Hemolytic anemia
B. Obstructive jaundice
C. Hepatitis
D. Hepatic cirrhosis

Chemistry/Correlate clinical and laboratory data/ Bilirubin/2

49. Which statement below regarding total and direct bilirubin levels is true?
A. Total bilirubin level is a less sensitive and specific marker of liver disease than the direct level.
B. Direct bilirubin exceeds 3.5 mg/dL in most cases of hemolytic anemia.
C. Direct bilirubin is normal in cholestatic liver disease.
D. The ratio of direct to total bilirubin exceeds 0.40 in hemolytic anemia.

Chemistry/Correlate clinical and laboratory data/Bilirubin/2

50. Which statement best characterizes serum bilirubin levels in the first week following delivery?
A. Serum bilirubin 24 hours after delivery should not exceed the upper reference limit for adults.
B. Jaundice is usually first seen 48–72 hours postpartum in neonatal hyperbilirubinemia.
C. Serum bilirubin above 5.0 mg/dL occurring 2–5 days after delivery indicates hemolytic or hepatic disease.
D. Conjugated bilirubin accounts for about 50% of the total bilirubin in neonates.

Chemistry/Correlate clinical and laboratory data/Bilirubin/2

Answers to Questions 46–50

46. **B** Conjugated bilirubin is increased in hepatitis and other causes of hepatic necrosis due to failure to re-excrete conjugated bilirubin reabsorbed from the intestine. Increased direct bilirubin can also be attributed to accompanying intrahepatic obstruction, which blocks the flow of bile.

47. **A** Obstruction prevents conjugated bilirubin from reaching the intestine resulting in decreased production, excretion, and absorption of urobilinogen. Conjugated bilirubin regurgitates into sinusoidal blood and enters the general circulation via the hepatic vein. The level of serum direct bilirubin (conjugated) becomes greater than unconjugated bilirubin.

48. **A** Conjugated bilirubin increases as a result of obstructive processes within the liver or biliary system or from failure of the enterohepatic circulation. Hemolytic anemia (prehepatic jaundice) presents a greater bilirubin load to a normal liver resulting in increased bilirubin excretion. When the rate of bilirubin formation exceeds the rate of excretion, the unconjugated bilirubin rises.

49. **A** Direct bilirubin measurement is a sensitive and specific marker for hepatic and posthepatic jaundice because it is not elevated by hemolytic anemia. In hemolytic anemia, the total bilirubin does not exceed 3.5 mg/dL, and the ratio of direct to total is less than 0.20. Unconjugated bilirubin is the major fraction in necrotic liver disease because microsomal enzymes are lost. Unconjugated bilirubin is elevated along with direct bilirubin in cholestasis because some necrosis takes place and some conjugated bilirubin is hydrolyzed back to unconjugated bilirubin.

50. **B** Bilirubin levels may reach as high as 2–3 mg/dL in the first 24 hours after birth owing to the trauma of delivery, such as resorption of a subdural hematoma. Neonatal hyperbilirubinemia occurs 2–3 days after birth due to increased hemolysis at birth and transient deficiency of the microsomal enzyme, UDP-glucuronyl transferase. Normally, levels rise to about 5–10 mg/dL but may be greater than 15 mg/dL, requiring therapy with UV light to photo-oxidize the bilirubin. Neonatal bilirubin is almost exclusively unconjugated.

51. A neonatal bilirubin assay performed at the nursery by bichromatic direct spectrophotometry is 4.0 mg/dL. Four hours later a second sample assayed for total bilirubin by the Jendrassik-Grof method gives a result of 3.0 mg/dL. Both samples are reported to be hemolyzed. What is the most likely explanation of these results?
   A. Hgb interference in the second assay
   B. δ-Bilirubin contributing to the result of the first assay
   C. Falsely high results from the first assay caused by direct bilirubin
   D. Physiological variation owing to premature hepatic microsomal enzymes

Chemistry/Apply knowledge to recognize sources of error/Bilirubin/3

52. Which reagent is used in the Jendrassik-Grof method to solubilize unconjugated bilirubin?
   A. 50% Methanol
   B. N-butanol
   C. Caffeine
   D. Acetic acid

Chemistry/Apply principles of basic laboratory procedures/Bilirubin/1

53. Which statement about colorimetric bilirubin methods is true?
   A. Direct bilirubin must react with diazo reagent under alkaline conditions.
   B. Most methods are based upon reaction with diazotized sulfanilic acid.
   C. Ascorbic acid can be used to eliminate interference caused by Hgb.
   D. The color of the azobilirubin product is independent of pH.

Chemistry/Apply principles of basic laboratory procedures/Bilirubin/1

54. Which statement below regarding bilirubin is true?
   A. Reserve albumin bilirubin binding can be measured by hematofluorometry.
   B. The albumin-bilirubin complex has a high affinity for a saphadex column.
   C. Albumin-bound bilirubin will cross the blood-brain barrier.
   D. All of the above.

Chemistry/Apply principles of special procedures/Bilirubin/2

55. Which statement below regarding the measurement of bilirubin by the Jendrassik-Grof method is correct?
   A. The same diluent is used for both total and direct assays to minimize differences in reactivity.
   B. Positive interference by Hgb is prevented by addition of HCl after the diazo reaction.
   C. The color of the azobilirubin product is intensified by addition of ascorbic acid.
   D. Fehling's reagent is added after the diazo reaction to form a blue azobilirubin pigment.

Chemistry/Apply principles of basic laboratory procedures/Bilirubin/2

Answers to Questions 51–55

51. **A** The Jendrassik-Grof method is based upon a diazo reaction that may be suppressed by Hgb. Because serum blanking and measurement at 600 nm correct for positive interference from Hgb, the results may be falsely low when significant hemolysis is present. Direct spectrophometric bilirubin methods employing bichromatic optics correct for the presence of Hgb. These are often called "neonatal bilirubin" tests. A commonly used approach is to measure absorbance at 454 nm and 540 nm. The absorbance contributed by Hgb at 540 nm is equal to the absorbance contributed by Hgb at 454 nm. Therefore, the absorbance difference will correct for free Hgb. Neonatal samples contain little or no direct or δ-bilirubin. They also lack carotene pigments that could interfere with the direct spectrophotometric measurement of bilirubin.

52. **C** A polarity modifier is required to make unconjugated bilirubin soluble in diazo reagent. The Malloy-Evelyn method uses 50% methanol to reduce the polarity of the diazo reagent. Caffeine is used in the Jendrassik-Grof method. This method is recommended because it is not falsely elevated by hemolysis and gives quantitative recovery of both conjugated and unconjugated bilirubin.

53. **B** Unconjugated bilirubin is poorly soluble in acid, and therefore, direct bilirubin is assayed using diazotized sulfanilic acid diluted in weak HCl. The direct diazo reaction should be measured after no longer than 3 minutes to prevent reaction of unconjugated bilirubin, or the diazo group can be reduced using ascorbate or hydroxylamine preventing any further reaction.

54. **A** Free bilirubin can be measured by determining the fluorescence of the albumin-bilirubin complex because free and bound bilirubin are in equilibrium. Reserve albumin binding capacity can also be estimated by addition of bilirubin to serum followed by column chromatography. Albumin-bound bilirubin is washed out of the column; then free bilirubin is detected by addition of diazo reagent.

55. **D** The Jendrassik-Grof method uses HCl as the diluent for the measurement of direct bilirubin because unconjugated bilirubin is poorly soluble at low pH. Total bilirubin is measured using an acetate buffer with caffeine added to increase the solubility of the unconjugated bilirubin. After addition of diazotized sulfanilic acid, the diazo group is reduced by ascorbic acid, and Fehling's reagent is added to alkalinize the diluent. At an alkaline pH the product changes from pink to blue shifting the absorbance maximum to 600 nm where Hgb does not contribute significantly to absorbance.

Calculations, Quality Control, and Statistics

1. How many grams of sodium hydroxide (NaOH) are required to prepare 150.0 mL of a 5.0% w/v solution?
   A. 1.5 g
   B. 4.0 g
   C. 7.5 g
   D. 15.0 g

   Clinical chemistry/Calculate/Solutions/2

2. How many milliliters of glacial acetic acid are needed to prepare 2.0 L of 10.0% v/v acetic acid?
   A. 10.0 mL
   B. 20.0 mL
   C. 100.0 mL
   D. 200.0 mL

   Clinical chemistry/Calculate/Solutions/2

3. A biuret reagent requires preparation of a stock solution containing 9.6 g of copper II sulfate ($CuSO_4$) per liter. How many grams of $CuSO_4 \cdot 5H_2O$ are needed to prepare 1.0 L of the stock solution?

   Atomic weights: H = 1.0; Cu = 63.6; O = 16.0; S = 32.1
   A. 5.4 g
   B. 6.1 g
   C. 15.0 g
   D. 17.0 g

   Clinical chemistry/Calculate/Reagent preparation/2

Answers to Questions 1–3

1. **C** A percent solution expressed in w/v (weight/volume) refers to grams of solute per 100.0 mL of solution. To calculate, multiply the percentage (as grams) by the volume needed (mL), then divide by 100.0 (mL).

   $$(5.0 \text{ g} \times 150.0 \text{ mL}) \div 100.0 \text{ mL} = 7.5 \text{ g}$$

   To prepare the solution, weigh 7.5 g of NaOH pellets and add to a 150.0-mL volumetric flask. Add sufficient deionized H_2O to dissolve the NaOH. After the solution cools, add deionized H_2O to the 150.0-mL line on the flask and mix again.

2. **D** The expression percent v/v refers to the volume of one liquid in mL present in 100.0 mL of solution. To calculate, multiply the percentage (as mL) by the volume required (mL), then divide by 100 (mL).

   $$(10.0 \text{ mL} \times 2000.0 \text{ mL}) \div 100.0 \text{ mL} = 200.0 \text{ mL}$$

   To prepare a 10.0% v/v solution of acetic acid, add approximately 1.0 L of deionized H_2O to a 2.0-L volumetric flask. Add 200.0 mL of glacial acetic acid and mix. Then, add sufficient deionized H_2O to bring the meniscus to the 2.0-L line and mix again.

3. **C** Determine the mass of $CuSO_4 \cdot 5H_2O$ containing 9.6 g of anhydrous $CuSO_4$. First, calculate the percentage of $CuSO_4$ in the hydrate, then divide the amount needed (9.6 g) by the percentage.

   $$\% \, CuSO_4 = \text{molecular weight } CuSO_4 \div$$
   $$\text{molecular weight } CuSO_4 \cdot 5H_2O \times 100$$
   $$= (159.7 \div 249.7) \times 100$$
   $$= 63.96\%$$
   $$\text{Grams } CuSO_4 \cdot 5H_2O = 9.6 \text{ g} \div 0.6396$$
   $$= 15.0 \text{ g}$$

   A convenient formula to use is:

   g hydrate = (MW hydrate ÷ MW anhydrous salt) × g anhydrous salt

4. How many milliliters of HNO_3 (purity 68.0%, specific gravity 1.42) is needed to prepare 1.0 L of a 2.0 N solution?

Atomic weights: H = 1.0; N = 14.0; O = 16.0
A. 89.5 mL
B. 126.0 mL
C. 130.5 mL
D. 180.0 mL

Clinical chemistry/Calculate/Reagent preparation/2

5. Convert 10.0 mg/dL calcium (atomic weight = 40.1) to International System of Units (SI).
A. 0.25
B. 0.40
C. 2.5
D. 0.4

Clinical chemistry/Calculate/SI unit conversion/2

6. Convert 2.0 mEq/L magnesium (atomic weight = 24.3) to milligrams per deciliter.
A. 0.8 mg/dL
B. 1.2 mg/dL
C. 2.4 mg/dL
D. 4.9 mg/dL

Clinical chemistry/Calculate/Unit conversion/2

7. How many milliliters of a 2,000.0 mg/dL glucose stock solution is needed to prepare 100.0 mL of a 150.0 mg/dL glucose working standard?
A. 1.5 mL
B. 7.5 mL
C. 15.0 mL
D. 25.0 mL

Clinical chemistry/Calculate/Solutions/2

Answers to Questions 4–7

4. C The molecular weight of HNO_3 is 63.0 g. Because the valance of the acid is 1 (1 mol of hydrogen is produced per mole of acid), the equivalent weight is also 63.0 g. The mass is calculated by multiplying the normality (2.0 N) by the equivalent weight (63.0 g) and volume (1.0 L); therefore, 126.0 g of acid are required. Because the purity is 68.0% and the specific gravity 1.42, the amount of HNO_3 in grams per milliliter is 0.68 × 1.42 g/mL or 0.9656 g/mL. The volume required to give 126.0 g is calculated by dividing the mass needed (grams) by the grams per milliliter.

$$mL\ HNO_3 = 126.0\ g \div 0.9656\ g/mL = 126.0\ g \times 1.0\ mL/0.9656\ g = 130.5\ mL$$

5. C The SI unit is the recommended method of reporting clinical laboratory results. The SI unit for all electrolytes is millimole per liter. To convert from milligrams per deciliter to millimoles per liter, multiply by 10 to convert to milligrams per liter, then divide by the atomic mass expressed in milligrams.

$$10.0\ mg/dL \times 10.0\ dL/1.0\ L = 100.0\ mg/L$$

$$100.0\ mg/L \times 1.0\ mmol/40.1\ mg = 2.5\ mmol/L$$

6. C To convert from milliequivalent per liter to milligrams per deciliter, first calculate the milliequivalent weight (equivalent weight expressed in milligrams), which is the atomic mass divided by the valence. Because magnesium is divalent, each mole has the charge equivalent of 2 mol of hydrogen. Then, multiply the milliequivalent per liter by the milliequivalent weight to convert to milligrams per liter. Next, divide by 10 to convert milligrams per liter to milligrams per deciliter.

$$\text{Milliequivalent weight Mg} = 24.3 \div 2$$
$$= 12.15\ mg/mEq$$
$$2.0\ mEq/L \times 12.15\ mg/mEq = 24.3\ mg/L$$
$$24.3\ mg/L \times 1.0\ L/10.0\ dL = 2.4\ mg/dL$$

7. B To calculate the volume of stock solution needed, divide the concentration of working standard by the concentration of stock standard, then multiply by the volume of working standard that is needed.

$$C_1 \times V_1 = C_2 \times V_2,$$
where C_1 = concentration of stock standard
V_1 = volume of stock standard
C_2 = concentration of working standard
V_2 = volume of working standard
$$2000.0\ mg/dL \times V_1 = 150.0\ mg/dL \times 100.0\ mL$$
$$V_1 = (150.0 \div 2000.0) \times 100.0\ mL$$
$$V_1 = 7.5\ mL$$

8. What is the pH of a buffer containing 40.0 mmol/L $NaHC_2O_4$ and 4.0 mmol/L $H_2C_2O_4$? ($pK_a = 1.25$)
A. 1.35
B. 2.25
C. 5.75
D. 6.12
Clinical chemistry/Calculate/pH/2

9. A solvent needed for HPLC requires a 20.0 mmol/L phosphoric acid buffer, pH 3.50, made by mixing KH_2PO_4 and H_3PO_4. How many grams of KH_2PO_4 is required to make 1.0 L of this buffer?

Formula weights: $KH_2PO_4 = 136.1$; $H_3PO_4 = 98.0$; pK_a $H_3PO_4 = 2.12$
A. 1.96 g
B. 2.61 g
C. 2.72 g
D. 19.2 g
Clinical chemisty/Calculate/Buffer/2

10. A procedure for cholesterol is calibrated with a serum-based cholesterol standard that was determined by the Abell-Kendall method to be 200.0 mg/dL. Assuming the same volume of sample and reagent are used, calculate the cholesterol concentration in the patient's sample from the following results.

Standard Concentration	Absorbance of Reagent Blank	Absorbance of Standard	Absorbance of Patient Serum
200 mg/dL	0.00	0.860	0.740

A. 123 mg/dL
B. 172 mg/dL
C. 232 mg/dL
D. 314 mg/dL
Clinical chemistry/Calculate/Beer's law/2

11. A glycerol kinase method for triglyceride calls for a serum blank in which normal saline is substituted for lipase reagent in order to measure endogenous glycerol. Given the following results, and assuming the same volume of sample and reagent are used for each test, calculate the triglyceride concentration in the patient's sample.
A. 119 mg/dL
B. 131 mg/dL
C. 156 mg/dL
D. 180 mg/dL
Clinical chemistry/Calculate/Beer's law/2

Answers to Questions 8–11

8. B The Henderson-Hasselbalch equation can be used to determine the pH of a buffer containing a weak acid and a salt of the acid.

$$pH = pK_a + \log \frac{salt}{acid}$$
$$= 1.25 + \log \frac{40.0 \text{ mmol/L}}{4.0 \text{ mmol/L}}$$
$$= 1.25 + \log 10$$
$$= 2.25$$

9. B The Henderson-Hasselbalch equation is used to calculate the ratio of salt to acid needed to give a pH of 3.50.

$pH = pK_a + \log(salt/acid)$
$3.50 = 2.12 + \log(KH_2PO_4/H_3PO_4)$
$1.38 = \log(KH_2PO_4/H_3PO_4)$
antilog $1.38 = KH_2PO_4/H_3PO_4$
$KH_2PO_4/H_3PO_4 = 23.99$

Rearranging gives $KH_2PO_4 = 23.99 \times H_3PO_4$. Because the phosphate in the buffer is 20.0 mmol/L, then $H_3PO_4 + KH_2PO_4$ must equal 20. Because $KH_2PO_4 = 23.99 \times H_3PO_4$ then:
$H_3PO_4 + (23.99 \times H_3PO_4) = 20.0$ mmol/L
$24.99 \times H_3PO_4 = 20.0$ mmol/L
$H_3PO_4 = 20.0/24.99 = 0.800$ mol/L
$KH_2PO_4 = 20.0 - 0.800 = 19.2$ mmol/L (0.0192 M)

To determine the grams required multiply the moles of KH_2PO_4 by the formula weight.
0.0192 mol/L $\times 136.1$ g/mol $= 2.613$ g

10. B $C_u = A_u/A_s \times C_s$ where C_u = concentration of unknown, A_u = absorbance of unknown, A_s = absorbance of standard, and C_s = concentration of standard.

$C_u = 0.74/0.86 \times 200$ mg/dL
$= 172$ mg/dL

11. B The serum blank absorbance is subtracted from the result for the patient's serum before applying the ratiometric formula to calculate concentration.
$C_u = [(A_u - A_{SB})/A_s] \times C_s$ where A_{SB}
$=$ absorbance of serum blank
$= (0.750 - 0.100)/0.620 \times 125$ mg/dL
$= 131$ mg/dL

Standard Concentration	Absorbance of Reagent Blank	Absorbance of Standard	Absorbance of Patient Serum	Absorbance of Serum Blank
125 mg/dL	0.000	0.62	0.750	0.100

12. A procedure for aspartate aminotransferase (AST) is performed manually because of a repeating error code for nonlinearity obtained on the laboratory's automated chemistry analyzer; 0.05 mL of serum and 1.0 mL of substrate are used. The reaction rate is measured at 30°C at 340 nm using a 1.0 cM light path, and the delta absorbance (ΔA) per minute is determined to be 0.382. Based upon a molar absorbtivity coefficient for NADH at 340 nm of 6.22×10^3 M^{-1} cM^{-1} L^{-1}, calculate the enzyme activity in international units (IUs) per liter.
   A. 26 IU/L
   B. 326 IU/L
   C. 1228 IU/L
   D. 1290 IU/L

   Clinical chemistry/Calculate/International units/2

13. Which of the following quality control (QC) rules would be broken 1 out of 20 times by chance alone?
   A. 1_{2s}
   B. 2_{2s}
   C. 1_{3s}
   D. 1_{4s}

   Chemistry/Evaluate laboratory data to assess validity/Accuracy of procedures/Quality control/1

14. Which of the following conditions is cause for rejecting an analytical run?
   A. Two consecutive controls greater than 2 *s* above or below the mean
   B. Three consecutive controls greater than 1 *s* above the mean
   C. Four controls steadily increasing in value but less than ±1 *s* from the mean
   D. All of the above

   Chemistry/Select course of action/Quality control/3

15. One of two controls within a run is above + 2 *s* and the other control is below −2 *s* from the mean. What do these results indicate?
   A. Poor precision has led to random error (RE).
   B. A systematic error (SE) is present.
   C. Proportional error is present.
   D. QC material is contaminated.

   Chemistry/Evaluate laboratory data to recognize problems/Quality control/2

16. Two consecutive controls are both beyond −2 *s* from the mean. How frequently would this occur on the basis of chance alone?
   A. 1:100
   B. 5:100
   C. 1:400
   D. 1:1600

   Chemistry/Evaluate laboratory data to assess validity/Accuracy of procedures/Quality control/2

Answers to Questions 12–16

12. **D** An IU is defined as 1 μmol of substrate consumed or product produced per minute. The micromoles of NADH consumed in this reaction are determined by dividing the change in absorbance per minute by the absorbance of 1 μmol of NADH. Because 1 mol/L/cm would have an absorbance of 6.22×10^3 absorbance units, then 1 μmol/mL/cm would produce an absorbance of 6.22. Therefore, dividing the ΔA per minute by 6.22 gives the micromoles of NADH consumed in the reaction. This is multiplied by the dilution of serum to determine the micromoles per milliliter, and multiplied by 1000 to convert to micromoles per liter.

$$IU/L = \frac{\Delta A/min \times TV(mL) \times 1000 \text{ mL/L}}{6.22(A/\mu mol/mL/cM) \times 1 \text{ cm} \times SV(mL)}$$

$$= \frac{\Delta A/min \times 1.05 \times 1000}{6.22 \times 0.05}$$

$$= \Delta A/min \times \frac{1050}{0.311}$$

$$= \Delta A/min \times 3376$$

$$= 0.382 \times 3376 = 1290 \text{ IU/L}$$

13. **A** The notation 1_{2s} means that one control is outside ±2 standard deviation units. QC results follow the bell-shaped curve called the Gaussian (normal) distribution. If a control is assayed 100 times, 68 out of 100 results would fall within +1 and −1 standard deviation (*s*) of the mean. Ninety-five out of 100 results would fall within +2 and −2 *s*. This leaves only 5 out of 100 results (1:20) that fall outside the ±2 *s* limit (99.7 out of 100 results fall within ±3 *s* of the mean).

14. **A** Rejecting a run when three consecutive controls fall between 1 and 2 *s* or when a trend of four increasing or decreasing control results occurs would lead to frequent rejection of valid analytical runs. Appropriate control limits are four consecutive controls above or below 1 *s* (4_{1s}) to detect a significant shift, and a cusum result exceeding the ±2.7 *s* limit to detect a significant trend.

15. **A** When control results deviate from the mean in opposite directions the run is affected by RE, which results from imprecision. An analytical run is rejected when two controls within the same run have an algebraic difference in excess of 4 *s* (R_{4s}).

16. **D** QC results follow a Gaussian or normal distribution. Ninety-five percent of the results fall within ±2 *s* of the mean; therefore, 2.5 out of 100 (1:40) are above +2 *s* and 2.5 out of 100 are below −2 *s*. The probability of two consecutive controls being beyond −2 *s* is the product of their individual probabilities. 1/40 × 1/40 = 1/1600 trials by chance.

17. The term R_4s means that:
  A. Four consecutive controls are greater than ± 1 standard deviation from the mean.
  B. Two consecutive controls in the same run are greater than 4 s units apart.
  C. Two consecutive controls in the same run are each greater than ± 4 s from the mean.
  D. There is a shift above the mean for four consecutive controls.

Chemistry/Evaluate laboratory data to assess validity/Accuracy of procedures/Quality control/2

18. A trend in QC results is most likely caused by:
  A. Deterioration of the reagent
  B. Miscalibration of the instrument
  C. Improper dilution of standards
  D. Electronic noise

Chemistry/Evaluate laboratory data to assess validity/Accuracy of procedures/Quality control/2

19. In most circumstances, when two controls within a run are both greater than ± 2 s from the mean, what action should be taken first?
  A. Recalibrate, then repeat controls followed by randomly selected patient samples if quality control is acceptable.
  B. Repeat the controls before taking any corrective action.
  C. Change the reagent lot, then recalibrate.
  D. Prepare fresh standards and recalibrate.

Chemistry/Evaluate laboratory data to take corrective action according to predetermined criteria/Quality control/3

20. When establishing QC limits, which practice below is *inappropriate?*
  A. Using last month's QC data to determine current target limits
  B. Exclusion of any QC results greater than ± 2 s from the mean
  C. Using control results from all shifts on which the assay is performed
  D. Using limits determined by reference laboratories using the same method

Chemistry/Apply principles of laboratory operations/Quality control/2

21. Which of the following assays has the poorest precision?

	Analyte	Mean (mmol/L)	Standard Deviation
A.	Ca	2.5	0.3
B.	K	4.0	0.4
C.	Na	140	4.0
D.	Cl	100	2.5

Chemistry/Calculate/Coefficient of variation/3

Answers to Questions 17–21

17. **B** The R_4s rule is applied when two consecutive controls have an algebraic difference exceeding 4 s, and only to controls within a run (level 1 − level 2) and not across different runs. The R_{4s} rule is sensitive to RE.

18. **A** A trend occurs when six or more consecutive quality control results either increase or decrease in the same direction; however, this is not cause for rejection until a multirule is broken. Trends are systematic errors (affecting accuracy) linked to an unstable reagent, calibrator, or instrument condition. For example, loss of volatile acid from a reagent causes a steady pH increase, preventing separation of analyte from protein. This results in lower QC results each day.

19. **A** When a 2_{2s} rule is broken an SE is present and corrective action is required (repeating just the QC will not correct the problem). If recalibration yields acceptable QC results, then at least three patient samples randomly chosen from the run must be repeated to determine the likelihood of analytical error in results from the run. Both sets of QC results must be reported and the corrective action documented in the QC log.

20. **B** Data between ± 2 and ± 3 s must be included in calculations of the next month's acceptable range. Elimination of these values would continuously reduce the distribution of QC results, making "out-of-control" situations a frequent occurrence.

21. **A** Although calcium has the lowest s, it represents the assay with poorest precision. Relative precision between different analytes or different levels of the same analyte must be evaluated by the coefficient of variation (CV) because standard deviation is dependent upon the mean. $CV = s \times 100/\text{Mean}$. This normalizes standard deviation to a mean of 100. The CV for calcium in the example is 12.0%.

22. Given the following data, calculate the coefficient of variation for glucose.

Analyte	Mean	Standard Deviation
Glucose	76 mg/dL	2.3

A. 3.0%
B. 4.6%
C. 7.6%
D. 33.0%

Clinical chemistry/Calculate/Statistics/2

23. Which of the following plots is best for detecting all types of QC errors?
A. Levy-Jennings
B. Tonks-Youden
C. Cusum
D. Linear regression

Chemistry/Evaluate laboratory data to recognize problems/Quality control/2

24. Which of the following plots is best for comparison of precision and accuracy among laboratories?
A. Levy-Jennings
B. Tonks-Youden
C. Cusum
D. Linear regression

Chemistry/Evaluate laboratory data to recognize problems/Quality control/2

25. Which plot will give the earliest indication of a trend?
A. Levy-Jennings
B. Tonks-Youden
C. Cusum
D. Histogram

Chemistry/Evaluate laboratory data to recognize problems/Quality control/2

26. All of the following are requirements for a QC material *except:*
A. Long-term stability.
B. The matrix is similar to the specimens being tested.
C. The concentration of analytes reflects the clinical range.
D. Analyte concentration must be independent of the method of assay.

Chemistry/Apply principles of basic laboratory procedures/Quality control/2

Answers to Questions 22–26

22. **A** The coefficient of variation is calculated by dividing the standard deviation by the mean and multiplying by 100.

$$CV = \frac{s}{\bar{x}} \times 100$$

$$= \frac{2.3}{76} \times 100 = 3.0\%$$

The CV is the most appropriate statistic to use when comparing the precision of samples that have different means. For example, when comparing the precision of the level 1 control to the level 2 control the coefficient of variation normalizes the variance to be independent of the mean. The control with the lower CV is the one for which the analysis is more precise.

23. **A** The Levy-Jennings plot is a graph of all QC results with concentration plotted on the y axis and run number on the x axis. The mean is at the center of the y axis, and concentrations corresponding to -2 and $+2$ s are highlighted. Results are evaluated for multirule violations across both levels and runs. Corrective action for shifts and trends can be taken before QC rules are broken.

24. **B** The Tonks-Youden plot is used for interlaboratory comparison of monthly means. The method mean for level 1 is at the center of the y axis and mean for level 2 at the center of the x axis. Lines are drawn from the means of both levels across the graph dividing it into four equal quadrants. If a laboratory's monthly means plot both in the lower left or upper right then SE exists in its method.

25. **C** Cusum points are the algebraic sum of the difference between each QC result and the mean. The y axis is the sum of differences and the x axis is the run number. The center of the y axis is 0. Because QC results follow a random distribution, the points should distribute about the zero line. Results are out of control when the slope exceeds 45° or a decision limit (e.g., ±2.7 s) is exceeded.

26. **D** Quality control materials are stable, made of the same components as the specimen, cover the dynamic linear range of the assay, and can be used for multiple analytes. The target mean for QC samples is determined from replicate assays by the user's method, not the "true" concentration of the analyte. Out-of-control results are linked to analytic performance rather than to the inherent accuracy of the method.

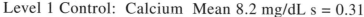

Level 1 Control: Calcium Mean 8.2 mg/dL s = 0.31

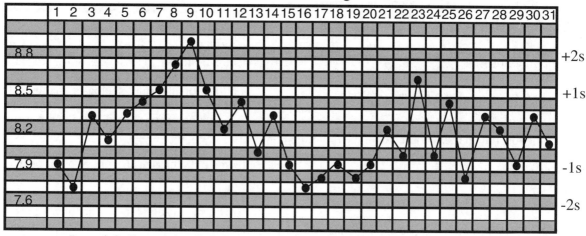

Level 2 Control: Calcium Mean 12.2 mg/dL s = 0.30

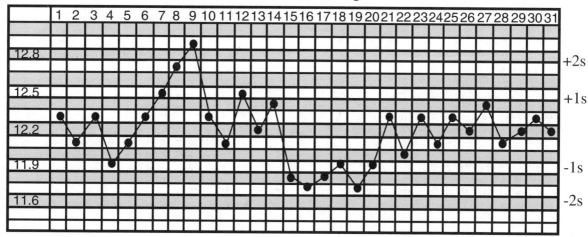

Questions 27–30 refer to the Levy-Jennings chart above.

27. Examine the Levy-Jennings chart and identify the QC problem that occurred during the first half of the month.
A. Shift
B. Trend
C. Random error
D. Kurtosis

Chemistry/Evaluate laboratory data to recognize problems/Quality control/3

28. Referring to the Levy-Jennings chart, what is the first day in the month when the run should be rejected and patient results should be repeated?
A. Day 6
B. Day 7
C. Day 8
D. Day 9

Chemistry/Evaluate laboratory data to recognize problems/Quality control/3

Answers to Questions 27–28

27. **B** A trend is characterized by six consecutive decreasing or increasing control results. The value for both controls becomes progressively higher from day 4 to day 9. Trends are caused by changes to the test system that increase over time, such as deterioration of reagents or calibrators, progressive changes in temperature, evaporation, light exposure, and bacterial contamination. A trend is a type of SE because all results are affected. Random error affects results in an unpredictable manner resulting in isolated or sporadic control errors. Control rules affected by RE are 1_{3s} and R_{4s}.

28. **D** Although the trend is apparent across QC levels by day 7, the patient results would not be rejected until day 9 when the 2_{2s} rule and 4_{1s} rule are broken. An advantage to plotting control data is that trends can be identified before results are out of control and patient data must be rejected. In this case, corrective steps should have been implemented by day 7 to avoid the delay and expense associated with having to repeat the analysis of patient samples.

29. Referring to the Levy-Jennings chart, what analytical error is present during the second half of the month?
A. Shift
B. Trend
C. Random error
D. Kurtosis

Chemistry/Evaluate laboratory data to recognize problems/Quality control/3

30. What is the first day in the second half of the month that patient results would be rejected?
A. Day 16
B. Day 17
C. Day 18
D. Day 19

Chemistry/Evaluate laboratory data to recognize problems/Quality control/3

31. Which of the following statistical tests is used to compare the means of two methods?
A. Student's *t* test
B. F distribution
C. Correlation coefficient (*r*)
D. Linear regression analysis

Chemistry/Evaluate laboratory data to assess the validity/Accuracy of procedures/Statistics/2

32. Two freezing point osmometers are compared by running 40 paired patient samples one time on each instrument, and the following results are obtained:

Instrument	Mean	Standard Deviation
Osmometer A	280 mOsm/kg	3.1
Osmometer B	294 mOsm/kg	2.8

If F = 2.8 at the 0.10 significance level (DF = 38), then what conclusion can be drawn regarding the precision of the two instruments?
A. There is no statistically significant difference in precision.
B. Osmometer A demonstrates better precision that is statistically significant.
C. Osmometer B demonstrates better precision that is statistically significant.
D. Precision cannot be evaluated statistically when single measurements are made on samples.

Chemistry/Evaluate laboratory data to assess the validity/Accuracy of procedures/Statistics/3

Answers to Questions 29–32

29. **A** A shift is characterized by six consecutive points lying on the same side of the mean. This occurs from day 15 to day 20. Shifts are caused by a change in the assay conditions that affect the accuracy of all results, such as a change in the concentration of the calibrator; change in reagent; a new lot of reagent that differs in composition; or improper temperature setting, wavelength, or sample volume. The term *kurtosis* refers to the degree of flatness or sharpness in the peak of a set of values having a Gaussian distribution.

30. **B** The 4_1s rule is broken across QC levels on day 17. This means that four consecutive controls are greater than $\pm 1\,s$ from the mean. QC rules that are sensitive to SE are applied across both runs and levels to increase the probability of error detection. These are 2_{2s}, 4_{1s}, and $10\,\bar{x}$.

31. **A** Student's *t* test is the ratio of mean difference to the standard error of the mean difference (bias/random error) and tests for a significant difference in means. The F test is the ratio of variances and determines if one method is significantly less precise. The correlation coefficient is a measure of the association between two variables and should be high in any method comparison. An *r* value less than 0.90 in method comparisons usually occurs when the range of results is too narrow.

32. **A** The F test determines whether there is a statistically significant difference in the variance of the two sampling distributions. Assuming the samples are collected and stored in the same way and the analysis is done by a technologist who is familiar with the instrument, then differences in variance can be attributed to a difference in instrument precision. The F test is calculated by dividing the variance $(s_1)^2$ of the instrument having the higher standard deviation by the variance $(s_2)^2$ of the instrument having the smaller standard deviation.

$$F = (s_1)^2 \div (s_2)^2 = (3.1)^2 \div (2.8)^2 = 9.61 \div 7.84 = 1.22$$

If the value of F is smaller than the critical value at the 0.10 level of significance, then the hypothesis (there is no significant difference in the variance of the two instruments) is accepted.

33. Two methods for total cholesterol are compared by running 40 paired patient samples one time on each instrument. The following results are obtained:

Instrument	Mean	Standard Deviation
Method x (reference method)	235 mg/dL	3.8
Method y (candidate method)	246 mg/dL	3.4

Assuming the samples are collected and stored in the same way and the analysis done by a technologist who is familiar with both methods, what is the bias of method y?
A. 0.4
B. 7.2
C. 10.6
D. 11.0

Chemistry/Evaluate laboratory data to assess the validity/Accuracy of procedures/Statistics/2

34. When the magnitude of error increases with increasing sample concentration it is called:
A. Constant error
B. Proportional error
C. Random error
D. Bias

Chemistry/Evaluate laboratory data to assess validity/Accuracy of procedures/Statistics/2

35. Serum samples collected from hospitalized patients over a 2-week period are split into two aliquots and analyzed for prostate specific antigen (PSA) by two methods. Each sample was assayed by both methods within 30 minutes of collection by a technologist familiar with both methods. The reference method is method x (upper reference limit = 4.0 μg/L). Linear regression analysis was performed by the least squares method, and results are as follows:

Linear Regression	Correlation Coefficient (r)	Standard Error of Estimate ($s_{y/x}$)
$y = 2.10 + 1.01x$	0.984	0.23

Which statement best characterizes the relationship between the methods?
A. There is a significant bias caused by constant error.
B. There is a significant proportional error.
C. There is no disagreement between the methods because the correlation coefficient approaches 1.0.
D. There are no SEs, but the RE of the new method is unacceptable.

Chemistry/Evaluate laboratory data to assess the validity/Accuracy of procedures/Statistics/2

Answers to Questions 33–35

33. D The bias is defined as the difference between the means of the two methods and is calculated using the formula: Bias = $\bar{y} - \bar{x}$. The bias is an estimate of SE. The student's t test is used to determine if bias is statistically significant. The t statistic is the ratio of bias to the standard error of the mean difference. The greater the bias, the higher the t score.

34. B Proportional error (slope or percent error) results in greater absolute error (deviation from the target value) at higher sample concentration. Constant error refers to a difference between the target value and the result, which is independent of sample concentration. For example, if both level 1 and level 2 controls for laboratory A average 5 mg/dL below the cumulative mean reported by all other laboratories using the same method, then laboratory A has a constant error of −5 mg/dL for that method.

35. A The linear regression analysis is the most useful statistic to compare paired patient results because it estimates the magnitude of specific errors. The y intercept of the regression line is a measure of constant error (bias), and the slope is a measure of proportional error. Together these represent the SE of the new method. The correlation coefficient is influenced by the range of the sample and the RE. Two methods that measure the same analyte will have a high correlation coefficient provided the concentrations are measured over a wide range, and this statistic should not be used to judge the acceptability of the new method. The standard error of estimate is a measure of the closeness of data points to the regression line and is an expression of RE.

36. A new method for BUN is evaluated by comparing the results of 40 paired patient samples to the urease-UV method. Normal and high controls were run on each shift for 5 days, five times per day. The results are as follows:

Linear Regression	Low Control	High Control
$y = -0.3 + 0.90x$	$\bar{x} = 14.2$ mg/dL; $s = 1.24$	$\bar{x} = 48.6$ mg/dL; $s = 1.12$

What is the total analytical error estimate for a sample having a concentration of 50 mg/dL?
A. -2.2 mg/dL
B. -2.8 mg/dL
C. -7.5 mg/dL
D. -10.0 mg/dL

Chemistry/Calculate/Method comparison statistics/3

37. In addition to the number of true-negatives (TN), which of the following measurements is needed to calculate specificity?
A. True-positives
B. Prevalence
C. False-negatives
D. False-positives

Chemistry/Calculation/Specificity/2

38. A new tumor marker for ovarian cancer is evaluated for sensitivity by testing serum samples from patients who have been diagnosed by staging biopsy as having malignant or benign lesions. The following results were obtained:
Number of malignant patients who are positive for CA 125 = 21 out of 24
Number of benign patients who are negative for CA 125 = 61 out of 62
What is the sensitivity of the new CA 125 test?
A. 98.4%
B. 95.3%
C. 87.5%
D. 85.0%

Clinical chemistry/Calculate/Sensitivity/2

39. A new test for prostatic cancer is found to have a sensitivity of 80.0% and a specificity of 84.0%. If the prevalence of prostate cancer is 4.0% in men over 42 years old, what is the predictive value of a positive test result (PV+) in this group?
A. 96.0%
B. 86.0%
C. 32.4%
D. 17.2%

Chemistry/Calculate/Predictive value/2

Answers to Questions 36–39

36. **C** Linear regression analysis gives an estimate of SE, which is equal to $(y - x_c)$ where x_c is the expected concentration, and y is the value predicted by the linear regression equation.
$$SE = [-0.3 + (0.9 \times 50 \text{ mg/dL})] - 50.0 \text{ mg/dL} = 44.7 - 50.0 = -5.3 \text{ mg/dL}$$

The standard deviation of the new method for the high control is used to estimate the RE because the mean of this control is nearest to the expected concentration of 50 mg/dL. RE is estimated by $\pm 1.96 \times s$.
$$RE = 1.96 \times 1.12 = \pm 2.2 \text{ mg/dL}$$

Total analytical error (TE) is equal to the sum of SE and RE.
$$TE = SE + RE = -5.3 \text{ mg/dL} + (-2.2 \text{ mg/dL}) = -7.5 \text{ mg/dL}$$

37. **D** The clinical specificity of a laboratory test is defined as the true-negatives divided by the sum of true-negatives and false-positives (FP).
$$\% \text{ Specificity} = \frac{TN \times 100}{TN + FP}$$

Specificity is defined as the percentage of disease-free people who have a negative test result. The probability of false-positives is calculated from the specificity as $1 - \dfrac{\text{specificity}}{100}$.

38. **C** Sensitivity is defined as the percentage of persons with the disease who have a positive test result. It is calculated as true-positives (TP) divided by the sum of TP and false-negatives (FN).
$$\% \text{ Sensitivity} = \frac{TP \times 100}{TP + FN}$$

Sensitivity = $(21 \times 100) \div (21 + 3) = 87.5\%$

39. **D** The predictive value of a positive test is defined as the percentage of persons with a positive test result (PV+) who will have the disease or condition. It is dependent upon the sensitivity of the test and the prevalence of the disease in the population tested. PV+ is calculated by multiplying the true-positives by 100, then dividing by the sum of true-positives and false-positives.
$$\% PV+ = \frac{TP \times 100}{(TP + FP)},$$ where TP equals (sensitivity × prevalence) and FP equals $(1 - \text{specificity}) \times (1 - \text{prevalence})$
$$= \frac{0.80 \times 0.04 \times 100}{(0.80 \times 0.04) + [(1 - 0.84) \times (1 - 0.04)]}$$
$$= \frac{0.032 \times 100}{0.032 + (0.96 \times 0.16)}$$
$$= 17.2\%$$

40. What measurement in addition to true-negatives and prevalence is required to calculate the predictive value of a negative test result (PV−)?
A. False-negatives
B. Variance
C. True-positives
D. False-positives

Chemistry/Calculate/Predictive value/2

Answer to Question 40

40. **A** The PV− is defined as the probability that a person with a negative test result is free of disease. A high PV− is a characteristic of a good screening test. The predictive value of a negative test is calculated by multiplying the true-negatives by 100, then dividing by the sum of the true-negatives and false-negatives.

$$\%PV- = \frac{TN \times 100}{(TN + FN)}$$

Creatinine, Uric Acid, BUN, and Ammonia

1. Creatinine is formed from the:
   A. Oxidation of creatine
   B. Oxidation of protein
   C. Deamination of dibasic amino acids
   D. Metabolism of purines

   Chemistry/Apply knowledge of fundamental biological characteristics/Biochemical/1

2. Creatinine is considered the substance of choice to measure endogenous renal clearance because:
   A. The rate of formation per day is independent of body size.
   B. It is completely filtered by the glomeruli.
   C. Plasma levels are highly dependent upon diet.
   D. Clearance is the same for both men and women.

   Chemistry/Apply knowledge of fundamental biological characteristics/Biochemical/1

3. Which statement regarding creatinine is true?
   A. Serum levels are elevated in early renal disease.
   B. High serum levels result from reduced glomerular filtration.
   C. Serum creatine has the same diagnostic utility as serum creatinine.
   D. Serum creatinine is a more sensitive measure of renal function than creatinine clearance.

   Chemistry/Calculate laboratory data with physiologic processes/Biochemical/2

4. Which of the formulas below is the correct expression for creatinine clearance?
   A. Creatinine clearance $= U/P \times V \times 1.73/A$
   B. Creatinine clearance $= P/V \times U \times A/1.73$
   C. Creatinine clearance $= P/V \times U \times 1.73/A$
   D. Creatinine clearance $= U/V \times P \times 1.73/A$

   Chemistry/Calculate/Creatinine clearance/1

Answers to Questions 1–4

1. **A** Creatinine is formed mainly in skeletal muscle from the oxidation of creatine. Creatinine is an anhydrous form of creatine formed at a rate of approximately 2% per day. Creatine can be converted to creatinine by addition of strong acid or alkali or by use of the enzyme creatine hydroxylase.

2. **B** Creatinine formation is dependent upon muscle mass and varies by less than 15% per day. It is not metabolized by the liver, or dependent on diet, and is 100% filtered by the glomeruli. It is not reabsorbed significantly but is secreted slightly, especially when filtrate flow is slow. It is the substance of choice for endogenous renal clearance tests.

3. **B** Serum creatinine is a specific but not a sensitive measure of glomerular function. About 60% of the filtration capacity of the kidneys is lost when serum creatinine becomes elevated. Because urine creatinine diminishes as serum creatinine increases in renal disease, the creatinine clearance is far more sensitive than serum creatinine in detecting glomerular disease.

4. **A** Creatinine clearance is the volume of plasma that contains the same quantity of creatinine that is excreted in the urine in 1 minute. It is calculated as the ratio of urine creatinine to plasma creatinine in milligrams per deciliter. This is multiplied by the volume of urine produced per minute and corrected for lean body mass by multiplying by 1.73/A, where A is the patient's body surface area in square meters.

5. Which of the following conditions is most likely to cause a falsely high creatinine clearance result?
   A. The patient uses the midstream void procedure when collecting his or her urine.
   B. The patient adds tap water to the urine container because he or she forgets to save one of the urine samples.
   C. The patient does not empty his or her bladder at the conclusion of the test.
   D. The patient empties his or her bladder at the start of the test and adds the urine to the collection.

   Chemistry/Identify source of error/Creatinine clearance/3

6. Given the following data, calculate the creatinine clearance.

   Serum creatinine = 1.2 mg/dL; urine creatinine = 120 mg/dL; urine volume = 1.75 L/day; surface area = 1.80 m^2
   A. Creatinine clearance = 16 mL/min
   B. Creatinine clearance = 117 mL/min
   C. Creatinine clearance = 126 mL/min
   D. Creatinine clearance = 168 mL/min

   Chemistry/Calculate/Creatinine clearance/2

7. In the creatinine clearance formula the term *1.73/A* is used to:
   A. Normalize clearance making it independent of muscle mass
   B. Correct clearance for creatinine that is secreted by the renal tubules
   C. Make the clearance measurement independent of filtrate flow rate
   D. Adjust clearance so that it is equal to inulin clearance

   Chemistry/Apply principles of special procedures/Creatinine clearance/1

8. Select the primary reagent used in the Jaffe method for creatinine.
   A. Alkaline copper II sulfate
   B. Saturated picric acid and NaOH
   C. Sodium nitroprusside and phenol
   D. Phosphotungstic acid

   Chemistry/Apply principles of general laboratory procedures/Biochemical/1

9. Which of the statements below regarding creatinine methods is true?
   A. The reaction of creatinine with alkaline picrate is highly specific.
   B. In persons with glomerular disease, enzymatic methods for creatinine are likely to give higher creatinine clearance results than the Jaffe method.
   C. Enzymatic methods generally give higher results for serum creatinine than methods based on Jaffe's reaction.
   D. When performing a creatinine clearance, the method used for serum should be enzymatic,

and the method used for urine should be based upon Jaffe's reaction.

Chemistry/Identify source of error/Biochemical/3

Answers to Questions 5–9

5. **D** Urine in the bladder should be eliminated and not saved at the start of the test because it represents urine formed prior to the test period. The other conditions (choices a–c) will result in falsely low urine creatinine or volume and, therefore, falsely lower clearance results. Error is introduced by incomplete emptying of the bladder when short times are used to measure clearance. A minimum 4-hour timed urine specimen should be collected (a 24-hour timed urine is the specimen of choice). When filtrate flow falls below 2 mL/min, error is introduced because tubular function has a greater effect upon urine creatinine, and some urine is likely to be retained in the bladder. The patient must be kept well hydrated during the test to prevent this.

6. **B** Creatinine clearance = urine creatinine ÷ serum creatinine × 1.75 L/day × 1 day/1440 min × 1000 mL/L × 1.73 m^2/1.80 m^2
   Creatinine clearance = 120 mg/dL ÷ 1.2 mg/dL × 1700 mL/1400 min × 1.73 m^2/1.80 m^2
   Creatinine clearance = 117 mL/min

7. **A** The term *1.73/A* corrects the clearance for variation in muscle mass as it relates to body size (surface area). The greater the muscle mass, the greater the creatinine clearance. Reference ranges are established for men, women, and children because each has a different percentage of lean muscle mass.

8. **B** The Jaffe method reaction uses saturated picric acid, which oxidizes creatinine in alkali, forming creatinine picrate. The reaction is nonspecific; ketones, ascorbate, proteins, and other reducing agents contribute to the final color. Alkaline $CuSO_4$ is used in the biuret method for protein, phenol-nitroprusside in the Berthelot reaction for ammonia, and phosphotungstic acid to measure uric acid.

9. **B** Enzymatic methods for creatinine are specific. Jaffe's reaction is nonspecific; proteins and other reducing substances may interfere (protein interference is eliminated by determining the rate of creatinine picrate formed between 25 and 120 seconds). When the serum creatinine is normal, the Jaffe method results in clearance values that compare well with the inulin clearance because serum creatinine is overestimated. However, in patients with poor renal function, the Jaffe method overestimates the creatinine clearance.

10. A sample of amniotic fluid collected for fetal lung maturity studies from a woman with a pregnancy compromised by hemolytic disease of the newborn (HDN) has a creatinine of 88 mg/dL. What is the most likely cause of this result?
   A. The specimen is contaminated with blood.
   B. Bilirubin has interfered with the measurement of creatinine.
   C. A random error occurred when the absorbance signal was being processed by the analyzer.
   D. The fluid is urine from accidental puncture of the urinary bladder.

Chemistry/Identify source of error/Biochemical/3

11. Urea is produced from:
   A. The catabolism of proteins and amino acids
   B. Oxidation of purines
   C. Oxidation of pyrimidines
   D. The breakdown of complex carbohydrates

Chemistry/Apply knowledge of fundamental biological characteristics/Biochemical/1

12. Urea concentration is calculated from the BUN by multiplying by a factor of:
   A. 0.5
   B. 2.14
   C. 6.45
   D. 14

Chemistry/Calculate/Biochemical/2

13. Which of the statements below about serum urea is true?
   A. Levels are independent of diet.
   B. Urea is not reabsorbed by the renal tubules.
   C. High BUN levels can result from necrotic liver disease.
   D. BUN is elevated in prerenal as well as renal failure.

Chemistry/Correlate laboratory data with physiologic processes/Biochemical/2

14. A patient's BUN is 60 mg/dL and serum creatinine is 3.0 mg/dL. These results suggest:
   A. Laboratory error measuring BUN
   B. Renal failure
   C. Prerenal failure
   D. Patient was not fasting

Chemistry/Evaluate laboratory data to determine possible inconsistent results/Biochemical/3

15. Urinary urea measurements may be used for calculation of:
   A. Glomerular filtration
   B. Renal blood flow
   C. Nitrogen balance
   D. All of the above

Chemistry/Correlate laboratory data with physiologic processes/Biochemical/2

Answers to Questions 10–15

10. **D** Creatinine levels in this range are found only in urine specimens. Adults usually excrete between 1.2 and 1.5 g of creatinine per day. For this reason, creatinine is routinely measured in 24-hour urine samples to determine the completeness of collection. A 24-hour urine with less than 0.8 g/day indicates that some of the urine was probably discarded. Creatinine is also used to evaluate fetal maturity. As gestation progresses, more creatinine is excreted into the amniotic fluid by the fetus. Although a level above 2 mg/dL is not a specific indicator of maturity, a level below 2 mg/dL indicates immaturity.

11. **A** Urea is generated by deamination of amino acids. Most is derived from the hepatic catabolism of proteins. Uric acid is produced by the catabolism of purines. Oxidation of pyrimidines produces orotic acid.

12. **B** BUN is multiplied by 2.14 to give the urea concentration in mg/dL.
$$BUN\ (mg/dL) = urea \times (\%\ N\ in\ urea \div 100)$$
$$Urea = BUN \times 1/(\%\ N\ in\ urea \div 100)$$
$$Urea = BUN \times (1/.467) = 2.14$$

13. **D** Urea is completely filtered by the glomeruli but reabsorbed by the renal tubules at a rate dependent upon filtrate flow and tubular status. Urea levels are a sensitive indicator of renal disease, becoming elevated by glomerular injury, tubular damage, or poor blood flow to the kidneys (prerenal failure). Serum urea (and BUN) levels are influenced by diet and are low in necrotic liver disease.

14. **C** BUN is affected by renal blood flow as well as by glomerular and tubular function. When blood flow to the kidneys is diminished by circulatory insufficiency (prerenal failure), glomerular filtration decreases and tubular reabsorption increases due to slower filtrate flow. Because urea is reabsorbed, BUN levels rise higher than creatinine. This causes the BUN:creatinine ratio to be greater than 10:1.

15. **C** Because BUN is handled by the tubules, serum levels are not specific for glomerular filtration rate. Urea clearance is influenced by diet and liver function as well as renal function. Protein intake minus excretion determines nitrogen balance. A negative balance (excretion exceeds intake) occurs in stress, starvation, fever, cachexia, and chronic illness.
$$Nitrogen\ balance =$$
$$(Protein\ intake\ in\ grams\ per\ deciliter \div 6.25) -$$
$$(Urine\ nitrogen\ in\ grams\ per\ day + 3)$$

16. BUN is determined electrochemically by coupling the urease reaction to measurement of:
A. Potential with an urea-selective electrode
B. The timed rate of increase in conductivity
C. The oxidation of ammonia
D. Carbon dioxide

Chemistry/Apply principles of special procedures/Biochemical/1

17. In the ultraviolet enzymatic method for BUN the urease reaction is coupled to a second enzymatic reaction using:
A. AST
B. Glutamate dehydrogenase
C. Glutamine synthetase
D. Alanine aminotransferase (ALT)

Chemistry/Apply principles of basic laboratory procedures/Biochemical/1

18. Which product is measured in the coupling step of the urease-UV method for BUN?
A. CO_2
B. Dinitrophenylhydrazine
C. Diphenylcarbazone
D. NAD^+

Chemistry/Apply principles of basic laboratory procedures/Biochemical/1

19. Which enzyme deficiency is responsible for phenylketonuria (PKU)?
A. Phenylalanine hydroxylase
B. Tyrosine transaminase
C. *p*-Hydroxyphenylpyruvic acid oxidase
D. Homogentisic acid oxidase

Chemistry/Apply knowledge of fundamental biological characteristics/Aminoaciduria/1

20. Which of the following conditions is classified as a renal-type aminoaciduria?
A. Fanconi's syndrome
B. Wilson's disease
C. Hepatitis
D. Homocystinuria

Chemistry/Correlate clinical and laboratory data/Aminoaciduria/2

Answers to Questions 16–20

16. **B** A conductivity electrode is used to measure the increase in conductance of the solution as urea is hydrolyzed by urease in the presence of sodium carbonate.

$$Urea + H_2O \rightarrow 2NH_3 + CO_2$$
$$2NH_3 + 2H_2O + Na_2CO_3 \rightarrow 2NH_4^+ + CO_3^{-2} + 2NaOH$$

Ammonium ions increase the conductance of the solution. The timed rate of current increase is proportional to the BUN concentration. NH_3-selective electrodes may also be used to measure BUN.

17. **B** BUN is most frequently measured by the urease-uv method in which the urease reaction is coupled to the glutamate dehydrogenase reaction generating NAD^+.

$$Urea + H_2O \xrightarrow{Urease} 2NH_3 + CO_2$$
$$2\text{-Oxoglutarate} + NH_3 + NADH +$$
$$H^+ \xrightarrow{GLD} Glutamate + NAD^+ + H_2O$$

When the urease reaction is performed under first-order conditions the decrease in absorbance at 340 nm is proportional to the urea concentration.

18. **D** In the urease-UV method, urease is used to hydrolyze urea, forming CO_2 and ammonia. Glutamate dehydrogenase catalyzes the oxidation of NADH, forming glutamate from 2-oxoglutarate and ammonia. The glutamate dehydrogenase reaction is used for measuring both BUN and ammonia.

19. **A** PKU is an overflow aminoaciduria resulting from the accumulation of phenylalanine. It is caused by a deficiency of phenylalanine hydroxylase, which converts phenylalanine to tyrosine. Excess phenylalanine accumulates in blood. This is transaminated, forming phenylpyruvic acid, which is excreted in the urine.

20. **A** Fanconi's disease is an inherited syndrome of anemia, mental retardation, rickets, and aminoaciduria. Because the aminoaciduria results from a defect in the renal tubule, it is classified as a (secondary inherited) renal-type aminoaciduria. Wilson's disease, inherited ceruloplasmin deficiency, causes hepatic failure. It is classified as a secondary inherited overflow-type because the aminoaciduria results from urea cycle failure. Hepatitis is classified as a secondary acquired overflow-type aminoaciduria. Homocystinuria is a primary inherited overflow-type aminoaciduria, and is caused by a deficiency of cystathionine synthase.

21. Which aminoaciduria results in the overflow of branched chain amino acids?
A. Hartnup's disease
B. Alkaptonuria
C. Homocystinuria
D. Maple syrup urine disease

Chemistry/Apply knowledge of fundamental biological characteristics/Aminoaciduria/1

22. Which of the following best describes the Guthrie test?
A. Bioassay for PKU dependent upon the phenylalanine requirement of *Bacillus subtilis*
B. Ion exchange HPLC and postcolumn reaction with ninhydrin
C. Two-dimensional TLC using ninhydrin staining
D. Reaction of phenylpyruvic acid with ferric chloride to form a blue-green complex

Chemistry/Apply principles of special procedures/Aminoaciduria/2

23. Blood ammonia levels are usually measured in order to evaluate:
A. Renal failure
B. Acid-base status
C. Hepatic coma
D. Gastrointestinal malabsorption

Chemistry/Correlate clinical and laboratory data/ Biochemical/2

24. Enzymatic measurement of ammonia requires which of the following substrates and coenzymes?

Substrate	**Coenzyme**
A. α-Ketoglutarate	NADH
B. Glutamate	NADH
C. Glutamine	ATP
D. Glutamine	NAD$^+$

Chemistry/Apply principles of basic laboratory procedures/Biochemical/1

25. Which statement about ammonia is true?
A. Normally most of the plasma ammonia is derived from intestinal absorption.
B. Ammonia-induced coma can result from acetaminophen poisoning.
C. Hepatic coma can result from Reye's syndrome.
D. All of the above.

Chemistry/Correlate clinical and laboratory data/ Biochemical/2

Answers to Questions 21–25

21. **D** Valine, leucine, and isoleucine accumulate due to branched chain decarboxylase deficiency in maple syrupuria. These are transaminated to ketoacids that are excreted giving urine a maple sugar odor. Alkaptonuria is caused by homogentisic acid oxidase deficiency causing homogentisic aciduria. Homocystinuria, is a no-threshold-type aminoaciduria that usually results from cystathionine synthase deficiency.

22. **A** All the methods above may be used to screen for PKU although the ferric chloride test is nonspecific and not sufficiently sensitive for newborns. The Guthrie test uses thienylalanine which inhibits the growth of *B. subtilis* unless excess phenylalanine is present. Guthrie assays using specific amino acid inhibitors are used to screen for maple syrup urine disease, tyrosinemia, lysinemia, and homocystinuria.

23. **C** Hepatic coma is caused by accumulation of ammonia in the brain as a result of liver failure. The ammonia increases central nervous system pH and is coupled to glutamate, a central nervous system neurotransmitter, forming glutamine. Blood and cerebrospinal fluid ammonia levels are used to distinguish encephalopathy caused by cirrhosis or other liver disease from nonhepatic causes and to monitor patients with hepatic coma.

24. **A** Enzymatic assays of ammonia utilize glutamate dehydrogenase (GLD). This enzyme forms glutamate from α-ketoglutarate (2-oxoglutarate) and ammonia, resulting in oxidation of NADH. The rate of absorbance decrease at 340 nm is proportional to ammonia concentration when the reaction rate is maintained under first-order conditions.

25. **D** Most of the ammonia absorbed from the intestines is transported to the liver via the portal vein and converted to urea. Blood ammonia levels will rise in any necrotic liver disease, including hepatitis, Reye's syndrome, and drug-induced injury. In cirrhosis shunting of portal blood to the general circulation accounts for the frequency of central nervous system complications.

26. SITUATION: A sample for ammonia assay is taken from an IV line that had been capped and injected with lithium heparin (called a heparin lock). The sample is drawn in a syringe containing lithium heparin, and immediately capped and iced. The plasma is separated and analyzed within 20 minutes of collection, and the result is 50 mg/dL higher than one measured 4 hours before. What is the most likely explanation of these results?
A. Significantly greater physiological variation is seen with patients having systemic, hepatic, and gastrointestinal diseases.
B. The syringe was contaminated with ammonia.
C. One of the two samples was collected from the wrong patient.
D. Stasis of blood in the line caused increased ammonia.

Chemistry/Evaluate sources of error/Specimen collection and handling/3

27. Uric acid is derived from the:
A. Oxidation of proteins
B. Catabolism of purines
C. Oxidation of pyrimidines
D. Reduction of catecholamines

Chemistry/Apply knowledge of fundamental biological characteristics/Biochemical/1

28. Which of the following conditions is associated with hyperuricemia?
A. Renal failure
B. Chronic liver disease
C. Xanthine oxidase deficiency
D. Paget's disease of the bone

Chemistry/Correlate clinical and laboratory data/Biochemical/2

29. Orders for uric acid are legitimate stat requests because:
A. Levels above 10 mg/dL cause urinary tract calculi.
B. Uric acid is hepatotoxic.
C. High levels induce aplastic anemia.
D. High levels cause joint pain.

Chemistry/Correlate clinical and laboratory data/Biochemical/2

30. Which uric acid method is associated with positive bias caused by reducing agents?
A. Uricase coupled to the Trinder reaction
B. UV uricase reaction coupled to catalase and alcohol dehydrogenase reactions
C. Measurement of the negative rate at 290 nm after addition of uricase
D. Phosphotungstic acid using a protein-free filtrate

Chemistry/Evaluate sources of error/Biochemical/2

Answers to Questions 26–30

26. **D** Falsely elevated blood ammonia levels are commonly caused by improper specimen collection. Venous stasis and prolonged storage cause peripheral deamination of amino acids causing a falsely high ammonia level. Plasma is the sample of choice since ammonia levels increase with storage. Lithium heparin and EDTA are acceptable anticoagulants; the anticoagulant used should be tested to make sure it is free of ammonia. A vacuum tube can be used if filled completely. Serum may be used provided the tube is iced immediately, and the serum is separated as soon as the sample clots. The patient should be fasting and must not have smoked for 8 hours because tobacco smoke can double the plasma ammonia level.

27. **B** Uric acid is the principal product of purine (adenosine and guanosine) metabolism. Oxidation of proteins yields urea along with CO_2, H_2O, and inorganic acids. Catecholamines are oxidized, forming vanillylmandelic acid (VMA) and homovanillic acid (HVA).

28. **A** Excessive retention of uric acid results from renal failure and diuretics (or other drugs) that block uric acid excretion. Hyperuricemia may result from overproduction of uric acid in primary essential gout or excessive cell turnover associated with malignancy and chemotherapy. Overproduction may also result from an enzyme deficiency in the pathway forming guanosine triphosphate (GTP) or adenosine monophosphate (AMP) (purine salvage). Hyperuricemia is also associated with ketoacidosis and lactate acidosis, hypertension, and hyperlipidemia. Xanthine oxidase converts xanthine to uric acid; therefore, a deficiency of this enzyme results in low serum levels of uric acid. Paget's disease of bone causes cyclic episodes of bone degeneration and regeneration and is associated with very high serum ALP and urinary calcium levels.

29. **A** Uric acid calculi form quickly when the serum uric acid level reaches 10 mg/dL. They are translucent compact stones that often lodge in the ureters causing postrenal failure.

30. **D** Uricase methods form allantoin, CO_2, and H_2O_2 from the oxidation of uric acid. When peroxide is used to oxidize a Trinder dye (e.g., a phenol derivative and 4-aminoantipyrine) some negative bias may occur when high levels of ascorbate or other reducing agents are present. Rate UV methods are free from this interference. Reduction of phosphotungstic acid by uric acid forms tungsten blue. This colorimetric reaction is nonspecific, resulting in falsely elevated uric acid caused by proteins and many other reducing substances.

Proteins, Electrophoresis, and Lipids

1. Kjeldahl's procedure for total protein is based upon the premise that:
   A. Proteins are negatively charged.
   B. The pK_a of proteins is the same.
   C. The nitrogen content of proteins is constant.
   D. Proteins have similar tyrosine and tryptophan content.

   Chemistry/Apply principles of special procedures/Proteins and enzymes/1

2. The term *biuret reaction* refers to:
   A. The reaction of phenolic groups with $CuSO_4$
   B. Coordinate bonds between Cu^{2+} and carboxyl and amino groups of biuret
   C. The protein error of indicator effect producing color when dyes bind protein
   D. The reaction of phosphomolybdic acid with protein

   Chemistry/Apply principles of basic laboratory procedures/Proteins and enzymes/1

3. Which statement about the biuret reaction for total protein is true?
   A. It is sensitive to protein levels below 0.1 mg/dL.
   B. It is suitable for urine, exudates, and transudates.
   C. Polypeptides and compounds with repeating imine groups react.
   D. Hemolysis will not interfere.

   Chemistry/Apply knowledge to identify sources of error/Proteins and enzymes/2

4. Which of the following protein methods has the highest analytical sensitivity?
   A. Refractometry
   B. Folin-Lowry
   C. Turbidimetry
   D. Direct ultraviolet absorption

   Chemistry/Apply knowledge of special procedures/Proteins and enzymes/2

Answers to Questions 1–4

1. **C** Kjeldahl's method measures the nitrogen content of proteins as ammonium ion by back titration following oxidation of proteins by sulfuric acid and heat. It assumes that proteins average 16% nitrogen by weight. Protein in grams per deciliter is calculated by multiplying protein nitrogen by 6.25.

2. **B** Biuret is a compound with two carbonyl groups and three amino groups and forms coordinate bonds with Cu^{2+} in the same manner as does protein.

3. **C** The biuret reaction is not sensitive to protein levels below 0.1 g/dL and, therefore, is not sensitive enough for assays of total protein in CSF, urine, or transudates. Slight hemolysis does not cause falsely high results. However, frankly hemolyzed samples contain sufficient globin to cause positive interference.

4. **B** The Folin-Lowry (Lowry's) method uses both biuret reagent and phosphotungstic/molybdic acids to oxidize the aromatic side groups on proteins. The aromatic residues will bind to Cu^{2+} in the biuret reagent, greatly increasing sensitivity.

5. Which of the following statements regarding proteins is true?
  A. Total protein and albumin are about 10% higher in ambulatory patients.
  B. Plasma total protein is about 15% higher than serum levels.
  C. Albumin normally accounts for about 40% of cerebrospinal fluid total protein.
  D. Transudative serous fluid protein is about two-thirds of the serum level.

Chemistry/Evaluate laboratory data to recognize health and disease states/Proteins and enzymes/2

6. Hyperalbuminemia is caused by:
  A. Dehydration syndromes
  B. Liver disease
  C. Burns
  D. Gastroenteropathy

Chemistry/Correlate clinical and laboratory data/Proteins and enzymes/2

7. High serum total protein but low albumin is usually seen in:
  A. Multiple myeloma
  B. Hepatic cirrhosis
  C. Glomerulonephritis
  D. Nephrotic syndrome

Chemistry/Correlate clinical and laboratory data/Proteins and enzymes/2

8. Which of the following conditions is most commonly associated with an elevated level of total protein?
  A. Glomerular disease
  B. Starvation
  C. Liver failure
  D. Malignancy

Chemistry/Correlate clinical and laboratory data/Proteins and enzymes/2

9. Which of the following dyes is the most specific for measurement of albumin?
  A. Bromcresol green (BCG)
  B. Bromcresol purple (BCP)
  C. Tetrabromosulfophthalein
  D. Tetrabromphenol blue

Chemistry/Apply principles of basic laboratory procedures/Proteins and enzymes/1

10. Which of the following factors is most likely to cause a falsely low result when using the BCG dye-binding assay for albumin?
  A. The presence of penicillin
  B. An incubation time of 120 seconds
  C. The presence of bilirubin
  D. Lipemia

Chemistry/Apply knowledge to recognize source of error/Proteins and enzymes/2

Answers to Questions 5–10

5. **A** Water pools in the vascular bed in nonambulatory patients lowering the total protein, albumin, hematocrit, and calcium. Plasma levels of total protein are about 0.2–0.4 g/dL higher than serum owing to fibrinogen. Cerebrospinal fluid albumin levels are normally 10–30 mg/dL which is approximately two-thirds of the CSF total protein. Transudates have a total protein below 3.0 g/dL and less than 50% of the serum total protein.

6. **A** A high serum albumin level is caused only by dehydration or administration of albumin. Liver disease, burns, gastroenteropathy, nephrosis, starvation, and malignancy cause hypoalbuminemia.

7. **A** In glomerulonephritis and nephrotic syndrome, both total protein and albumin are low due to loss of proteins through the glomeruli. Acute glomerulonephritis gives rise to the delayed response pattern of chronic inflammation. Nephrotic syndrome is characterized by high α-2 macroglobulin. In hepatic cirrhosis decreased hepatic production of protein results in low total protein and albumin.

8. **D** Malignant disease is usually associated with increased immunoglobulin and acute phase protein production. However, nutrients required for protein synthesis are consumed causing reduced hepatic albumin production. Glomerular damage causes albumin and other low molecular weight proteins to be lost through the kidneys. Liver failure and starvation result in decreased protein synthesis.

9. **B** Tetrabromphenol blue and tetrabromosulfophthalein are dyes that change pK_a in the presence of protein. Although they have greater affinity for albumin than globulins, they are not sufficiently specific to apply to measurement of serum albumin. BCG and BCP are anionic dyes that undergo a spectral shift when they bind albumin at acid pH. BCP is more specific for albumin than BCG. However, BCG is the method used most often because BCP produces a much smaller absorbance signal than BCG, making it less sensitive. The reactivity of BCG with globulins requires a longer incubation time than with albumin, and reaction times are kept at 30 seconds or less to increase specificity. Both dyes are free of interference from bilirubin.

10. **A** BCG and BCP are not significantly affected by bilirubin or hemolysis although negative interference caused by free Hgb has been reported with some BCG methods. Lipemic samples may cause positive interference, which can be eliminated by serum blanking. Incubation times as long as 2 minutes result in positive interference from globulins, which react with the dye. Penicillin and some other anionic drugs bind to albumin at the same site as the dye causing falsely low results.

11. At pH 8.6 proteins are _____ charged and migrate toward the _____.
    A. Negatively   Anode
    B. Positively   Cathode
    C. Positively   Anode
    D. Negatively   Cathode

    Chemistry/Apply knowledge of fundamental biological characteristics/Electrophoresis/1

12. Electrophoretic movement of proteins toward the anode will be made to *decrease* by increasing the:
    A. Buffer pH
    B. Ionic strength of the buffer
    C. Current
    D. Voltage

    Chemistry/Apply principles of basic laboratory procedures/Electrophoresis/2

13. At pH 8.6, the cathodal movement of γ globulins is caused by:
    A. Electroendosmosis
    B. Wick flow
    C. A net positive charge
    D. Cathodal sample application

    Chemistry/Apply principles of basic laboratory procedures/Electrophoresis/2

14. Which of the conditions below will prevent any migration of proteins across an electrophoretic support medium such as agarose?
    A. Using too high a voltage
    B. Excessive current during the procedure
    C. Loss of contact between a buffer chamber and the medium
    D. Evaporation of solvent from the surface of the medium.

    Chemistry/Apply principles of basic laboratory procedures/Electrophoresis/2

15. Which of the proteins listed below has the highest *pI*?
    A. Albumin
    B. Transferrin
    C. Ceruloplasmin
    D. IgG

    Chemistry/Apply knowledge of fundamental biological characteristics/Electrophoresis/1

16. Which of the proteins listed below migrates in the β region at pH 8.6?
    A. Haptoglobin
    B. Orosomucoprotein
    C. Antichymotrypsin
    D. Transferrin

    Chemistry/Apply knowledge of fundamental biological characteristics/Electrophoresis/1

Answers to Questions 11–16

11. **A** Proteins are amphoteric owing to ionization of acidic and basic side chains of amino acids. When the pH of the solution equals the isoelectric point (*pI*), the protein will have no net charge and is insoluble. When the pH of the solution is above the *pI*, the protein will have a net negative charge. Anions migrate toward the anode (positive electrode).

12. **B** *Electrophoresis* is the migration of charged molecules in an electric field. Increasing the strength of the field by increasing voltage (or current) increases migration. However, increasing ionic strength decreases the migration of proteins. Counterions (cations) in the buffer move with the proteins reducing their electromagnetic attraction for the anode.

13. **A** Agarose and cellulose acetate contain fixed anions (e.g., acetate) that attract counterions when hydrated with buffer. When voltage is applied the cations migrate to the cathode creating an osmotic force that draws H_2O with them. This force, called *electroendosmosis*, opposes protein migration toward the anode and may cause some γ globulins to be displaced toward the cathode.

14. **C** Movement of proteins is dependent upon the presence of a salt bridge that allows current to flow via transport of ions to the electrodes across the support medium. If the salt bridge is not intact, there will be no migration, even if voltage is maintained across the electrodes. For agarose and cellulose acetate, heat causes evaporation of solvent from the buffer. This increases the ionic strength causing current to rise during the run. Excessive heat can damage the support medium and denature proteins. Power = E (voltage) × I (current) × t (time); since $E = I \times R$ (resistance), heat is proportional to the square of current ($P = I^2 \times R \times t$). Constant current mode is used for long runs to prevent heat damage.

15. **D** Albumin is the fastest migrating protein toward the anode at pH 8.6 followed by α_1-, α_2-, β-, and γ-globulins. Because albumin is fastest, it has the greatest net negative charge and lowest *pI* (about 4.6). γ-Globulins are predominantly immunoglobulins and have the highest *pI* (about 7.2).

16. **D** Transferrin, β lipoprotein, C3, and C4 (fibrinogen if plasma is used) are the dominant proteins in the β-globulin region. Haptoglobin and α_2-macroglobulin are the principal proteins in the α_2-fraction. α_1-Antitrypsin and orosomucoprotein (α_1-acid glycoprotein) make up most of the α_1-fraction. Immunoglobulins dominate the γ region.

17. Which of the following is one advantage of high-resolution (HR) agarose electrophoresis over lower current electrophoresis?

A. High-resolution procedures detect monoclonal and oligoclonal bands at a lower concentration.

B. A smaller sample volume is used.

C. Results are obtained more rapidly.

D. More samples can be applied to the support medium.

Chemistry/Apply principles of special procedures/Electrophoresis/2

18. Which of the following conditions is associated with "β-γ bridging"?

A. Multiple myeloma

B. Malignancy

C. Hepatic cirrhosis

D. Rheumatoid arthritis

Chemistry/Correlate clinical and laboratory data/Electrophoresis/2

19. Which support medium can be used to determine the molecular weight of a protein?

A. Cellulose acetate

B. Polyacrylamide gel

C. Agar gel

D. Agarose gel

Chemistry/Apply principles of special procedures/Electrophoresis/2

20. Which of the following stains is used for lipoprotein electrophoresis?

A. Oil Red O

B. Coomassie Brilliant Blue

C. Amido Black

D. Ponceau S

Chemistry/Select reagents/Media/ Blood products/Electrophoresis/1

21. Which of the following serum protein electrophoresis results suggests an acute inflammatory process?

| | | Globulins | | |
Albumin	α_1	α_2	β	γ
A. Decreased	Increased	Decreased	Normal	Normal
B. Normal	Increased	Normal	Increased	Increased
C. Decreased	Increased	Increased	Normal	Normal
D. Increased	Increased	Increased	increased	Increased

Chemistry/Correlate clinical and laboratory data/Electrophoresis/2

22. Which of the conditions below is usually associated with an acute inflammatory pattern?

A. Myocardial infarction (MI)

B. Malignancy

C. Rheumatoid arthritis

D. Hepatitis

Chemistry/Correlate clinical and laboratory data/Electrophoresis/2

Answers to Questions 17–22

17. **A** HR agarose procedures use higher current and a cooling device to resolve 12 or more bands. Advantages include phenotyping of α_1-antitrypsin (detection of Z and S variants), detection of β_2 microglobulin in urine indicating tubular proteinuria (often associated with drug-induced nephrosis), and greater sensitivity detecting monoclonal gammopathies, immune complexes, and oligoclonal bands in CSF associated with multiple sclerosis.

18. **C** Hepatic cirrhosis produces a polyclonal gammopathy associated with a high IgA level. This obliterates the valley between β and γ zones. Malignancy and rheumatoid arthritis produce polyclonal gammopathies classified as chronic inflammatory or delayed response patterns. Multiple myeloma produces a zone of restricted mobility usually in the γ, but sometimes in the β or α_2-region.

19. **B** Polyacrylamide and starch gels separate by molecular sieving as well as charge. Sodium dodecyl sulfate (SDS), is a nonionic detergent that binds to proteins neutralizing charge. Polyacrylamide gel electrophoresis (PAGE) after treating with SDS separates proteins on the basis of molecular size. The smaller proteins become trapped in the pores of the gel and migrate more slowly.

20. **A** Oil Red O and Sudan Black B stain neutral fats and are used to stain lipoproteins as well as fat in urine or stool. The other stains are used for proteins. Coomassie Brilliant Blue is more sensitive than Ponceau S or Amido Black, and all three stains have slightly greater affinity for albumin than globulins. In addition, silver nitrate may be used to stain CSF proteins because it has far greater sensitivity than the other stains.

21. **C** Acute inflammation is characterized by increased production of acute phase proteins. These include α_1-antitrypsin, α_1-acid glycoprotein, α_1-antichymotrypsin, and haptoglobin. Albumin is slightly decreased. γ- and β-fractions are normal.

22. **A** MI produces a pattern of acute inflammation usually associated with tissue injury. This pattern results from production of acute phase proteins including α_1-antitrypsin, α_1-antichymotrypsin, and haptoglobin. It is also seen in early infection, pregnancy, and early nephritis. Malignancy, rheumatoid arthritis, and hepatitis are associated with a chronic inflammatory pattern. This differs from the acute pattern by the addition of a polyclonal gammopathy.

23. The electrophoretic pattern shown in the densito-
metric tracing below most likely indicates:
A. α_1-Antitrypsin deficiency
B. Infection
C. Nephrosis
D. Systemic sclerosis

*Chemistry/Evaluate laboratory data to recognize
health and disease states/Proteins and enzymes/2*

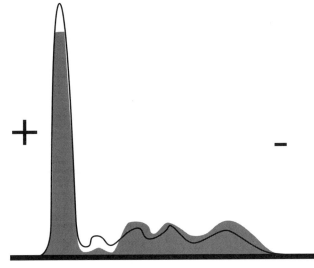

24. Quantitative determination of Hgb A_2 is best
performed by:
A. Column chromatography
B. Alkali denaturation
C. Electrophoresis
D. Direct bichromatic spectrophotometry

*Chemistry/Apply principles of basic laboratory pro-
cedures/Hemoglobin/1*

25. Hgb F concentration is usually measured by:
A. Alkali denaturation of Hgb A and Hgb A_2
B. Specific Hgb F peroxidase reaction
C. Turbidimetric assay of Hgb F after precipitation
with ammonium sulfate
D. Ion exchange chromatography

*Chemistry/Apply principles of special
procedures/Hemoglobin/1*

26. Select the correct order of Hgb migration on
cellulose acetate at pH 8.6.
A. $- C \rightarrow F \rightarrow S \rightarrow A +$
B. $- S \rightarrow C \rightarrow A \rightarrow F +$
C. $- C \rightarrow S \rightarrow F \rightarrow A +$
D. $- S \rightarrow F \rightarrow A \rightarrow C +$

*Chemistry/Apply principles of special
procedures/Electrophoresis/2*

27. Which of the following abnormal Hgbs migrates to
the same position as Hgb S on cellulose acetate or
agarose at pH 8.6?

A. Hgb C
B. Hgb D_{Punjab}
C. Hgb O
D. Hgb E

*Chemistry/Apply principles of special
procedures/Electrophoresis/2*

Answers to Questions 23–27

23. **A** This pattern shows a marked decrease in the
α_1-globulin (slightly less then one-fifth of the
expected peak area). Staining of the α_1-globulin
fraction is predominately determined by the
α_1-antitrypsin level. A value of less than 20% of
normal (0.2–0.4 g/dL) is usually caused by homozygous α_1-antitrypsin deficiency. There is a
slight decrease in albumin and increase in the α_2-
fraction. Patients with α_1-antitrypsin deficiency
often display elevations in the α_2-globulin and γ-
globulin fraction because the condition is
associated with chronic emphysema and
hepatic cirrhosis.

24. **A** Hgb A_2 is most often measured by anion
exchange column chromatography. Because Hgbs
A and F have a greater negative charge than Hgb
A_2, they are retained on the column after Hgb A_2 is
eluted using glycine and potassium cyanide. The
Hgb elutes as cyanmethemoglobin and is
measured at 415 nm. Hgb F is measured by alkali
denaturation. Ammonium sulfate precipitates Hgb
A and Hgb A_2, but Hgb F remains soluble.

25. **A** Hgb is reacted with Drabkin's reagent to form
cyanmethemoglobin. The cyanmethemoglobin derivatives of Hgb A and Hgb A_2 are denatured by
NaOH and then precipitated using 40%
ammonium sulfate. Hgb F is alkali-resistant and
remains in solution. The absorbance of the supernatant is measured at 540 nm.

26. **C** Hgb A_2 is the slowest of the normal Hgbs, and
Hgb A is the fastest. Hgb F migrates just behind
Hgb A. Hgb S migrates midway between Hgb A_2
and Hgb A. Hgbs C, C_{Harlem} (Georgetown), O, and E
migrate with Hgb A_2. Hgbs G and D_{Punjab} and Hgb
$_{Lepore}$ migrate with Hgb S.

27. **B** Hgb D migrates with Hgb S on cellulose acetate
or agarose at pH 8.6–9.2. Hgb S may be differentiated from Hgb D using citrate (acid) agar at pH
6.2. Using this technique, Hgb S migrates further
toward the anode than Hgb D. Hgb C, E, O, and
C_{Harlem} migrate to the same position as Hgb A_2 on
cellulose acetate at pH 8.6–9.2.

28. Which Hgb is a β-δ chain hybrid and migrates to the same position as Hgb S at pH 8.6?
A. Hgb C $_{Harlem}$
B. Hgb $_{Lepore}$
C. Hgb G $_{Philadelphia}$
D. Hgb D $_{Punjab}$

Chemistry/Apply principles of special procedures/Electrophoresis/2

29. Select the correct order of Hgb migration on citrate agar at pH 6.2.
A. $- F \rightarrow S \rightarrow C \rightarrow A +$
B. $- F \rightarrow A \rightarrow S \rightarrow C +$
C. $- A \rightarrow S \rightarrow F \rightarrow C +$
D. $- A \rightarrow C \rightarrow S \rightarrow F +$

Chemistry/Apply principles of special procedures/Electrophoresis/2

30. Which Hgb separates from Hgb S on citrate (acid) agar, but not agarose or cellulose acetate?
A. Hgb D $_{Punjab}$
B. Hgb E
C. Hgb C $_{Harlem}$ (Georgetown)
D. Hgb O

Chemistry/Evaluate laboratory data to verify test results/Electrophoresis/2

31. Which of the following statements regarding the identification of monoclonal proteins by immuno-electrophoresis (IEP) or immunofixation electrophoresis (IFE) is true?
A. The monoclonal band must be present in the γ region.
B. When testing for a monoclonal gammopathy both serum and urine must be examined.
C. A diagnosis of monoclonal gammopathy is based upon quantitation of IgG, IgA, and IgM.
D. A monoclonal band always indicates a malignant disorder.

Chemistry/Correlate clinical and laboratory data/Immunoelectrophoresis/2

32. Which statement best describes IEP?
A. Proteins are separated by electrophoresis followed by overlay of anti-immunoglobulin.
B. Proteins react with monospecific antisera followed by electrophoresis.
C. Antisera are electrophoresed, then diffused against patient's serum.
D. Serum is electrophoresed; the separated immunoglobulins diffuse against specific antisera.

Chemistry/Apply knowledge of special procedures/Immunoelectrophoresis/2

Answers to Questions 28–32

28. B Hgb $_{Lepore}$ results from translocation of β and δ globin genes resulting in a polypeptide chain that migrates midway between Hgb A$_2$ and Hgb A. The chain is transcribed more slowly than the β polypeptide chain causing the quantity of Hgb $_{Lepore}$ to be less than 15%. Hgb $_{Lepore}$ is suspected when Hgb migrating in the "S" zone comprises less than 20% of the total Hgb. In Hgb S trait, the AS phenotype produces 20–40% Hgb S.

29. B Hgb C and Hgb S bind to sulfated pectins in agar gel, forming a complex that is negatively charged. Hgb C migrates furthest toward the anode followed by Hgb S. Hgbs A, A$_2$, E, G, and $_{Lepore}$ migrate slightly toward the cathode. Hgb F migrates furthest toward the cathode.

30. A Hgbs O, E, and C $_{Harlem}$ migrate to the same position as Hgbs A$_2$ and C on agarose (or cellulose acetate) at pH 8.6. Hgb D $_{Punjab}$ migrates to the same position as Hgb S on agarose, but moves with Hgb A on citrate agar. Agarose is a purified form of agar; it lacks the sulfated pectins required to separate Hgbs D and G from Hgb S, and Hgbs E, C $_{Harlem}$, and O from Hgb C. Hgb C $_{Harlem}$ is a sickling Hgb and it migrates to the same position as Hgb S on citrate (acid) agar.

31. B Quantitation of IgG, IgA, IgM, or IgD indicates the concentration of each class of immunoglobulin but does not distinguish monoclonal from polyclonal gammopathies. Monoclonal characteristics are determined by demonstrating restricted electrophoretic mobility, indicating that all immunoglobulins in the band are of the same amino acid sequence. Monoclonal light chains are seen in about 40% of monoclonal gammopathies. In up to 25% of multiple myeloma patients, a heavy chain gene deletion results in production of monoclonal light chains only. Because these are filtered by the glomerulus, the procedure must be performed on urine as well as serum. Some patients with a monoclonal protein fail to develop malignant plasma cell proliferation. This state is referred to as a monoclonal gammopathy of undetermined significance.

32. D IEP requires protein electrophoresis to separate immunoglobulins followed by immunodiffusion to identify them via precipitation with specific antisera. IFE is a rapid alternative used to identify monoclonal bands. Specific antisera are spread over the agarose gel after electrophoresis. Precipitin bands can be visualized by washing and staining the gel after an hour's incubation.

33. In double immunodiffusion reactions the precipitin band is:
A. Invisible before the equivalence point is reached
B. Concave to the protein of greatest molecular weight
C. Closest to the well containing the highest level of antigen
D. Located in an area of antibody excess

Chemistry/Apply knowledge of special procedures/Immunodiffusion/1

34. Which statement regarding IEP is true?
A. Serum containing a monoclonal protein should have a κ:λ ratio of 0.5.
B. A monoclonal arc seen with monospecific antiserum should not be seen with polyvalent (total) anti-immunoglobulin serum.
C. CSF should be concentrated 50- to100-fold before performing IEP.
D. When oligoclonal bands are seen in the CSF, they must also be present in serum to indicate multiple sclerosis.

Chemistry/Apply knowledge of special procedures/Immunoelectrophoresis/2

35. Which of the following statements regarding IEP is true?
A. Oligoclonal banding is seen in the CSF of more than 90% of multiple sclerosis cases.
B. The Bence Jones protein heat test is specific for monoclonal light chains.
C. Light chains found in urine are always derived from monoclonal protein.
D. The IgA band is usually cathodal to the IgG precipitin band.

Chemistry/Correlate clinical and laboratory data/ Immunoelectrophoresis/2

36. Which isoenzyme of creatine kinase (CK) has the fastest electrophoretic mobility at pH 8.6?
A. MM
B. MB
C. BB
D. Macro CK

Chemistry/Apply principles of special procedures/Electrophoresis/1

37. Macro CK-1 results from:
A. Formation of a complex between CK-1 (BB) and immunoglobulin
B. A polymer of CK-1 (BB)
C. Enzymatic conversion of an isoform of CK-3 (MM)
D. An aggregate of CK-3 (MM)

Chemistry/Apply knowledge to identify sources of error/Electrophoresis/1

Answers to Questions 33–37

33. B In double immunodiffusion (Ouchterlony), the molecules of lower molecular weight move fastest through the gel causing a visible precipitin arc when antigen and antibody approach equivalence. At equivalence the precipitin arc remains stationary. If the concentration of antisera is constant, the distance of the precipitin arc from the antigen well is proportional to antigen concentration.

34. C Any monoclonal precipitin band formed when heavy or light chain specific antiserum reacts with the sample should also be found in the same position when the sample is tested against polyvalent antihuman Ig. Normally, immunoglobulins with κ light chains outnumber those with λ chains 2:1. In a monoclonal gammopathy this ratio always heavily favors the light chain type of M protein. A diagnosis of multiple sclerosis is usually confirmed by demonstration of oligoclonal banding in the CSF, which is *not* present in the serum. CSF is usually concentrated 50–100 times to increase sensitivity.

35. A The α heavy chain is more acidic than γ or μ chains, giving IgA a greater net negative charge at alkaline pH. The IgA precipitin arc is anodal to the IgG or IgM arc. In hepatic cirrhosis the β-γ bridging observed on serum protein electrophoresis results from increased IgA. Light chains in the form of Fab fragments are often found in increased amounts in the urine of patients with polyclonal gammopathies, especially from patients with an autoimmune disease. These can cause a positive Bence Jones test and will produce a polyclonal (spread-out) appearance on IEP or IFE films.

36. C CK isoenzymes are dimers composed of M and B subunits. The B subunit is more acidic resulting in CK-1 (BB) migrating the farthest toward the anode followed by CK-2 (MB), then CK-3 (MM). CK-1 migrates in the prealbumin zone, CK-2 after albumin, and CK-3 between the β and γ zones. It is important to recognize the yellow fluorescence of albumin so that it is not confused with CK-1.

37. A Macro CK-1 is rarely found in the serum (most often seen in elderly patients) and has no clinical significance. When present, macro CK-1 can be recognized by electrophoresis and is located between CK-2 and CK-3. It may coelute with CK-2 (MB) when column chromatography is used to measure CK isoenzymes.

38. Select the polypeptide chain combination designated LD-5.
A. M_4
B. M_2H_2
C. MH_3
D. H_4

Chemistry/Apply knowledge of fundamental biological characteristics/Isoenzyme/1

39. In reference to serum protein bands, select the position of the LD-1 band following electrophoresis of LD isoenzymes at pH 8.6.
A. Anodal to albumin
B. Between albumin and α_1-globulin
C. Between α_2- and β-globulin
D. Between β- and γ-globulin

Chemistry/Apply principles of special procedures/Electrophoresis/1

40. Detection of LD and CK isoenzyme bands following electrophoresis is facilitated by:
A. Adding substrates to the gel and measuring catalytic activity
B. Precipitation using antisera against the polypeptide chains of the enzyme
C. Staining with a dye specific for the isoenzymes
D. Elution of other proteins from the gel followed by precipitation with sulfosalicylic acid

Chemistry/Apply principles of special procedures/Electrophoresis/1

41. Select the order of mobility of lipoproteins electrophoresed on cellulose acetate or agarose at pH 8.6.
A. $-$ Chylomicrons $\rightarrow$ pre-β $\rightarrow$ β $\rightarrow$ α $+$
B. $-$ β $\rightarrow$ pre-β $\rightarrow$ α $\rightarrow$ chylomicrons $+$
C. $-$ Chylomicrons $\rightarrow$ β $\rightarrow$ pre-β $\rightarrow$ α $+$
D. $-$ α $\rightarrow$ β $\rightarrow$ pre-β $\rightarrow$ chylomicrons $+$

Chemistry/Apply principles of special procedures/Electrophoresis/1

42. Following ultracentrifugation of plasma, which fraction correlates with pre-β lipoprotein?
A. Very low-density lipoprotein (VLDL)
B. Low-density lipoprotein (LDL)
C. High-density lipoprotein (HDL)
D. Chylomicrons

Chemistry/Apply principles of special procedures/Lipoproteins/2

43. Select the lipoprotein fraction that carries most of the endogenous triglycerides.
A. VLDL
B. LDL
C. HDL
D. Chylomicrons

Chemistry/Correlate laboratory data with physiologic processes/Lipoproteins/2

44. The protein composition of HDL is what percentage by weight?
A. Less than 2%
B. 25%
C. 50%
D. 90%

Chemistry/Correlate laboratory data with physiological processes/Lipoproteins/1

Answers to Questions 38–44

38. **A** Lactate dehydrogenase (LD) is a tetramer that can comprise two polypeptide chains designated H (heart) and M (muscle). These can assemble in five ways, giving the five isoenzymes named LD-1 (H_4), LD-2 (H_3M), LD-3 (H_2M_2), LD-4 (HM_3), and LD-5 (M_4).

39. **B** The H chain is more negative than the M chain at pH 8.6, permitting LD-1 to migrate farthest toward the anode. LD-1 is located between the albumin and α_1 zones, LD-2 between the α_1 and α_2 zones, LD-3 between the α_2 and β zones, LD-4 in the fast γ, and LD-5 in the slow γ zone.

40. **A** Quantitation of isoenzymes is made after electrophoresis by saturating the pores of agarose or cellulose acetate with substrate and incubating at 37°–45°C. Bands form on the gel where the isoenzymes are located on the medium. Densitometric scanning allows relative (%) concentration to be calculated. Measuring the fluorescence of NADH permits detection equivalent to about 2–3 IU/L enzyme activity.

41. **C** Although pre-β lipoprotein is lower in density than β lipoprotein, it migrates faster on agarose or cellulose acetate owing to its more negative apoprotein composition. When lipoproteins are separated on polyacrylamide gel, pre-β moves slower than β lipoprotein. Molecular sieving causes migration to correlate with lipoprotein density when PAGE is used.

42. **A** The VLDL migrates in the pre-β zone. The LDL is made in the liver by enzymatic cleavage of VLDL. The VLDL is about 50% triglyceride, but LDL is only 10% triglyceride by weight. The LDL is more dense than VLDL, but less negatively charged, causing it to migrate in the β region.

43. **A** The VLDL is formed in the liver largely from chylomicron remnants and hepatic-derived triglycerides. Therefore, the VLDL transports the majority of endogenous triglycerides, while the triglycerides of chylomicrons are derived entirely from dietary absorption.

44. **C** About 50% of the weight of HDL is protein, largely Apo A-I and Apo A-II. The HDL is about 30% phospholipid and 20% cholesterol by weight. The HDL binds and esterifies free cholesterol from cells and transports it to the liver where it can be eliminated in the bile.

45. Broad (floating) β lipoprotein occurs in type _____
lipoproteinemia and consists of _____.
A. I   Chylomicrons
B. II   VLDL
C. III   IDL
D. IV   VLDL

*Chemistry/Correlate clinical and laboratory data/
Lipoproteins/2*

46. Which of the following is associated with Tangier
disease?
A. Apoprotein C-II deficiency
B. Heparin-activated capillary lipoprotein lipase
deficiency
C. Apoprotein C-II activated lipase
D. Apoprotein A-I deficiency

*Chemistry/Correlate clinical and laboratory data/
Lipoproteins/2*

47. Which of the following formulas correctly estimates
the VLDL cholesterol?
A. Serum triglycerides divided by 5
B. Total cholesterol minus HDL cholesterol
C. Total cholesterol multiplied by 0.25
D. LDL cholesterol multiplied by 0.25

Chemistry/Calculate/Lipoproteins/1

48. Select the cutoff for serum total cholesterol recom-
mended by the National Cholesterol Education
Program.
A. 200 mg/dL
B. 250 mg/dL
C. 300 mg/dL
D. 300 mg/dL for adult men and 250 mg/dL for
adult women

*Chemistry/Evaluate laboratory data to recognize
health and disease states/Lipids/1*

49. Select the cutoff for serum LDL cholesterol recom-
mended by the National Cholesterol Education
Program.
A. 80 mg/dL
B. 160 mg/dL
C. 190 mg/dL
D. 220 mg/dL

*Chemistry/Evaluate laboratory data to recognize
health and disease states/Lipids/1*

50. Which apoprotein is *inversely* related to risk for
coronary heart disease?
A. Apoprotein A-I
B. Apoprotein B
C. Apoprotein C-II
D. Apoprotein E-IV

*Chemistry/Correlate clinical and laboratory data/
Lipoproteins/2*

Answers to Questions 45–50

45. **C** Floating β is a rare hyperlipoproteinemia
inherited as an autosomal recessive trait. It results
from a failure to convert VLDL to LDL causing IDL
to accumulate. Defective clearance of IDL is
thought to result from deficiency of Apo E-III. The
IDL has a density of about 1.006–1.020 causing it to
float on the 1.063 density potassium bromide
solution used to recover LDL by ultracentrifugation.

46. **D** Deficiency of peripheral (blood) lipoprotein
lipase is the cause of type I and is also associated
with type V hyperlipoproteinemia. Deficiencies of
heparin activated lipase, Apo C-II activated lipase,
and Apo C-II have been described. All result in
decreased hydrolysis of chylomicrons leading to
chylomicronemia. Deficiency of Apo A-I is seen in
Tangier disease, a familial hypocholesterolemia
with deficient or absent HDL.

47. **A** In a patient without chylomicronemia and a
triglyceride level below 400 mg/dL, the serum
triglycerides reflect the amount of plasma VLDL.
Because the ratio of cholesterol to triglyceride in
VLDL is between 1:5 and 1:6, the serum triglyceride
divided by 5 estimates the cholesterol in VLDL.
Some laboratories prefer to use triglyceride divided
by 6 instead of triglyceride divided by 5 to estimate
VLDL cholesterol. In patients with hypertriglyc-
eridemia, the LDL cholesterol should be measured
rather than calculated. This can be done by ultracentrifugation, or by a "direct" LDL cholesterol
assay. The "direct" assay uses polyclonal antibodies
bound to latex beads to precipitate lipoproteins
containing apo-AI and apo-E, leaving the LDL
fraction in the supernatant.

48. **A** The 50th percentile for total cholesterol, 200
mg/dL, is the recommended cutoff for total cholesterol screening. Patients with a serum cholesterol
exceeding 200 mg/dL are evaluated for risk factors
and LDL cholesterol before determining whether
follow-up tests, or dietary or drug intervention may
be needed.

49. **B** When total cholesterol exceeds 200 mg/dL, the
LDL cholesterol is used to determine whether intervention is appropriate. An LDL cholesterol
greater than 160 mg/dL and two risk factors for
coronary heart disease indicate a need for dietary
intervention. An LDL cholesterol greater than 200
mg/dL indicates the need for drug intervention.

50. **A** Apoprotein A-I and Apo A-II are the principal
apoproteins of HDL, and low Apo A-I has a high
correlation with atherosclerosis. Conversely, Apo
B100 is the principal apoprotein of LDL, and an
elevated level is a major risk factor in developing
coronary heart disease. Apoprotein assays are not
recommended as screening tests because they are
not as well standardized as total cholesterol
assays.

51. Which of the following secondary hyperlipoproteinemias is most consistently associated with type II lipoprotein phenotype?
A. Hypothyroidism
B. Hepatobiliary obstruction
C. Oral contraceptive therapy
D. Diabetes mellitus

*Chemistry/Correlate clinical and laboratory data/
Lipoproteins/2*

52. Which of the following diseases is caused by a deficiency of sphingomyelinase?
A. Gaucher's disease
B. Fabry's disease
C. Niemann-Pick disease
D. Tay-Sachs disease

*Chemistry/Correlate clinical and laboratory data/
Lipids/2*

53. Which method is considered the candidate reference method for triglyceride measurement?
A. Glycerol kinase-ultraviolet
B. CDC modification of Van Handel and Zilversmit
C. Hantzsch condensation
D. Glycerol kinase coupled to peroxidase

*Chemistry/Apply principles of basic laboratory
procedures/Lipids/1*

54. Which of the following enzymes is common to all enzymatic methods for triglyceride measurement?
A. Glycerol phosphate oxidase
B. Glycerol phosphate dehydrogenase
C. Glycerol kinase
D. Pyruvate kinase

*Chemistry/Apply principles of basic laboratory
procedures/Lipids/2*

Answers to Questions 51–54

51. **A** The conditions listed are very commonly encountered causes of secondary hyperlipoproteinemia. Oral contraceptives, pregnancy, and estrogens may cause hyperlipoproteinemia, which is usually a phenocopy of type IV (high VLDL and endogenous triglycerides). Hypothyroidism and obstructive hepatobiliary diseases are usually associated with type II (high LDL and hypercholesterolemia). Diabetes mellitus and chronic pancreatitis may produce phenocopies of type I, IV, or V.

52. **C** The diseases mentioned result from inborn errors of lipid metabolism (lipidoses) caused by deficiency of an enzyme needed for lipid degradation. Specific lipids accumulate in the lysosomes. Niemann-Pick disease results from a deficiency of sphingomyelinase; Gaucher's from β-glucocerebrosidase; Fabry's (sex-linked) from α-galactosidase A; Tay-Sachs from N acetylglucosaminidase A.

53. **B** Enzymatic methods for triglyceride measurement are widely used because they eliminate the need for extraction and saponification. However, they are subject to positive interference from endogenous glycerol and variations in the efficiency of lipase, which can result in under or overestimation of triglycerides. The most accurate method for triglyceride assay is the nonenzymatic method based upon reaction of formaldehyde with chromotropic acid. In this method, extraction with silicic acid and chloroform separates triglycerides from lipoproteins, phospholipids, and glycerol. Saponification with alcoholic potassium hydroxide (KOH) produces glycerol, which is oxidized to formaldehyde by periodate. The formaldehyde reacts with chromotropic acid to form a pink product. The Centers for Disease Control and Prevention (CDC) method uses a 2:1 ratio of unsaturated (triolein) to saturated (tripalmitin) triglycerides to calibrate the assay because this represents the ratio normally found in serum.

54. **C** All enzymatic triglyceride methods require lipase to hydrolyze triglycerides, and glycerol kinase to phosphorylate glycerol, forming glycerol-3-phosphate. The two most common methods measure the glycerol-3-phosphate produced.

$$\text{Glycerol-3-phosphate} + NAD^+ \xrightarrow{\text{Glycerol phosphate dehydrogenase}} \text{dihydroxyacetone phosphate} + NADH + H^+$$

$$\text{2. Glycerol-3-phosphate} + O_2 \xrightarrow{\text{Glycerol phosphate oxidase}} \text{dihydroxyacetone phosphate} + H_2O_2$$

$$H_2O_2 + \text{phenol} + \text{4-aminophenazone} \xrightarrow{\text{Peroxidase}} \text{quinone imine dye} + H_2O$$

55. Select the reagent needed in the coupling enzyme reaction used to generate a colored product in the cholesterol oxidase method for cholesterol.
A. Cholestahexaene
B. H_2O_2
C. Phenol
D. Cholest-4-ene-3-one

Chemistry/Apply knowledge of basic laboratory procedures/Lipids/2

56. Which of the following substances causes interference with the oxidation of cholesterol in the Liebermann-Burchard reaction?
A. Acetic acid
B. Sulfuric acid
C. Acetic anhydride
D. H_2O

Chemistry/Apply knowledge of basic laboratory procedures/Lipids/1

57. Which of the following methods for HDL cholesterol is the reference method?
A. Manganese-heparin
B. Magnesium-phosphotungstate
C. Magnesium-dextran
D. Ultracentrifugation

Chemistry/Apply knowledge of basic laboratory procedures/Lipids/1

58. Cholesterol esterase is used in enzymatic assays to:
A. Oxidize cholesterol to form peroxide
B. Hydrolyze fatty acids bound to the third carbon atom of cholesterol
C. Separate cholesterol from apoproteins A-I and A-II by hydrolysis
D. Reduce NAD^+ to NADH

Chemistry/Apply knowledge of basic laboratory procedures/Lipids/2

59. HDL cholesterol is measured on a 12-hour fasting serum sample from a patient with a triglyceride level of 950 mg/dL. The HDL is performed by the magnesium-dextran method, and the result is 48 mg/dL. The serum is diluted 1:2 with saline, and the assay is repeated by the same method. The new result is 32 mg/dL. What is the most likely explanation of this difference?
A. An error was made in performing the dilution.
B. The calculation of HDL cholesterol did not make allowance for the dilution.
C. The diluent used should have been magnesium chloride and sodium phosphotungstate.
D. High triglycerides prevented complete precipitation of VLDL in the undiluted sample.

Chemistry/Apply knowledge to recognize sources of error/Lipids/3

Answers to Questions 55–59

55. **C** Cholesterol oxidase catalyzes the oxidation of free cholesterol at the C3-OH group, forming cholest-4-ene-3-one and H_2O_2. The peroxide is used in a peroxidase reaction to oxidize a dye (e.g., 4-aminophenazone), which couples to phenol, forming a red quinone imine complex. The same coupling (indicator) reaction is used in the Trinder glucose oxidase method.

56. **D** The Liebermann-Burchard reaction depends upon dehydration of cholesterol and oxidation by sulfuric acid to form cholestahexaene sulfonic acid. For complete dehydration the reagent must be anhydrous. The Liebermann-Burchard reaction is nonspecific and is used only in the Abell-Kendall method after cholesterol is extracted to remove interferents and saponified to form free cholesterol.

57. **D** Ultracentrifugation of plasma in a potassium bromide solution with a density of 1.063 is used to separate HDL from LDL and VLDL. The HDL fraction is transferred from the bottom of the tube and assayed for cholesterol content by the Abell-Kendall method. The remaining three methods rely upon selective precipitation or magnetic removal of lipoproteins containing apoprotein B using a polyanionic solution. Magnesium-dextran and magnesium-phosphotungstate tend to give slightly lower results than manganese-heparin because they precipitate some HDL. A "direct HDL" can also be performed using cholesterol esterase and oxidase enzymes that are conjugated to polyethylene glycol. In the presence of sulfated cyclodextrin, the polyethylene glycol (PEG)-modified enzymes display greatly reduced catalytic activity against the cholesterol of LDL, VLDL, and chylomicrons. The method is sufficiently selective to measure HDL cholesterol.

58. **B** Approximately two-thirds of the serum cholesterol has a fatty acid esterified to the hydroxyl group of the third carbon atom of the cholesterol molecule. Cholesterol esterase hydrolyzes fatty acids and is required because cholesterol oxidase cannot utilize esterified cholesterol as a substrate.

59. **D** When serum triglycerides are elevated (>400 mg/dL), incomplete removal of lipoproteins containing apoprotein B is the most commonly encountered source of error. In this instance the HDL cholesterol should be determined by ultracentrifugation or the specimen diluted with saline before analysis. An alternative approach is to process the supernatant a second time with the pretreatment reagents provided the dilution does not result in an absorbance that is below the detection limit. Calculations of LDL cholesterol are subject to error as well when triglycerides are greater than 400 mg/dL.

60. What is the purpose of the saponification step used in the Abell-Kendall method for cholesterol measurement?
A. Remove phospholipids
B. Reduce sterol molecules structurally similar to cholesterol
C. Convert cholesterol esters to free cholesterol
D. Remove proteins that can interfere with color formation

Chemistry/Apply knowledge of basic laboratory procedures/Lipids/2

61. Lipoprotein (a), or Lp(a), is significant when elevated in serum because it:
A. Is an independent risk factor for atherosclerosis
B. Blocks the clearance of VLDLs
C. Displaces apo-A1 from HDLs
D. Is linked closely to a gene for obesity

Chemistry/Apply knowledge of fundamental biological characteristics/Lipoproteins/1

62. Which type of dietary fatty acid is *not* associated with an increase in serum LDL cholesterol production?
A. Monosaturated *trans* fatty acids
B. Saturated fatty acids
C. Monosaturated *cis* fatty acids
D. Monosaturated *trans* Ω-9 fatty acids

Chemistry/Apply knowledge of fundamental biological characteristics/Fatty acids/1

63. What is the clinical utility of testing for serum prealbumin?
A. Low levels are associated with increased free cortisol.
B. High levels are an indicator of acute inflammation.
C. Serial low levels indicate compromised nutritional status.
D. Levels correlate with glomerular injury in patients with diabetes mellitus.

Chemistry/Apply knowledge of fundamental biological characteristics/Proteins/1

64. Which serum protein should be measured in a patient suspected of having Wilson's disease?
A. Hemopexin
B. α_1-Antitrypsin
C. Haptoglobin
D. Ceruloplasmin

Chemistry/Apply knowledge of fundamental biological characteristics/Proteins/2

Answers to Questions 60–64

60. **C** Saponification is performed to hydrolyze the fatty acid esters of cholesterol, forming free cholesterol. This is required because the Liebermann-Burchard reagent reacts more intensely with cholesterol esters than with free cholesterol. Saponification is followed by extraction of cholesterol in petroleum ether to separate it from proteins and interfering substances. The Abell-Kendall method remains the reference method because differences in esterase activity and interference in the peroxidase step are potential sources of error in enzymatic assays.

61. **A** Lp(a) is a complex of apoB-100 and protein (a) formed by a disulfide bridge. The complex is structurally similar to plasminogen and is thought to promote coronary heart disease by interfering with the normal fibrinolytic process.

62. **C** Polyunsaturated and *cis* monosaturated fatty acids are not associated with increased production of LDL cholesterol. On the other hand, saturated and *trans* monosaturated fatty acids are both associated with increased LDL. *Cis* fatty acids are those in which the H atoms belonging to the double-bonded carbons are on the same side of the molecule. Ω-9 (n-9) fatty acids are those with a double bond located 9 carbons from the terminal methyl group. Ω Fatty acids are associated with increased cholesterol, if the hydrogens attached to the double-bonded carbons are in the *trans* position.

63. **C** Prealbumin (also called transthyretin) is a small protein with a half-life of only 2 days. Serum levels fall rapidly in patients with deficient protein nutrition. As a result, prealbumin is used to detect malnutrition and to measure the patient's response to dietary supplementation. The cutoff used to identify nutritional deficiency in elderly patients is usually 11 mg/dL.

64. **D** α_1-Antitrypsin, haptoglobin, and ceruloplasmin are acute phase proteins and will be increased in inflammatory diseases. Ceruloplasmin is an α_2-globulin that binds the majority of the serum copper. Levels are low in almost all patients with Wilson's disease, an autosomal recessive disorder caused by accumulation of copper in liver, brain, kidney, and other tissues. Low ceruloplasmin may occur in patients with nephrosis, malnutrition, and hepatobiliary disease. Therefore, the diagnosis of Wilson's disease is made by demonstrating decreased ceruloplasmin, increased serum and urinary copper, and the presence of Kayser-Fleischer rings (brown deposits at the edge of the cornea).

65. A patient with hemolytic-uremic syndrome associated with septicemia has a haptoglobin level that is normal although the plasma free Hgb is elevated and hemoglobinuria is present. Which test would be more appropriate than haptoglobin to measure this patient's hemolytic episode?
A. Hemopexin
B. α_1-Antitrypsin
C. C-reactive protein
D. Transferrin

Chemistry/Apply knowledge to recognize inconsistent laboratory results/Proteins/3

Answer to Question 65

65. **A** Hemopexin is a small globulin that binds to free heme. Haptoglobin is an α_2-globulin that binds to free Hgb and disappears from the serum when intravascular hemolysis produces more than 3 g of free plasma Hgb. However, haptoglobin is an acute phase protein, and hepatic production and release are increased in response to acute infections. The normal serum haptoglobin is most likely the result of increased synthesis and would not accurately estimate the hemolytic episode in this patient.

Clinical Enzymology

1. An IU of enzyme activity is the quantity of enzyme that:
   A. Converts 1 μmol of substrate to product per liter
   B. Forms 1 mg of product per deciliter
   C. Converts 1 mmol of substrate to product per minute
   D. Forms 1 mmol of product per liter

   Chemistry/Apply principles of basic laboratory procedures/Enzymes/1

2. Which statement below describes a nonkinetic enzyme assay?
   A. Initial absorbance is measured followed by a second reading after 5 minutes.
   B. Absorbance is measured at 10-second intervals for 100 seconds.
   C. Absorbance is monitored continuously for 1 minute using a chart recorder.
   D. Reflectance is measured from a xenon source lamp pulsing at 60 Hz.

   Chemistry/Apply principles of basic laboratory procedures/Enzymes/2

3. Which of the following statements regarding enzymatic reactions is true?
   A. The enzyme shifts the equilibrium of the reaction to the right.
   B. The enzyme alters the equilibrium constant of the reaction.
   C. The enzyme increases the rate of the reaction.
   D. The enzyme alters the energy difference between reactants and products.

   Chemistry/Apply knowledge of fundamental biological characteristics/Enzymes/1

4. Which statement about enzymes is true?
   A. An enzyme alters the Gibb's free energy of the reaction.
   B. Enzymes cause a reaction with a positive free energy to occur spontaneously.
   C. An enzyme's natural substrate has the highest Km.
   D. A competitive inhibitor will alter the apparent Km of the reaction.

   Chemistry/Apply knowledge of fundamental biological characteristics/Enzymes/2

Answers to Questions 1–4

1. **C** The IU is a rate expressed in micromoles per minute. Activity is reported as IUs per liter (IU/L) or mIU/mL. The SI unit for enzyme activity is the katal (1 katal converts 1 mol of substrate to product in 1 second).

2. **A** A kinetic assay uses several evenly spaced absorbance measurements to calculate the change in absorbance per unit time. A constant change in absorbance per unit of time occurs only when the rate of the reaction is zero order (independent of substrate concentration). Enzyme activity is proportional to rate only under zero-order conditions.

3. **C** An enzyme will accelerate the rate of a reaction, reducing the time required to reach equilibrium. The concentration of reactants and products at equilibrium will be the same with or without the enzyme.

4. **D** Enzymes alter the energy of activation by forming a metastable intermediate, the enzyme substrate complex. Enzymes do not alter the free energy or direction of a reaction. Competitive inhibitors bind to the active site where the enzyme binds substrate and are overcome by increasing the substrate concentration.

5. Which substrate concentration is needed to achieve zero-order conditions?
A. Greater than $99 \times Km$
B. $[S] = Km$
C. Less than $10 \times Km$
D. $[S] = 0$

Chemistry/Select reagents/Enzymes/3

6. Which statement below is true?
A. Apoenzyme + prosthetic group = holoenzyme.
B. A coenzyme is an inorganic molecule required for activity.
C. Cofactors are as tightly bound to the enzyme as a prosthetic group.
D. All of the above.

Chemistry/Apply fundamental biological characteristics/Enzymes/2

7. Which of the following statements about enzymatic reactions is true?
A. NADH has absorbance maximas at 340 and 366 nm.
B. Enzyme concentration must be in excess to achieve zero-order kinetics.
C. Rate is proportional to substrate concentration in a zero-order reaction.
D. Accumulation of the product increases the reaction rate.

Chemistry/Apply principles of basic laboratory procedures/Enzymes/2

8. The increase in the level of serum enzymes used to detect cholestatic liver disease is caused mainly by:
A. Enzyme release from dead cells
B. Leakage from cells with altered membrane permeability
C. Decreased perfusion of the tissue
D. Increased production and secretion by cells

Chemistry/Correlate laboratory data with physiologic processes/Enzymes/2

9. Which enzyme below is considered most tissue-specific?
A. CK
B. Amylase
C. ALP
D. Alcohol dehydrogenase

Chemistry/Correlate clinical and laboratory data/Enzymes/2

10. Which of the following enzymes is activated by calcium ions?
A. CK
B. Amylase
C. ALP
D. LD

Chemistry/Apply knowledge of fundamental biological characteristics/Enzymes/2

Answers to Questions 5–10

5. **A** A zero-order reaction rate is independent of substrate concentration because there is sufficient substrate to saturate the enzyme. $V = V_{max} \times [S]/Km + [S]$ where V = velocity, V_{max} = maximum velocity, $[S]$ = substrate concentration, and Km = substrate concentration required to give $1/2$ V_{max}. If $[S] >>> Km$, then the Km can be ignored. $V = V_{max} \times [S]/[S]$ or velocity approaches maximum and is independent of substrate concentration.

6. **A** A coenzyme is an organic molecule required for full enzyme activity. A prosthetic group is a coenzyme that is tightly bound to the apoenzyme and is required for activity. Cofactors are inorganic atoms or molecules needed for full catalytic activity. Pyridoxyl-5′-phosphate is a prosthetic group for ALT and AST. Consequently, patients with low levels of pyridoxal-5′-phosphate (P-5′-P) (vitamin B_6 deficiency) may have reduced transaminase activity *in vitro*.

7. **A** Most enzymes are measured by monitoring the rate of absorbance change at 340 nm as NADH is produced or consumed. This rate will be proportional to enzyme activity when substrate is in excess. When the enzyme is present in excess, the initial reaction rate will be proportional to substrate concentration. This condition, called a first-order reaction, is needed when the enzyme is used as a reagent to measure a specific analyte.

8. **D** The amount of enzyme in the serum can be increased by necrosis, altered permeability, secretion, or synthesis. It is also dependent upon tissue perfusion, enzyme half-life, molecular size, and location of the enzyme within the cell. Most enzymes are liberated by necrosis, but a few, such as ALP and γ-glutamyltransferase, are produced and secreted at a greater rate in obstructive liver disease.

9. **D** No enzyme is truly tissue specific and diagnostic accuracy depends upon recognizing the pattern of change produced by different diseases. This includes the quantity of enzyme released, characteristic rise and return to normal, the isoenzyme(s) released, and the concomitant changes of other enzymes. Alanine aminotransferase and alcohol dehydrogenase are primarily increased in necrotic liver disease.

10. **B** Most enzymes require metals as activators or cofactors. CK and ALP require Mg^{2+} for full activity, and amylase requires Ca^{2+}. Metals required for activity should be components of the substrate used for enzyme analysis. The substrate must also contain anions required (e.g., Cl^- for amylase) and should not contain inhibiting cations or anions (e.g., Zn^{2+} and Mn^{2+} for CK).

11. Which statement about methods for measuring LD is true?
    A. The formation of pyruvate from lactate (forward reaction) generates NAD^+.
    B. The pyruvate to lactate reaction proceeds at about twice the rate as the forward reaction.
    C. The lactate to pyruvate reaction is optimized at pH 7.4.
    D. The negative rate reaction is preferred.

    Chemistry/Apply principles of basic laboratory dehydrogenase/2

12. Which of the following enzymes is a transferase?
    A. ALP
    B. CK
    C. Amylase
    D. LD

    Chemistry/Apply knowledge of fundamental biological characteristics/Enzymes/2

13. Which LD isoenzyme was originally described as α hydroxybutyrate dehydrogenase (HBDH)?
    A. LD-1
    B. LD-2
    C. LD-4
    D. LD-5

    Chemistry/Apply knowledge of fundamental biological characteristics/Lactate dehydrogenase/1

14. Which condition produces the highest elevation of serum LD?
    A. Pernicious anemia
    B. Myocardial infarction
    C. Acute hepatitis
    D. Muscular dystrophy

    Chemistry/Correlate clinical and laboratory data/Lactate dehydrogenase/2

15. Following an AMI, activity of LD usually peaks:
    A. Within 1 day postinfarction and returns to normal after 3 days
    B. Twenty-four to 36 hours postinfarction and returns to normal after 3 days
    C. Forty-eight hours postinfarction and returns to normal after 4 days
    D. Three days postinfarction and returns to normal after 1 week

    Chemistry/Correlate clinical and laboratory data/Creatine kinase/2

16. Which statement regarding LD isoenzymes is true?
    A. An LD-1:LD-2 ratio greater than 1.0 is specific evidence of AMI.
    B. Malignancy usually causes an increase in LD-2, LD-3, LD-4.
    C. Hepatic injury is associated with increases in LD-4 and LD-5.
    D. LD-3 is normally the isoenzyme in highest concentration in serum.

    Chemistry/Evaluate laboratory data to recognize health and disease states/Lactate dehydrogenase/2

Answers to Questions 11–16

11. **B** Although the rate of the reverse reaction (P → L) is faster, the L → P reaction is more popular because it produces a positive rate (generates NADH), is not subject to product inhibition, and is highly linear. The pH optimum for the forward reaction is approximately 8.8.

12. **B** Enzymes are identified by a numeric system called the EC (Enzyme Commission) number. The first number refers to the class of the enzyme. There are six classes; in order these are oxidoreductases, transferases, hydrolases, lyases, isomerases, and ligases. Dehydrogenases are oxidoreductases whereas kinases and transaminases are transferases. CK is EC number 2.7.3.2, which distinguishes it from other kinases.

13. **A** LD-1 has a relatively low *Km* for the substrate α hydroxybutyrate, and oxidizes it, forming α ketobutyrate and NADH. The HBDH activity was measured as an aid to diagnosis of MI but has been replaced by measurements of LD-1 based upon electrophoresis or immunoassay.

14. **A** Serum LD levels are highest in pernicious anemia reaching 10–50 times the upper reference limit (URL) as a result of intramedullary hemolysis. Moderate elevations (2–10 × URL) are seen in acute myocardial infarction (AMI), necrotic liver disease, and muscular dystrophy. Slight increases (2–3 ×URL) are seen in obstructive liver disease.

15. **D** CK is the first enzyme to rise above the reference range after an AMI, peaking 18–36 hours and returning to normal within 3 days. AST follows, peaking 24–48 hours postinfarction and returning to normal in 4–5 days. This pattern of CK → AST → LD is specific for AMI but has been replaced by serial measurements of myoglobin, troponin I, and CK-MB, which usually can detect and confirm the AMI within 6–8 hours. The troponins are three proteins (T, I, and C) that comprise the thin filaments of cardiac and skeletal muscle fibers. Both troponin I (TNI) and troponin T(TNT) have unique sequences that differ between cardiac and skeletal muscle. Antibodies specific for the cardiac isoforms can be used to measure their concentration in serum.

16. **C** LD-1 is not a specific marker for MI and is increased in hemolytic anemia, renal infarction, crush injury, and the late stages of muscular dystrophy. Malignancy causes variable LD isoenzyme increases appearing most often as a zone 3 pattern (high LD-4 and LD-5). Hepatic injury causes increases in LD-4 and LD-5, which normally account for less than 15% of the total LD activity. LD-2 is the fraction in highest concentration in normal serum, accounting for approximately 25%–40% of total LD activity.

17. In which type of liver disease would you expect the greatest elevation of LD?
A. Toxic hepatitis
B. Alcoholic hepatitis
C. Cirrhosis
D. Acute viral hepatitis

Chemistry/Correlate clinical and laboratory data/Lactate dehydrogenase/2

18. The LD pleural fluid:serum ratio for a transudative fluid is usually:
A. 3:1 or higher
B. 2:1
C. 1:1
D. 1:2 or less

Chemistry/Correlate clinical and laboratory data/Lactate dehydrogenase/2

19. Which of the following conditions will interfere with the measurement of LD?
A. Slight hemolysis during sample collection
B. Storage at 4°C for 3 days
C. Storage at room temperture for 16 hours
D. Use of plasma collected in heparin

Chemistry/Apply knowledge to recognize sources of error/Lactate dehydrogenase/3

20. In the Oliver-Rosalki method the reverse reaction is used to measure CK activity. The enzyme(s) used in the coupling reactions is (are):
A. Hexokinase and G-6-PD
B. Pyruvate kinase and LD
C. Luciferase
D. Adenylate kinase

Chemistry/Apply knowledge of basic laboratory procedures/Creatine kinase/2

21. In the Oliver-Rosalki method for CK, adenosine monophosphate (AMP) is added to the substrate in order to:
A. Inhibit adenylate kinase
B. Block the oxidation of glutathione
C. Increase the amount of ADP that is available
D. Block the action of diadenosine pentaphosphate

Chemistry/Apply principles of basic laboratory procedures/Creatine kinase/2

Answers to Questions 17–21

17. **A** Liver disease produces an elevated LD-4 and LD-5. Levels may reach up to 10 times the URL in toxic hepatitis and in hepatoma. However, LD levels are lower in viral hepatitis (2–5 × URL) and only slightly elevated in cirrhosis (2–3 × URL).

18. **D** The LD activity of body fluids is normally less than serum, and a fluid:serum LD greater than 1:2 is highly suggestive of an exudative process. High LD in chest fluid is often caused by lung malignancy, metastatic carcinoma, Hodgkin's disease, and leukemia.

19. **A** RBCs are rich in LD-1 and LD-2, and even slight hemolysis will falsely elevate results. Hemolytic, megaloblastic, and pernicious anemias are associated with LD levels of 10–50 times the URL. LD is stable for 2 days at room temperature or 1 week at 4°C; however, freezing causes deterioration of LD-5. The activity of LD is inhibited by EDTA, which binds divalent cations; serum or heparinized plasma should be used.

20. **A** The Oliver-Rosalki method for CK is based upon the formation of ATP from creatine phosphate. Hexokinase catalyzes the phosphorylation of glucose by ATP. This produces glucose-6-PO_4 and adenosine diphosphate (ADP). The glucose-6-PO_4 is oxidized to 6-phosphogluconate as $NADP^+$ is reduced to NADPH.

$$ATP + glucose \xrightarrow{Hexokinase} ADP + glucose\text{-}6\text{-}PO_4$$

$$glucose\text{-}6\text{-}PO_4 + NADP^+ \xrightarrow{G\text{-}6\text{-}PD} 6\text{-}phosphogluconate$$

$$+ NADPH + H^+$$

21. **A** Positive interference in the Oliver-Rosalki method can occur when adenylate kinase is present in the serum from hemolysis or damaged tissue. Adenylate kinase hydrolyzes ADP, forming AMP and ATP (2 ADP $\xrightarrow{AK}$ AMP + ATP). This reaction is inhibited by adding AMP and diadenosine pentaphosphate (Ap$_5$A) to the substrate.

22. SITUATION: A specimen for CK performed on an automated analyzer using an optimized Oliver-Rosalki method gives an error flag indicating substrate depletion. The sample is diluted 1:2 and 1:4 by the serial dilution technique and reassayed. After correcting for the dilution, the results are as follows:

1:2 Dilution = 3000 IU/L; 1:4 Dilution = 3600 IU/L

Dilutions are made a second time and assayed again but give identical results. What is the most likely explanation?
A. The serum became contaminated prior to making the 1:4 dilution.
B. The wrong pipet was used to make one of the dilutions.
C. An endogenous competitive inhibitor is present in the serum.
D. An error has been made in calculating the enzyme activity of one of the two dilutions.

Chemistry/Apply knowledge to recognize sources of error/Creatine kinase/3

23. SITUATION: A physician calls to request a CK on a sample already sent to the laboratory for coagulation studies. The sample is 4-hour-old citrated blood and has been stored at 4°C. The plasma shows very slight hemolysis. What is the best course of action and the reason for it?
A. Perform the CK assay on the sample because no interferent is present.
B. Reject the sample because it is slightly hemolyzed.
C. Reject the sample because it has been stored too long.
D. Reject the sample because the citrate will interfere.

Chemistry/Apply knowledge to recognize sources of error/Creatine kinase/3

24. Which of the statements below regarding total CK is true?
A. Levels are unaffected by strenuous exercise.
B. Levels are unaffected by repeated intramuscular injections.
C. Highest levels are seen in Duchenne's muscular dystrophy.
D. The enzyme is highly specific for heart injury.

Chemistry/Evaluate laboratory data to recognize health and disease states/Creatine kinase/2

25. Which of the following statements regarding the clinical use of CK-MB (CK-2) is true?
A. CK-MB becomes elevated before myoglobin and TNI after an AMI.
B. CK-MB levels are normal in cases of cardiac ischemia.
C. Mass unit assays are more sensitive than electrophoretic methods.

D. An elevated CK-MB is always accompanied by an elevated total CK.

Chemistry/Correlate clinical and laboratory data/Creatine kinase/2

Answers to Questions 22–25

22. **C** When a competitive inhibitor is present in the serum, a dilution of the sample will cause an increase in the reaction rate by reducing the concentration of the inhibitor. Dilution of serum frequently increases the activity of CK and amylase. The same effect will occur when a smaller volume of serum is used in the assay because less inhibitor will be present in the reaction mixture.

23. **D** CK activity is lost with excessive storage, the most labile isoenzyme being CK-1. However, CK in serum is stable at room temperature for about 4 hours and up to 1 week at 4°C provided that an optimized method is used. Slight hemolysis does not interfere because CK is absent from RBCs. More significant hemolysis may cause positive interference by contributing ATP, glucose-6-PO_4, and adenylate kinase to the serum. Calcium chelators remove magnesium as well as calcium and should not be used.

24. **C** Total CK is neither sensitive nor specific for AMI. An infarct can occur without causing an elevated total CK. Exercise and intramuscular injections cause a significant increase in total CK. Crush injuries and muscular dystrophy can increase the total CK up to 50 times the URL.

25. **C** Serum myoglobin becomes abnormal within 3 hours after an AMI before TNI and CK-MB. Immunochemical methods for measuring CK-MB are more sensitive than electrophoresis (fluorescent densitometry) and are as sensitive as TNI if a cutoff of 6 μg/L is used. TNI and CK-MB become abnormal 4–6 hours after an AMI and peak within 8 hours. TNI remains elevated for approximately 1 week after an AMI, is not increased in crush injury, and is not as likely to be elevated by renal failure as is CK-MB. There is usually less than 5 U/L CK-MB in the serum of healthy adults, while the total CK ranges from 10 to 110 U/L. Consequently, an abnormal CK-MB can occur in the absence of an elevated total CK.

26. Isoforms of CK are:
   A. Isoenzymes of CK formed from variants of the B subunit
   B. Formed in the circulation by hydrolysis of lysine from CK-MM and CK-MB
   C. Formed only when blood is collected in heparin
   D. Artifacts of electrophoresis caused by attachment to albumin

   Chemistry/Apply knowledge of fundamental biological characteristics/Creatine kinase/2

27. A patient's CK-MB is reported as 18 μg/L and the total CK as 560 IU/L. What is the CK relative index (CKI)?
   A. 0.10%
   B. 3.2%
   C. 10.0%
   D. 30.0%

   Chemistry/Correlate clinical and laboratory data/Creatine kinase/2

28. Differentiation of MI and non-MI causes of increased serum CK-MB is based upon all of the following *except*:
   A. Whether the increase is persistent or transient
   B. Whether the percent as well as IU/L CK-MB is increased
   C. The presence of high levels of other cardiac markers
   D. The serum level of total CK

   Chemistry/Evaluate laboratory data to recognize health and disease states/Creatine kinase/2

29. Which statement about the isoenzymes of CK is true?
   A. Macro CK-1 is formed by immunoglobulins binding to CK-BB.
   B. Macro CK-2 is mitochondrial and composed of different subunits than CK-2.
   C. Double antibody sandwich assays are specific for CK-MB.
   D. All of the above.

   Chemistry/Apply knowledge to identify sources of error/Creatine kinase/2

30. Which of the following statements about the aminotransferases (AST and ALT) is true?
   A. Isoenzymes of AST and ALT are not found in humans.
   B. Both transfer an amino group to α ketoglutarate.
   C. Both require NADP+ as a coenzyme.
   D. Both utilize four carbon amino acids as substrates.

   Chemistry/Apply knowledge of fundamental biological characteristics/Aminotransferase/2

Answers to Questions 26–30

26. **B** Isoforms are modified forms of isoenzymes and exist for CK-MM and MB. They result from the hydrolysis of lysine from the M peptide by carboxypeptidases in the plasma. Removal of lysine results in faster electrophoretic mobility. The isoforms of CK-MM are CK-MM1, CK-MM2, and CK-MM3. Isoforms of CK-MB are designated CK-MB1 and CK-MB2. CK-MM3 and CK-MB2 are the unmodified tissue isoforms and rise within 4 hours after AMI.

27. **B** The CKI is an expression of the percentage of the total CK that is attributed to CK-MB.

$$CKI = \frac{CK\text{-}MB \text{ in } \mu g/L \text{ or } U/L}{Total\ CK \text{ in } IU/L} \times 100$$

The reference range is 0%–4%. Values above 4% point to an increase in CK-MB from cardiac muscle.

28. **D** CK-MB rises 4–6 hours postinfarction and peaks in 16–20 hours. LD-1 rises about 8–12 hours postinfarction and peaks within 2 days. CK-MB returns to normal within 1–3 days, but LD-1 remains elevated for 7–10 days. A sequential rise and fall of CK-MB and LD-1 is a specific marker for AMI. TNT and TNI are also cardiac specific markers. They may become elevated sooner than CK-MB and remain elevated for 7–14 days following an AMI. Absolute CK-MB increases are evaluated cautiously, when CK-MB is less than 5% because noncardiac sources may be responsible.

29. **D** Atypical CK isoenzymes include macro and mitochondrial forms. These have slower electrophoretic mobility than CK-MB and do not interfere with electrophoretic assays. Macro CK-1 will interfere with isoenzyme separation by column chromatography. CK-BB and adenylate kinase interfere with immunoinhibition assays using only a single antibody that blocks the M subunit, but immunologic assays using antibodies to two sites (one to the M and the other to the B subunit) are specific for CK-MB.

30. **B** ALT catalyzes the transfer of an amino group from alanine, a three-carbon amino acid, to α ketoglutarate (2-oxoglutarate), forming pyruvate. AST catalyzes the transfer of an amino group from aspartate (four carbons) to α-ketoglutarate, forming oxaloacetate. The reactions are highly reversible and regulate the flow of aspartate into the urea cycle. Both transaminases require P-5'-P as an intermediate amino acceptor (coenzyme). Cytoplasmic and mitochondrial isoenzymes are produced but are not differentiated in clinical practice.

31. Select the products formed from the forward reaction of AST.
A. Alanine and α-ketoglutarate
B. Oxaloacetate and glutamate
C. Aspartate and glutamine
D. Glutamate and NADH

Chemistry/Apply knowledge of fundamental biological characteristics/Aminotransferase/1

32. Select the products formed from the forward reaction of ALT.
A. Aspartate and alanine
B. Alanine and α-ketoglutarate
C. Pyruvate and glutamate
D. Glutamine and NAD⁺

Chemistry/Apply knowledge of fundamental biological characteristics/Aminotransferase/1

33. Which of the statements below regarding the methods of Henry for AST and ALT is correct?
A. Hemolysis will cause positive interference in both AST and ALT assays.
B. Loss of activity occurs if samples are frozen at −20°C.
C. The absorbance at the start of the reaction should not exceed 1.0 A.
D. Reaction rates are unaffected by addition of P-5′-P to the substrate.

Chemistry/Apply principles of basic laboratory procedures/Aminotransferase/2

34. Select the coupling enzyme used in the kinetic AST reaction of Henry.
A. LD
B. Malate dehydrogenase
C. Glutamate dehydrogenase
D. G-6-PD

Chemistry/Apply principles of basic laboratory procedures/Aminotransferase/1

35. What is the purpose of LD in the kinetic method of Henry for AST?
A. Forms NADH enabling the reaction to be monitored at 340 nm
B. Rapidly exhausts endogenous pyruvate in the lag phase
C. Reduces oxaloacetate preventing product inhibition
D. Generates lactate, which activates AST

Chemistry/Select reagents/Aminotransferase/2

36. Which statement below regarding the naming of transaminases is true?
A. Serum glutamic oxaloacetic transaminase (SGOT) is the older abbreviation for ALT.
B. Serum glutamic pyruvic transaminase (SGPT) is the older abbreviation for AST.
C. SGPT is the older abbreviation for ALT.
D. SGOT is the newer abbreviation for AST.

Chemistry/Apply knowledge of fundamental biological characteristics/Aminotransferase/1

Answers to Questions 31–36

31. **B** AST forms oxaloacetate and glutamate from aspartate and α-ketoglutarate (2-oxoglutarate). Both transaminases use α-ketoglutarate and glutamate as a common substrate and product pair. Both aspartate and alanine can be used to generate glutamate in the central nervous system where it acts as a neurotransmitter.

32. **C** Because glutamate is a common product for transaminases, pyruvate (a three-carbon ketoacid) and glutamate would be generated from the transamination reaction between alanine and α-ketoglutarate.

33. **A** RBCs are rich in AST and to a lesser extent in ALT. Hemolysis causes positive interference in both assays although the affect on AST is greater. Samples are stable for up to 24 hours at room temperature and up to 3 days at 4°C, and should be frozen if kept longer. The starting absorbance should be at least 1.5 A for both assays. Substrates with lower concentrations of NADH are subject to NADH depletion during the lag phase due to side reactions or high transaminase activity. When P-5′-P is added, a significant increase in activity sometimes occurs because some of the enzyme in the serum is in the inactive apoenzyme form.

34. **B** The method of Henry for AST uses malate dehydrogenase (MD) to reduce oxaloacetate to malate. The electrons come from NADH forming NAD⁺.

$$\text{Aspartate} + \text{α-ketoglutarate} \xrightarrow{\text{AST}} \text{Oxaloacetate} + \text{Glutamate}$$

$$\text{Oxaloacetate} + \text{NADH} + \text{H}^+ \xrightarrow{\text{MD}} \text{Malate} + \text{NAD}^+$$

35. **B** Patients with liver disease often have high levels of pyruvate and LD. The LD can catalyze the reaction of pyruvate with NADH in the substrate, forming NAD⁺ and lactate. This would give a falsely high rate for AST because NAD⁺ is the product measured. Adding LD to the substrate causes pyruvate to be depleted in the first 30 seconds, before AST and MD reactions reach steady state.

36. **C** SGOT refers to the products measured in the *in vitro* reaction, and is more correctly named AST for the four-carbon amino acid substrate aspartate. SGPT is the older name referring to the products of the reaction for ALT. SGPT is more correctly named ALT for the 3-carbon amino acid substrate alanine.

37. Which statement accurately describes serum transaminase levels in AMI?
   A. ALT is increased 5- to 10-fold after an AMI.
   B. AST peaks 24–48 hours after an AMI and returns to normal within 4–6 days.
   C. AST levels are usually 20–50 times the upper limit of normal after an AMI.
   D. Isoenzymes of AST are of greater diagnostic utility than the total enzyme level.

Chemistry/Correlate clinical and laboratory data/Aminotransaminases/2

38. Which condition gives rise to the highest serum level of transaminases?
   A. Acute hepatitis
   B. Alcoholic cirrhosis
   C. Obstructive biliary disease
   D. Diffuse intrahepatic cholestasis

Chemistry/Correlate clinical and laboratory data/Aminotransferase/2

39. In which liver disease is the DeRitis ratio (ALT:AST) usually greater than 1.0?
   A. Acute hepatitis
   B. Chronic hepatitis
   C. Hepatic cirrhosis
   D. Hepatic carcinoma

Chemistry/Evaluate laboratory data to recognize health and disease states/Aminotransferase/2

40. Which of the following liver diseases produces the highest levels of transaminases?
   A. Hepatic cirrhosis
   B. Obstructive jaundice
   C. Chronic hepatitis
   D. Alcoholic hepatitis

Chemistry/Correlate clinical and laboratory data/Aminotransferase/2

41. Which of the following statements regarding transaminases is true?
   A. ALT is often increased in muscular disease, pancreatitis, and lymphoma.
   B. ALT is increased in infectious mononucleosis, but AST is usually normal.
   C. ALT is far more specific for liver diseases than is AST.
   D. Substrate depletion seldom occurs in assays of serum from hepatitis cases.

Chemistry/Correlate clinical and laboratory data/Aminotransaminases/2

42. Select the most sensitive marker for alcoholic liver disease.
   A. GLD
   B. ALT
   C. AST
   D. γ-Glutamyltransferase (GGT)

Chemistry/Correlate clinical and laboratory data/Enzymes/2

Answers to Questions 37–42

37. **B** ALT may be slightly elevated after an AMI. AST levels can reach up to 10 times the URL after AMI, but elevations of this range are also seen in patients with muscular dystrophy, crush injury, obstructive jaundice, pulmonary embolism, infectious mononucleosis, and cancer of the liver.

38. **A** The transaminases usually reach 20–50 times the URL in acute viral and toxic hepatitis. Both transaminases are moderately increased (5–10 × URL) in infectious mononucleosis, diffuse intrahepatic obstruction, lymphoma, and cancer of the liver, and slightly increased (2–5 × URL) in cirrhosis and extrahepatic obstruction.

39. **A** ALT prevails over AST in acute hepatitis; however, AST is greater than ALT in chronic hepatitis, carcinoma, and cirrhosis of the liver. Activity of both transaminases is influenced by serum vitamin B_6 (P-5'-P) levels. Because vitamin B_6 is needed for activity, apparent levels will be lower in patients with vitamin B_6 deficiency unless P-5'-P has been added to the substrate.

40. **C** Elevation of transaminases is greatest in acute hepatitis (20–50 × URL). Levels are moderately elevated (5–10 × URL) in chronic hepatitis and hepatic cancer. They are slightly elevated (2–5 × URL) in hepatic cirrhosis, alcoholic hepatitis, and obstructive jaundice.

41. **C** ALT is far more specific for liver disease than AST. Both transaminases are moderately increased in infectious mononucleosis. High ALT may result from nonhepatic causes such as AMI, muscle injury or disease, and severe hemolysis, but nonhepatic sources can be ruled out by a high direct bilirubin. Elevated ALT (e.g., >65 IU/L) is used along with immunologic tests for hepatitis to disqualify blood donors. AST is increased in muscle disease, MI, pancreatitis, and lymphoma.

42. **D** Although AST and ALT are elevated in alcoholic hepatitis, GGT is the most sensitive indicator of alcoholic liver disease. Levels of GGT can reach in excess of 25 times the URL in alcoholic hepatitis. It is also markedly elevated in obstructive jaundice; a high GGT supports the inference that liver is the tissue source of an elevated ALP.

43. Which enzyme is *least* useful in differentiating necrotic from obstructive jaundice?
A. GGT
B. ALT
C. 5′ Nucleotidase
D. LD

Chemistry/Correlate clinical and laboratory data/ Enzymes/2

44. Which of the statements below about the phosphatases is true?
A. They hydrolyze adenosine triphosphate and related compounds.
B. They are divided into two classes based upon pH needed for activity.
C. They exhibit a high specificity for substrate.
D. They are activated by P_i.

Chemistry/Apply knowledge of fundamental biological characteristics/Phosphatases/1

45. Which of the following statements regarding ALP is true?
A. In normal adults the primary tissue source is fast-twitch skeletal muscle.
B. Geriatric patients have a lower serum ALP than other adults.
C. Serum ALP levels are lower in children than in adults.
D. Pregnant women have a higher level of serum ALP than other adults.

Chemistry/Correlate clinical and laboratory data/ Phosphatases/2

46. Which isoenzymes of ALP are inhibited by L-phenylalanine?
A. Intestinal and placental
B. Bone and intestinal
C. Liver and placental
D. Renal and liver

Chemistry/Apply principles of special procedures/ Phosphatases/1

47. Which isoenzyme of ALP is most heat-stable?
A. Bone
B. Liver
C. Intestinal
D. Placental

Chemistry/Apply knowledge of fundamental biological characteristics/Phosphatases/1

48. Which isoenzyme of ALP migrates farthest toward the anode when electrophoresed at pH 8.6?
A. Placental
B. Bone
C. Liver
D. Intestinal

Chemistry/Apply principles of special procedures/ Phosphatases/1

Answers to Questions 43–48

43. D GGT and 5′ nucleotidase are markedly elevated in both intra- and posthepatic obstruction. ALT is slightly elevated in obstructive jaundice but is markedly elevated in necrotic jaundice. Although LD is usually greater in necrotic jaundice ($5–10 \times$ N) than in obstructive jaundice ($<2 \times$ N), elevations in these ranges overlap frequently in hepatic disease and result from many other causes.

44. B Phosphatases are classified as either alkaline or acid depending upon the pH needed for optimum activity. The phosphatases hydrolyze a wide range of monophosphoric acid esters. ALP is inhibited by phosphorus (product inhibition). The International Federation of Clinical Chemistry (IFCC) recommended method employs 2-amino-2-methyl-1-propanol, a buffer that binds P_i.

45. D ALP is higher in children than in adults due to bone growth. Children and geriatric patients have higher serum ALP due to increased bone isoenzyme. Serum ALP levels are often two- or threefold higher than the URL in the third term of pregnancy. In nonpregnant normal adults serum ALP is derived from liver and bone. Liver, bone, placental, renal, and intestinal isoenzymes of ALP can be separated by electrophoresis, and many other ALP isoenzymes have been identified by isofocusing. RBCs, leukocytes, and the prostate are the primary sources of acid phosphatase isoenzymes.

46. A Liver and bone isoenzymes are difficult to separate by agarose electrophoresis, and many laboratories use heat stability and selective inhibitors to help identify the tissue source when ALP is elevated. Phenylalanine inhibits placental and intestinal forms; $3M$ urea inhibits bone ALP.

47. D Placental (and Regan isoenzyme associated with malignancy) is the only isoenzyme that retains activity when serum is heated to 65°C for 10 minutes. Heat inactivation is used primarily to distinguish liver ALP from bone ALP. If less than 20% activity remains after heating serum to 56°C for 10 minutes, then bone ALP is most likely present.

48. C Liver ALP isoenzymes migrate farthest toward the anode, but fast and slow variants occur. The slow liver ALP band is difficult to distinguish from placental and bone ALP. The order from cathode to anode is:

−Renal→Intestinal→Bone→Placental→Liver +

49. Which isoenzyme of ALP is inhibited by urea?
A. Placental
B. Bone
C. Liver
D. Intestinal

Chemistry/Apply principles of special procedures/Phosphatases/1

50. Which of the following statements regarding ALP is true?
A. Isoenzymes of ALP are antigenically distinct and can be identified by specific antibodies.
B. Highest serum levels are seen in intrahepatic obstruction.
C. Elevated serum ALP seen with elevated GGT suggests a hepatic source.
D. When jaundice is present, an elevated ALP suggests acute hepatitis.

Chemistry/Correlate clinical and laboratory data/Phosphatases/2

51. In which condition would an elevated serum ALP be likely to occur?
A. Squamous cell carcinoma
B. Hepatoma
C. Leukemia
D. All of the above

Chemistry/Correlate clinical and laboratory data/Phosphatases/2

52. Which condition is *least* likely to be associated with increased serum ALP?
A. Osteomalacia
B. Pancreatic disease
C. Hyperparathyroidism and hyperthyroidism
D. Osteoporosis

Chemistry/Correlate clinical and laboratory data/Phosphatases/2

53. Which substrate is used in the Bowers-McComb method for ALP?
A. *p*-Nitrophenyl phosphate
B. β-Glycerophosphate
C. Phenylphosphate
D. α-Naphthylphosphate

Chemistry/Apply principles of basic laboratory procedures/Phosphatases/2

54. Which of the following is used in the IFCC recommended method for ALP?
A. Multipoint or continuous measure of absorbance increase at 405 nm
B. Use of 2-amino-2-methyl-1-propanol buffer to chelate phosphorus
C. Addition of Zn^{2+} and HEDTA to chelate the excess Zn^{2+}
D. All of the above

Chemistry/Apply principles of basic laboratory procedures/Phosphatases/2

Answers to Questions 49–54

49. **B** Bone ALP isoenzyme is inhibited by urea, and placental and intestinal ALP are inhibited by phenylalanine. Bone ALP can be distinguished from liver ALP by coupling two methods. For example, loss of ALP activity by heating to 56°C for 10 minutes and by addition of 3*M* urea points to ALP derived from bone.

50. **C** ALP isoenzymes can result from different genes or from modification of a common gene product in the tissues. Some differ in carbohydrate content rather than protein content and cannot be identified by immunologic methods. Highest levels of ALP are seen in Paget's disease of bone where ALP can be as high as 25 times the URL. GGT in serum is derived from the hepatobiliary system and is increased in alcoholic hepatitis and hepatobiliary obstruction. It is not increased in diseases of bone or in pregnancy. When the increase in GGT is twofold higher than the increase in ALP, the liver is assumed to be the source of the elevated ALP. Serum ALP is a sensitive marker for extrahepatic obstruction, which causes an increase of approximately 10 times the URL. A lesser increase is seen in intrahepatic obstruction. ALP is only mildly elevated in acute hepatitis as a result of accompanying obstruction.

51. **D** In addition to obstructive jaundice and bone diseases, ALP is a tumor marker for several malignancies. In most cases the ALP is the product of fetal gene activation and resembles placental ALP (e.g., Regan isoenzyme). Leukemia and Hodgkin's disease may cause an elevated leukocyte- or bone-derived ALP.

52. **D** ALP is elevated in osteomalacia (ricketts), bone cancer, and bone disease secondary to hyperthyroidism and hyperparathyroidism, but it is high in less than 30% of osteoporosis patients. Pancreatic disease associated with biliary obstruction, such as cancer at the head of the pancreas, is associated with elevated ALP.

53. **A** The method of Bowers-McComb (Szasz modification) is the IFCC recommended method for ALP. This method uses 2-amino-2-methyl-1-propanol, pH 10.15, and measures the increase in absorbance at 405 nm as *p*-nitrophenyl phosphate is hydrolyzed to *p*-nitrophenol.

54. **D** As with most other enzymes, ALP should be measured by a kinetic (continuous monitoring) method to ensure that the reaction rate is constant and remains zero order. AMP buffer chelates phosphorus preventing product inhibition; Zn^{2+} and Mg^{2+} are added to the substrate to activate ALP. HEDTA chelates the excess Zn^{2+}, which is inhibitory at high concentrations.

55. Which of the following buffers inhibits prostatic acid phosphatase (PAP)?
A. Citrate
B. TRIS (tris[hydroxymethyl]aminomethane)
C. Tartrate
D. Diethanolamine

Chemistry/Apply principles of special procedures/ Phosphatases/1

56. SITUATION: Blood in a red-stoppered tube for acid phosphatase (ACP) is brought to the laboratory on ice and allowed to clot. The serum is separated and refrigerated for 2 hours before an enzymatic assay is performed. The result is 2.4 IU/L (reference range 0.5–2.0 IU/L). The result is questioned and the sample is sent to a reference laboratory for analysis by RIA. The result of the immunologic assay is 7.2 µg/L (URL = 3.0 µg/L). What is the most likely explanation of these results?
A. An analytical error was made in the enzymatic assay.
B. Positive interference in the RIA was caused by a cross-reaction with nonprostatic ACP.
C. Some of the ACP was inactive due to improper sample processing.
D. The sample should not have been stored below 18°C.

Chemistry/Apply knowledge to identify sources of error/Phosphatases/3

57. SITUATION: Serum from a 50-year-old man was analyzed for both PAP and PSA following a digital rectal exam of the prostate. The PAP result is 6.0 µg/L (URL = 3.0 µg/L), and the PSA is 2.0 µg/L (URL = 4.0 µg/L). Both tests are repeated on the same sample and the results remain unchanged. What is the most likely explanation?
A. The PAP is falsely elevated by prostatic irritation.
B. The patient has benign prostatic hypertrophy.
C. The patient has an infection of the prostate.
D. The PSA is falsely low because it is not as sensitive as the PAP.

Chemistry/Apply knowledge to identify sources of error/Phosphatases/3

58. Which of the following statements regarding acid phosphatase is true?
A. Enzymatic methods must utilize a tartrate buffer to inhibit nonprostatic ACP.
B. The pH optimum for PAP is 6.5.
C. Serum with a high ALP will show positive interference.
D. ACP is useful in confirming the presence of seminal fluid in a vaginal sample.

Chemistry/Apply knowledge of fundamental biological characteristics/Enzyme/2

59. All of the following statements regarding amylase are true *except:*
A. It requires Ca^{2+} for full activity.

B. Activity will vary with the lot of starch used.
C. Amyloclastic methods measure the residual starch.
D. Overrange samples are diluted in deionized water.

Chemistry/Apply knowledge to identify sources of error/Enzyme/2

Answers to Questions 55–59

55. **C** Acid phosphatase is sometimes used along with PSA to screen for cancer of the prostate, and is used to monitor for recurrence in patients who are being treated with antiandrogen therapy. Tests for acid phosphatase must utilize a substrate that is specific for prostatic isoenzyme or an immunochemical assay that detects only PAP. Tartrate inhibits the prostatic isoenzyme, and therefore, PAP can be determined by subtracting the acid phosphatase activity of serum with tartrate added from the activity without tartrate.

56. **C** Acid phosphatase is very labile and should be collected on ice and acidified prior to storage. As the pH rises, some of the enzyme becomes inactive, which will falsely lower results when catalytic activity is measured. Acid phosphatase can be measured by RIA or EIA using an antibody specific for PAP. The immunologic assay measures the mass of enzyme and is not as affected by a change in pH. RIA may be slightly more sensitive than kinetic assays in detecting stage A or B prostatic cancer, and is considered more sensitive analytically because it detects PAP that may be inactive as a result of improper storage.

57. **A** The PSA test is clinically more sensitive than PAP in detecting stages A and B prostatic cancer. The PSA also has the advantage of being stable in storage and is not elevated by trauma associated with digital rectal exam. However, both PAP and PSA may be elevated in prostatic infections and benign prostatic hypertrophy.

58. **D** An ACP greater than 50 IU/L in a vaginal sample is taken as evidence of the presence of seminal fluid. The serum level of nonprostatic acid phosphatase is increased by hemolysis, leukemia, and some diseases of bone. However, these nonprostatic isoenzymes exhibit a high *Km* for commercial ACP substrates, making these assays almost entirely specific for prostatic isoenzyme in the absence of frank hemolysis. Tartrate is an inhibitor of the prostatic isoenzyme. The pH optimum for ACP assays ranges from 4.7 to 5.4. ALP is not active in this pH range.

59. **D** Chloride ions are required for amylase activity. Samples with high activity should be diluted with NaCl to prevent inactivation.

60. Which of the following amylase methods is typically based upon a rate reaction?
A. Somogyi
B. Dye-starch
C. Starch-Iodine
D. Turbidimetric

Chemistry/Apply knowledge of basic laboratory procedures/Enzyme/1

61. How soon following acute abdominal pain due to pancreatitis is the serum amylase expected to rise?
A. 1–2 hours
B. 2–12 hours
C. 3–4 days
D. 5–6 days

Chemistry/Correlate clinical and laboratory data/Enzymes/2

62. Which of the statements below regarding the diagnosis of pancreatitis is correct?
A. Amylase and lipase are as predictive in chronic as in acute pancreatitis.
B. Diagnostic sensitivity is increased by assaying both amylase and lipase.
C. Measuring the urinary amylase:creatinine ratio is useful only when patients have renal failure.
D. Serum lipase peaks several hours before amylase after an episode of acute pancreatitis.

Chemistry/Correlate clinical and laboratory data/Enzymes/2

63. Which of the following conditions is associated with a high serum amylase?
A. Mumps
B. Intestinal obstruction
C. Alcoholic liver disease
D. All of the above

Chemistry/Correlate clinical and laboratory data/Enzymes/2

Answers to Questions 60–63

60. **D** The Somogyi method measures the formation of maltose after incubating serum and starch for 30 minutes at 37°C. Dye-starch or chromolytic methods measure the amount of dye released from starch after incubation with serum. The amount of dye released is determined by comparison to pure dye standards. Turbidimetric methods determine the clearing of starch as a negative rate reaction.

61. **B** Serum amylase usually peaks 2–12 hours following acute abdominal pain resulting from pancreatitis. Levels reach 2–6 times the URL and return to normal within 3–4 days. Urinary amylase peaks concurrently with serum but rises higher and remains elevated for up to 1 week.

62. **B** Serum lipase peaks about the same time as amylase but remains abnormal for about 1 week following an episode of acute pancreatitis. In acute pancreatitis the rate of urinary amylase excretion increases, and the urinary amylase:creatinine ratio or the amylase:creatinine clearance ratio are helpful in diagnosing some cases of pancreatitis. The normal A:C clearance ratio is 1%–4%. In acute pancreatitis the ratio is usually above 4% and can be as high as 15%. In chronic pancreatitis, acinar cell degeneration often occurs, resulting in loss of amylase and lipase production. This lowers the sensitivity of amylase and lipase in detecting chronic disease to below 50%. Patients with chronic disease have pancreatic insufficiency giving rise to abnormal triolein ^{131}I and β carotene absorption, increased fecal fat, and decreased fecal trypsin.

63. **D** Both salivary and pancreatic amylases designated S-type and P-type, respectively, are present in normal serum. High amylase occurs in mumps, ectopic pregnancy, biliary obstruction, peptic ulcers, alcoholism, malignancies, and other non-pancreatic diseases. Isoenzyme assay can be used to rule out mumps, malignancy, and ectopic pregnancy, which give rise to high S-type amylase.

64. Which of the statements below regarding amylase methods is true?
- A. Dilution of serum may result in lower than expected activity.
- B. Methods generating NADH are preferred because they have higher sensitivity.
- C. Synthetic substrates can be conjugated to *p*-nitrophenol (PNP) for a kinetic assay.
- D. The reference range is consistent from method to method.

Chemistry/Apply knowledge to identify sources of error/Enzymes/2

65. The reference method for lipase uses olive oil as the substrate because:
- A. Other esterases can hydrolyze triglyceride and synthetic diglycerides.
- B. The reaction product can be coupled to NADH generating reactions.
- C. Synthetic substrates are less soluble than olive oil in aqueous reagents.
- D. Triglyceride substrates cause product inhibition.

Chemistry/Apply knowledge of basic laboratory procedures/Enzymes/2

66. Lipase is assayed along with amylase because:
- A. Lipase is not increased in mumps.
- B. Lipase remains elevated longer than amylase in acute pancreatitis.
- C. Neither amylase or lipase is consistently elevated in chronic pancreatitis.
- D. All of the above.

Chemistry/Correlate clinical and laboratory data/Enzymes/2

67. The reference method for serum lipase is based upon:
- A. Assay of triglycerides following incubation of serum with olive oil
- B. Rate turbidimetry
- C. Titration of fatty acids with dilute NaOH following controlled incubation of serum with olive oil
- D. Immunochemical assay

Chemistry/Apply principles of basic laboratory procedures/Enzymes/1

68. Which of the following enzymes is usually *depressed* in liver disease?
- A. Leucine aminopeptidase (LAP)
- B. GLD
- C. Pseudocholinesterase
- D. Aldolase

Chemistry/Correlate clinical and laboratory data/Enzymes/2

Answers to Questions 64–68

64. **C** Many endogenous inhibitors of amylase, such as wheat germ, are found in serum. Diluted samples often show higher than expected activity caused by dilution of the inhibitor. Units of amylase activity vary widely depending upon the method of assay and calibration. Synthetic substrates such as maltotetrose or 4-nitrophenol maltohepatoside can be used for kinetic assays. Maltotetrose is hydrolyzed to maltose by amylase, and the maltose hydrolyzed by α-glucosidase or maltose phosphorylase, forming glucose or glucose-1-phosphate, respectively. These can be measured by coupling to NADH generating reactions. However, some enzymatic methods have unfavorable kinetics, such as negative interference caused by LD and pyruvate, long lag phases caused by endogenous glucose, or nonlinear rates. Methods using *p*-nitrophenol can be performed kinetically without these interferences. The substrate, maltohepatoside esterified to *p*-nitrophenol, is "blocked" so that α-glucosidase will not hydrolyze the PNP until the substrate is split by amylase, forming maltotriose. The PNP generated increases the absorbance at 410 nm in proportion to amylase activity.

65. **A** Triglycerides may be hydrolyzed by nonspecific esterases in serum as well as lipase. Lipase acts only at an interface of oil and H_2O and requires bile salts and colipase for activity. Colipase is a protein secreted by the pancreas.

66. **D** Lipase adds both sensitivity and specificity to the diagnosis of acute pancreatitis. Lipase elevation is of greater magnitude ($2–10 \times N$) and duration than amylase in acute pancreatitis. When the lipase method is optimized by inclusion of colipase and bile salts, the test is more sensitive and specific than serum amylase for detection of acute pancreatitis.

67. **C** The reference method of Cherry and Crandall is based upon the titration of fatty acids formed by the hydrolysis of an emulsion of olive oil after incubation for 24 hours at 37°C. Because most of the activity occurs within the first 3 hours, the incubation time may be shortened to as little as 1 hour without loss of clinical utility.

68. **C** Levels of pseudocholinesterase are decreased in patients with liver disease as a result of depressed synthesis. In cirrhosis and hepatoma there is a 50%–70% reduction in serum level and a 30%–50% reduction in hepatitis. LAP is increased in both necrotic and obstructive jaundice. GLD is increased in necrotic jaundice, and aldolase in necrotic jaundice and muscle disease.

69. A serum ALP level greater than twice the elevation of GGT suggests:
A. Misidentification of the specimen
B. Focal intrahepatic obstruction
C. Acute alcoholic hepatitis
D. Bone disease or malignancy

Chemistry/Evaluate laboratory data to recognize health and disease states/Enzymes/2

70. Which of the following enzymes is usually increased in acute lymphocytic leukemia (ALL)?
A. ALT
B. Acid phosphatase
C. Terminal deoxynucleotidyl transferase (TdT)
D. Cholinesterase

Chemistry/Correlate clinical and laboratory data/Enzymes/2

Answers to Questions 69–70

69. **D** In obstructive jaundice, GGT is elevated more than ALP. A disproportionate increase in ALP points to a nonhepatic source of ALP, often bone disease. GGT is the most sensitive marker of acute alcoholic hepatitis, rising about fivefold higher than ALP or transaminases.

70. **C** TdT is found in the blasts of all patients with T-cell ALL, and most who have null-cell or pre-B-cell ALL. Patients with B-cell ALL are TdT-negative.

Clinical Endocrinology

1. Which of the following hormones is often decreased by approximately 25% in the serum of pregnant women who have a fetus with Down syndrome?
   A. Estriol (E_3)
   B. Human chorionic gonadotropin (HCG)
   C. Progesterone
   D. Estradiol (E_2)

   Chemistry/Correlate laboratory data with physiologic processes/Endocrine/2

2. SIADH causes:
   A. High serum vasopressin
   B. Hyponatremia
   C. Urine osmolality to be higher than plasma
   D. All of the above

   Chemistry/Correlate clinical and laboratory data/ Endocrine/2

3. Select the hormone that is associated with galactorrhea, pituitary adenoma, and amenorrhea.
   A. E_2
   B. Progesterone
   C. Follicle-stimulating hormone (FSH)
   D. Prolactin

   Chemistry/Correlate clinical and laboratory data/ Endocrine/2

4. Zollinger-Ellison (Z-E) syndrome is characterized by great (e.g., 20-fold) elevation of:
   A. Gastrin
   B. Cholecystokinin
   C. Pepsin
   D. Glucagon

   Chemistry/Correlate clinical and laboratory data/Gastric/2

Answers to Questions 1–4

1. **A** E_3 is produced in the placenta and fetal liver from dehydroepiandosterone derived from the mother and fetal liver. E_3 is the major estrogen produced during pregnancy, and levels rise throughout gestation. Serum free E_3 is often lower than expected for the gestational age in a pregnancy associated with Down syndrome. The combination of low serum free E_3, low α-fetoprotein (AFP), and high HCG is used as a screening test to detect Down syndrome. When one of the three markers is abnormal, amniocentesis should be performed for the diagnosis of Down syndrome by karyotyping. The three markers have a combined sensitivity (detection rate) of near 65%.

2. **D** SIADH results in excessive secretion of ADH, causing fluid retention, hyponatremia, and hypokalemia. It is suspected when urine osmolality is higher than plasma, but urine sodium concentration is normal. Patients with sodium depletion have a urine osmolality higher than plasma but a low urine sodium.

3. **D** Serum prolactin may be increased from hypothalamic dysfunction or pituitary adenoma. When levels are greater than five times the URL a pituitary tumor is suspected. Prolactin is measured by RIA or enzyme immunoassay (EIA).

4. **A** Z-E syndrome is caused by a pancreatic or intestinal tumor secreting gastrin (gastrinoma), and results in greatly increased gastric acid production. Basal acid output (BAO) and peak acid output (PAO) are greatly elevated and the BAO/PAO exceeds 0.6.

5. Which statement about multiple endocrine neoplasia (MEN) is true?
  A. It is associated with hyperplasia or neoplasia of at least two endocrine organs.
  B. Insulinoma is always present when the pituitary is involved.
  C. It is inherited as an autosomal recessive disorder.
  D. Plasma hormone levels from affected organs are elevated at least tenfold.

Chemistry/Correlate clinical and laboratory data/ Endocrine/2

6. Select the main estrogen produced by the ovaries and used to evaluate ovarian function.
  A. E_3
  B. E_2
  C. Epiestriol
  D. Hydroxyestrone

Chemistry/Apply knowledge of fundamental biological characteristics/Estrogen/1

7. Which statement best describes the relationship between luteinizing hormone (LH) and FSH in cases of dysmenorrhea?
  A. Both are usually increased when there is pituitary adenoma.
  B. Increases in both hormones and a decrease in estrogen signal a pituitary cause of ovarian failure.
  C. Both hormones normally peak 1–2 days before ovulation.
  D. In menopause, the LH level at the midcycle peak is higher than the level of FSH.

Chemistry/Correlate clinical and laboratory data/ Endocrine/2

8. When pituitary adenoma is the cause of decreased estrogen production, an increase of which hormone is most frequently responsible?
  A. Prolactin
  B. FSH
  C. LH
  D. Thyroid-stimulating hormone (TSH)

Chemistry/Correlate clinical and laboratory data/ Endocrine/2

Answers to Questions 5–8

5. **A** Multiple endocrine neoplasia syndrome is inherited as an autosomal dominant disease involving excess production of hormones from several endocrine glands. MEN I results from adenomas (usually benign) of at least two glands, including the pituitary, adrenal cortex, parathyroid, and pancreas. The parathyroid gland is the organ most commonly involved, and in those patients an elevated Ca_i is an early sign. The pancreas is the next most frequently involved organ, but the hormone most commonly oversecreted is gastrin (not insulin). MEN II usually results from pheochromocytoma and thyroid carcinoma. MEN II-B is a variant of MEN II showing the addition of neurofibroma.

6. **B** E_2 is the major estrogen produced by the ovaries and gives rise to both estrone (E_1) and E_3. E_2 is used to evaluate both ovarian function and menstrual cycle dysfunction.

7. **C** In women, serum or urine LH and FSH are measured along with estrogen and progesterone to evaluate the cause of menstrual cycle abnormalities and anovulation. Both hormones show a pronounced serum peak 1–2 days prior to ovulation and urine peak 20–44 hours before ovulation. Normally the LH peak is sharper and greater than the FSH peak; however, in menopause, the FSH usually becomes higher than LH. In patients with primary ovarian failure, the LH and FSH are elevated because low estrogen levels stimulate release of luteinizing hormone-releasing hormone (LHRH) from the hypothalamus. Conversely, in pituitary failure, levels of FSH and LH are reduced, and this reduction causes a deficiency of estrogen production by the ovaries.

8. **A** Prolactinoma can result in anovulation because high levels of prolactin suppress release of LHRH, causing suppression of growth hormone (GH), FSH, and estrogen. Prolactinoma is the most commonly occurring pituitary tumor accounting for 40%–60%. Adenomas producing FSH have a frequency of about 20%, while those pituitary tumors secreting LH and TSH are rare.

9. Which of the following statements is correct in assessing GH deficiency?
A. Pituitary failure may involve one, several, or all adenohypophyseal hormones; but GH deficiency is usually found.
B. A normal random serum level of GH in a child under 6 years old rules out GH deficiency.
C. Administration of arginine, insulin, or glucagon will suppress GH release.
D. GH levels in the blood show little variation within a 24-hour period.

Chemistry/Apply knowledge of fundamental biological characteristics/Endocrine/2

10. Which statement best describes the level of GH in patients with pituitary adenoma associated with acromegaly?
A. The fasting GH level is always elevated at least twofold.
B. Some patients will require a glucose suppression test to establish a diagnosis.
C. A normal fasting GH level rules out acromegaly.
D. Patients produce a lower concentration of insulin-like growth factor I (IGF-1) than expected from their GH level.

Chemistry/Correlate clinical and laboratory data/Endocrine/2

11. Hyperparathyroidism is most consistently associated with:
A. Hypocalcemia
B. Hypocalciuria
C. Hypophosphatemia
D. Metabolic alkalosis

Chemistry/Correlate clinical and laboratory data/Endocrine/2

12. Which statement regarding the use of PTH is true?
A. Determination of serum PTH level is the best screening test for disorders of calcium metabolism.
B. PTH levels differentiate primary and secondary causes of hypoparathyroidism.
C. PTH levels differentiate primary and secondary causes of hypocalcemia.
D. PTH levels are low in patients with pseudohypoparathyroidism.

Chemistry/Correlate clinical and laboratory data/Endocrine/2

Answers to Questions 9–12

9. **A** Because GH is the most abundant pituitary hormone, it may be used as a screening test for pituitary failure in adults. Pituitary hormone deficiencies are rare and are evaluated by measuring those hormones associated with the specific type of target organ dysfunction. GH secretion peaks during sleep, and pulsed increases are seen following exercise and meals. In adults, a deficiency of GH can be ruled out by demonstrating normal or high levels on two successive tests. In children, there is extensive overlap between normal and low GH levels, and a stimulation (provocative) test is usually needed to establish a diagnosis of deficiency. Exercise is often used to stimulate GH release. If GH levels are greater than 6 μg/L after vigorous exercise then deficiency is ruled out. In addition to exercise, drugs such as arginine, insulin, propranolol, and glucagon can be used to stimulate GH release. Deficiency is documented by registering a subnormal response to two stimulating agents.

10. **B** Approximately 90% of patients with acromegaly will have an elevated fasting GH level, but 10% will not. In addition, a single measurement is not sufficient to establish a diagnosis of acromegaly because various metabolic and nutritional factors can cause an elevated serum GH in the absence of pituitary disease. The glucose suppression test is used to diagnose acromegaly. An oral dose of 100 g of glucose will suppress the serum GH level at 1 hour (postadministration) to below 1 μg/L in normal patients, but not in patients with acromegaly. Patients with acromegaly also have high levels of IGF-1, also called somatomedin C, which is overproduced by the liver in response to excess release of GH.

11. **C** Hyperparathyroidism causes increased resorption of calcium and decreased renal retention of phosphate. Increased serum calcium leads to increased urinary excretion. The distal collecting tubule of the nephron reabsorbs less bicarbonate as well as phosphate, resulting in acidosis.

12. **C** Serum Ca_i is the best screening test to determine if a disorder of calcium metabolism is present, and will distinguish primary hyperparathyroidism (high Ca_i) and secondary hyperparathyroidism (low Ca_i). PTH levels are used to distinguish primary and secondary causes of hypocalcemia. Serum PTH is low in primary hypocalcemia (which results from parathyroid gland disease), but is high in secondary hypocalcemia (e.g., renal failure). Serum PTH is also used for the early diagnosis of secondary hypocalcemia because PTH levels rise prior to a decrease in the serum Ca_i. Serum PTH is used to help distinguish primary hyperparathyroidism (high PTH) and hypercalcemia of malignancy (usually low PTH), and pseudohypoparathyroidism from primary hypoparathyroidism. Pseudohypoparathyroidism results from a deficient response to PTH and is associated with normal or elevated serum PTH.

13. The best method of analysis for serum PTH involves using antibodies that detect:
A. The amino-terminal fragment of PTH
B. The carboxy-terminal end of PTH
C. Both the amino-terminal fragment and intact PTH
D. All fragments of PTH as well as intact hormone

Chemistry/Apply principles of special procedures/Hormone assays/1

14. Which of the following is most often elevated in hypercalcemia associated with malignancy?
A. Parathyroid-derived PTH
B. Ectopic PTH
C. Parathyroid hormone-related protein (PTHRP)
D. Calcitonin

Chemistry/Apply principles of special procedures/Hormone assays/1

15. Steroids with a dihydroxyacetone group at C17 are classified as:
A. Androgens
B. 17-Hydroxycorticosteroids
C. 17-Ketosteroids
D. Estrogens

Chemistry/Apply knowledge of fundamental biological characteristics/Adrenal/1

16. Which statement below regarding adrenal cortical dysfunction is true?
A. Patients with Cushing's syndrome usually have hyperkalemia.
B. Cushing's syndrome is associated with glucose intolerance.
C. Addison's disease is associated with hypernatremia.
D. Addison's disease is caused by elevated levels of cortisol.

Chemistry/Correlate clinical and laboratory data/Adrenal/2

Answers to Questions 13–16

13. **C** PTH is a polypeptide made up of 84 amino acids. The biological activity of the hormone resides in the N-terminal portion of the polypeptide, but the hormone is rapidly degraded producing N-terminal, middle, and C-terminal fragments. Fragments lacking the N-terminal portion are inactive. Immunoassays for PTH using antibodies to different portions of the polypeptide will give different results. The assay of choice is a two-site double antibody sandwich method that measures only intact PTH and active fragments. Methods that use single antibodies may detect inactive as well as active PTH fragments and are not as specific for parathyroid disease.

14. **C** PTHRP is a peptide produced by many tissues and normally present in the blood at a very low level. The peptide has an N-terminal sequence of 8 amino acids that are the same as found in PTH and which will stimulate the PTH receptors of bone. Some malignancies (e.g., squamous, renal, bladder, and ovarian cancers) secrete PTHRP, causing hypercalcemia associated malignancy. Because the region shared with PTH is small and poorly immunoreactive, the peptide does not crossreact in most assays for PTH. For this reason, and because tumors producing ectopic PTH are rare, almost all patients who have an elevated Ca_i and elevated PTH have primary hyperparathyroidism. The immunoassay for PTHRP will frequently be elevated in patients who have not yet been diagnosed with malignancy but have an elevated Ca_i, without an elevated serum PTH. Calcitonin is a hormone produced in the medulla of the thyroid that opposes the action of PTH. However, calcitonin levels do not greatly influence the serum calcium. Assay of calcitonin is used exclusively to diagnose medullary thyroid cancer, which produces very high serum levels.

15. **B** Steroids having a dihydroxyacetone group at C17 are called Porter-Silber chromogens because they react in the Porter-Silber reaction for 17-hydroxycorticosteroids. All are C21 steroids, of which the major one is cortisol. The Porter-Silber reaction for 17-hydroxysteroids is based upon the coupling of phenylhydrazine in sulfuric acid with the dihydroxyacetone group of C21 adrenal corticosteroids forming a yellow product. Only those 17-hydroxysteroids with the dihydroxyacetone group at C17 will react.

16. **B** Patient's with Cushing's syndrome have elevated levels of cortisol and other adrenal corticosteroids. This causes the characteristic cushingoid appearance that includes obesity, acne, and humpback posture. Osteoporosis, hypertension, hypokalemia, and glycosuria are characteristics. Addison's disease results from adrenal hypoplasia and produces the opposite symptoms including hypotension, hyperkalemia, and hypoglycemia.

17. Which of the following statements about cortisol in Cushing's syndrome is true?
A. Twenty-four-hour urinary free cortisol is a more sensitive test than plasma total cortisol.
B. Patients with Cushing's disease show pronounced diurnal variation in serum cortisol.
C. Urinary free cortisol is increased by a high serum cortisol-binding protein concentration.
D. An elevated serum total cortisol level is diagnostic of Cushing's syndrome.

Chemistry/Apply knowledge to identify sources of error/Cortisol/2

18. Which of the following diseases is characterized by primary hyperaldosteronism caused by adrenal adenoma, carcinoma, or hyperplasia?
A. Cushing's disease
B. Addison's disease
C. Conn's disease
D. Pheochromocytoma

Chemistry/Correlate clinical and laboratory data/Endocrine/2

19. Which of the following is the most common cause of Cushing's syndrome?
A. Pituitary adenoma
B. Adrenal hyperplasia
C. Overuse of corticosteroids
D. Ectopic adrenocorticotropic hormone (ACTH) production by tumors

Chemistry/Correlate clinical and laboratory data/Adrenal/2

20. Which of the following is the mechanism causing Cushing's disease?
A. Excess secretion of pituitary ACTH
B. Adrenal adenoma
C. Treatment with corticosteroids
D. Ectopic ACTH production by tumors

Chemistry/Apply knowledge of fundamental biological characteristics/Adrenal/2

21. In which situation is the test for 17-ketogenic steroids still of clinical utility?
A. Evaluation of adrenal function in pregnancy
B. In patients with a borderline positive overnight dexamethasone suppression test
C. Evaluation of congenital adrenal hyperplasia
D. Differentiation of Cushing's syndrome from disease

Chemistry/Select course of action/Adrenal/2

Answers to Questions 17–21

17. **A** Serum cortisol can be increased by factors such as stress, medications, and cortisol-binding protein, and the cortisol level of normal patients will overlap those seen in Cushing's syndrome because of pulse variation. When cortisol levels become elevated, cortisol-binding protein becomes saturated, and free (unbound) cortisol is filtered by the glomeruli. Most is reabsorbed, but a significant amount reaches the urine as free cortisol. Twenty-four hour urinary free cortisol avoids the diurnal variation that may affect plasma free cortisol levels and is a more sensitive test than serum total or free cortisol.

18. **C** Conn's syndrome is characterized by hypertension, hypokalemia, and hypernatremia with increased plasma and urine aldosterone and decreased renin. Cushing's syndrome results from excessive production of cortisol, and Addison's disease from deficient production of adrenal corticosteroids. Pheochromocytoma is a tumor of chromaffin cells (usually adrenal) that produces catecholamines.

19. **C** The most common cause of Cushing's syndrome is the administration of medications with cortisol or glucocorticoid activity. Excluding iatrogenic causes, approximately 60%–70% of Cushing's syndrome results from hypothalamic-pituitary misregulation and is called Cushing's disease. Adrenal adenoma or carcinoma (non-ACTH-mediated Cushing's syndrome) make up about 20% of cases, and ectopic ACTH production accounts for 10%–20%.

20. **A** Cushing's disease refers to adrenal hyperplasia resulting from misregulation of the hypothalamic-pituitary axis. It is usually caused by small pituitary adenomas. Cushing's syndrome may be caused by Cushing's disease, adrenal adenoma or carcinoma, ectopic ACTH-producing tumors, or excessive corticosteroid administration. The cause of Cushing's syndrome can be differentiated using ACTH, dexamethasone suppression, and metyrapone stimulation tests.

21. **C** Congenital adrenal hyperplasia (CAH) (adrenogenital syndrome) results from a deficiency of an enzyme required for synthesis of cortisol. Approximately 90% of cases are caused by a deficiency of 21-hydroxylase blocking conversion of 17-hydroxyprogesterone to 11-deoxycortisol. Most other cases are caused by 11-hydroxylase deficiency, which blocks conversion of 11-deoxycortisol to cortisol. Precursors of cortisol, usually either 17-hydroxyprogesterone or 11-deoxycortisol are increased. This results in low serum cortisol levels, but high 17-ketogenic steroids. The two most common features of CAH are salt-wasting caused by increased mineralocorticoid activity and virilization due to increased androgens.

22. Which test is used to distinguish ACTH-mediated Cushing's syndrome from adrenal adenoma or carcinoma?
   A. Overnight dexamethasone suppression
   B. Petrosal sinus sampling
   C. Serum ACTH
   D. Twenty-four-hour urinary free cortisol

Chemistry/Select course of action/Adrenal/2

23. Which is the most widely used screening test for Cushing's syndrome?
   A. Overnight dexamethasone suppression test
   B. Corticotropin-releasing hormone stimulation test
   C. Petrosal sinus sampling
   D. Metyrapone stimulation test

Chemistry/Select course of action/Adrenal/2

24. Which test is the most specific for establishing a diagnosis of Cushing's disease (pituitary Cushing's)?
   A. Low dose dexamethasone suppression
   B. High dose dexamethasone suppression
   C. Twenty-four-hour urinary free cortisol
   D. Petrosal sinus sampling following corticotropin-releasing hormone stimulation

Chemistry/Correlate clinical and laboratory data/Adrenal/2

25. Which statement below about the diagnosis of Addison's disease is true?
   A. Patients with primary Addison's show a normal response to ACTH stimulation.
   B. Primary and secondary Addison's can often be differentiated by plasma ACTH.
   C. Twenty-four-hour urinary free cortisol is normal in Addison's disease.
   D. Pituitary ACTH reserves are normal in secondary Addison's disease.

Chemistry/Correlate clinical and laboratory data/Adrenal/2

Answers to Questions 22–25

22. **C** Serum ACTH assays are very helpful in distinguishing the cause of Cushing's syndrome. Patients with adrenal tumors have values approaching zero. Patients with ectopic ACTH tumors have values greater than 200 pg/dL. Fifty percent of patients with Cushing's disease have high 8 AM ACTH levels (between 100–200 pg/dL). The high dose dexamethasone suppression test and the metyrapone stimulation test are also useful. Patients with pituitary Cushing's show more than 50% suppression of cortisol release after receiving an 8-mg dose of dexamethasone, but patients with adrenal tumors or ACTH-producing tumors do not. Metyrapone blocks cortisol formation by inhibiting 11-hydroxylase. This causes an increase in ACTH output in normal patients and patients with pituitary Cushing's. Patients with adrenal tumors and those with ectopic ACTH tumors show no increase above the baseline.

23. **A** Dexamethasone is a synthetic corticosteroid that exhibits 30-fold greater negative feedback on the hypothalamus than cortisol. When an oral dose of 1 mg of the drug is given to a patient at 11 PM, the 8 AM serum total cortisol level should be below 5.0 μg/dL. Patients with Cushing's syndrome almost always exceed this cutoff. Therefore, a normal response to dexamethasone excludes Cushing's syndrome with a sensitivity of about 98%.

24. **D** Although dexamethasone suppression tests have a high sensitivity, some patients without Cushing's syndrome have indeterminate results (e.g., values between 5 and 10 μg/dL) or abnormal results owing to medications or other conditions. When corticotropin-releasing hormone is given intravenously, patients with pituitary Cushing's have an exaggerated ACTH response. Samples are drawn from the sinuses draining the pituitary gland and from the peripheral blood. In patients with pituitary tumors, the ACTH will be several times higher in the sinus samples than in the peripheral blood samples.

25. **B** ACTH (Cortrosyn) stimulation is used as a screening test for Addison's disease. A 250-μg dose of Cortrosyn is given intravenously. Normal patients show a 2–5 times increase in serum cortisol. A subnormal response occurs in both primary and secondary Addison's disease. Plasma ACTH is high in primary but is low in secondary Addison's disease. Patients with secondary Addison's (pituitary failure) do not respond to metyrapone because the ACTH reserve is diminished.

26. Which of the statements below regarding the catecholamines is true?
A. They are derived from tryptophan.
B. They are produced by the zona glomerulosa of the adrenal cortex.
C. Plasma levels show both diurnal and pulsed variation.
D. They are excreted in urine primarily as free catecholamines.

Chemistry/Apply knowledge of fundamental biological characteristics/Catecholamines/2

27. Which assay using 24-hour urine is considered the best single screening test for pheochromocytoma?
A. Total urinary catecholamines
B. VMA
C. Homovanillic acid (HVA)
D. Metanephrines

Chemistry/Correlate clinical and laboratory data/ Catecholamines/2

28. Which metabolite is most often increased in carcinoid tumors of the intestine?
A. 5-Hydroxyindolacetic acid (5-HIAA)
B. 3-Methoxy-4-hydroxyphenylglycol (MHPG)
C. 3-Methoxydopamine
D. HVA

Chemistry/Correlate clinical and laboratory data/ Endocrine/1

29. Which statement regarding the measurement of urinary catecholamines is true?
A. An increased excretion of total urinary catecholamines is specific for pheochromocytoma.
B. Twenty-four-hour urinary catecholamine assay avoids pulse variations associated with measurement of plasma catecholamines.
C. Total urinary catecholamine measurement provides greater specificity than measurement of urinary free catecholamines.
D. Total urinary catecholamines are not affected by exercise.

Chemistry/Apply knowledge to identify sources of error/Catecholamines/2

30. Which method used to measure catecholamines is the *least* specific?
A. Measurement of fluorescence following oxidation by potassium ferricyanide.
B. Measurement of free catecholamines by HPLC with electrochemical detection.
C. Measure of radioactivity after conversion by catechol-*O*-methyltransferase (COMT) to tritiated metanephrines.
D. RIA followed by measurement and subtraction of metanephrines.

Chemistry/Apply principles of special procedures/Catecholamines/2

Answers to Questions 26–30

26. **C** Catecholamines, epinephrine and norepinephrine and dopamine, are produced from the amino acid tyrosine by the chromaffin cells of the adrenal medulla. Plasma and urinary catecholamines are measured in order to diagnose pheochromocytoma. Symptoms include hypertension, headache, sweating, and other endocrine involvement. Plasma catecholamines are oxidized rapidly to metanephrines and VMA; only about 2% is excreted as free catecholamines.

27. **D** Catecholamines are metabolized to metanephrines and VMA. Urinary catecholamines are increased by exercise and dietary ingestion. Measurement of 24-hour urinary metanephrine is about 95% sensitive for pheochromocytoma, and is the best single test. Specificity and sensitivity for detecting pheochromocytoma approach 100% when both VMA and metanephrines are measured.

28. **A** 5-HIAA is a product of serotonin catabolism. Excess levels are found in urine of patients with carcinoid tumors composed of argentaffin cells. Carcinoid tumors are usually found in the intestine or lung.

29. **B** Measurement of total urinary catecholamines is not a specific test for pheochromocytoma. Urine levels may be increased by exercise and in muscular diseases. Catecholamines in urine may also be derived from dietary sources rather than endogenous production. Most catecholamines are excreted as the glucuronide, and the urinary free catecholamines increase only when there is increased secretion. Measurement of free hormone in urine is equal in clinical sensitivity and specificity to measurement of metanephrines. Twenty-four hour urine is the sample of choice because plasma levels are subject to pulse variation and affected by the patient's psychological and metabolic condition at the time of sampling.

30. **A** Most laboratories measuring catecholamines use HPLC with electrochemical detection because the trihydroxyindol reaction is not specific. HPLC-ECD separates catecholamines by reverse phase chromatography, then detects them by oxidizing the aromatic ring at +0.8 V to a quinone ring. Current is proportional to epinephrine and norepinephrine concentration. Fluorescent methods employing ferricyanide (trihydroxyindole method) or ethylenediamine (EDA method) show interference by Aldomet and several other drugs. The radioenzymatic assay of catecholamines is a specific alternative to HPLC but requires a liquid scintillation counter. The method uses the enzyme COMT to transfer a tritiated methyl group from S-adenosyl methionine to the catecholamines. This results in formation of radiolabeled metanephrines that are measured.

31. Which statement about sample collection for catecholamines and metabolites is true?
    A. Blood for catecholamines is collected with the patient resting and supine.
    B. Twenty-four–hour urine for VMA, catecholamines, or metanephrines is collected in 20 mL of 6 *N* HCl.
    C. Twenty-four–hour urine creatinine should be measured with VMA, HVA, or metanephrines.
    D. All of the above.

    Chemistry/Apply principles of special procedures/ Specimen collection and handling/2

32. Which statement below applies to both measurement of VMA and metanephrines in urine?
    A. Both can be oxidized to vanillin and measured at 360 nm without interference from dietary compounds.
    B. Both can be measured immunochemically after hydrolysis and derivitization.
    C. Both require acid hydrolysis prior to measurement.
    D. Both can be measured by specific HPLC and GC-MS assays.

    Chemistry/Apply principles of special procedures/Catecholamines/2

33. Urinary HVA is most often assayed to detect:
    A. Pheochromocytoma
    B. Neuroblastoma
    C. Adrenal medullary carcinoma
    D. Psychiatric disorders such as manic depression

    Chemistry/Correlate laboratory and clinical data/Catecholamines/1

34. Thyroid hormones are derived from the amino acid:
    A. Phenylalanine
    B. Methionine
    C. Tyrosine
    D. Histidine

    Chemistry/Apply knowledge of fundamental biological characteristics/Thyroid/1

35. Which statement regarding thyroid hormones is true?
    A. Circulating levels of T_3 and T_4 are about equal.
    B. T_3 is about 10 times more active than T_4.
    C. The rate of formation of monoiodotyrosine and diiodotyrosine is about equal.
    D. All of the above.

    Chemistry/Apply knowledge of fundamental biological characteristics/Thyroid/2

Answers to Questions 31–35

31. **D** Stress and exercise induce catecholamine elevation and, therefore, patients must be resting supine for at least 30 minutes prior to blood collection. Many drugs contain epinephrine, which may falsely elevate catecholamine measurements. In addition, many drugs inhibit monoamine oxidase, which is needed to convert metanephrines to VMA. Therefore, medications should be removed prior to testing whenever possible. Twenty-four–hour urine samples are preserved with HCl because catecholamines and their metabolites are rapidly oxidized when pH is greater than 2. Renal clearance affects excretion of catecholamine metabolites; it is preferable to report VMA, HVA, and metanephrines in micrograms per milligram creatinine.

32. **D** VMA and metanephrines can both be measured as vanillin after oxidation with periodate. However, these methods are affected by dietary sources of vanillin; coffee, chocolate, bananas, and vanilla must be excluded from the diet. For this reason, VMA is commonly measured by extraction with ethyl acetate and absorption onto a silica gel column that is washed with a 1:1 mixture of ethanol:ethyl acetate to remove interfering substances. The VMA is eluted with H_2O and reacted with a diazo reagent to produce a purple color. Metanephrines may be measured by competitive ELISA after hydrolysis and conversion to an N-acyl-metanephrine, which is immunoreactive. Metanephrines can be measured by HPLC using a fluorescence detector, and VMA can be measured by HPLC using an electrochemical detector.

33. **B** HVA is the major metabolite of dopa, and urinary HVA is elevated in more than 75% of neuroblastoma patients. MHPG is the major metabolite of norepinephrine in the central nervous system. Urinary levels of MHPG have been shown to correlate with manic-depressive status being low in depression and elevated during the manic phase.

34. **C** Thyroid hormones are derived from the enzymatic modification of tyrosine residues on thyroglobulin. Tyrosine is halogenated enzymatically with iodine, forming monoiodotyrosine (MIT) and diiodotyrosine (DIT). Enzymatic coupling of these residues form T_3 (3,5,3'-triiodothyronine) and T_4 (3,5,3',5'-tetraiodothyronine). These are hydrolyzed from thyroglobulin, forming active hormones.

35. **B** The rate of DIT synthesis is twice that of MIT and the rate of coupling favors formation of T_4. Levels of T_4 are about 50 times those of T_3, but T_3 is approximately 10 times more active physiologically. Eighty percent of circulating T_3 is derived from enzymatic conversion of T_4 by T_4 5'-deiodinase.

36. Which of the statements below regarding thyroid hormones is true?
A. Both protein-bound and free T_3 and T_4 are physiologically active.
B. Total T_3 and T_4 are influenced by the level of thyroxine binding globulin.
C. Variation in thyroxine-binding protein levels affects both free T_3 and T_4.
D. An elevated serum total T_4 and T_3 is diagnostic of hyperthyroidism.

Chemistry/Apply knowledge of fundamental biological characteristics/Thyroid/2

37. Which of the following conditions will increase total T_4 by increasing TBG?
A. Acute illness
B. Anabolic steroid use
C. Nephrotic syndrome
D. Pregnancy or estrogens

Chemistry/Correlate clinical and laboratory data/Thyroid/2

38. Select the most appropriate single screening test for thyroid disease.
A. Free thyroxine index
B. Total T_3 assay
C. Total T_4
D. TSH assay

Chemistry/Correlate clinical and laboratory data/Thyroid/2

39. The serum TSH level is *decreased* in:
A. Primary hyperthyrodism
B. Primary hypothyroidism
C. Secondary hyperthyroidism
D. Euthyroid sick syndrome

Chemistry/Correlate clinical and laboratory data/Thyroid/1

40. Which assay is the most specific and sensitive test for diagnosing thyroid disease?
A. Free T_3 assay
B. Free thyroxine index
C. Thyrotropin-releasing hormone (TRH) stimulation test
D. TBG assay

Chemistry/Correlate clinical and laboratory data/Thyroid/2

41. Which of the following statements is true regarding reverse T_3 (rT_3)?
A. Formed in the blood by degradation of T_4
B. Physiologically active, but less than T_3
C. Decreased in euthyroid sick syndrome
D. Interferes with the measurement of serum T_3 by RIA

Chemistry/Apply knowledge of fundamental biological characteristics/Thyroid/2

Answers to Questions 36–41

36. **B** Total serum T_4 and T_3 are dependent upon both thyroid function and the amount of thyroxine-binding proteins such as thyroxine-binding globulin (TBG). Total T_4 or T_3 may be abnormal in a patient with normal thyroid function, if TBG levels are abnormal. For this reason, free T_3 and T_4 are more specific indicators of thyroid function than are measurements of total hormone.

37. **D** Pregnancy and estrogens are the most common cause of increased TBG. Other causes include hepatitis, morphine, and clofibrate therapy. Acute illness, anabolic steroids, and nephrotic syndrome decrease the level of TBG. Pregnancy causes an elevated serum total T_4 but does not affect free T_4 or thyroid status.

38. **D** TSH is produced by the anterior pituitary in response to low levels of free T_4 or T_3. A normal TSH rules out thyroid disease. TSH is low in primary hyperthyroidism and high in primary hypothyroidism.

39. **A** Low TSH and a high T_3 (and usually T_4) occur in primary hyperthyroidism. A high TSH and low T_4 occur in primary hypothyroidism but can also occur in an acutely ill patient without thyroid disease, the euthyroid sick syndrome. Secondary hyperthyroidism is caused by pituitary hyperfunction resulting in increased serum TSH.

40. **C** TRH stimulation test is used to confirm borderline cases of abnormal thyroid function. In normal patients, intravenous injection of 500 µg of TRH causes a peak TSH response within 30 minutes. In patients with primary hypothyroidism, there is an exaggerated response (>30 U/L). Patients with hyperthyroidism do not show the expected rise in TSH after TRH stimulation.

41. **A** Reverse T_3 is formed from the deiodination of T_4 in the blood. It is an inactive isomer of T_3, ($3,3',5'$-triiodothyronine). Reverse T_3 is increased in acute and chronic illness and is used to identify patients with euthyroid sick syndrome.

42. Which statement regarding the free thyroxine index (FTI) is true?
  A. The FTI is proportional to total thyroxine divided by the unsaturated thyroxine-binding globulin (UTBG).
  B. A euthyroid patient has a normal FTI even when T_4 is affected by TBG.
  C. The FTI is high in hyperthyroidism and low in hypothyroidism.
  D. All of the above.

Chemistry/Correlate clinical and laboratory data/Thyroid/2

43. T_3 resin uptake (T_3U or T Uptake) is a measure of:
  A. The unoccupied binding sites on TBG
  B. The ability of the thyroid gland to take up radio-labeled iodine
  C. The binding of T_3 to thyroxine receptors
  D. The plasma level of free T_3

Chemistry/Apply knowledge of fundamental biological characteristics/Thyroid/2

44. A patient has an elevated serum T_3 and free T_4 and a low serum TSH. What is the most likely cause of these results?
  A. Primary hyperthyroidism
  B. Secondary hyperthyroidism
  C. Euthyroid with increased thyroxine-binding proteins
  D. Euthyroid sick syndrome

Chemistry/Correlate clinical and laboratory data/Thyroid/3

Answers to Questions 42–44

42. **D** The FTI is an indirect measure of free T_4. Bound T_4 is in equilibrium with free T_4 and UTBG (Bound $T_4 \rightarrow$ Free T_4 + UTBG). Free T_4 increases when the ratio of bound T_4:UTBG increases. Because bound T_4 comprises more than 99.9% of the total T_4, free T_4 is proportional to total T_4/UTBG).

43. **A** The T Uptake test determines the available binding sites on TBG or the UTBG. Most laboratories use a nonisotopic method for measuring T uptake. Nonisotopic tests usually use anti-T_4 to detect the T_4 not bound by TBG. For example, excess T_4 is mixed with serum to saturate thyroxine-binding proteins. The T_4 not bound by TBG and other proteins competes with fluorescent-labeled T_4 for a limited amount of anti-T_4. The amount of fluorescence in the antigen-antibody complexes will be proportional to the UTBG of the serum. Most laboratories report the T Uptake result as a ratio called the thyroid hormone-binding ratio (THBR). When the signal measured is inversely proportional to UTBG (e.g., EMIT) the ratio is determined by dividing the patient's result by the normal serum control. When the signal is proportional to UTBG (e.g., FPIA) the ratio is determined by dividing the normal serum control by the patient's result. (In either case, FTI = $T_4 \times$ THBR). The THBR has a reference interval of 0.85–1.15. Patients with a high UTBG, such as those with hypothyroidism, have a low THBR, T_3U, or T Uptake.

44. **A** A low TSH is almost always caused by either primary hyperthyroidism (suppression via high free thyroid hormone) or secondary hypothyroidism (decreased pituitary function). In rare cases, it can be induced by medications. In this patient, high levels of T_3 and free T_4 are causing the low TSH, indicating primary hyperthyroidism. In secondary hyperthyroidism the TSH will be elevated in addition to at least the T_3. Patients with an increased thyroxine-binding protein level will have an increase in T_3 but not free T_4 or TSH, and will also have an increased UTBG. Patients with euthyroid sick syndrome usually have a low T_3 or T_4 but a normal or slightly elevated TSH.

45. A serum thyroid panel reveals an increase in total T_4, normal TSH, and low THBR (increased UTBG). What is the most likely cause of these results?
A. Primary hyperthyroidism
B. Secondary hyperthyroidism
C. Euthyroid with increased thyroxine-binding protein
D. Subclinical hypothyroidisim

Chemistry/Correlate clinical and laboratory data/Thyroid/3

Answer to Question 45

45. **C** Patients with a normal TSH are euthyroid, and most commonly an increase in total T_4 in these patients is caused by an increase in TBG. An increase in TBG causes an increase in total T_4 but not free T_4. Subclinical hypothyroidism is usually associated with a high TSH, but normal free T_3 and T_4. When TSH is indeterminate, the diagnosis is made by demonstrating an exaggerated response to the TRH stimulation test.

Toxicology and Therapeutic Drug Monitoring

1. In which of the cases below is qualitative analysis of the drug usually adequate?
   A. To determine whether the dose of a drug with a low therapeutic index is likely to be toxic
   B. To determine whether a patient is complying with the physician's instructions
   C. To adjust dose if individual differences or disease alter expected response
   D. To determine whether the patient has been taking amphetamines

   Chemistry/Apply knowledge of fundamental biological characteristics/Therapeutic drug monitoring/1

2. The term *pharmacokinetics* refers to the:
   A. Relationship between drug dose and the drug blood level
   B. Concentration of drug at its sites of action
   C. Relationship between blood concentration and therapeutic response
   D. The relationship between blood and tissue drug levels

   Chemistry/Apply knowledge of fundamental biological characteristics/1

3. The term *pharmacodynamics* is an expression of the relationship between:
   A. Dose and physiological effect
   B. Drug concentration at target sites and physiological effect
   C. Time and serum drug concentration
   D. Blood and tissue drug levels

   Chemistry/Apply knowledge of fundamental biological characteristics/Therapeutic drug monitoring/1

Answers to Questions 1–3

1. **D** The purpose of therapeutic drug monitoring is to achieve a therapeutic blood drug level rapidly and minimize the risk of drug toxicity caused by overdose. Therapeutic drug monitoring is a quantitative procedure performed for drugs with a narrow therapeutic index (ratio of the concentration producing the desired effect to the concentration producing toxicity). Drug groups that require monitoring because of high risk of toxicity include aminoglycoside antibiotics, anticonvulsants, antiarrhythmics, antiasthmatics, and psychoactive drugs. When testing for abuse substances the goal is usually to determine whether the drug is present or absent. The most common approach is to compare the result to a cutoff determined by measuring a standard containing the lowest level of drug that is considered significant.

2. **A** Pharmacokinetics is the mathematical expression of the relationship between drug dose and drug blood level. When the appropriate formula is applied to quantitative measures of drug dose, absorption, distribution, and elimination the blood concentration can be accurately determined.

3. **B** Pharmacodynamics is the relationship between the drug concentration at the receptor site (tissue concentration) and the response of the tissue to that drug. For example, the relationship between lidocaine concentration in the heart muscle and the duration of the action potential of Purkinje fibers.

4. Select the five pharmacological parameters that determine serum drug concentration.
  A. Absorption, anabolism, perfusion, bioactivation, excretion
  B. Liberation, equilibration, biotransformation, re-absorption, elimination
  C. Liberation, absorption, distribution, metabolism, excretion
  D. Ingestion, conjugation, integration, metabolism, elimination

Chemistry/Apply knowledge of fundamental biological characteristics/Therapeutic drug monitoring/1

5. Which route of administration is associated with 100% bioavailability?
  A. Sublingual
  B. Intramuscular
  C. Oral
  D. Intravenous

Chemistry/Apply knowledge of fundamental biological characteristics/Therapeutic drug monitoring/2

6. The phrase *first pass hepatic metabolism* means that:
  A. One hundred percent of a drug is excreted by the liver.
  B. All drug is inactivated by hepatic enzymes after one pass through the liver.
  C. Some drug is metabolized from the portal circulation reducing bioavailability.
  D. The drug must be metabolized in the liver to an active form.

Chemistry/Apply knowledge of fundamental biological characteristics/Therapeutic drug monitoring/2

7. Which formula can be used to estimate dosage needed to give a desired steady-state blood level?
  A. Dose per hour = clearance (milligrams per hour) $\times$ average concentration at steady state $\div$ f
  B. Dose per day = fraction absorbed $-$ fraction excreted
  C. Dose = fraction absorbed $\times$ (1/protein-bound fraction)
  D. Dose per day = half-life $\times$ log V_d (volume distribution)

Chemistry/Calculate/Therapeutic drug monitoring/2

8. Which statement is true regarding the volume distribution (V_d) of a drug?
  A. V_d is equal to the clearance divided by the elimination rate constant (K).
  B. V_d is the theoretical volume in liters into which the drug distributes.
  C. The higher the V_d, the higher the dose needed to reach the target blood level.
  D. All of the above.

Chemistry/Apply knowledge of fundamental biological characteristics/Therapeutic drug monitoring/2

9. For drugs with first-order elimination which statement about drug clearance is true?
  A. Clearance = elimination rate $\div$ serum level.
  B. It is most often performed by the liver.
  C. It is directly related to half-life.
  D. Clearance rate is independent of dose.

Chemistry/Apply knowledge of fundamental biological characteristics/Therapeutic drug monitoring/2

Answers to Questions 4–9

4. **C** *Liberation* is the release of the drug and *absorption* is the transport of drug from the site of administration to the blood. The percent of drug absorption and the rate of absorption determine the bioavailable fraction, *f*. This is the fraction of the dose that reaches the blood.

5. **D** When a drug is administered intravenously, all the drug enters the bloodstream, and therefore, the bioavailable fraction is 1.0.

6. **C** Drugs given orally enter the blood via the portal circulation and are transported directly to the liver. Some drugs are excreted by the liver, and a fraction will be lost by hepatic excretion before the drug reaches the general circulation. An example is propranolol, a β-blocker that reduces heart rate and hypertension. The bioavailable fraction is 0.2–0.4 when given orally.

7. **A** After a patient receives a loading dose to rapidly bring the drug level up to the desired therapeutic range, a maintenance dose must be given at consistent intervals to maintain the blood drug level at the desired concentration. The dose per hour is determined by multiplying the clearance per hour by the desired average steady-state concentration, then dividing by *f* (bioavailable fraction).

8. **D** The V_d of a drug represents the dilution of the drug after it has been distributed in the body. The V_d is used to estimate the peak drug blood level expected after a loading dose is given. The peak blood level equals the dose multiplied by f/V_d.

9. **A** First-order elimination represents a linear relationship between the amount of drug eliminated per hour and the blood level of drug. For drugs following linear kinetics, clearance equals the elimination rate divided by the drug concentration in blood. When clearance (in milligrams per hour) and *f* are known, the dose per hour needed to give a desired average drug level at steady state can be calculated.

10. Which statement about steady-state drug levels is true?
   A. The absorbed drug must be greater than the amount excreted.
   B. Steady state can be measured after two elimination half-lives.
   C. Constant intravenous infusion will give the same minima and maxima as an oral dose.
   D. Oral dosing intervals give peaks and troughs in the dose-response curve.

   Chemistry/Apply knowledge of fundamental biological characteristics/Therapeutic drug monitoring/2

11. If too small a peak-trough difference is seen for a drug given orally then:
   A. The dose should be decreased.
   B. Time between doses should be decreased.
   C. Dose interval should be increased.
   D. Dose per day and time between doses should be decreased.

   Chemistry/Select course of action/Therapeutic drug monitoring/3

12. If the peak level is appropriate but the trough level too low at steady state, then the dose interval should:
   A. Be lengthened without changing the dose per day
   B. Be lengthened and dose rate decreased
   C. Not be changed but dose per day increased
   D. Be shortened, but dose per day not changed

   Chemistry/Select source of action/Therapeutic drug monitoring/3

13. If the steady-state drug level is too high the best course of action is to:
   A. Decrease the dose
   B. Decrease the dose interval
   C. Decrease the dose and decrease the dose interval
   D. Change the route of administration

   Chemistry/Select course of action/Therapeutic drug monitoring/3

14. When should blood samples for trough drug levels be collected?
   A. 30 minutes after peak levels
   B. 45 minutes before the next dose
   C. 1–2 hours after the last dose
   D. Immediately before the next dose is given

   Chemistry/Apply knowledge to recognize sources of error/Sample collection and handling/1

15. Blood sample collection time for peak drug levels:
   A. Varies with the drug depending on its rate of absorption
   B. Is independent of drug formulation
   C. Is independent of the route of administration
   D. Is 30 minutes after a bolus intravenous injection is completed

Chemistry/Apply knowledge to recognize sources of error/Sample collection and handling/2

Answers to Questions 10–15

10. **D** When drugs are infused intravenously, both the distribution and elimination rates are constant. This eliminates the peaks and troughs seen in the dose-response curve. Peak and trough levels are characteristics of intermittent dosing regimens. The steady state is reached when drug in the next dose is sufficient only to replace the drug eliminated since the last dose. Steady state can be measured after five drug half-lives because blood levels will have reached 97% of steady state.

11. **C** Increasing the dosing interval will reduce the trough concentration of the drug, and increasing the dose will increase the peak concentration of the drug resulting in a greater peak-trough difference. The peak-trough ratio is usually adjusted to 2 with dose interval set to equal the drug half-life. Under these conditions both peak and trough levels often fall within the therapeutic range.

12. **D** Increasing the dose rate may result in peak drug levels in the toxic range. Decreasing the dosing interval will raise the trough level so that it is maintained in the therapeutic range. The trough level is affected by the drug clearance rate. If clearance increases, then trough level decreases.

13. **A** Decreasing both dose and dosing interval will have offsetting effects on peak and trough blood levels. The appropriate dose can be calculated if the clearance or V_d and f are known.

14. **D** The trough concentration of a drug is the lowest concentration obtained in the dosing interval. This occurs immediately before the absorption of the next dose given. Trough levels are usually collected just before the next dose is given.

15. **A** The peak concentration of a drug is the highest concentration obtained in the dosing interval. For oral drugs the time of peak concentration is dependent upon their rates of absorption and elimination and is determined by serial blood measurements. Peak levels for oral drugs are usually drawn 1–2 hours after administration of the dose. For drugs given intravenously, peak levels are measured immediately after the infusion is completed.

16. Which could account for drug toxicity following a normally prescribed dose?
   A. Decreased renal clearance caused by kidney disease
   B. Discontinuance of another drug
   C. Altered serum protein binding caused by disease
   D. All of the above

Chemistry/Apply knowledge of fundamental biological characteristics/Therapeutic drug monitoring/2

17. Select the elimination model that best describes most oral drugs.
   A. One compartment, linear first-order elimination
   B. Michaelis-Menton or concentration-dependent elimination
   C. Two compartment with a biphasic elimination curve
   D. Logarithmic elimination

Chemistry/Apply knowledge of fundamental biological characteristics/Therapeutic drug monitoring/2

18. Drugs rapidly infused intravenously usually follow which elimination model?
   A. One compartment, first order
   B. One compartment, logarithmic
   C. Biphasic or two compartment with serum level rapidly falling in the first phase
   D. Michaelis-Menton or concentration-dependent elimination

Chemistry/Apply knowledge of fundamental biological characteristics/Therapeutic drug monitoring/2

19. Which fact must be considered when evaluating a patient who displays signs of drug toxicity?
   A. Drug metabolites (e.g., N-acetylprocainamide) may need to be measured as well as parent drug.
   B. If the concentration of total drug is within therapeutic limits, the concentration of free drug cannot be toxic.
   C. If the drug has a wide therapeutic index, then it will not be toxic.
   D. A drug level cannot be toxic if the trough is within the published therapeutic range.

Chemistry/Apply knowledge of fundamental biological characteristics/Therapeutic drug monitoring/2

20. When a therapeutic drug is suspected of causing toxicity, which specimen is the most appropriate for an initial investigation?
   A. Trough blood sample
   B. Peak blood sample
   C. Urine at the time of symptoms
   D. Gastric fluid at the time of symptoms

Chemistry/Select course of action/Therapeutic drug monitoring/3

Answers to Questions 16–20

16. **D** Therapeutic drug monitoring is necessary for drugs that have a narrow therapeutic index. Individual differences alter pharmacokinetics causing lack of correlation between dose and drug blood level. These include age, diet, ingestion with or without food, genetic factors, exercise, smoking, pregnancy, metabolism of other drugs, protein binding, and disease states.

17. **A** Most drugs given orally distribute uniformly through the tissues reaching rapid equilibrium, so both blood and tissues can be viewed as a single compartment. Elimination according to Michaelis-Menton kinetics is nonlinear because at high concentrations, the hepatic enzyme system becomes saturated, reducing the elimination efficiency.

18. **C** Drugs rapidly infused intravenously follow a two-compartment model of elimination. The central compartment is the blood and tissues that are well perfused. The second consists of tissues for which distribution of drug is time-dependent. In determining the loading dose the desired serum concentration should be multiplied by the volume of the central compartment to avoid toxic levels.

19. **A** Altered drug pharmacokinetics may result in toxicity even when the dose of drug is within the accepted therapeutic range. Two common causes of this are the presence of unmeasured metabolites that are physiologically active, and the presence of a higher than expected concentration of free drug. Because only free drug is physiologically active, decreased binding protein or factors that shift the equilibrium favoring more unbound drug can result in toxicity when the total drug concentration is within the therapeutic range. Some drugs with a wide therapeutic index are potentially toxic because they may be ingested in great excess with little or no initial toxicity. For example, acetaminophen overdose does not usually become apparent until 3–5 days after the overdose. This creates the potential for hepatic damage to occur from continued use, especially in patients who have decreased hepatic or renal function because the drug half-life is extended.

20. **B** When a drug is suspected of toxicity, the peak blood sample (sample after absorption and distribution are complete) should be obtained because it is most likely to exceed the therapeutic limit. If the peak level is above the upper therapeutic limit, then toxicity is confirmed, and the drug dose is lowered. If the peak drug concentration is within the therapeutic range, toxicity is less likely, but cannot be ruled out. A high concentration of free drug, the presence of active metabolites, and abnormal response to the drug are causes of drug toxicity that may occur when the blood drug level is within the published therapeutic range.

21. For a drug that follows first-order pharmacokinetics, adjustment of dosage to achieve the desired blood level can be made using which formula?

A. $\text{New dose} = \dfrac{\text{current dose}}{\text{concentration at steady state}}$
   $\times \text{desired concentration}$

B. $\text{New dose} = \dfrac{\text{current dose}}{\text{desired concentration}}$
   $\times \text{concentration at steady state}$

C. $\text{New dose} = \dfrac{\text{concentration at steady state}}{\text{desired concentration}}$
   $\times \text{half-life}$

D. $\text{New dose} = \dfrac{\text{concentration at steady state}}{\text{current dose}}$
   $\times \text{desired concentration}$

Chemistry/Apply knowledge of fundamental biological characteristics/Therapeutic drug monitoring/2

22. For which drug group are both peak and trough measurements usually required?
A. Antiarrhythmics
B. Analgesics
C. Tricyclic antidepressants
D. Aminoglycoside antibiotics

Chemistry/Select course of action/Therapeutic drug monitoring/2

23. Which of the following statements about TLC for drug screening is true?
A. Acidic drugs are extracted in an alkaline nonpolar solvent.
B. A drug is identified by comparing its R_f value and staining to standards.
C. Testing must be performed using a urine sample.
D. Opiates and other alkaloids are extracted at an acid pH.

Chemistry/Apply principles of special procedures/Chromatography/2

24. The EMIT for drugs of abuse uses an:
A. Antibody conjugated to a drug
B. Enzyme conjugated to an antibody
C. Enzyme conjugated to a drug
D. Antibody bound to a solid phase

Chemistry/Apply principles of special procedures/Biochemical theory and principle/2

25. Which statement about EMIT is true?
A. Enzyme activity is inversely proportional to drug level.
B. Formation of NADH is monitored at 340 nm.
C. ALP is the commonly used conjugate.
D. Assay use is restricted to serum.

Chemistry/Apply principles of special procedures/Biochemical theory and principle/2

Answers to Questions 21–25

21. **A** Most drugs follow first-order pharmacokinetics, meaning the clearance of drug is linearly related to the drug dose. The dose of such drugs can be adjusted by multiplying the ratio of the current dose to blood concentration by the desired drug concentration provided the blood concentration is measured at steady state.

22. **D** Aminoglycoside antibiotics cause damage to the eighth cranial nerve at toxic levels resulting in hearing loss. When given at subtherapeutic doses they fail to resolve infection. Most drugs falling in the other classes have a narrow peak-trough difference but are highly toxic when blood levels exceed the therapeutic range. Usually, these can be safely monitored by measuring trough levels.

23. **B** TLC can be performed on urine, serum, or gastric fluid and qualitatively identifies most drugs. Each has a characteristic R_f, which is the ratio of the distance migrated by the drug to the solvent. The R_f of the sample must match the R_f of the drug standard. Extraction of drugs for TLC is highly pH-dependent. The pH must be adjusted to reduce the solubility (ionization) of the drug in the aqueous phase. Alkaline drugs (e.g., opiates) are extracted at pH 9.0 and acidic drugs (e.g., barbiturates) at pH 4.5.

24. **C** In EMIT, enzyme-labeled drug competes with drug in the sample for a limited amount of reagent antibodies. When antibody binds to the enzyme-drug conjugate it blocks the catalytic site of the enzyme. Enzyme activity is directly proportional to sample drug concentration because the quantity of unbound drug-enzyme conjugate will be highest when drug is present in the sample.

25. **B** EMIT is a homogenous immunoassay meaning that free antigen does not have to be separated from bound antigen. Most EMIT assays use a two-reagent system. Reagent A contains substrate (usually glucose-6-PO_4), coenzyme (NAD^+), and antibody to the drug. Reagent B contains enzyme-labeled drug (usually G-6-PD-drug) and buffer. The enzyme activity of the low standard is used as the cutoff.

26. Which statement below regarding FPIA is true?
  A. Plane-polarized fluorescence is directly related to the drug level.
  B. β-Galactosidase is commonly used to label the antigen.
  C. Separation of free and bound labeled antigen is not required.
  D. Assays are based upon the double antibody sandwich method.

Chemistry/Apply principles of special procedures/ Biochemical theory and principle/2

27. Which statement about measurement of carboxy-hemoglobin is true?
  A. Blood can be treated with alkaline dithionite to form deoxyhemoglobin.
  B. Carboxyhemoglobin absorbance peaks are at approximately 540 and 570 nm.
  C. Correction for deoxyhemoglobin can be made by bichromatic analysis at 541:555 nm.
  D. All of the above.

Chemistry/Apply principles of special procedures/ Carboxyhemoglobin/2

28. Which of the following statements about blood alcohol measurement is correct?
  A. Alcohol levels greater than 0.05% w/v correlate with intoxication.
  B. The skin puncture site should be disinfected with isopropanol.
  C. The reference method is based upon enzymatic oxidation of ethanol by alcohol dehydrogenase.
  D. Gas chromatography methods require extraction of ethanol from serum.

Chemistry/Apply principles of special procedures/ Ethanol/2

29. Which drug can be detected with ferric chloride in perchloric-nitric acids?
  A. Phenothiazines
  B. Acetaminophen
  C. Morphine
  D. Maprobamate

Chemistry/Apply principles of special procedures/ Toxicology/1

Answers to Questions 26–29

26. **C** Fluorescein-labeled drug, serum, and antibody are mixed and placed in the light path of a fluorometer. When drug-fluorescein conjugate is bound by antibody its rotation slows causing plane polarized fluorescence. Unbound conjugate emits unpolarized green light, which is not detected. Antibody-bound conjugate (polarized fluorescence) is inversely related to serum drug concentration.

27. **D** Bichromatic analysis of carboxyhemoglobin is performed after treatment with alkaline dithionite to reduce oxyhemoglobin to deoxyhemoglobin. This removes the 540 nm absorbance peak of oxyhemoglobin, which interferes with the carboxyhemoglobin absorbance peak at 541 nm. The ratio of absorbance at 541:555 nm is directly proportional to carboxyhemoglobin concentration. Percent carboxyhemoglobin can also be determined from simultaneous absorbance measurements at 548, 568, and 578 nm.

28. **A** Alcohol dehydrogenase is not specific for ethanol, and *in vitro* interference can occur with some ADH methods when skin is disinfected with other alcohols. For this reason, and to avoid interference with the interpretation of chromatograms for volatiles, blood samples are collected after disinfecting the skin site with benzalkonium chloride or other nonalcohol antiseptic. GLC is the legally accepted method of ethanol analysis. The low boiling point of ethanol permits direct analysis on blood or plasma diluted with water containing 1-propanol or other suitable internal standard.

29. **A** Ferric ions react with phenothiazine tranquilizers forming an intense purple complex. The reaction is nonspecific but useful as a screening test. Ferric ions react with many metabolites and drugs in urine including salicylate (purple), phenylpyruvic acid (green), and acetoacetic acid (pink). Acetaminophen in urine is detected by boiling to form *p*-amphenol. This reacts with *o*-cresol, forming indophenol blue.

30. Which specimen is the sample of choice for lead screening?
A. Whole blood
B. Hair
C. Serum
D. Urine

Chemistry/Apply principles of special procedures/ Lead/1

Answer to Question 30

30. **A** Lead accumulates in RBCs, bones, and neural tissues, and whole blood, hair, and urine are suitable for demonstrating lead toxicity. Greatest sensitivity is obtained by using whole blood, which can detect exposure over time. Because lead is rapidly eliminated from plasma, serum or plasma should not be used to test for lead exposure. Lead binds to sulfhydryl groups of proteins such as delta-aminolevulinic acid (Δ-ALA) dehydratase and ferrochelatase and interferes with heme synthesis. This results in increased free erythrocyte protoporphyrin, erythrocyte zinc protoporphyrin, urinary coproporphyrin III, and δ aminolevulinic acid, which are also useful markers for lead poisoning. When screening for lead poisoning in children, the method of choice is graphite furnace atomic absorption spectrophotometry. This method has a sensitivity of 1.0 μg/dL, which is required to accurately demonstrate normal levels in children. The CDC cutoff for normal lead in children is less than 10.0 μg/dL.

Clinical Chemistry Problem Solving

1. Which of the procedures below can be used to evaluate a new glucose method for proportional error?
   A. Compare the standard deviation of 40 patient samples to the hexokinase method.
   B. Measure a mixture made from equal parts of normal and high QC sera.
   C. Add 5.0 mg of glucose to 1.0 mL of a serum of known concentration and measure.
   D. Compare the mean of 40 normal samples to the hexokinase method.

   Chemistry/Select course of action/Method evaluation/3

2. Which of two instruments can be assumed to have the narrower bandpass? Assume that wavelength is accurately calibrated.
   A. The instrument giving the highest absorbance for a solution of 0.1 mmol/L NADH at 340 nm
   B. The instrument giving the lowest %T for a solution of nickel sulfate at 700 nm
   C. The instrument giving the highest %T reading for 1.0% v/v HCl at 350 nm
   D. The instrument giving the most linear plot of absorbance versus concentration

   Chemistry/Select course of action/ Spectrophotometry/3

3. A lipemic sample gives a sodium of 130 mmol/L by flame photometry and 142 mmol/L using a direct (undiluted) ion-selective electrode (ISE). Assuming acceptable QC, which of the following is the most appropriate course of action?
   A. Report a sodium result of 136 mmol/L.
   B. Ultracentrifuge the sample and repeat by ISE.
   C. Dilute the sample 1:4 and repeat by ISE.
   D. Report the ISE result.

   Chemistry/Select course of action/Electrolytes/3

Answers to Questions 1–3

1. **C** Proportional error is percentage deviation from the expected result, and affects the slope of the calibration curve. It causes a greater absolute error (loss of accuracy) as concentration increases. It is measured by a recovery study in which a sample is spiked with known amounts of analyte. In the example, the concentration should increase by 500 mg/dL.

2. **A** Bandpass is defined by the range of wavelengths passed through the sample at the specified wavelength setting. It can be measured using any solution having a narrow absorbance peak (e.g., NADH at 340 nm). The instrument producing the purest monochromatic light will have the highest absorbance reading.

3. **D** Lipemic samples give lower results for sodium (pseudohyponatremia) by flame photometry or prediluted ISE methods because the H_2O phase is mostly diluent and a significant component of the sample volume is displaced by lipid. Direct ISEs measure sodium in the plasma water, more accurately reflecting patient status.

4. SITUATION: A 2_{2S} QC error occurs for serum calcium by atomic absorption. Fresh standards prepared in 5.0% w/v albumin are found to be linear, but repeating the controls with fresh material does not improve the QC results. Select the most likely cause of this problem.
A. Matrix effect caused by a viscosity difference between the standards and QC sera
B. Chemical interference caused incomplete atomization
C. Incomplete deconjugation of protein-bound calcium
D. Ionization interference caused by excessive heat

Chemistry/Evaluate laboratory data to recognize problems/Atomic absorption/3

5. SITUATION: A serum osmolality measured in the emergency room is 326 mOsm/kg. Two hours later, chemistry results are:

Na = 135 mmol/L; BUN = 18 mg/dL; glucose = 72 mg/dL; measured osmolality = 318 mOsm/kg

What do these results suggest?
A. Laboratory error in electrolyte or glucose measurement
B. Drug or alcohol intoxication
C. Specimen misidentification
D. Successful rehydration of the patient

Chemistry/Evaluate laboratory data to determine possible inconsistent results/Osmolality/3

6. When calibrating a pH meter, unstable readings occur for both pH 7.00 and 4.00 calibrators, although both can be set to within 0.1 pH unit. Select the most appropriate course of action.
A. Measure the pH of the sample and report to the nearest 0.1 pH.
B. Replace both calibrators with unopened buffers and recalibrate.
C. Examine the reference electrode junction for salt crystals.
D. Move the electrodes to another pH meter and calibrate.

Chemistry/Select course of action/pH/3

7. A method calls for extracting an acidic drug from urine with an anion exchange column. The pK_a of the drug is 6.5. Extraction is enhanced by adjusting the sample pH to:
A. 8.5
B. 6.5
C. 5.5
D. 4.5

Chemistry/Select course of action/ Chromatography/3

8. SITUATION: A patient who has a positive urinalysis for glucose and ketones has a glycosylated Hgb of 4.0%. A fasting glucose performed the previous day was 180 mg/dL. Assuming acceptable QC you would:

A. Report the glycosylated Hgb.
B. Request a new specimen and repeat the glycosylated Hgb.
C. Perform a Hgb electrophoresis on the sample.
D. Perform a glucose measurement on the sample.

Chemistry/Evaluate laboratory data to determine possible inconsistent results/Glycosylated hemoglobin/3

Answers to Questions 4–8

4. **B** Poor recovery of calcium by atomic absorption is often caused by failure to break thermostable bonds between calcium and phosphate (a form of chemical interference). This may be caused by failure to add lanthanum to the diluent or by low atomizer temperature.

5. **B** The *osmolal gap* is the difference between calculated and measured osmolality. Here the osmolal gap is 38 mOsm/kg. When the osmolal gap is greater than 12 mOsm/kg, an unmeasured solute is present or an analytical error occurred when measuring the osmolality, electrolytes, urea, or glucose. The reference range for serum osmolality is 280–295 mOsm/kg. Both measurements are above the URL. These results point to the presence of an unmeasured solute. A significant osmolal gap in samples from emergency room patients usually results from alcohol or drug consumption. The difference in osmolality between the two samples is 8 mOsm/kg and can be explained by alcohol metabolism.

6. **C** Noise in pH measurements often results from a blocked junction between the reservoir of the reference electrode and test solution. This occurs when salt crystals collect at the junction or when KCl concentration in the reservoir increases due to evaporation of water. The fluid in the reference electrode should be replaced with warm deionized water. After the crystals have dissolved, the water is replaced with fresh reference electrolyte solution.

7. **A** Extraction of a negatively charged drug onto an anion exchange (positively charged) column is optimal when more than 99% of the drug is in the form of anion. The extraction pH should be 2 pH units above the pK_a of an acidic drug. When pH = pK_a the drug will be 50% ionized, and when pH is greater than pK_a the majority of drug is anionic.

8. **B** The glycosylated Hgb is within normal limits (2%–8%), but the fasting glucose indicates frank diabetes mellitus. Although the glycosylated Hgb reflects the average blood glucose 2–3 months earlier, the value reported is inconsistent with the other laboratory results. A high probability of sample misidentification or analytical error necessitates that the test be repeated.

9. Quality control results for uric acid are as follows:

	Run 1	Run 2	Run 3	Run 4	Mean	s
					Expected Results	
QC1	3.5	3.8	4.1	4.2 mg/dL	3.6 mg/dL	0.40
QC2	6.8	7.2	7.4	7.5 mg/dL	7.0 mg/dL	0.25

Results should be reported from:
A. Run 1 only
B. Runs 1 and 2
C. Runs 1, 2, and 3
D. Runs 1, 2, 3, and 4

Chemistry/Select course of action/Quality control/3

10. SITUATION: A peak blood level for orally administered theophylline (therapeutic range 8–20 mg/L) measured at 8 AM is 5.0 mg/L. The preceding trough level was 4.6 mg/L. What is the most likely explanation of these results?
A. Laboratory error made on peak measurement.
B. Specimen for peak level was collected from wrong patient
C. Blood for peak level was drawn too soon.
D. Elimination rate has reached maximum.

Chemistry/Apply knowledge to recognize sources of error/Therapeutic drug monitoring/3

11. SITUATION: A patient breathing room air has the following arterial blood gas and electrolyte results:

pH = 7.54; P_{CO_2} = 18.5 mm Hg; P_{O_2} = 145 mm Hg; HCO_3 = 18 mmol/L

Na = 135 mmol/L; K = 4.6 mmol/L; Cl = 98 mmol/L; T_{CO_2} = 26 mmol/L

The best explanation for these results is:
A. Blood for electrolytes was drawn above an IV.
B. Serum sample was hemolyzed.
C. Venous blood was sampled for arterial blood gases.
D. Blood gas sample was exposed to air.

Chemistry/Evaluate laboratory data to determine possible inconsistent results/Blood gases/3

12. SITUATION: Laboratory results on a patient from the emergency room are:

Glucose = 1100 mg/dL; Na = 155 mmol/L; K = 1.2 mmol/L; Cl = 115 mmol/L; T_{CO_2} = 3.0 mmol/L

What is the most likely explanation of these results?
A. Sample drawn above an IV
B. Metabolic acidosis with increased anion gap
C. Diabetic ketoacidosis
D. Laboratory error measuring electrolytes caused by hyperglycemia

Chemistry/Evaluate laboratory data to recognize problems/Specimen collection/3

13. SITUATION: Results of CK isoenzymes by electrophoresis are reported as CK-1 0%; CK-2 45%; CK-3

55%. The patient's biochemical profile showed elevated bilirubin and ALP, but normal total CK. The most likely explanation is:
A. Massive MI secondary to hepatic congestion.
B. Mitochondrial CK of hepatic origin is present.
C. Fluorescent albumin-bilirubin complex was mistaken for CK-2.
D. CK-1 denatured by heat has migrated with CK-2.

Chemistry/Evaluate laboratory data to assess validity/Accuracy of procedures/CK isoenzymes/3

Answers to Questions 9–13

9. **C** Although no single result exceeds the 2s limit, the 4_{1S} rule is broken on Run 4. This means that both QC1 and QC2 exceeded +1s on Run 3 and Run 4.

10. **C** Sample collection time is critical for accurate therapeutic drug monitoring. Blood for trough levels must be collected immediately before the next dose. Blood collection time for peak levels must not occur prior to complete absorption and distribution of drug. This usually requires 1–2 hours for orally administered drugs. The therapeutic range for theophylline is 8–20 mg/L. These results are most consistent with a peak sample having been drawn prior to complete absorption of the drug.

11. **D** A patient breathing room air cannot have an arterial P_{O_2} greater than 105 mm Hg because alveolar P_{O_2} is 110 mm Hg when IP_{O_2} = 150 mm Hg. Exposure to air caused loss of CO_2 gas and increased pH. This patient's blood gas values do not correlate with T_{CO_2}.

12. **A** These results are consistent with dilution of venous blood by intravenous fluid containing 5% dextrose and normal saline. The intravenous fluid is free of potassium and bicarbonate, accounting for the low level of these electrolytes (incompatible with life).

13. **C** A CK-MB level of 45% should be questioned because no tissue has that much CK-MB. Albumin-bilirubin complex migrates between CK-1 and CK-2, and care must be taken not to confuse the fluorescent albumin band with CK-1 or CK-2.

14. SITUATION: A patient has the following electrolyte results:

Na = 130 mmol/L; K = 4.8 mmol/L; Cl = 105 mmol/L; TCO_2 = 26 mmol/L

Assuming acceptable QC, select the best course of action.
A. Report these results.
B. Check the albumin, total protein, Ca, P, and Mg results; if normal, repeat the sodium test.
C. Request a new sample.
D. Recalibrate and repeat the potassium test.

Chemistry/Evaluate laboratory data to check for sources of error/Anion gap/3

15. A stat plasma lithium determined using an ion-selective electrode is measured at 14.0 mmol/L. Select the most appropriate course of action.
A. Immediately report this result.
B. Check sample for hemolysis.
C. Call for a new specimen.
D. Rerun the lithium calibrators.

Chemistry/Select course of action/Therapeutic drug monitoring/3

16. A chromatogram for blood alcohol (GC) gives broad trailing peaks and increased retention times for ethanol and internal standard. This is most likely caused by:
A. A contaminated injection syringe
B. Water contamination of the column packing
C. Carrier gas flow rate that is too fast
D. Oven temperature that is too high

Chemistry/Evaluate laboratory data to recognize problems/Gas chromatography/3

17. SITUATION: An amylase result is 550 U/L. A 1:4 dilution of the specimen in NaCl gives 180 U/L (before mathematical correction). The dilution is repeated with the same results. The technologist should:
A. Report the amylase as 550 U/L.
B. Report the amylase as 720 U/L.
C. Report the amylase as 900 U/L.
D. Dilute the sample 1:10 in distilled water and repeat.

Chemistry/Select course of action/Amylase/3

18. SITUATION: A patient's biochemistry results are:

ALT = 55 IU/L; AST = 165 IU/L; glucose = 87 mg/dL; LD = 340 IU/L; Na = 142 mmol/L; K = 6.8 mmol/L; Ca = 8.4 mg/dL; P_i = 7.2 mg/dL

Select the best course of action.
A. Report results along with an estimate of the degree of hemolysis.
B. Repeat LD but report all other results.
C. Request a new sample.
D. Dilute the serum 1:2 and repeat AST and LD.

Chemistry/Select course of action/Hemolysis/3

19. A blood sample is left on a phlebotomy tray for 4 hours before it is delivered to the laboratory. Which group of tests could be performed?
A. Glucose, Na, K, Cl, TCO_2
B. Uric acid, BUN, creatinine
C. Total and direct bilirubin
D. CK, ALT, ALP, ACP

Chemistry/Apply knowledge of fundamental biological characteristics/Sample collections and handling/3

Answers to Questions 14–19

14. **B** The anion gap of this sample is only 6 mmol/L. This may result from laboratory error, retention of an unmeasured cation (e.g., calcium), or low level of unmeasured anion such as phosphorus or albumin. The sodium is inappropriately low for the chloride and bicarbonate and should be repeated if no biochemical cause is apparent.

15. **C** Lithium in excess of 2.0 mmol/L is toxic (in some laboratories 1.5 mmol/L is the upper therapeutic limit). A level of 14 mmol/L would not occur unless the sample were contaminated with lithium. This would most likely result from collection in a green-stoppered tube containing the lithium salt of heparin.

16. **B** Increased oven temperature or gas flow rate will shorten retention times and decrease peak widths. Syringe contamination may cause the appearance of ghost peaks. Water in a PEG column such as Carbowax used for measuring volatiles causes longer retention times and loss of resolution.

17. **B** A 1:4 dilution refers to 1 part serum and 3 parts diluent; the result is multiplied by 4 to determine the serum concentration. Serum may contain wheat germ gluten or other natural amylase inhibitors that, when diluted, result in increased enzyme activity. Serum for amylase should always be diluted with normal saline because chloride ions are needed for amylase activity.

18. **A** Results indicate a moderately hemolyzed sample. Because sodium, calcium, and glucose are not significantly affected, results should be reported along with an estimate of visible hemolysis. The physician may reorder affected tests of interest.

19. **B** Glucose in serum is metabolized by cells at a rate of about 7% per hour. Bilirubin levels will fall if the sample is exposed to sunlight. Hemolysis will adversely affect enzyme levels. Uric acid, BUN, and creatinine are least likely to be affected.

20. An HPLC assay for procainamide gives an internal standard peak that is 15% greater in area and height for sample 1 than sample 2. The technologist should suspect that:
A. The column pressure increased while sample 2 was being analyzed.
B. Less recovery from sample 2 occurred in the extraction step.
C. The pH of the mobile phase increased during chromatography of sample 2.
D. There was more procainamide in sample 1 than sample 2.

Chemistry/Apply principles of special procedures/Liquid chromatography/3

21. After staining a silica gel plate to determine the L/S ratio the technologist notes that the lipid standards both migrated 1 cm faster than usual. The technologist should:
A. Repeat the separation on a new silica gel plate.
B. Check the pH of the developing solvent.
C. Prepare fresh developing solvent and repeat the assay.
D. Reduce solvent migration time for all subsequent runs.

Chemistry/Select course of action/Thin layer chromatography/3

22. A quantitative urine glucose was determined to be 160 mg/dL by the Trinder glucose oxidase method. The sample was refrigerated overnight. The next day, the glucose is repeated and found to be 240 mg/dL using a polarographic method. What is the most likely cause of this discrepancy?
A. Poor precision when performing one of the methods
B. Contamination resulting from overnight storage
C. High levels of reducing substances interfering with the Trinder reaction
D. Positive interference in the polarographic method caused by hematuria

Chemistry/Evaluate laboratory data to determine possible inconsistent results/Glucose/3

23. SITUATION: Results of an iron profile are:

Serum Fe = 40 μg/dL; TIBC = 400 μg/dL; ferritin = 40μg/L (reference range 15–200); transferrin = 310 mg/dL

These results indicate:
A. Error in calculation of TIBC
B. Serum iron falls before ferritin in iron deficiency
C. A defect in iron transport and not Fe deficiency
D. Excess release of ferritin caused by injury

Chemistry/Evaluate laboratory data to determine possible inconsistent results/Iron deficiency/3

24. SITUATION: Results of an iron profile are:

Serum Fe = 40 μg/dL; TIBC = 400 μg/dL; ferritin = 50 μg/L

All of the following tests are useful in establishing a diagnosis of Fe deficiency *except:*
A. Protein electrophoresis
B. Erythrocyte zinc protoporphyrin
C. Serum transferrin
D. Hgb electrophoresis

Chemistry/Evaluate laboratory and clinical data to specify additional tests/Iron deficiency/3

Answers to Questions 20–24

20. **B** The internal standard compensates for variation in extraction, evaporation, reconstitution, and injection volume. The same amount of internal standard is added to all samples and standards prior to assay. Increased column pH or pressure usually alters retention time, and may not affect peak quantitation.

21. **C** TLC plates migrate in solvent until the front comes to 1 cm of the top of the plate. Separation of lipids on silica gel is based upon adsorption. Higher R_f values indicate greater solubility of lipids in the developing solvent. This may be caused by evaporation of H_2O, lowering the polarity of the solvent.

22. **C** Urine often contains high levels of ascorbate and other reducing substances. These may cause significant negative bias when measuring glucose using a peroxidase coupled method. The reductants complete with chromogen for H_2O_2.

23. **D** Serum ferritin levels fall before iron or TIBC in iron deficiency, and a low level of serum ferritin is diagnostic. However, low tissue levels of ferritin may be masked by increased release into the blood in liver disease, infection, and acute inflammation. Although this patient's serum ferritin is within reference limits, serum iron is low and percent saturation is only 10%. These results point to iron deficiency.

24. **D** Electrophoresis may show an elevated β-globulin (transferrin) characteristic of iron deficiency or inflammation that would help explain a normal ferritin. Zinc protoporphyrin is elevated in iron deficiency and in lead poisoning. Hemoglobinopathies and thalassemias are not associated with iron deficiency.

25. Serum protein and IEP are ordered on a patient. The former is performed, but there is no evidence of a monoclonal protein. Select the best course of action.
A. Perform quantitative Ig G, A, M.
B. Perform the IEP on the serum.
C. Report the result; request a urine sample for protein electrophoresis.
D. Perform IFE on the serum.

Chemistry/Evaluate laboratory data to recognize and report the need for additional tests/Immunoelectrophoresis/3

26. SITUATION: Hgb electrophoresis is performed and all of the Hgbs have greater anodal mobility than usual. A fast Hgb is at the edge of the gel and bands are blurred. The voltage is set correctly, but the current reading on the ammeter is too low. Select the course of action that would correct this problem.
A. Reduce the voltage.
B. Dilute the buffer and adjust the pH.
C. Prepare fresh buffer and repeat the test.
D. Reduce the running time.

Chemistry/Select course of action/Electrophoresis/3

27. A technologist is asked to use the serum from a clot tube left over from a chemistry profile run at 8 AM for a stat Ca_I at 11 AM. The technologist should:
A. Perform the assay on the 8 AM sample.
B. Perform the test only if the serum container was tightly capped.
C. Perform the assay on the 8 AM sample only if it was refrigerated.
D. Request a new sample.

Chemistry/Select course of action/Ionized calcium/3

28. SITUATION: A patient's biochemistry results are:

Na = 125 mmol/L; Cl = 106 mmol/L; K = 4.5 mmol/L; TCO_2 = 19 mmol/L; chol = 240 mg/dL; triglyceride = 640 mg/dL; glucose = 107 mg/dL; AST = 16 IU/L; ALT = 11 IU/L; amylase = 200 U/L

Select the most likely cause of these results.
A. The sample is hemolyzed.
B. Serum was not separated from cells in sufficient time.
C. Lipemia is causing *in vitro* interference.
D. The specimen is contaminated.

Chemistry/Evaluate laboratory data to recognize problems/Lipemia/3

29. A gastric fluid from a patient suspected of having taken an overdose of amphetamine is sent to the laboratory for analysis. The technologist should:
A. Perform an EMIT assay for amphetamine.
B. Refuse the sample and request serum or urine.
C. Dilute 1:10 with H_2O and filter; perform TLC for amphetamines.

D. Titrate to pH 7.0, then follow procedure for measuring amphetamine in urine.

Chemistry/Select course of action/Toxicology/3

30. SITUATION: Results of biochemistry tests are:

Na = 138 mmol/L; K = 4.2 mmol/L; Cl = 94 mmol/L; TCO_2 = 20 mmol/L; glucose = 100 mg/dL; T bili = 1.2 mg/dL; BUN = 6.8 mg/dL; creat = 1.0 mg/dL; albumin = 4.9 g/dL; T protein = 5.1 g/dL

What should be done next?
A. Request a new specimen.
B. Repeat the total protein.
C. Repeat all tests.
D. Perform a protein electrophoresis.

Chemistry/Evaluate laboratory data to determine possible inconsistent results/Total protein/3

Answers to Questions 25–30

25. **C** An area of restricted mobility should be identified on serum protein electrophoresis before IEP is performed. About one out of four patients with multiple myeloma have monoclonal free λ or κ chains in urine only, and therefore, urine electrophoresis should be included in initial testing.

26. **C** Increased mobility, decreased resolution, and low current result from low ionic strength. Reducing voltage will slow migration but will not improve resolution. Diluting the buffer will reduce the current resulting in poorer resolution.

27. **D** Ca_I is pH-dependent. Heparinized blood is preferred because it can be assayed immediately. Serum may be used, but the specimen must remain tightly capped while clotting and centrifuging, and analyzed as soon as possible.

28. **C** The triglyceride level is about five times normal causing the sample to be lipemic. This will cause pseudohyponatremia (unbalanced electrolytes). Lipemia may cause a falsely high rate reaction when amylase is measured by turbidimetry; however, the high amylase may be associated with pancreatitis, which results in hyperlipidemia.

29. **C** The gastric sample can be measured by TLC. It should not be used in place of serum or urine without documentation of acceptability by the reagent manufacturer or laboratory. Some immunochemical assays for amphetamines may cross-react with phenylpropanolamine (a decongestant) requiring positives to be confirmed by a second method.

30. **B** All results are normal except total protein. The albumin level cannot be 96% of the total protein, and a random error in total protein measurement is assumed.

31. The chart below compares the monthly total bilirubin mean of Laboratory A to the monthly mean of Laboratory B, which uses the same control materials, analyzer, and method.

	Level 1 Control		Level 2 Control	
	Mean	CV	Mean	CV
Lab A	1.1 mg/dL	2.1%	6.7 mg/dL	3.2%
Lab B	1.4 mg/dL	2.2%	7.0 mg/dL	3.6%

Both laboratories performed controls at the beginning of each shift using commercially prepared liquid QC serum stored at −20°C. Which of the following conditions would explain these differences?
A. Improper handling of the control material by Laboratory A resulted in loss of bilirubin due to photodegradation.
B. The laboratories used a different source of bilirubin calibrator.
C. Laboratory B obtained higher results because its precision was poorer.
D. Carryover from another reagent falsely elevated the results of Laboratory B.

Chemistry/Evaluate data to determine possible sources of error/Quality Control/3

32. After installing a new analyzer and reviewing the results of patients for 1 month, the lead technologist notices a greater frequency of patients with abnormally high triglyceride results. Analysis of all chemistry profiles run the next day indicated that triglyceride results are abnormal whenever the test is run immediately after any sample that is measured for lipase. These observations point to which type of error?
A. Specificity of the triglyceride reagents
B. Precision in pipeting of lipemic samples
C. Bias caused by sequence of analysis
D. Reagent carryover

Chemistry/Evaluate data to determine possible sources of error/Automation/3

33. SITUATION: A digoxin result from a stable patient with a normal electrocardiogram (EKG) is reported as 7.4 ng/mL (URL 2.6 ng/mL) using an immunofluorescent method. Renal function tests were normal and the patient was not taking any other medications. The assay was repeated and results were the same. The sample was frozen and sent to a reference laboratory for confirmation. The result was 1.6 ng/mL measured by a competitive RIA procedure. Which best explains the discrepancy in results?
A. The fluorescent immunoassay was performed improperly.
B. Digoxin was lower by the RIA method because it is less sensitive.

C. An interfering substance was present that cross-reacted with the antibody in the fluorescent immunoassay.
D. Freezing the specimen caused lower results by converting the digoxin to an inactive metabolite.

Chemistry/Evaluate data to determine possible sources of error/Therapeutic drug monitoring/3

Answers to Questions 31–33

31. **B** Interlaboratory variation in bilirubin results is often caused by differences in the assigned value of the calibrator used. Bilirubin calibrators are either serum-based material that have been reference assayed or unconjugated bilirubin stabilized by addition of alkali and albumin. Calibrator differences result in SE or bias and is suspected when the laboratory's mean shows bias when compared to the mean of all other laboratories reporting that method. When suspected, the molar absorbtivity of the azobilirubin reaction product should be measured and the theoretical bilirubin calculated. Photodegradation generally results in a greater loss of bilirubin at higher concentration and also contributes to random error. Note that the bias between Laboratory A and Laboratory B is constant and that Laboratory A has the lower CV.

32. **D** Carryover errors are usually attributed to interference caused by a sample with a very high concentration of analyte preceding a normal sample. However, reagent carryover may also occur on automated systems that use common reagent delivery lines or reusable cuvets. In the case of lipase methods, triglycerides used in the reagent may coat the reagent lines or cuvets interfering with the triglyceride measurements that directly follow.

33. **C** An error was suspected because there was a discrepancy between the test result and the patient's clinical status (i.e., signs of digoxin toxicity such as ventricular arrhythmia were not present.) Some substances termed DLIFs (digoxin-like immunologic factors) can cross-react with antibodies used to measure digoxin. The extent of interference varies with the source of antidigoxin used. In addition, falsely elevated digoxin results may result from accidental ingestion of plant poisons such as oleandrin and from administration of Digibind, a Fab fragment against digoxin that is used to reverse digoxin toxicity.

34. The following results are reported on an adult male patient being evaluated for chest pain:

Time	Myoglobin (Cutoff = 100)	Troponin I (Cutoff = 0.5)	CK-MB (Cutoff = 10)
Admission	12 μg/L	3.1 μg/L	18 μg/L
3 hours postadmission	360 μg/L	3.8 μg/L	30 μg/L
6 hours postadmission	300 μg/L	4.0 μg/L	40 μg/L

What is the most likely cause of these results?
A. The wrong sample was assayed for the first myoglobin.
B. The patient did not suffer an MI until after admission.
C. Hemolysis caused interference with the 3-hour and 6-hour myoglobin result.
D. The patient is suffering from unstable angina.

Chemistry/Evaluate data to determine possible sources of error/Cardiac markers/ 3

35. Analysis of normal and abnormal QCs performed at the beginning of the evening shift revealed a 2_{2s} error across levels for triglyceride. Both controls were within the 3 s limit. The controls were assayed again, and one control was within the acceptable range and the other was slightly above the 2 s limit. No further action was taken and the patient results that were part of the run were reported. Which statement best describes this situation?
A. Appropriate operating procedures were followed.
B. Remedial evaluation should have been taken, but otherwise, the actions were appropriate.
C. Remedial action should have been considered and controls repeated with a fresh aliquot; at least three of the patient samples should have been repeated.
D. The controls should have been run twice before reporting results.

Chemistry/Evaluate data to determine possible sources of error/Quality control/3

36. SITUATION: CK-MB is measured on an automated analyzer using a single antibody immunoinhibition method. The result is 12 μg/L (URL = 10 μg/L). The assay is repeated on the same sample using a double antibody immunoprecipitation method, and the result is 9 μg/L (URL = 10 μg/L). What is the most likely explanation for these results?
A. Deterioration of CK-MB during storage.
B. Differences in the affinity of the antibody against the M subunit used in the tests.
C. The immunoinhibition method has a higher variance.
D. The presence of CK-1 in the sample.

Chemistry/Evaluate data to determine possible sources of error/Cardiac markers/3

Answers to Questions 34–36

34. **A** Myoglobin is the first cardiac marker to rise outside the URL following an MI (2–3 hours) followed by TNI (4–6 hours) and CK-MB (4–8 hours). The admission TNI and CK-MB are both elevated, and they continue to rise in all three samples. Because TNI and CK-MB peak 8–12 hours post-MI and 12–18 hours post-MI, respectively, the infarction occurred within the last 8–12 hours. The myoglobin remains elevated for 24 hours post-MI and should have been elevated in the admission sample.

35. **C** Quality control limits are chosen to achieve a low probability of false rejection. For example, a 2_{2s} error occurs only once in 1600 occurrences by chance. Therefore, such an error can be assumed to be significant. However, this does not mean the error will occur if the controls are repeated again. The error detection rate (power function) of the 2_{2s} rule is only about 30% for a single run. This means that there is a greater chance the repeated controls will be within range than outside acceptable limits. Therefore controls should never be repeated until the test system is evaluated for potential sources of error. If no errors are apparent, it is permissible to repeat the controls using fresh materials; however, at least three samples chosen randomly (or the entire run if there are less than three samples) should also be repeated and the differences evaluated before releasing the results.

36. **D** Single antibody immunoinhibition methods measure the activity of the B subunit of CK-MB after neutralizing the M subunit with anti-M. Methods employing antibodies to both M and B subunits are specific for CK-MB because both antibodies must bind to generate a measurement signal. Single antibody assays are used as a screening test only. Results that are below the URL may be reported as normal. Results above the URL should be confirmed by a specific method for CK-MB or other specific biochemical marker for MI, such as TNI.

37. Which set of the following laboratory results is most likely from a patient who has suffered an AMI? Reference intervals are in parenthesis.

Total CK (10–110 U/L)	CK-MB (1–10 μg/L)	CK index (1%–4%)
A. 600 U/L	16 μg/L	2.7%
B. 170 U/L	14 μg/L	8.2%
C. 160 U/L	4 μg/L	2.5 %
D. 50 U/L	2 μg/L	4.0 %

Chemistry/Evaluate laboratory data to explain inconsistent results/Enzymes/3

38. Hemoglobin electrophoresis performed on agarose at pH 8.8 gives the following results:

A_2 Position	S Position	F Position	A Position
35%	30%	5%	30%

All components of the Hgb C,S,F,A control hemolysate were within the acceptable range. What is the most likely cause of this patient's result?
A. Hgb $_{Lepore}$
B. Hgb S-β-thalassemia (Hgb S/β$^+$)
C. Hgb SC disease posttransfusion
D. Specimen contamination

Chemistry/Evaluate laboratory data to explain inconsistent results/Enzymes/3

Answers to Questions 37–38

37. **B** Results shown in C and D can be excluded because the CK-MB is not increased. Results shown in A and B have CK-MB levels above the URL. However, patient A has a CK index under 4.0% and a five- to tenfold elevation of total CK. These results indicate release of a small of amount of CK-MB from skeletal muscle rather than from cardiac muscle. In order to increase the sensitivity of CK-MB, some laboratories use an URL of 6 μg/L. This cutoff can detect about two-thirds of AMI cases within 3 hours of the infarct but requires evaluation of the CK index and other cardiac markers to avoid a high number of false positives.

38. **C** Hemoglobin $_{Lepore}$ results from a hybridization of the β and δ genes and produces a pattern that is similar to Hgb S trait (AS), except that the quantity of Hgb S is below 20%. Hemoglobin S-β-thalassemia minor results in an increase in Hgb A_2 (and possibly Hgb F) because there is reduced transcription of the structurally normal β chain. However, the Hgb S should be greater than the Hgb A, and the amount at the Hgb A_2 is far too high. The concentration of Hgb at the A_2 position is too high to result from contamination or to be considered as Hgb A_2. This pattern appears to express two abnormal Hgbs (Hgb S and C) as well as the normal adult Hgb A. Because inheritance of two abnormal β genes prohibits formation of normal Hgb A, this pattern would occur only if the patient has been transfused with normal RBCs. Hemoglobin SC disease usually produces almost equal amounts of Hgb C and S (and usually a slight increase in Hgb F), and is the most likely cause of these results. This could be confirmed by citrate agar electrophoresis or isofocusing to identify the abnormal Hgbs, and review of the patient's medical record for evidence of recent blood transfusion.

Na	K	Cl	HCO$_3$	BUN	Glucose	Creatinine	Uric Acid
140 mmol/L	5.8 mmol/L	102 mmol/L	18 mmol/L	2.6 mg/dL	20 mg/dL	DL	DL
132 mmol/L	4.8 mmol/L	98 mmol/L	24 mmol/L	DL	DL	DL	DL

39. Two consecutive serum samples give the results shown above for a metabolic function profile.

DL = Detection limit flag (absorbance below detectable limit)

The instrument is a random access analyzer that uses two sample probes. The first probe aspirates a variable amount of serum for the spectrophotometric chemistry tests, and the second probe makes a 1:50 dilution of serum for electrolyte measurements. What is the most likely cause of these results?
A. Both patients have renal failure.
B. There is an insufficient amount of sample in both serum tubes.
C. There is a fibrin strand in the probe used for the spectrophotometric chemistry tests.
D. The same patient's sample was accidentally run twice.

Chemistry/Evaluate data to determine possible sources of error/Automation/3

40. SITUATION: A blood sample in a red-stoppered tube is delivered to the laboratory for electrolytes, calcium, and phosphorus. The tube is approximately half full and is accompanied by a purple-stoppered tube for a complete blood count that is approximately three-quarters full. The chemistry results are as follows:

Na	K	Cl	HCO$_3$	Ca	InP
135	11.2	103	14	2.6	3.8
mmol/L	mmol/L	mmol/L	mmol/L	mg/dL	mg/dL

What is the most likely explanation of these serum calcium results?
A. Severe hemolysis during sample collection.
B. Laboratory error in the calcium measurement.
C. The wrong order of draw was used for vacuum tube collection.
D. Some anticoagulated blood was added to the red-stoppered tube.

Chemistry/Evaluate data to determine possible sources of error/Electrolytes/3

41. SITUATION: A patient previously diagnosed with primary hypothyroidism and started on thyroxine replacement therapy is seen for follow-up testing after 2 weeks. The serum free T$_4$ is normal but the TSH is still elevated. What is the most likely explanation for these results?
A. Laboratory error in measurement of free T$_4$.
B. Laboratory error in measurement of TSH.
C. *In vitro* drug interference with the free T$_4$ assay.

D. Results are consistent with a euthyroid patient in the early phase of therapy.

Chemistry/Evaluate laboratory data to explain inconsistent results/Endocrinology/3

Answers to Questions 39–41

39. **C** Electrolyte results for both patients are within the physiological range but are distinctly different. The first results indicate a high potassium and increased anion gap, and one would expect the BUN, uric acid, and creatinine to be elevated. However, the results for BUN and glucose are unlikely for any patient, and the creatinine and uric acid signals are below the detection limit of the analyzer indicating that little or no sample was added because the sample probe is partially obstructed or the serum level is too low. The results for the second sample are below detection limits for all spectrophotometric tests, which may be the result of complete probe obstruction or the inability to generate a detectable signal with the trace quantity of serum that was added. Because all of the low or undetectable signals are for tests sampled by the first probe, the only explanation is that the probe is obstructed or malfunctioning.

40. **D** The potassium and the calcium results are above and below physiological limit values, respectively. Although hemolysis could explain the high potassium, hemolysis does not cause a significant change in serum calcium. The wrong order of draw could result in falsely low calcium value but would not be sufficient to cause a result that is incompatible with life (and does not explain a grossly elevated potassium). The results and the condition of the tubes indicate that blood from a full tube collected in K$_3$ EDTA was added to the clot tube chelating the calcium and increasing the potassium.

41. **D** Results of thyroid tests (especially in hospitalized patients) may sometimes appear discrepant because medications and nonthyroid illnesses can affect test results. The pituitary is slow to respond to thyroxine replacement, and 6–8 weeks are usually required before TSH levels fall back to normal. In the early stage of therapy the patient should be monitored by the free T$_4$ result. This patient's free T$_4$ is normal, indicating that replacement therapy is adequate. The high TSH sometimes seen in treated patients is referred to as *pituitary lag.*

42. SITUATION: A 6-year-old being treated with phenytoin was recently placed on valproic acid for better control of seizures. After displaying signs of phenytoin toxicity including ataxia, a stat phenytoin is determined to be 15.0 mg/L (reference range 10–20 mg/L). A peak blood level drawn 5 hours after the last dose is 18.0 mg/L. The valproic acid measured at the same time is within therapeutic limits. Quality control is within acceptable limits for all tests, but the accuracy of the results is questioned by the physician. What is the most appropriate next course of action?
A. Repeat the valproic acid level using the last specimen.
B. Repeat the phenytoin on both trough and peak samples using a different method.
C. Recommend measurement of free phenytoin using the last specimen.
D. Recommend a second trough level be measured.

Chemistry/Evaluate laboratory data to explain inconsistent results/TDM/3

43. The following results are obtained from three consecutive serum samples using an automated random access analyzer that samples directly from a bar-coded tube. Calibration and QC performed at the start of the shift are within the acceptable range, and no error codes are reported by the analyzer for any tests on the three samples. Upon results verification, what is the most appropriate course of action?
A. Report the results and proceed with other tests since no analytical problems are noted.
B. Repeat the controls before continuing with further testing, but report the results.
C. Check sample identification prior to reporting.
D. Do not report BUN results for these patients or continue BUN testing.

Chemistry/Evaluate laboratory data to explain inconsistent results/Automation/3

Answers to Questions 42–43

42. **C** Phenytoin levels must be monitored closely because toxic drug levels can occur unexpectedly due to changing pharmacokinetics. Phenytoin follows a nonlinear rate of elimination, which means that clearance decreases as blood levels increase. At high blood levels, saturation of the hepatic hydroxylating enzymes can occur, causing an abrupt increase in the blood level from a small increase in dose. The drug half-life estimated from the two drug levels is approximately 15 hours, which is within the range expected for children, so decreased clearance is not likely the problem. Valproic acid competes with phenytoin for binding sites on albumin. Free phenytoin is the physiologically active fraction and is normally very low, so small changes in protein binding can cause a large change in free drug. For example, a 5% fall in protein binding caused by valproic acid can increase the free phenytoin level by 50%. This patient's free phenytoin level should be measured, and the dose of phenytoin reduced to produce a free drug level that is within the therapeutic range.

43. **D** BUN is elevated five- to tenfold for three consecutive patients in the absence of any other laboratory evidence of renal disease. The glucose results show conclusively that the samples are not from the same patient. Therefore, the BUN results must be caused by a SE and should not be reported. Further testing for BUN should cease until the analytical components of the BUN assay are completely evaluated and the cause of these results identified and corrected. This is demonstrated by successful recalibration and performance of controls within acceptable limits. Following this, the BUN assay should be repeated on the three samples along with all other specimens with a spurious BUN result that have occurred since the start of the shift.

Na	K	Cl	HCO$_3$	BUN	Glucose	Creatinine	Uric Acid
140 mmol/L	3.6 mmol/L	100 mmol/L	28 mmol/L	130 mg/dL	110 mg/dL	1.2 mg/dL	4.8 mg/dL
148 mmol/L	4.2 mmol/L	110 mmol/L	24 mmol/L	135 mg/dL	86 mg/dL	0.8 mg/dL	3.9 mg/dL
138 mmol/L	4.0 mmol/L	105 mmol/L	22 mmol/L	142 mg/dL	190 mg/dL	1.0 mg/dL	4.6 mg/dL

44. An AFP measured on a 30-year-old pregnant woman at approximately 12 weeks gestation is 2.5 multiples of the median (MOM). What course of action is most appropriate?
A. Repeat the serum AFP in 2 weeks.
B. Recommend AFP assay on amniotic fluid.
C. Repeat the AFP using the same sample by another method.
D. Repeat the AFP using the sample by the same method.

Chemistry/Select course of action/AFP/3

45. SITUATION: Biochemistry tests are performed 24 hours apart on a patient and a δ-check flag is reported for inorganic phosphorus by the laboratory information system. Given the results below, identify the most likely cause.
A. Results suggest altered metabolic status caused by poor insulin control.
B. The patient was not fasting when the sample was collected on day 2.
C. The samples were drawn from two different patients.
D. The δ-check limit is invalid when samples are collected 24 or more hours apart.

Chemistry/Evaluate data to determine possible sources of error/Automation/3

Answers to Questions 44–45

44. **A** The analytical sensitivity of immunochemical AFP tests is approximately 5 ng/mL. The maternal serum AFP at 12 weeks' gestation is barely above the analytical detection limit. Therefore, to achieve the needed sensitivity, the test should be repeated at 14 weeks. If the result is still equal to or greater than 2.5 MOM, then ultrasound should be performed to verify last menstrual period dating. AFP normally first becomes detectable in maternal serum at week 12 and increases by 15% per week through the 26th week. Levels of 2.5 MOM or greater are associated with spina bifida but also occur in ventral wall and abdominal wall defects, fetal death, Turner's syndrome, trisomy 13, congenital hypothyroidism, tyrosinemia, and several other fetal conditions. A positive serum test should always be repeated, and if positive again, followed by ultrasound. If ultrasound does not explain the elevation, amniotic fluid testing including AFP and acetylcholinesterase is usually recommended.

45. **B** The δ check compares the difference of the patient's two most recent laboratory results within a 3-day period to a δ limit usually determined as a percentage difference. The purpose of the δ check is to detect sample identification errors. A δ-check flag can also be caused by random analytical errors and interfering substances such as hemolysis, icterus, and lipemia, and by metabolic changes associated with disease or treatment. Therefore, results should be carefully considered before determining the cause. In this case, hemolysis and icterus can be ruled out because enzymes sensitive to hemolysis interference (AST, ALT, and LD) and bilirubin are within normal limits. Tests showing a significant difference are P_i, ALP, triglycerides, and glucose. These four tests are elevated by diet (the ALP from postprandial secretion of intestinal ALP). All other tests show a high level of agreement between days, and the differences are attributable to normal physiological and analytical variation.

	AST U/L	ALT U/L	ALP U/L	LD U/L	CK U/L	GGT U/L	TP g/dL	ALB g/dL	TBIL mg/dL	GLU mg/dL	TG mg/dL	CA mg/dL	InP mg/dL	BUN mg/dL
Day 1	20	15	40	100	15	40	8.2	3.6	0.8	84	140	8.7	4.2	16
Day 2	22	14	65	90	20	36	8.3	3.8	1.0	128	190	8.8	5.2	26

BIBLIOGRAPHY

1. Bennington, JL (ed): Dictionary and Encyclopedia of Laboratory Medicine and Technology. WB Saunders, Philadelphia, 1984.
2. Burtis, CA and Ashwood, ER (eds): Tietz Textbook of Clinical Chemistry. WB Saunders, Philadelphia, 1994.
3. Henry, JB (ed): Clinical Diagnosis and Management by Laboratory Methods. WB Saunders, Philadelphia, 1996.
4. Kaplan, LA and Pesce, AJ (eds): Clinical Chemistry Theory Analysis and Correlation. CV Mosby, St. Louis, 1996.

CHAPTER FIVE

Urinalysis and Body Fluids

Routine Physical and Biochemical Urine Tests

1. Which statement below regarding renal function is true?
   A. Glomeruli are far more permeable to H_2O and salt than other capillaries.
   B. The collecting tubule reabsorbs sodium and secretes potassium in response to antidiuretic hormone (ADH).
   C. The collecting tubule is permeable to H_2O only in the presence of aldosterone.
   D. The thick ascending limb is highly permeable to H_2O and urea.

   Body fluids/Apply knowledge of fundamental biological characteristics/Urine/1

2. Which statement regarding normal salt and H_2O handling by the nephron is correct?
   A. The ascending limb of the tubule is highly permeable to salt but not H_2O.
   B. The stimulus for ADH release is low arterial pressure in the afferent arteriole.
   C. The descending limb of the tubule is impermeable to urea but highly permeable to salt.
   D. Renin is released in response to high plasma osmolality.

   Body fluids/Apply knowledge of fundamental biological characteristics/Urine/1

3. Which statement concerning renal tubular function is true?
   A. In salt deprivation the kidneys will conserve sodium at the expense of potassium.
   B. Potassium is not excreted when serum concentration is below 3.5 mmol/L.
   C. No substance can be excreted into urine at a rate that exceeds the glomerular filtration rate.
   D. The amount of phenolsulphonphthalein (PSP) dye excreted in urine after 15 minutes is dependent mainly on renal blood flow.

   Body fluids/Correlate laboratory data with physiological processes/Urine electrolytes/2

Answers to Questions 1–3

1. **A** The formation of plasma ultrafiltrate depends upon high hydrostatic pressure and permeability of the glomeruli. Aldosterone is released when effective arterial pressure falls, and ADH when plasma osmolality becomes too high. The collecting tubule reabsorbs sodium and secretes potassium in response to aldosterone, and is permeable to H_2O only in the presence of ADH. The thick ascending limb is permeable to salt but not to H_2O or urea.

2. **A** The tubules are able to concentrate the filtrate because the descending limb is highly permeable to H_2O and urea but not to salt, and the ascending limb is permeable to salt. Salt leaving the ascending limb creates a hypertonic interstitium that forces H_2O from the descending limb. Renin is released in response to low hydrostatic pressure in the afferent arteriole, which stimulates the juxtaglomerular cells. ADH is released by the posterior pituitary in response to high plasma osmolality.

3. **A** Potassium is not a threshold substance and will be secreted by the tubules even when plasma potassium levels are low. Patients on diuretics or who have hypovolemia become hypokalemic for this reason. The PSP dye excretion test is sometimes used to measure renal tubular function. In the first 15 minutes following administration of PSP, the amount of dye excreted into the urine is mainly dependent upon tubular secretion. As the blood level falls, the amount excreted becomes dependent upon renal blood flow. Some substances (e.g., penicillin) can be excreted at a rate exceeding glomerular filtration because the tubules secrete the drug.

4. Which of the following is *inappropriate* when collecting urine for routine bacteriologic culture?
   A. The container must be sterile.
   B. The midstream void technique must be used.
   C. The collected sample must be plated within 2 hours unless refrigerated.
   D. The sample may be held at 2°–8°C for up to 48 hours prior to plating.

   Body fluids/Apply knowledge to identify sources of error/Specimen collecting and handling/2

5. Which statement about sample collection for routine urinalysis is true?
   A. Preservative tablets should be used for collecting random urine specimens.
   B. Containers may be washed and reused if rinsed in deionized H_2O.
   C. Samples may be stored at room temperature for up to 2 hours.
   D. Random samples are acceptable when renal disease is suspected.

   Body fluids/Apply knowledge to identify sources of error/Specimen collection and handling/2

6. Which urine color is correlated correctly with the pigment-producing substance?
   A. Smoky red urine with homogentisic acid
   B. Dark amber urine with myoglobin
   C. Deep yellow urine and yellow foam with bilirubin
   D. Red-brown urine with biliverdin

   Body fluids/Correlate laboratory data with physiological processes/Urine color/2

7. Which of the following substances will cause urine to produce red fluorescence when examined with an ultraviolet lamp (360 nm)?
   A. Myoglobin
   B. Porphobilinogen (PBG)
   C. Urobilin
   D. Coproporphyrin

   Body fluids/Correlate clinical and laboratory data/Urine porphyrins/2

8. Which of the conditions below is associated with normal urine color but produces red fluorescence when urine is examined with an ultraviolet (Wood's) lamp?
   A. Acute intermittent porphyria
   B. Lead poisoning
   C. Erythropoietic porphyria
   D. Porphyria cutanea tarda

   Body fluids/Correlate clinical and laboratory data/Urine color/2

Answers to Questions 4–8

4. **D** Urine specimens should be plated and incubated within 2 hours of collection (some laboratories use a 1-hour time limit), and within 24 hours if the sample is refrigerated at 2°–8°C immediately following collection. No additives are permitted when urine is collected for culture.

5. **D** The first morning voided sample is the most sensitive for screening purposes because formed elements are concentrated, but random samples are satisfactory because glomerular bleeding, albuminuria, and cast formation may occur at any time. Perservative tablets should be avoided because they may cause chemical interference with dry reagent strip and turbidimetric protein tests. Samples should be refrigerated if not tested within 30 minutes of collection.

6. **C** Homogentisic acid causes a dark brown or black-colored urine. Myoglobin causes a red to red-brown color in urine, and biliverdin causes a green or yellow-green color. In addition to metabolic diseases and renal disease, abnormal color can be caused by drugs (e.g., Gantrisin, Pyridium), dyes excreted by the kidneys (e.g., PSP), and natural or artificial food coloring (e.g., beets).

7. **D** Myoglobin causes a positive test for blood but does not cause urine to fluoresce. PBG causes urine to become dark (orange to orange-brown) on standing but does not fluoresce. It reacts with *p*-dimethylaminobenzaldehyde (Watson-Schwartz test) and is not extracted into butanol or chloroform. Uroporphyrin and coproporphyrin produce red or orange-red fluorescence. Unlike hemoglobin, porphyrins lack peroxidase activity. Urobilin is an oxidation product of urobilinogen. It turns the urine orange to orange-brown but does not produce fluorescence.

8. **B** Lead poisoning blocks the synthesis of heme causing accumulation of PBG and coproporphyrin III in urine. However, uroporphyrin levels are not sufficiently elevated to cause red pigmentation of the urine. There is sufficient coproporphyrin to cause a positive test for fluorescence. Acute intermittent porphyria is the most common inherited porphyria and produces increased urinary delta-aminolevulinic acid (Δ-ALA), and PBG. The PBG turns the urine orange to orange-brown upon standing. Erythropoietic porphyria and porphyria cutanea tarda produce large amounts of uroporphyrin causing the urine to be red or port wine-colored.

9. A brown or black pigment in urine can be caused by:
A. Gantrisin
B. Phenolsulfonphthalein
C. Rifampin
D. Melanin

Body fluids/Correlate clinical and laboratory data/Urine color/2

10. Urine that is dark red or port wine in color may be caused by:
A. Lead poisoning
B. Porphyria cutanea tarda
C. Alkaptonuria
D. Hemolytic anemia

Body fluids/Correlate clinical and laboratory data/Urine color/2

11. Which of the following tests is affected *least* by standing or improperly stored urine?
A. Glucose
B. Protein
C. pH
D. Bilirubin

Body fluids/Apply knowledge to identify sources of error/Urine/Specimen collection and handling/2

12. Which type of urine sample is needed for a D-xylose absorption test on an adult patient?
A. 24-hour urine sample collected with 20 mL of 6 N HCl
B. 2-hour timed postprandial urine preserved with boric acid
C. 5-hour timed urine kept under refrigeration
D. Random urine preserved with formalin

Body fluids/Apply principles of basic laboratory procedures/Urine/Specimen collection and handling/2

13. Which of the following is *inappropriate* when collecting a 24-hour urine sample for catecholamines?
A. Urine in the bladder is voided and discarded at the start of the test.
B. At 24 hours any urine in the bladder is voided and added to the collection.
C. All urine should be collected in a single container that is kept refrigerated.
D. Hydrochloric acid (HCl) is added to the container after the 24-hour urine volume is measured.

Body fluids/Apply knowledge to identify sources of error/Urinary catecholamines/2

14. Urine production of less than 400 mL/day is:
A. Consistent with normal renal function and H_2O balance
B. Termed isosthenuria
C. Defined as oliguria

D. Associated with diabetes mellitus

Body fluids/Correlate clinical and laboratory data/Urine volume/2

Answers to Questions 9–14

9. **D** Excretion of melanin in malignant melanoma and homogentisic acid in alkaptonuria cause the urine to turn black on standing. Other substances that may cause brown or black-colored urine are methemoglobin, PBG, porphobilin, and urobilin. Gantrisin, PSP dye, and rifampin are three examples of drugs that cause a red or orange-red color in urine.

10. **B** Porphyria cutanea tarda and erythropoietic porphyria produce sufficient uroporphyrins to cause dark red urine. Acute intermittent porphyria produces large amounts of PBG, which may be oxidized to porphobilin, turning the urine orange to orange-brown.

11. **B** Standing urine may become alkaline due to loss of volatile acids and ammonia production. Bilirubin glucuronides may become hydrolyzed to unconjugated bilirubin or oxidized to biliverdin, resulting in a false-negative dry reagent strip test. Glucose can be consumed by glycolysis or oxidation by cells.

12. **C** The D-xylose absorption test is used to distinguish pancreatic insufficiency from intestinal malabsorption. The test requires a blood sample taken 2 hours after oral administration of 25 g of D-xylose, and a 5-hour timed urine sample. Tests requiring a 24-hour urine sample include catecholamines, vanillyl mandelic acid (VMA), metanephrines, cortisol, and estriol.

13. **D** When collecting a 24-hour urine sample the bladder must be emptied of urine at the start of the test and discarded. The bladder must be emptied at the conclusion of the test and the urine added to the collection. In order to prevent degradation of catecholamines (also VMA, metanephrines, and cortisol) during storage, the urine should be kept at or below pH 2. HCl (10 mL of 6 N HCl) must be added to the container prior to the collection to prevent oxidative loss of these analytes.

14. **C** Normal daily urine excretion is usually 600–1600 mL/day. Isosthenuria refers to urine of constant specific gravity (SG) of 1.010, which is the SG of the glomerular filtrate. Glycosuria causes retention of H_2O within the tubule resulting in dehydration and polyuria rather than oliguria.

15. Which of the following contributes to SG, but *not* to osmolality?
A. Protein
B. Salt
C. Urea
D. Glucose

Body fluids/Evaluate laboratory data to determine possible inconsistent results/Specific gravity/2

16. Urine with a SG consistently between 1.002 and 1.003 indicates:
A. Acute glomerulonephritis
B. Renal tubular failure
C. Diabetes insipidus
D. Addison's disease

Body fluids/Evaluate laboratory data to recognize health and disease states/Specific gravity/2

17. In which of the following conditions is the urine SG likely to be *below* 1.025?
A. Diabetes mellitus
B. Drug overdose
C. Chronic renal failure
D. Prerenal failure

Body fluids/Evaluate data to recognize health and disease states/Specific gravity/2

18. Which statement below regarding methods for measuring SG is true?
A. To correct a urinometer subtract 0.001 per each 3°C below 15.5°C.
B. Colorimetric SG tests are falsely elevated when a large quantity of glucose is present.
C. Colorimetric SG readings are falsely elevated when pH is alkaline.
D. Refractometry should be performed before the urine is centrifuged.

Body fluids/Apply knowledge to identify sources of error/Specific gravity/2

19. What is the principle of the colorimetric reagent strip determination of SG in urine?
A. Ionic strength alters the pK_a of a polyelectrolyte.
B. Sodium and other cations are chelated by a ligand that changes color.
C. Anions displace a pH indicator from a mordant, making it water-soluble.
D. Ionized solutes catalyze oxidation of an azo dye.

Body fluids/Apply principles of basic laboratory procedures/Specific gravity/1

20. Which statement below regarding urine pH is true?
A. High-protein diets promote an alkaline urine pH.
B. pH tends to decrease as urine is stored.
C. Contamination should be suspected if urine pH is less than 4.5.
D. Bacteriuria is most often associated with a low urine pH.

Body fluids/Correlate clinical and laboratory data/Urine pH/2

Answers to Questions 15–20

15. **A** All substances that dissolve in the urine contribute to osmotic pressure or osmolality. This includes nonionized solutes such as urea, uric acid, and glucose as well as salts, but not colloids such as protein and lipids.

16. **C** In severe renal diseases the tubules fail to concentrate the filtrate. Salt and H_2O equilibrate by diffusion causing an SG of about 1.010. If the SG of urine is below that of plasma, free H_2O is lost. This results from failure to produce ADH (diabetes insipidus) or scarring of the renal medulla.

17. **C** Glucose and drug metabolites increase the SG of urine. In prerenal failure the tubules are undamaged. Ineffective arterial pressure stimulates aldosterone release. This increases sodium reabsorption, which stimulates ADH release. Water and salt are retained, and the urine-plasma osmolar ratio (U:P) exceeds 2:1. Chronic renal failure is associated with nocturia, polyuria, and low SG caused by scarring of the collecting tubules.

18. **A** Cells and undissolved solutes refract light and will cause falsely high SG readings by refractometry if urine is not centrifuged. The density of urine increases at low temperature causing less fluid to be displaced by the urinometer. Colorimetric SG tests are less sensitive to nonionized compounds, and are negatively biased when large quantities of glucose or urea (nonelectrolytes) are present. Colorimetric SG readings are approximately 0.005 lower when pH is greater than 6.5.

19. **A** A polyelectrolyte with malic acid residues will ionize in proportion to the ionic strength of urine. This causes the pH indicator, bromthymol blue, to react as if it were in a more acidic solution. The indicator will be blue at low SG and green at higher SG.

20. **C** Bacteriuria is usually associated with an alkaline pH caused by the production of ammonia from urea. Extended storage may result in loss of volatile acids causing increased pH. A high-protein diet promotes excretion of inorganic acids. The tubular maximum for H^+ secretion occurs when urine pH reaches 4.5, the lowest urinary pH that the kidneys can produce.

21. In renal tubular acidosis the pH of urine is:
   A. Consistently acid
   B. Consistently alkaline
   C. Neutral
   D. Variable, depending upon diet

Body fluids/Correlate clinical and laboratory data/Urine pH/2

22. The normal daily urine output for an adult is approximately:
   A. 0.2–0.5 L
   B. 0.6–1.6 L
   C. 2.7–3.0 L
   D. 3.2–3.5 L

Body fluids/Apply knowledge of fundamental biological characteristics/Urine/1

23. The SG of the filtrate in Bowman's space is approximately:
   A. 1.000–1.002
   B. 1.004–1.006
   C. 1.008–1.010
   D. 1.012–1.014

Body fluids/Apply knowledge of fundamental biological characteristics/Urine/1

24. A patient with partially compensated respiratory alkalosis would have a urine pH of:
   A. 4.5–5.5
   B. 5.5–6.5
   C. 6.5–7.5
   D. 7.5–8.5

Body fluids/Correlate clinical and laboratory data/Urine pH/2

25. Which of the following is most likely to cause a false-positive dry reagent strip test for protein?
   A. Urine of high SG
   B. Highly buffered alkaline urine
   C. Bence Jones proteinuria
   D. Salicylates

Body fluids/Apply knowledge to identify sources of error/Urinary protein/2

26. When testing for urinary protein with sulfosalicylic acid (SSA) which condition may produce a false-positive result?
   A. Highly buffered alkaline urine
   B. The presence of x-ray contrast media
   C. Increased urinary SG
   D. The presence of red blood cells (RBCs)

Body fluids/Apply knowledge to identify sources of error/Urinary protein/2

Answers to Questions 21–26

21. **B** Renal tubular acidosis results from a defect in the renal tubular reabsorption of bicarbonate. Hydrogen ions are not secreted when bicarbonate ions are not reabsorbed. Wasting of sodium bicarbonate ($NaHCO_3$) and potassium bicarbonate ($KHCO_3$) results in alkaline urine and hypokalemia in association with acidosis.

22. **B** Under conditions of normal fluid intake, the reference range for urine volume is 0.6–1.6 L per day. Urine output will vary widely with fluid intake. In cases of fluid deprivation almost all filtrate will be reabsorbed resulting in daily excretion as low as 500 mL. When fluid intake is excessive, up to 2.0 L of urine may be voided. Urine output beyond these extremes is considered abnormal.

23. **C** The SG of the filtrate in Bowman's space approximates the SG of the plasma because sodium, chloride, glucose, urea, and other main solutes are completely filtered by the glomeruli. This corresponds to an osmolality of approximately 280 mOsm/kg.

24. **D** Urine pH is determined by diet, acid-base balance, water balance, and renal function. In partially compensated respiratory alkalosis, the kidneys reabsorb less bicarbonate which results in lower net acid excretion. The loss of bicarbonate helps to compensate for alkalosis and causes urine pH to be alkaline.

25. **B** In addition to highly buffered alkaline urine a false-positive dry reagent test may be caused by quaternary ammonium compounds which increase urine pH. Because the dry reagent strip tests are insensitive to globulins a false negative is likely in the case of Bence Jones proteinuria. Positive interference by drugs is uncommon for dry reagent strip protein tests but is common for turbidimetric tests. High urinary SG will suppress the color reaction of the strip protein tests. Some pigmented drugs such as Gantrisin may cause difficulty in reading the reaction pad, resulting in a false-positive protein.

26. **B** Turbidimetric assays are used to test urine suspected of giving a false-positive dry reagent strip test for albumin because the urine is highly alkaline (pH $\geq$8.0) or contains pigmentation that interferes with reading the protein test pad. In addition, SSA tests are used when screening urine for an increased concentration of globulins because dry reagent strip tests are insensitive to globulins. Sulfosalicylic acid is less specific but more sensitive for albuminuria than dry reagent strip tests. Iodinated dyes, penicillin, salicylate, and tolbutamide may result in false-positives. Trace turbidity is difficult to determine when urine is cloudy due to bacteriuria, mucus, or crystals. Alkaline urine may titrate SSA reducing its sensitivity.

27. A discrepancy between the urine SG determined by measuring refractive index and urine osmolality would be most likely to occur:
   A. After catheterization of the urinary tract
   B. In diabetes mellitus
   C. After an intravenous pyelogram (IVP)
   D. In uremia

   Body fluids/Evaluate data to determine possible inconsistent results/Specific gravity/2

28. Which of the following is likely to result in a false-negative dry reagent strip test for proteinuria?
   A. Penicillin
   B. Aspirin
   C. Amorphous phosphates
   D. Bence Jones protein

   Body fluids/Apply knowledge to identify sources of error/Urinary protein/1

29. Daily loss of protein in urine normally does not exceed:
   A. 30 mg
   B. 50 mg
   C. 100 mg
   D. 150 mg

   Body fluids/Apply knowledge of fundamental biological characteristics/Urinary protein/1

30. Which of the following is *least* likely to cause a false-positive result with turbidimetric protein tests?
   A. Tolbutamide
   B. X-ray contrast media
   C. Penicillin or sulfa antibiotics
   D. Ascorbic acid

   Body fluids/Apply knowledge to identify sources of error/Urinary protein/2

31. Which statement best describes the clinical utility of tests for microalbuminuria?
   A. Testing may detect early renal involvement in diabetes mellitus.
   B. Microalbuminuria refers to a specific subfraction of albumin found only in persons with diabetic nephropathy.
   C. A positive test result indicates the presence of orthostatic albuminuria.
   D. Testing should be part of the routine urinalysis.

   Body fluids/Correlate clinical and laboratory data/Urinary protein/2

32. Which of the conditions below is *least* likely to be detected by dry reagent strip tests for proteinuria?
   A. Orthostatic albuminuria
   B. Chronic renal failure
   C. Pyelonephritis
   D. Renal tubular proteinuria

   Body fluids/Apply principles of basic laboratory procedures/Urine protein/2

Answers to Questions 27–32

27. **C** The IVP dye contains iodine and is highly refractile. This increases the refractive index of urine, causing falsely high measurement of solute concentration. Refractive index is affected by the size and shape of solutes and undissolved solids such as protein. Osmolality is the most specific measure of total solute concentration because it is affected only by the number of dissolved solutes.

28. **D** Dry reagent strip tests using tetrabromphenol blue or tetrachlorophenol tetrabromosulfophthalein are insensitive to globulins and may not detect immunoglobulin light chains. Turbidimetric methods such as 3% SSA will often detect Bence Jones protein but may give a false-positive reaction with penicillin, tolbutamide, salicylates, and x-ray contrast dyes containing iodine. Amorphous phosphates may precipitate in refrigerated urine making interpretation of turbidimetric tests difficult.

29. **D** Small amounts of albumin and other low molecular weight proteins such as amylase, β-microglobulins, and immunoglobulin fragments are excreted in the urine. Proteinuria does not normally exceed 30 mg/dL or 150 mg/day. The detection limit of the SSA test to albumin is approximately 1.5 mg/dL, and for dry reagent strip tests is approximately 5 mg/dL. Therefore trace positives by either method may occur in the absence of renal disease.

30. **D** Although ascorbic acid (vitamin C) may interfere with tests for glucose, blood, bilirubin, and nitrite it does not cause either a false-negative or positive reaction for protein.

31. **A** In diabetes, an early sign of renal involvement is an increased rate of albumin excretion approaching 300 μg/mL. This may be significant even when urine albumin concentration remains within normal limits. Consequently, tests for microalbuminuria are too sensitive for use in routine urinalysis but are useful in screening diabetics for increased urinary albumin excretion.

32. **D** The detection limit (sensitivity) of dry reagent strip protein tests is approximately 5 mg/dL albumin and is sufficient to detect urinary albumin levels found in orthostatic albuminuria and renal diseases, with the exception of tubular proteinuria. Renal tubular proteinuria results from failure of damaged tubules to reabsorb β-microglobulin. Dry reagent strip tests for proteinuria are insensitive to globulins and do not detect small quantities of hemoglobin, myoglobin, or microglobulins. Protein electrophoresis is used to detect β_2-microglobulinuria.

33. The normal renal threshold for glucose is:
  A. 70–85 mg/dL
  B. 100–115 mg/dL
  C. 130–145 mg/dL
  D. 165–180 mg/dL

  Body fluids/Apply knowledge of fundamental biological characteristics/Urine glucose/1

34. In which of the following conditions is glycosuria most likely?
  A. Addison's disease
  B. Hypothyroidism
  C. Pregnancy
  D. Hypopituitarism

  Body fluids/Correlate clinical and laboratory data/Urine glucose/2

35. In addition to ascorbate the glucose oxidase reaction may be inhibited by:
  A. Acetoacetic acid (AAA)
  B. ε-Aminocaproic acid
  C. Creatinine
  D. All of the above

  Body fluids/Apply knowledge to identify sources of error/Urine glucose/1

36. A positive glucose oxidase test and a negative test for reducing sugars indicates:
  A. True glycosuria
  B. False-positive reagent strip test
  C. False-negative reducing test caused by ascorbate
  D. Galactosuria

  Body fluids/Evaluate laboratory data to determine possible inconsistent results/Urine glucose/2

37. A negative glucose oxidase test and a positive test for reducing sugars in urine indicates:
  A. True glycosuria
  B. A false-negative glucose oxidase reaction
  C. The presence of a nonglucose reducing sugar such as galactose
  D. A trace quantity of glucose

  Body fluids/Evaluate laboratory data to determine possible inconsistent results/Urine glucose/2

38. In what condition may urinary ketone tests underestimate ketosis?
  A. Acidosis
  B. Hemolytic anemia
  C. Renal failure
  D. Excessive use of vitamin C

  Body fluids/Apply knowledge to identify sources of error/Urinary ketones/2

39. AAA is detected in urine by reaction with:
  A. Sodium nitroprusside
  B. o-Toluidine
  C. m-Dinitrobenzene
  D. m-Dinitrophenylhydrazine

Body fluids/Apply principles of basic laboratory procedures/Urinary ketones/1

Answers to Questions 33–39

33. **D** The renal threshold is the concentration of a substance (e.g., glucose) in blood that must be exceeded before it can be detected in the urine. Threshold substances require a carrier to transport them from the tubular lumen to the vasa recta. When the carrier becomes saturated the tubular maximum is reached causing the substance to be excreted in the urine.

34. **C** In addition to diabetes mellitus glycosuria may occur in other endocrine diseases, pregnancy, in response to drugs that affect glucose tolerance or renal threshold, and several other conditions, especially those involving the liver or central nervous system (CNS). Cushing's disease and hyperthyroidism cause impaired glucose tolerance and cause hyperglycemia. Increased estrogens produced in pregnancy lower the renal threshold for glucose and may impair glucose tolerance. Hyperpituitarism causes hyperglycemia mediated by increased release of growth hormone.

35. **A** AAA and salicylates may inhibit the glucose oxidase reaction by the same mechanism as ascorbate. These reducing agents compete with the chromogen for hydrogen peroxide. Low SG may increase and high SG decrease the color reaction for glucose in urine.

36. **A** Glucose oxidase is specific for β-D-glucose. Therefore a positive reaction is always considered significant unless contamination is evident. A reducing test should not be used to confirm a positive glucose oxidase test because it is not as specific or as sensitive.

37. **C** Reducing tests utilize alkaline copper sulfate and heat to oxidize glucose. Other reducing substances, including several sugars and antibiotics, may react making the test inappropriate as a screening test for glucose. A positive test for reducing sugars seen with a negative glucose oxidase test may occur in lactose, galactose, and fructosuria and other disorders of carbohydrate metabolism.

38. **A** Tests for urinary ketone bodies are sensitive to AAA. They react weakly with acetone and do not react with β hydroxybutyric acid. Acidosis favors formation of β hydroxybutyric acid and may cause a falsely low estimate of serum or urine ketones in diabetic ketoacidosis.

39. **A** Urinary ketones are detected using alkaline sodium nitroprusside or nitroferricyanide. L-Dopa may cause a false-positive with the former and phenylpyruvic acid (PKU) and some antibiotics with the latter.

40. Nondiabetic ketonuria can occur in all of the following *except:*
    A. Pregnancy
    B. Renal failure
    C. Starvation
    D. Lactate acidosis

    Body fluids/Correlate clinical and laboratory data/Urinary ketones/2

41. Which of the following statements regarding the tablet (Acetest) and classical nitroprusside reaction for ketones is true?
    A. The reaction is most sensitive to acetone.
    B. Nitroprusside reacts with acetone, AAA, and β hydroxybutyric acid.
    C. It may be falsely positive in phenylketonuria.
    D. The reaction is not sensitive enough to detect serum ketones.

    Body fluids/Apply knowledge to identify sources of error/Urinary ketones/2

42. Gerhardt's test for AAA is based upon:
    A. Oxidation of AAA to acetone by peroxide
    B. Boiling urine to convert AAA to acetone
    C. Reduction of AAA to β hydroxybutyric acid using ascorbic acid
    D. Reaction of AAA with nitroferricyanide

    Body fluids/Apply principles of special procedures/Urinary ketones/1

43. Hemoglobin in urine can be differentiated from myoglobin using:
    A. 80% ammonium sulfate to precipitate hemoglobin
    B. Sodium dithionite to reduce hemoglobin
    C. *o*-Dianisidine instead of benzidine as the color indicator
    D. Microscopic examination

    Body fluids/Select methods/Hemoglobinuria/2

44. Which of the following conditions is associated with a negative blood test and an increase in urine urobilinogen?
    A. Calculi of the kidney or bladder
    B. Malignancy of the kidney or urinary system
    C. Crush injury
    D. Extravascular hemolytic anemia

    Body fluids/Correlate clinical and laboratory data/Hematuria/2

45. A positive blood test and a negative microscopic examination for RBCs can occur when:
    A. Urine is hypotonic or alkaline.
    B. Myoglobinuria is present.
    C. Intravascular hemolytic anemia is present.
    D. All of the above.

    Body fluids/Evaluate laboratory data to determine possible inconsistent results/Hematuria/2

Answers to Questions 40–45

40. **B** Ketonuria results from excessive oxidation of fats forming acetyl coenzyme A (CoA). In addition to diabetes mellitus, ketonuria occurs in starvation, carbohydrate restriction, alkalosis, lactate acidosis, and von Gierke disease (glycogen stores cannot be utilized). Ketonuria also occurs in pregnancy, associated with increased vomiting and cyclic fever.

41. **C** The tablet nitroprusside test is sensitive to 5–10 mg/dL AAA. Both tablet and dry reagent strip tests for ketones are less sensitive to acetone than AAA and do not detect β hydroxybutyric acid. High levels of phenylpyruvic acid (phenylketonuria) will cause a false-positive reaction in the tablet and classical nitroprusside reactions but do not usually interfere with the dry reagent strip test for ketones. To determine serum ketones, serial dilutions of serum are added to tablets. The highest dilution giving a trace positive is multiplied by 10 mg/dL to estimate ketones. Normal serum will be negative (reference range 0–3 mg/dL), but ketosis is readily detected.

42. **B** In Gerhardt's test, ferric chloride ($FeCl_3$) reacts with AAA to give a red color. Because the reaction is nonspecific, the presence of AAA is confirmed by boiling a sample of urine and repeating the test. Boiling oxidizes acetoacetic to acetone, which evaporates causing the reaction with $FeCl_3$ to become negative.

43. **A** Both hemoglobin and myoglobin have peroxidase activity and cause a positive blood test. However, myoglobin is soluble in 80% w/v ammonium sulfate in urine, but hemoglobin precipitates. A positive blood reaction with supernatant after addition of ammonium sulfate and sodium hydroxide (NaOH) confirms the presence of myoglobin.

44. **D** A positive test for blood can occur from renal or lower urinary tract bleeding, intravascular hemolytic anemia, and transfusion reaction. Extravascular hemolysis results in increased bilirubin production rather than plasma hemoglobin. This may cause increased urobilinogen in urine but not a positive blood reaction.

45. **D** The blood test detects intact RBCs, hemoglobinuria, and myoglobinuria. Red cells will lyse in alkaline or hypotonic urine resulting in a positive blood test but negative microscopic examination for RBCs. However, the presence of more than 4–5 RBCs per high power field (HPF) should correlate with a positive blood test (nonhemolyzed trace).

46. Which statement about the dry reagent strip blood test is true?

A. Tests for blood are based upon its reaction with peroxidase.

B. A blood reaction is often positive in the absence of visible red color.

C. A nonhemolyzed trace is present when there are 1–2 RBCs per HPF.

D. Salicylates cause a false-positive reaction.

Body fluids/Apply principles of basic laboratory procedures/Hematuria/2

47. Which of the following statements regarding the dry reagent strip test for bilirubin is true?

A. A positive test is seen in prehepatic, hepatic, and posthepatic jaundice.

B. The test detects only conjugated bilirubin.

C. Standing urine may become falsely positive due to bacterial contamination.

D. High levels of ascorbate will cause positive interference.

Body fluids/Apply knowledge to recognize sources of error/Urine bilirubin/2

48. Which of the following reagents is used to detect urobilinogen in urine?

A. *p*-Dinitrobenzene

B. *p*-Aminosalicylate

C. *p*-Dimethylaminobenzaldehyde

D. *p*-Dichloroaniline

Body fluids/Apply principles of basic laboratory procedures/Urine urobilinogen/1

49. Which of the following statements regarding urinary urobilinogen is true?

A. Diurnal variation occurs with highest levels seen in the early morning.

B. High levels occurring with a positive bilirubin test indicate obstructive jaundice.

C. Dry reagent strip tests do not detect decreased levels.

D. False-positive results may occur if urine is stored for more than 2 hours.

Body fluids/Correlate clinical and laboratory data/Urine bilirubin/2

Answers to Questions 46–49

46. **B** The blood reaction uses anhydrous peroxide and benzidine. Hemoglobin has peroxidase activity and catalyzes the oxidation of benzidine by peroxide. The reaction is sensitive to submilligram levels of free hemoglobin, whereas visible hemolysis does not occur unless free hemoglobin exceeds 20 mg/dL. The test detects approximately 4–5 intact RBCs per HPF as a nonhemolyzed trace. Greater than three RBCs per HPF is abnormal.

47. **B** Only the conjugated form of bilirubin is excreted into the urine. Urinary bilirubin is positive in necrotic and obstructive jaundice but not in prehepatic jaundice, which results in a high level of serum unconjugated bilirubin. The highest levels of urinary bilirubin occur in obstructive jaundice, which causes decreased urinary urobilinogen. Very few drugs have been reported to interfere with urine bilirubin tests, which are based upon formation of azobilirubin by reaction with a diazonium salt. Positive interference by rifampin and chlorpromazine have been reported. Urine must be fresh because sunlight destroys bilirubin. Bacteria may cause hydrolysis of glucuronides forming unconjugated bilirubin, which does not react with the diazonium reagent. Ascorbate inhibits the reaction by reducing the diazo reagent.

48. **C** Urobilinogen reacts with Ehrlich's aldehyde reagent (*p*-dimethylaminobenzaldehyde in HCl) to form a pink color. Dry reagent strips use either *p*-dimethylaminobenzaldehyde or 4-methoxybenzene diazonium tetrafluoroborate to detect urobilinogen. The former reagent may react with PBG, salicylate, and sulfonamides giving falsely high results. False-positive results may occur in the presence of Pyridium and Gantrisin, which color the urine orange-red. Formalin may cause a false-negative reaction.

49. **C** Urobilinogen exhibits diurnal variation, and highest levels are seen in the afternoon. A 2-hour postprandial afternoon sample is the sample of choice for detecting increased urine urobilinogen. Urobilinogen is formed by bacterial reduction of conjugated bilirubin in the bowel. In obstructive jaundice, delivery of bilirubin into the intestine is blocked resulting in decreased fecal, serum, and urine urobilinogen. However, the dry reagent strip tests are not sensitive enough to detect abnormally low levels. Urobilinogen is rapidly oxidized to urobilin, which does not react with dry reagent strip tests.

50. Which statement about the Watson-Schwartz test is true?
A. Urobilinogen is water-soluble and gives a pink color in the upper layer.
B. Urobilinogen is extracted in chloroform and gives a pink color in the lower layer.
C. PBG is extracted in *n*-butanol.
D. Dietary indoles cannot be separated from PBG.

Body fluids/Apply principles of special procedures/ Urine urobilinogen/2

51. Which of the following statements regarding the test for nitrite in urine is true?
A. It detects more than 95% of clinically significant bacteriuria.
B. Formation of nitrite is unaffected by the urine pH.
C. The test is dependent upon an adequate dietary nitrate content.
D. A positive test differentiates bacteriuria from *in vitro* bacterial contamination.

Body fluids/Apply knowledge to recognize sources of error/Nitrite/2

52. Which statement about the dry reagent strip test for leukocytes is true?
A. The test detects only intact white blood cells (WBCs).
B. The reaction is based upon the hydrolysis of substrate by WBC esterases.
C. Several antibiotics may give a false-positive reaction.
D. The test is sensitive to 2–3 WBCs per HPF.

Body fluids/Apply principles of basic laboratory procedures/Leukocytes/2

53. Select the clearance test that can be used to measure renal blood flow:
A. Urea
B. Inulin
C. Creatinine
D. *p*-Aminohippuric acid (PAH)

Body fluids/Apply knowledge of fundamental biological characteristics/PAH/1

54. Which of the following statements about creatinine clearance is correct?
A. Dietary restrictions are required during the 24 hours preceding the test.
B. Fluid intake must be restricted to below 600 mL in the 6 hours preceding the test.
C. Creatinine clearance is mainly determined by renal tubular function.
D. Creatinine clearance is dependent upon lean body mass.

Body fluids/Apply knowledge of fundamental biological characteristics/Creatinine clearance/1

Answers to Questions 50–54

50. **B** The Watson-Schwartz test differentiates urobilinogen and indole derivatives from PBG. A pink color extracted by chloroform will be in the lower layer and is caused by the urobilinogen-aldehyde product. Dietary indoles may react and will extract in the chloroform layer. Melanogens and most drugs are extracted into *n*-butanol. PBG remains in the aqueous layer after extraction with both chloroform and *n*-butanol. A pink color forming in the aqueous phase that remains in the aqueous phase after addition of *n*-butanol is caused by PBG.

51. **C** The nitrite test is dependent upon the activity of bacterial reductase, and false-negatives have been reported when urine is highly acidic. Nitrite is formed by reduction of diet-derived nitrates and reacts with *p*-arsanilic acid or sulfanilamide to form a diazonium compound. This reacts with benzoquinoline to form a pink azo dye. False negatives also occur in the presence of ascorbate, which reduces the diazonium product. Nitrite is positive in about 70% of clinically significant bacterial infections of the urinary tract. Sensitivity is limited by the requirements for dietary nitrate and 3–4 hour storage time in the bladder. In addition, the causative bacteria must be able to reduce nitrate.

52. **B** PMNs in urine are detected by the presence of esterases that hydrolyze an ester such as indoxylcarbonic acid. The product reacts with a diazonium salt to give a purple color. The test detects esterases in urine as well as intact WBCs but is not sensitive to less than 5–10 WBCs per HPF. Several antibiotics, high protein, and high SG inhibit the esterase reaction. Formalin may cause a false-positive result.

53. **D** PAH is secreted by the renal tubules. When infused at a rate giving a blood level below the tubular maximum, excretion is dependent upon blood flow to the kidneys. Inulin and creatinine clearance are dependent upon glomerular filtration rate and urea clearance on the glomerular filtration rate, tubular function, and nitrogen metabolism.

54. **D** Although some creatinine is derived from the diet, it is rapidly filtered by the glomeruli, and time variations are reduced by collection of urine for at least 4 hours. Creatinine is produced from oxidation of creatine at a constant rate of about 2% per day. It is filtered completely and not significantly reabsorbed. However, creatinine secretion by the tubules is increased when filtrate flow is slow, and patients must be given at least 600 mL of H_2O at the start of the test and kept well hydrated throughout. Body size determines how much creatinine is produced, and clearance must be normalized to eliminate this variable.

55. A male patient's creatinine clearance is 75 mL/min. This indicates:
- A. Normal glomerular filtration rate.
- B. The patient is uremic and will be hyperkalemic.
- C. Renal tubular dysfunction.
- D. Reduced glomerular filtration without uremia.

Body fluids/Correlate clinical and laboratory data/Creatinine clearance/2

56. Which of the following tests is a specific measure of glomerular filtration?
- A. PSP dye excretion
- B. Fishberg concentration test
- C. Mosenthaul dilution test
- D. Inulin clearance

Body fluids/Correlate laboratory data with physiological processes/Renal function/1

57. Which of the following statements regarding creatinine clearance is true?
- A. As renal failure progresses the creatinine clearance more accurately reflects the true glomerular filtration rate.
- B. Results are slightly higher than inulin clearance due to tubular secretion.
- C. Creatinine clearance results are independent of the method of creatinine assay.
- D. Creatinine clearance may be normal when serum creatinine is increased.

Body fluids/Apply knowledge to recognize sources of error/Creatinine clearance/2

58. Which statement regarding urea is true?
- A. Urea is 100% filtered by the glomeruli.
- B. Blood urea levels are independent of diet.
- C. Urea is not significantly reabsorbed by the tubules.
- D. Urea excretion is a specific measure of glomerular function.

Body fluids/Correlate laboratory data with physiological processes/Urea/1

59. Given the following data calculate the creatinine clearance.

Serum creatinine = 1.5 mg/dL; urine creatinine = 102 mg/dL; urine volume = 1.7 mL/min; body surface area = 1.73 m^2
- A. 47 mL/min
- B. 97 mL/ min
- C. 100 mL/ min
- D. 116 mL/ min

Body fluids/Calculate/Creatinine clearance/2

60. Given the following data calculate the creatinine clearance.

Serum creatinine = 2.4 mg/dL; urine creatinine = 105 mg/dL; urine volume = 1.4 L/day; surface area = 1.80 m^2
- A. 41 mL/min
- B. 78 mL/min
- C. 87 mL/min

- D. 110 mL/min

Body fluids/Calculate/Creatinine clearance/2

Answers to Questions 55–60

55. D Normal creatinine clearance in men is 107–140 mL/min. Men have a slightly higher clearance than women (87–107 mL/min) due to greater lean body mass. Values below the lower reference limit, but above 60 mL/min indicate glomerular damage but not of severity sufficient to cause uremia.

56. D Inulin clearance is a research tool used to determine the glomerular filtration rate. The other three tests are measures of tubular function but are used infrequently because they are associated with significant health risks. The amount of PSP dye excreted after 15 minutes is dependent upon tubular secretion. The Fishberg concentration test measures the ability to concentrate urine after deprivation of H$_2$O. The Mosenthaul test measures the ability to excrete free H$_2$O after excessive H$_2$O intake.

57. B Creatinine clearance tends to overestimate the glomerular filtration rate when compared to inulin clearance. When Jaffe's reaction is used to measure creatinine, the presence of nonspecific reactants in the serum tends to compensate for this, and results agree more closely than when creatinine is measured by an enzymatic method. However, as renal failure progresses, the relative contribution of nonspecific substances decreases. The tubules secrete more creatinine as glomerular filtration slows. These two factors combine to cause significant overestimation of the glomerular filtration rate as glomerular function deteriorates.

58. A Serum urea and blood urea nitrogen (BUN) levels are affected by diet, hepatic function, tubular function, and filtrate flow as well as the glomerular filtration rate. BUN rises higher than serum creatinine in prerenal failure because the tubules reabsorb 30%–40% of the filtered urea. BUN is a sensitive indicator of renal disease but is not specific for glomerular function.

59. D The clearance formula is U ÷ P × V × 1.73/A, where U = urine creatinine (mg/dL), P = plasma creatinine (mg/dL), V = urine volume (mL/min), and 1.73 = mean body surface area (m^2)

102 mg/dL ÷ 1.5 mg/dL × 1.7 mL/min × (1.73 m^2 ÷ 1.73 m^2) = 115.6 mL/min

60. A Convert volume in liters per day to milliliters per minute by multiplying 1000/1440.

1.4 L/day × 1000 mL/L × 1 day/24 hr × 1 hr/60 min = 1400 mL/1440 min = 1 mL/min

Creatinine clearance = 105 mg/dL ÷ 2.4 mg/dL × 1 mL/min × (1.73 m^2 ÷ 1.8 m^2) = 41 mL/min

Urine Microscopy and Clinical Correlations

1. Which of the following dyes are used in Stern-heimer-Malbin stain?
   A. Hematoxylin and eosin
   B. Crystal violet and safranin
   C. Methylene blue and eosin
   D. Methylene blue and safranin

   Body fluids/Apply principles of basic laboratory procedures/Staining/1

2. Which of the following statements regarding WBCs in urinary sediment is true?
   A. "Glitter cells" seen in the urinary sediment are a sign of renal disease.
   B. Bacteriuria in the absence of WBCs indicates lower urinary tract infection (UTI).
   C. WBCs other than PMNs are not found in urinary sediment.
   D. WBC casts indicate that pyuria is of renal rather than lower urinary origin.

   Body fluids/Correlate clinical and laboratory data/Urinary sediment/2

3. Which description of sediment staining with Stern-heimer-Malbin is correct?
   A. Transitional epithelium: cytoplasm pale blue, nucleus dark blue
   B. Renal epithelium: cytoplasm light blue, nucleus dark purple
   C. Glitter cells: cytoplasm dark blue, nucleus dark purple
   D. Squamous epithelium: cytoplasm pink, nucleus pale blue

   Body fluids/Apply knowledge of fundamental biological characteristics/Staining/2

Answers to Questions 1–3

1. **B** Sternheimer-Malbin is a supravital stain used to help differentiate renal tubular epithelium from transitional cells and PMNs. The mononuclear cells are clearly distinguished from both live and dead PMNs. Transitional cells appear mostly blue, but renal cells take up both dyes resulting in an azurophilic appearance (orange-purple cytoplasm and dark purple nucleus).

2. **D** The majority of WBCs in the urinary sediment will be PMNs. Eosinophils and monocunclear cells will occassionally be seen. Mononuclear cells are especially likely in patients with chronic inflammatory diseases and in renal transplant rejection where they may account for as many as 30% of the WBCs. Glitter cells are PMNs with highly refractile granules exhibiting Brownian movement. They are seen only when urine SG is below 1.020. These cells resist staining with Sternheimer-Malbin and are considered to be living (fresh) WBCs. When seen in large numbers they indicate urinary tract injury (with pseudopod extensions they point to infection). The presence of bacteria in urine in the absence of PMNs usually results from contamination by vaginal or skin flora that multiply *in vitro*, especially in unrefrigerated specimens. The presence of WBC casts is always significant, and when associated with pyuria and bacteriuria, indicates renal involvement in the infection.

3. **A** Live WBCs exclude Sternheimer-Malbin stain while dead cells stain with a deeply blue-purple nucleus and pale orange-blue cytoplasm. Renal epithelium have an orange-purple cytoplasm and dark purple nucleus. Squamous epithelium have a blue or purple cytoplasm and an orange-purple nucleus. Red cells stain very pale pink or not at all and hyaline casts stain faintly pink.

4. SITUATION: A 5-mL urine specimen is submitted for routine urinalysis and analyzed immediately. The SG of the sample is 1.012 and the pH is 6.5. The dry reagent strip test for blood is a large positive (3+) and the microscopic examination shows 11–20 RBCs per HPF. The leukocyte esterase reaction is a small positive (1+), and the microscopic examination shows 0–5 WBCs per HPF. What is the most likely cause of these results?

A. Myoglobin is present in the sample.
B. Free hemoglobin is present.
C. Insufficient volume causing microscopic results to be under estimated.
D. Some WBCs have been misidentified as RBCs.

Body fluids/Apply knowledge to identify sources of error/Urinalysis/3

5. Which of the following statements regarding epithelial cells in the urinary system is correct?

A. Caudate epithelial cells originate from the upper urethra.
B. Transitional cells originate from the upper urethra, ureters, bladder, or renal pelvis.
C. Cells from the proximal renal tubule are usually round in shape.
D. Squamous epithelium line the vagina, urethra, and wall of the urinary bladder.

Body fluids/Apply knowledge of fundamental biological characteristics/Urine sediment/2

6. Which of the statements regarding examination of unstained sediment is true?

A. Renal cells can be differentiated reliably from WBCs.
B. Large numbers of transitional cells are often seen after catheterization.
C. Neoplastic cells from the bladder are not found in urinary sediment.
D. RBCs are easily differentiated from nonbudding yeast.

Body fluids/Correlate clinical and laboratory data/Urine sediment/2

7. Which of the following statements regarding cells found in urinary sediment is true?

A. Transitional cells resist swelling in hypotonic urine.
B. Renal tubular cells are often polyhedral and have an eccentric round nucleus.
C. Trichomonads have an oval shape with a prominent nucleus and a single anterior flagellum.
D. Clumps of bacteria are frequently mistaken for blood casts.

Body fluids/Apply knowledge of fundamental biological characteristics/Urine sediment/2

Answers to Questions 4–7

4. C Given the SG and pH, most RBCs and WBCs will be intact. Both the RBC and WBC counts are lower than expected from the dry reagent strip results. Myoglobin or free hemoglobin may account for the poor correlation between the blood reaction and the RBC count but does not explain the lower than expected WBC count. Microscopic reference ranges are based upon concentrating a uniform volume of sediment from 12 mL of urine. When less urine is used, falsely low results will be obtained unless corrective action is taken. The specimen should be diluted with normal saline to 12 mL, then centrifuged at $450 \times g$ for 5 minutes. Sediment should be prepared according to the established procedure and the results multiplied by the dilution factor (in this case, $12 \div 5$ or 2.4).

5. B Caudate cells are transitional epithelium that have a sawtooth-shaped tail and are found in the urinary bladder and the pelvis of the kidney. Transitional epithelium line the upper two-thirds of the urethra and the ureters as well as the urinary bladder and renal pelvis. Renal tubular cells may be columnar, polyhedral, or oval depending upon the portion of the tubule from which they originate. Cells from the proximal tubule are columnar and have a distinctive brush border. Squamous epithelium line the vagina and lower third of the urethra.

6. B Renal cells and PMNs are about the same size and can be confused in unstained sediment. Catheterization often releases large clumps or sheets of transitional and squamous cells. These should be distinguished from neoplastic cells derived from the urinary bladder. When cells appear atypical (e.g., large cells in metaphase) they should be referred to a pathologist for cytological examination. Nonbudding yeast cells are approximately the same in size and appearance as RBCs. When RBCs are initially seen in the absence of a positive blood test, the probability of a falsely positive microscopic examination is very high. The microscopic examination should be reviewed for the presence of yeast.

7. B Transitional epithelial cells readily take up H_2O and appear much larger than renal cells or WBCs when urine is hypotonic. Transitional cells are considered a normal component of the sediment unless present in large numbers and associated with signs of inflammation such as mucus and PMNs, or presenting features of malignant cells. In contrast renal cells are significant when seen conclusively in the sediment. They are often teardrop, polyhedral, or elongated cells with a round eccentric nucleus. Conclusive identification requires staining. *Trichomonas vaginalis* displays an indistinct nucleus and two pairs of prominent anterior flagella. Amorphous urate crystals deposited on the slide may be mistaken for granular or blood casts.

8. Which of the following statements regarding RBCs in the urinary sediment is true?
 A. Yeast cells will lyse in dilute acetic acid but RBCs will not.
 B. RBCs are often swollen in hypertonic urine.
 C. RBCs of glomerular origin often appear dysmorphic.
 D. Yeast cells will tumble when the cover glass is touched but RBCs will not.

Body fluids/Apply knowledge of fundamental biological characteristics/Urine sediment/2

9. Renal tubular epithelial cells are shed into the urine in largest numbers in which condition?
 A. Malignant renal disease
 B. Acute glomerulonephritis
 C. Nephrotic syndrome
 D. Cytomegalovirus (CMV) infection of the kidney

Body fluids/Evaluate laboratory data to recognize health and disease states/Urinary sediment/2

10. The ova of which parasite may be found in the urinary sediment?
 A. *T. vaginalis*
 B. *Entamoeba histolytica*
 C. *Schistosoma hematobium*
 D. *Trichuris trichiura*

Body fluids/Apply knowledge of fundamental biological characteristics/Urinary sediment/1

11. Oval fat bodies are often seen in:
 A. Chronic glomerulonephritis
 B. Nephrotic syndrome
 C. Acute tubular nephrosis
 D. Renal failure of any cause

Body fluids/Correlate clinical and laboratory data/Urine sediment/2

12. All of the following statements regarding urinary casts are true *except:*
 A. Many hyaline casts may appear in sediment after jogging or exercise.
 B. An occasional granular cast may be seen in a normal sediment.
 C. Casts can be seen in significant numbers even when protein tests are negative.
 D. Hyaline casts will dissolve readily in alkaline urine.

Body fluids/Apply knowledge to recognize sources of error/Urine casts/2

13. Which condition promotes the formation of casts in the urine?
 A. Chronic production of alkaline urine
 B. Polyuria
 C. Reduced filtrate formation
 D. Low urine SG

Body fluids/Apply knowledge of fundamental characteristics/Urine casts/2

Answers to Questions 8–13

8. **C** RBCs are difficult to distinguish from nonbudding yeast in unstained sediment. RBCs tumble when the cover glass is touched and will lyse when the sediment is reconstituted in normal saline containing 2% v/v acetic acid. A nonhemolyzed trace blood reaction confirms the presence of RBCs. RBCs have a granular appearance in hypertonic urine due to crenation. The RBC membrane becomes distorted when passing through the glomerulus, often appearing scalloped, serrated, or invaginated. Such cells are termed *dysmorphic* RBCs and are associated with glomerulonephritis.

9. **D** Although seen in glomerulonephritis and pyelonephritis, the largest numbers of renal tubular cells appear in urine in association with viral infections of the kidney. Renal epithelium may show characteristic viral inclusions associated with CMV and rubella. High numbers of renal epithelium are also found in the sediment of patients with drug-induced tubular nephrosis and some cases of heavy metal poisoning. Renal tumors do not usually shed cells into the urine.

10. **C** Ova of *S. hematobium* are most often recovered from urine because the adult trematodes colonize the blood vessels of the urinary bladder. The eggs are approximately 150×60 μm and are nonoperculated. They are yellowish and have a prominent terminal spine.

11. **B** Oval fat bodies are degenerated renal tubular epithelium that have reabsorbed cholesterol from the filtrate. Although they can occur in any inflammatory disease of the tubules, they are commonly seen in the nephrotic syndrome, which is characterized by marked proteinuria and hyperlipidemia.

12. **C** Proteinuria accompanies cylindruria because protein is the principle component of casts. After strenuous exercise, hyaline casts may be present in the sediment in significant numbers but will disappear after resting for at least 24 hours.

13. **C** Cast formation is promoted by an acid filtrate, high solute concentration, slow movement of filtrate, and reduced filtrate formation. The appearance of a cast is dependent upon the location and time spent in the tubule as well as the chemical and cellular composition of the filtrate.

14. The mucoprotein that forms the matrix of a hyaline cast is called:
A. Bence Jones protein
B. β-Microglobulin
C. Tamm-Horsfall protein
D. Arginine-rich glycoprotein

Body fluids/Apply knowledge of fundamental biological characteristics/Urine casts/1

15. "Pseudocasts" are often caused by:
A. A dirty cover glass or slide
B. Bacterial contamination
C. Amorphous urates
D. Mucus in the urine

Body fluids/Apply knowledge to identify sources of error/Urine casts/2

16. Which of the following statements regarding urinary casts is correct?
A. Fine granular casts are more significant than coarse granular casts.
B. Cylinduria is always clinically significant.
C. The appearance of cylindroids signals the onset of end-stage renal disease.
D. Broad casts are associated with severe renal tubular obstruction.

Body fluids/Apply knowledge of fundamental biological characteristics/Urine casts/2

17. A sediment with moderate hematuria and RBC casts most likely results from:
A. Chronic pyelonephritis
B. Nephrotic syndrome
C. Acute glomerulonephritis
D. Lower urinary tract obstruction

Body fluids/Correlate clinical and laboratory data/Urine sediment/2

18. Urine sediment characterized by pyuria with bacterial and WBC casts indicates:
A. Nephrotic syndrome
B. Pyelonephritis
C. Polycystic kidney disease
D. Cystitis

Body fluids/Correlate clinical and laboratory data/Urine sediment/2

19. Which type of casts signals the presence of chronic renal failure?
A. Blood casts
B. Fine granular casts
C. Waxy casts
D. Fatty casts

Body fluids/Apply knowledge of fundamental biological characteristics/Urine casts/2

Answers to Questions 14–19

14. C Hyaline casts are composed of a mucoprotein called Tamm-Horsfall protein. In addition, casts may contain cells, immunoglobulins, light chains, cellular proteins, fat, bacteria, and crystalloids.

15. C Pseudocasts are formed by amorphous urates that may deposit in uniform cylindrical shapes as the sediment settles under the cover glass. They may be mistaken for granular or blood casts. However, they are highly refractile and lack the well-defined borders of true casts.

16. D There is no clinical difference between fine and coarse granular casts. Granular casts may form by degeneration of cellular casts, but some show no evidence of cellular origin. Granular casts may form from inclusion of urinary calculi, but some are of unknown etiology. Cylinduria refers to the presence of casts in the urine. Hyaline casts may be seen in small numbers in normal patients and in large numbers following strenuous exercise and long-distance running. Hyaline casts may also be increased in patients taking certain drugs such as diuretics. Broad casts form in dilated or distal tubules and indicate chronic renal failure or severe obstruction. Waxy casts form when there is prolonged stasis in the tubules and signal end-stage renal failure. Cylindroids are casts with tails and have no special clinical significance.

17. C Red-cell casts indicate the renal orgin of hematuria. Urinary obstruction may be associated with hematuria from ruptured vessels, but not casts. WBCs and WBC casts predominate in pyelonephritis. Sediment in chronic glomerulonephritis is variable, but usually exhibits moderate to severe intermittant hematuria. In addition pyuria and cylinduria (with granular, blood, waxy, and epithelial casts) are frequent. In nephrotic syndrome the sediment may be unremarkable except for the presence of oval fat bodies and hyaline casts. In some cases, fatty, waxy, and epithelial cell casts may also be found.

18. B Pyelonephritis results from bacterial infection of the renal pelvis and interstitium. It is characterized by polyuria resulting from failure of the tubules to reabsorb fluid. Obstruction of tubules and compression by WBCs may reduce glomerular filtration as well as H_2O reabsorption. The finding of WBC casts helps to differentiate pyelonephritis from urinary tract infection.

19. C Waxy casts form from the degeneration of cellular casts. Because the casts must remain lodged in the tubule long enough for the granular protein matrix to waxify, they are associated with chronic or end-stage renal failure. Both waxy and broad casts form in chronic renal failure when there is severe stasis, and they are associated with a poor prognosis.

20. SITUATION: Urinalysis of a sample from a patient suspected of having a transfusion reaction reveals small yellow-brown crystals in the microscopic examination. Dry reagent strip tests are normal with the exception of a positive blood reaction (moderate) and trace positive protein. The pH of the urine is 6.5. What test should be performed to positively identify the crystals?
A. Confirmatory test for bilirubin
B. Cyanide-nitroprusside test
C. Polarizing microscopy
D. Prussian blue stain

Body fluids/Select course of action/Urine sediment/3

21. When examining urinary sediment, which of the following is considered an abnormal finding?
A. 0–2 RBCs per HPF
B. 0–1 hyaline casts per low power field (LPF)
C. 0–1 renal cell casts per LPF
D. 2–5 WBCs per HPF

Body fluids/Evaluate laboratory data to recognize health and disease states/Urinary sediment/2

22. SITUATION: A urine sample with a pH of 6.0 produces an abundance of pink sediment after centrifugation that appears as densely packed yellow-brown granules under the microscope. The crystals are so dense that no other formed elements can be evaluated. What is the best course of action?
A. Request a new urine specimen.
B. Suspend the sediment in prewarmed saline, then repeat centrifugation.
C. Acidify a 12-mL aliquot with three drops of glacial acetic acid and heat to 56°C for 5 minutes before centrifuging.
D. Add five drops of 1*N* HCl to the sediment and examine.

Body fluids/Select course of action/Urine sediment/3

23. Hexagonal uric acid crystals can be distinguished from cystine crystals because:
A. Uric acid is insoluble in HCl and cystine is soluble.
B. Cystine gives a positive nitroprusside test after reduction with sodium cyanide (NaCN).
C. Cystine crystals are colorless.
D. All of the above.

Body fluids/Apply principles of special procedures/Urine crystals/2

24. The presence of tyrosine and leucine crystals together in a urine sediment usually indicates:
A. Renal failure
B. Chronic liver disease
C. Hemolytic anemia
D. Hartnup disease

Body fluids/Correlate clinical and laboratory data/Urine crystals/2

25. Which of the following crystals is considered nonpathological?

A. Hemosiderin
B. Bilirubin
C. Ammonium biruate
D. Cholesterol

Body fluids/Evaluate laboratory data to recognize health and disease states/Urine crystals/2

Answers to Questions 20–25

20. **D** A positive blood test and trace protein occurring with a normal test for urobilinogen and an absence of RBCs are consistent with an intravascular transfusion reaction. Small yellow-brown granular crystals at an acid pH may be uric acid, bilirubin, or hemosiderin. Bilirubin crystals are ruled out by the negative dry reagent strip test for bilirubin. Potassium ferrocyanide is used in the Prussian blue staining reaction to detect hemosiderin deposits in urinary sediment. Hemosiderin is associated with hemochromatosis and increased RBC destruction. Causes of urinary hemosiderin include transfusion reaction, hemolytic anemia, and pernicious anemia.

21. **C** Epithelial casts are rarely seen but indicate a disease process affecting the renal tubules. They are associated with diseases causing necrosis of the tubules such as hepatitis, CMV, and other viral infections, and mercury and ethylene glycol toxicity. Even a rare cellular cast is considered clinically significant.

22. **B** Urates are yellow-brown granules and form in acid or neutral urine. They often form following refrigeration of urine and can be dissolved by addition of warm saline or dilute NaOH. Amorphous phosphates are colorless and form in neutral or alkaline urine. They dissolve in dilute acetic acid but precipitate if heated.

23. **D** Flat six-sided uric acid crystals may be mistaken for cystine crystals. Cystine transmits polarized light and is soluble in dilute HCl. Uric acid is insoluble in HCl and is less anisotropic. Cystine is reduced by NaCN forming cystiene. The -SH group of cystiene reacts with nitroprusside to form a red color.

24. **B** Tyrosine crystals may occur in tyrosinosis, an overflow aminoaciduria, or in tyrosinemia. However, when seen along with leucine crystals, the cause is chronic liver disease, usually cirrhosis of the liver. Tyrosine usually forms fine brown or yellow needles, and leucine forms yellow spheres with concentric rings.

25. **C** Abnormal crystals are those that result from a pathological process. Hemosiderin crystals result from intravascular RBC destruction. Bilirubin crystals are found in severe necrotic and obstructive liver diseases, and cholesterol crystals in nephrotic syndrome, diabetes mellitus, and hypercholesterolemias.

26. At which pH are ammonium biurate crystals usually found in urine?
    A. Acid urine only
    B. Acid or neutral urine
    C. Neutral or alkaline urine
    D. Alkaline urine only

    Body fluids/Correlate laboratory data with physiological processes/Urine crystals/2

27. Which crystal appears in urine as a long, thin hexagonal plate, and is linked to ingestion of large amounts of benzoic acid?
    A. Cystine
    B. Hippuric acid
    C. Oxalic acid
    D. Uric acid

    Body fluids/Correlate laboratory data with physiological processes/Urine crystals/2

28. Which of the following crystals is seen commonly in alkaline and neutral urine?
    A. Calcium oxalate
    B. Uric acid
    C. Magnesium ammonium phosphate
    D. Cholesterol

    Body fluids/Correlate laboratory data with physiological processes/Urine crystals/1

29. Small yellow needles are seen in the sediment of a urine sample with a pH of 6.0. Which of the following crystals can be ruled out?
    A. Sulfa crystals
    B. Bilirubin crystals
    C. Uric acid crystals
    D. Cholesterol crystals

    Body fluids/Apply knowledge of fundamental biological characteristics/Urine crystals/2

30. Oval fat bodies are derived from:
    A. Renal tubular epithelium
    B. Transitional epithelium
    C. Degenerated WBCs
    D. Mucoprotein matrix

    Body fluids/Apply knowledge of fundamental biological characteristics/Urine sediment/1

31. Oval fat bodies are often associated with:
    A. Lipoid nephrosis
    B. Acute glomerulonephritis
    C. Aminoaciduria
    D. Pyelonephritis

    Body fluids/Correlate clinical and laboratory data/Urine sediment/2

32. Urine of constant low SG ranging from 1.008 to 1.010 most likely indicates:
    A. Addison's disease
    B. Renal tubular failure
    C. Prerenal failure
    D. Diabetes insipidus

Body fluids/Evaluate laboratory data to recognize health and disease states/Specific gravity/2

Answers to Questions 26–32

26. **D** Ammonium biurate is often called a "thornapple" crystal because it forms a dark brown spiny sphere. Calcium carbonate is another common crystal that is seen only in alkaline urine. Sodium urate and uric acid form in acid or neutral urine.

27. **B** Hippuric acid forms long, flat six-sided plates. It results from the metabolism of benzoic acid and resembles the "coffin lid" appearance of triple phosphate. It may occur normally as a result of ingestion of vegetables preserved with benzoic acid.

28. **C** Magnesium ammonium phosphate, also called triple phosphate, may be present in neutral or alkaline urine. Crystals containing phosphates do not occur in acid urine.

29. **D** Cholesterol crystals are colorless rectangular plates that often have a notched corner and appear stacked in a stair-step arrangement. Cholesterol crystals are highly anisotropic and can be positively identified using a polarizing microscope. Bilirubin, sulfa, or uric acid crystals may occur as small yellow or yellow-brown needles or rods in neutral or acid urine. Bilirubin crystals should be suspected when the dry reagent strip test for bilirubin is positive and cells in the sediment are dark yellow (bile-stained). Sulfa crystals are soluble in acetone, concentrated HCl, and NaOH. They can be confirmed by the lignin test in which one drop of sediment and one drop of 10% HCl react with newsprint to produce a yellow-orange color.

30. **A** Oval fat bodies form from degenerated renal epithelial cells that have reabsorbed cholesterol from the filtrate. They stain with Oil Red O or Sudan III. The fat globules within the cells give a maltese cross effect when examined under polarized light.

31. **A** The term *lipoid nephrosis* is a synonym for idiopathic nephrotic syndrome. Like other causes of nephrotic syndrome, it is associated with gross proteinuria, edema, and hyperlipidemia; however, the idiopathic form is also associated with hematuria.

32. **B** The SG of the filtrate in Bowman's space is approximately 1.010. Urine produced consistently with an SG of 1.010 has the same osmolality of the plasma and results from failure of the tubules to modify the filtrate.

33. Which of the following characterizes prerenal failure and helps to differentiate it from acute renal failure caused by renal disease?
A. BUN:creatinine ratio of 20:1 or higher
B. Urine-plasma (U:P) osmolal ratio greater than 2:1
C. Low daily excretion of sodium
D. All of the above

Body fluids/Correlate clinical and laboratory data/Renal disease/2

34. Which of the following conditions characterizes chronic glomerulonephritis and helps to differentiate it from acute glomerulonephritis?
A. Hematuria
B. Polyuria
C. Hypertension
D. Azotemia

Body fluids/Correlate clinical and laboratory data/Renal disease/2

35. Which of the following conditions is seen in acute renal failure and helps to differentiate it from prerenal failure?
A. Hyperkalemia and uremia
B. Oliguria and edema
C. Low creatinine clearance
D. Abnormal urinary sediment

Body fluids/Correlate clinical and laboratory data/Renal disease/2

36. Which of the following conditions characterizes acute renal failure and helps to differentiate it from chronic renal failure?
A. Hyperkalemia
B. Hematuria
C. Cylinduria
D. Proteinuria

Body fluids/Correlate clinical and laboratory data/Renal disease/2

37. The serum concentration of which analyte is likely to be decreased in untreated cases of acute renal failure?
A. Hydrogen ions
B. Inorganic phosphorus
C. Calcium
D. Uric acid

Body fluids/Correlate clinical and laboratory data/Renal disease/2

38. Which condition below is associated with the greatest proteinuria?
A. Acute glomerulonephritis
B. Chronic glomerulonephritis
C. Nephrotic syndrome
D. Acute pyelonephritis

Body fluids/Correlate clinical and laboratory data/Renal disease/2

Answers to Questions 33–38

33. **D** Prerenal failure is caused by deficient renal blood flow. The tubules are undamaged and will reabsorb more BUN than normal because filtrate flow is slow. Under the influence of aldosterone they reabsorb sodium and concentrate the urine. The BUN:creatinine ratio and U:P osmolal ratio are very high and sodium output low. In renal disease, the BUN:creatinine ratio is 10 or less, the U:P osmolal ratio approaches 1.0, and the daily sodium excretion is high.

34. **B** Acute glomerulonephritis results in severe compression of the glomerular vessels. This reduces filtration causing a progression from oliguria to anuria. In contrast, polyuria is associated with chronic glomerulonephritis, which causes scarring of the collecting tubules. Both acute and chronic glomerulonephritis cause low urine osmolality, azotemia, acidosis, hypertension, proteinuria, and hematuria.

35. **D** Reduced glomerular filtration as evidenced by low creatinine clearance characterizes both prerenal and acute renal failure. This results in retention of fluid causing edema, reduced urine volume, hypertension, uremia, and hyperkalemia in both prerenal and acute renal failure. The kidneys are not damaged in prerenal failure and, therefore, the microscopic examination is usually normal.

36. **A** In acute renal failure, reduced glomerular filtration coupled with decreased tubular secretion results in hyperkalemia. In chronic renal failure, scarring of the collecting tubules prevents salt and H_2O reabsorption. This results in normal or low serum potassium despite reduced glomerular filtration. The sediment in chronic renal failure is characterized by intermittent heavy hematuria and proteinuria.

37. **C** Decreased glomerular filtration in renal failure results in high serum creatinine, BUN, and uric acid. Failure of the tubules results in retention of hydrogen ions and phosphates causing acidosis and an increased anion gap. The tubules fail to respond to parathyroid hormone resulting in excessive loss of calcium in urine. Serum sodium is usually normal or slightly increased while hyperkalemia is a constant finding in acute renal failure.

38. **C** Although all four conditions are associated with proteinuria, it is greatest in the nephrotic syndrome. Urinary albumin loss is typically in excess of 4 g/day causing dry reagent strip protein tests to give 3+ to 4+ reactions. In contrast to glomerulonephritis and pyelonephritis, the urinary sediment in nephrotic syndrome is not usually characterized by either hematuria or pyuria. Various casts, lipid laden renal epithelial cells, and oval fat bodies are usually found.

39. Which of the following conditions is known to cause glomerulonephritis?
A. Diabetes mellitus
B. Autoimmune damage following recent respiratory infection with group A *Streptococcus*
C. Systemic lupus erythematosus (SLE)
D. All of the above

Body fluids/Apply knowledge of fundamental biological characteristics/Renal disease/2

40. Acute pyelonephritis is commonly caused by:
A. Bacterial infection of medullary interstitium
B. Circulatory failure
C. Renal calculi
D. Antigen-antibody reactions within the glomeruli

Body fluids/Apply knowledge of fundamental biological characteristics/Renal disease/2

41. All of the following are characteristics of the nephrotic syndrome *except:*
A. Hyperlipidemia
B. Hypoalbuminemia
C. Hematuria and pyuria
D. Severe edema

Body fluids/Correlate clinical and laboratory data/Renal disease/2

42. Which of the following conditions is a characteristic finding in patients with obstructive renal disease?
A. Polyuria
B. Azotemia
C. Dehydration
D. Alkalosis

Body fluids/Correlate laboratory data with physiological processes/Renal disease/2

43. Whewellite and weddellite kidney stones are composed of:
A. Magnesium ammonium phosphate
B. Calcium oxalate
C. Calcium phosphate
D. Calcium carbonate

Body fluids/Apply knowledge of fundamental biological characteristics/Renal calculi/1

44. Which of the following abnormal crystals is often associated with formation of renal calculi?
A. Cystine
B. Ampicillin
C. Tyrosine
D. Leucine

Body fluids/Correlate clinical and laboratory data/Renal calculi/2

Answers to Questions 39–44

39. **D** Insulin deficiency produces sclerotic vascular damage to the glomeruli often resulting in crescentic glomerulonephritis. Group A *Streptococcus* and SLE result in immunologically mediated damage to the glomeruli usually causing membranous or membranoproliferative glomerulonephritis.

40. **A** Acute pyelonephritis is caused by infection of the medullary interstitium usually by coliforms that enter from the lower urinary tract. *Escherichia coli* is the most commonly implicated bacterium.

41. **C** Although casts may be present, the urinary sediment in nephrotic syndrome is not characterized by RBCs and WBCs or by RBC, blood, and WBC casts. In nephrotic syndrome, unlike renal failure, the creatinine clearance and serum potassium are usually normal. Nephrotic syndrome often follows the anuric phase of acute glomerulonephritis indicating a reversal of the inflammatory process.

42. **B** Obstructive renal disease may result from renal or urinary tract calculi, benign prostatic hypertrophy, chronic urinary tract infection, or urogenital malignancy. Obstruction causes the hydrostatic pressure in Bowman's space to increase. This pressure opposes glomerular filtration. If the hydrostatic pressure in Bowman's space equals the hydrostatic pressure in the glomeruli, then filtrate will not be produced resulting in anuria. Postrenal failure produces many of the same serum abnormalities as acute renal failure, including hyperkalemia, acidosis, edema, and azotemia. The urinary sediment will often be abnormal as well. Bacteriuria and pyuria are common, and hematuria may result from rupture of the vasa recta or other blood vessels.

43. **B** Over three-fourths of urinary tract stones are composed of calcium salts, and hyperparathyroidism is commonly associated with calcium stones. Stones composed of magnesium ammonium phosphate are called *struvite* and lodge in the renal pelvis, causing a characteristic "staghorn" appearance on radiographic examination. Stones mainly composed of calcium phosphate are called *hydroxyapatite* or *bushite* depending upon the calcium composition. Stones of $CaCO_3$ are called *carbonate apatite*.

44. **A** Cystinuria is caused by an autosomal recessive defect in the tubular reabsorption of dibasic amino acids (a renal type aminoaciduria). Cystine crystals are highly insoluble and form kidney stones. Tyrosine crystals form fine dark sheaves or needles and may result from liver disease or tyrosinosis, an overflow aminoaciduria. Leucine crystals form yellow spheres with concentric rings and are seen in chronic liver disease. Ampicillin forms long colorless prisms in sheaves in some patients being treated with high doses.

45. Which statement about renal calculi is true?
  A. Calcium oxalate and calcium phosphate account for about three-fourths of all stones.
  B. Uric acid stones cannot be seen by x-ray and occur in chronic acid urine.
  C. Triple phosphate stones are found in the renal pelvis as "staghorn" calculi.
  D. All of the above.

Body fluids/Apply knowledge of fundamental biological characteristics/Renal calculi/2

Answer to Question 45

45. **D** Calcium oxalate is the most common component of urinary stones and can form calculi in urine of any pH. Oxalates are hard, dark, and coarse stones. Uric acid stones are always pigmented yellow to reddish brown. Stones made of primarily calcium phosphate (as hydroxyapatite) are light and crumble easily.

Cerebrospinal, Serous, and Synovial Fluids

1. Cerebrospinal fluid (CSF) is formed by ultrafiltration of plasma through the:
   A. Choroid plexus
   B. Sagittal sinus
   C. Anterior cerebral lymphatics
   D. Arachnoid membrane

   Body fluids/Apply knowledge of fundamental biological characteristics/Cerebrospinal fluid/1

2. Which statement below regarding CSF is true?
   A. Normal values for mononuclear cells are higher for infants than adults.
   B. Absolute neutrophilia is not significant if the total WBC count is less than $25/\mu L$.
   C. The first aliquot of CSF should be sent to the microbiology laboratory.
   D. Neutrophils compose the majority of WBCs in normal CSF.

   Body fluids/Apply principles of basic laboratory procedures/Cerebrospinal fluid/2

3. When collecting CSF a difference between opening and closing fluid pressure greater than 100 mm H_2O indicates:
   A. Low CSF volume
   B. Subarachnoid hemorrhage
   C. Meningitis
   D. Hydrocephalus

   Body fluids/Correlate laboratory data with physiological processes/Cerebrospinal fluid/2

Answers to Questions 1–3

1. **A** CSF is formed by ultrafiltration of plasma though the choroid plexus, a tuft of capillaries in the pia mater located in the third and fourth ventricles. Endothelium of the choroid plexus vessels and ependymal cells lining the ventricles act as a barrier to the passage of proteins, drugs, and metabolites. Glucose in CSF is about one-third the plasma glucose. Total protein in CSF is only 15–45 mg/dL, while chloride levels are 10%–15% higher than plasma. Approximately 500 mL of ultrafiltrate are produced per day, the bulk of which is returned to the circulation via the sagittal sinus. The normal volume of CSF in adults is 90–150 mL (10–60 mL for small children).

2. **A** Lymphocytes account for 40%–80% of WBCs in adults; however, in infants, monocytes may predominate. In the CSF of adults the PMNs should be less than 10% and less than $5/\mu L$. Disease may be present when the WBC count is normal, if the majority of WBCs are PMNs. The first aliquot is sent to the chemistry department because it may be contaminated with blood or skin flora.

3. **A** Normal CSF volume in adults is 90–150 mL. When volume is low, an abnormally high difference is observed between opening and closing pressure. Low opening pressure is caused by reduced volume or block above the puncture site. High opening pressure may result from high CSF volume, CNS hemorrhage, or malignancy.

4. Which of the following findings is consistent with a subarachnoid hemorrhage rather than a traumatic tap?
A. Clearing of the fluid as it is aspirated
B. A clear supernatant after centrifugation
C. Xanthochromia
D. Presence of a clot in the sample

Body fluids/Evaluate laboratory data to recognize health and disease states/Cerebrospinal fluid/2

5. The term used to denote a high WBC count in the CSF is:
A. Empyemia
B. Neutrophilia
C. Pleocytosis
D. Hyperpycorrhachia

Body fluids/Apply knowledge of fundamental biological characteristics/Cerebrospinal fluid/1

6. Which of the adult CSF values in the table below are consistent with bacterial meningitis?

Body fluids/Evaluate laboratory data to recognize health and disease states/Cerebrospinal fluid/2

7. Given the following data, determine the corrected CSF WBC count.

	CSF Values	**Peripheral Blood Values**
RBCs	6000/μL	4.0×10^6/μL
WBCs	150/μL	5.0×10^3/μL

A. 8 WBC/μL
B. 142 WBC/μL
C. 120 WBC/μL
D. 145 WBC/μL

Body fluids/Calculate/CSF hematology/2

8. SITUATION: What is the most likely cause of the following CSF results?

CSF glucose 20 mg/dL; CSF protein 100 mg/dL; CSF lactate 50 mg/dL
A. Viral meningitis
B. Viral encephalitis
C. Cryptococcal meningitis
D. Acute bacterial meningitis

Body fluids/Evaluate laboratory data to recognize health and disease states/Cerebrospinal fluid/2

Answers to Questions 4–8

4. **C** Xanthochromia is pigmentation of CSF caused by subarachnoid hemorrhage, high CSF protein, free hemoglobin, or bilirubin. The bilirubin may be caused by hepatic disease, CNS hemorrhage, or prior traumatic tap. In subarachnoid hemorrhage the fluid will be pink if the RBC count is greater than 500/μL and will turn yellow in about 12 hours. Granulocyte infiltration occurs immediately afterward and disappears after 24 hours. It is followed by an increase in macrophages showing evidence of erythrophagocytosis that remains for up to 2 weeks.

5. **C** *Pleocytosis* refers to an increase in WBCs within the CSF. Bacterial meningitis causes a neutrophilic pleocytosis, viral meningitis a lymphocytic pleocytosis, tuberculous and fungal meningitis a mixed cell pleocytosis. Other causes of pleocytosis include multiple sclerosis, cerebral hemorrhage or infarction, and leukemia.

6. **C** Normal WBC counts for CSF are 0–5/μL for adults and 0–30/μL for children. Neutrophils predominate the differential in bacterial meningitis while lymphocytes predominate in viral meningitis. Hemorrhage and traumatic tap will also cause increased PMNs, and WBC counts should be corrected using the CSF RBC count.

7. **B** Corrected WBC count = WBCs in CSF − [(Blood WBCs × CSF RBCs) ÷ Blood RBCs]

Corrected WBC count = 150/μL − [(5000/μL WBCs × 6000/μL RBCs) ÷ 4,000,000/μL RBCs]

Corrected WBC count = 150/μL − 7.5/μL

Corrected WBC count = 142/μL

8. **D** Acute bacterial meningitis causes increased production of immunoglobulins in CSF. Glucose levels are below normal due to consumption by PMNs and bacteria. Lactate levels rise due to increased pressure and hypoxia. When associated with increased PMNs and lactate dehydrogenase–5 (LD-5), these findings point to bacterial meningitis.

WBCs	Lymphocytes	Monocytes	Eosinophils	Neutrophils	Neuroectodermal cells
A. 50/μL	44%	55%	0%	0%	1%
B. 300/μL	75%	21%	3%	0%	1%
C. 2000/μL	5%	15%	0%	80%	0%
D. 2500/μL	0%	50%	0%	10%	0%

9. Which of the following is associated with *low* CSF glucose and *high* protein?
A. Multiple sclerosis
B. Malignancy
C. Subarachnoid hemorrhage
D. All of the above

Body fluids/Correlate clinical and laboratory data/Cerebrospinal fluid/2

10. The limulus lysate test on CSF is a sensitive assay for:
A. Demyelinating diseases of the spinal cord
B. Cryptococcal meningitis
C. Gram-negative bacterial endotoxin
D. Open neural tube defects

Body fluids/Apply principles of special procedures/Cerebrospinal fluid/1

11. Which of the following results is consistent with fungal meningitis?
A. Normal CSF glucose
B. Pleocytosis of mixed cellularity
C. Normal CSF protein
D. High CSF lactate

Body fluids/Correlate clinical and laboratory data/Cerebrospinal fluid/2

12. In what suspected condition should a wet prep using a warm slide be examined?
A. Cryptococcal meningitis
B. Amoebic meningoencephalitis
C. Mycobacterium tuberculosis infection
D. Neurosyphilis

Body fluids/Select course of action/Cerebrospinal fluid/3

13. Which of the following CSF test results is most commonly increased in patients with multiple sclerosis?
A. Glutamine
B. Lactate
C. IgG index
D. Ammonia

Body fluids/Correlate clinical and laboratory data/Cerebrospinal fluid/2

14. Which of the following is an *inappropriate* procedure for performing routine CSF analysis?
A. A differential is done only if the total WBC count is greater than 10/μL.
B. A differential should be done on a stained CSF concentrate.
C. A minimum of 30 WBCs should be differentiated.
D. A wright-stained slide should be examined rather than a chamber differential.

Body fluids/Apply principles of standard operating procedures/Cerebrospinal fluid/2

Answers to Questions 9–14

9. **D** Low glucose in malignancy and multiple sclerosis results from increased utilization. Glucose is reduced in subarachnoid hemorrhage due to release of glycolytic enzymes from RBCs. All three conditions result in high CSF protein, but multiple sclerosis is associated with an increased IgG index because of local production of IgG.

10. **C** Hemolymph extracted from the horseshoe crab *Limulus polyphemus* will coagulate in the presence of minute amounts of gram-negative endotoxin. An India ink prep and latex agglutination test are used to rapidly identify *Cryptococcus neoformans* in CSF. Assay of myelin basic protein and oligoclonal banding are sensitive tests for multiple sclerosis.

11. **B** In fungal meningitis the glucose will be low and the total protein elevated; however, unlike bacterial meningitis, the lactate is usually below 35 mg/dL. Fungal meningitis usually produces a pleocytosis of mixed cellularity consisting of lymphocytes, PMNs, monocytes, and eosinophils. In some cases lymphocytes predominate while in others PMNs make up the majority of WBCs.

12. **B** Amoeba in CSF appear very similar to monocytes in stained films but can be differentiated by their characteristic pseudopod mobility in a wet prep on a prewarmed slide. *Naegleria fowleri* and *Acanthamoeba* species are causative agents of primary amoebic meningoencephalitis.

13. **C** IgG Index = $\dfrac{(CSF\ IgG \div serum\ IgG)}{(CSF\ albumin \div serum\ albumin)}$

An IgG-albumin index is the ratio of CSF IgG:serum IgG divided by the CSF albumin:serum albumin. Values greater than 0.85 indicate CSF IgG production as seen in multiple sclerosis, or increased CSF production combined with increased permeability as seen in infection. Multiple sclerosis is characterized by the presence of oligoclonal banding in the CSF in more than 90% of patients with active disease. The total protein and myelin basic protein are increased and the glucose is decreased. Reye's syndrome results in hepatic failure, causing high CSF levels of ammonia and glutamine. CSF lactate is usually normal in patients with multiple sclerosis.

14. **A** A relative (percent) increase in PMNs may be significant even when the WBC count does not exceed the upper limit of normal. Cytocentrifugation should be used to concentrate the cells followed by staining with Wright's stain.

15. Which cell is present in the CSF in greater numbers in newborns than in older children or adults?
    A. Eosinophils
    B. Lymphocytes
    C. Monocytes
    D. Neutrophils

    Body fluids/Correlate clinical and laboratory data/Cerebrospinal fluid/2

16. Neutrophilic pleocytosis is associated with:
    A. Cerebral infarction
    B. Malignancy
    C. Myelography
    D. All of the above

    Body fluids/Correlate clinical and laboratory data/Cerebrospinal fluid/2

17. Which statement about CSF protein is true?
    A. An abnormal serum protein electrophoretic pattern does not affect the CSF pattern.
    B. The upper reference limit for CSF total protein in newborns is one-half adult levels.
    C. CSF IgG is increased in panencephalitis, malignancy, and neurosyphilis.
    D. Antibodies to *Treponema pallidum* disappear after successful antibiotic therapy.

    Body fluids/Correlate clinical and laboratory data/Cerebrospinal fluid/2

18. Which of the following statements regarding routine microbiologic examination of CSF is true?
    A. A Gram stain should always be performed on a sediment of CSF.
    B. The Gram stain is positive in more than 70% of cases of acute meningitis.
    C. India ink and acid fast stains are indicated if monocytosis is present in CSF.
    D. All of the above.

    Body fluids/Apply knowledge of standard operating procedures/Cerebrospinal fluid/2

19. Which organism is the most frequent cause of bacterial meningitis in neonates?
    A. *Neisseria meningitidis*
    B. Group B *Streptococcus*
    C. *Streptococcus pneumoniae*
    D. *Klebsiella pneumoniae*

    Body fluids/Correlate clinical and laboratory data/Cerebrospinal fluid/2

20. Which statement about LD in CSF is true?
    A. LD is greatly elevated in bacterial but not viral meningitis.
    B. LD-5 predominates in bacterial meningitis, but LD-1 is highest in normal CSF.
    C. CSF LD is increased in malignancy, hemorrhage, lymphoma, and leukemia.
    D. All of the above.

Body fluids/Correlate clinical and laboratory data/Cerebrospinal fluid/2

Answers to Questions 15–20

15. **C** In newborns the upper reference limit (URL) for WBCs is 30/μL (URL for adults is 5/μL) with the majority of WBCs being monocytes or macrophages. In normal neonates, monocytes (including macrophages and histiocytes) account for about 75% of the WBCs, lymphocytes for about 20%, and PMNs for about 3%. In normal adults, lymphocytes account for about 60% of the WBCs, monocytes for about 35%, and PMNs for about 2%.

16. **D** Neutrophils may appear in CSF from many causes making it necessary to correlate results of chemical assays with hematologic findings. Low glucose and high protein occur in both malignancy and bacterial meningitis. LD isoenzymes and lactate may be helpful in distinguishing malignancy from bacterial meningitis.

17. **C** Although the blood-brain barrier excludes most plasma proteins, abnormal serum proteins can cause parallel CSF electrophoretic patterns. Therefore, an abnormal CSF pattern indicates CNS disease only if not duplicated by the serum pattern. Normal CSF total protein in newborns may be up to two times higher than adult levels. Antibodies to *T. pallidum* remain in CSF after treatment, but nontreponemal antibodies disappear. Consequently, the Venereal Disease Research Laboratory (VDRL) is recommended in combination with the FTA-ABS test for diagnosing active tertiary syphilis.

18. **D** Culture should be performed on the sediment of the second or third aliquot of the CSF after it is centrifuged. Blood and chocolate agar and broth should always be used, and if sterile, held a minimum of 3 days. Blood cultures should be done because septicemia occurs in about one-half of bacterial meningitis cases.

19. **B** Group B *Streptococcus* and *E. coli* are the two most common isolates in neonates. *Hemophilus influenzae, S. pneumoniae,* and *N. meningitidis* are the most common isolates in children. *S. pneumoniae* is the most frequent isolate in the elderly.

20. **D** LD activity in CSF is elevated in several disorders and after a traumatic tap. Isoenzymes help to distinguish the cause. LD-5 predominates in bacterial meningitis. When LD is high in viral meningitis, the dominate isoenzyme is LD-2 from lymphocytes. In lymphocytic leukemia LD-3 from lymphoblasts predominates.

21. Which of the following statements regarding serous fluids is true?
A. The normal volume of pleural fluid is 30–50 mL.
B. Mesothelial cells, PMNs, lymphocytes, and macrophages may be present in normal fluids.
C. X-ray can detect a 10% increase in the volume of a serous fluid.
D. Normal serous fluids are colorless.

Body fluids/Correlate clinical and laboratory data/Serous fluid/2

22. The term *effusion* refers to:
A. A chest fluid that is purulent
B. A serous fluid that is chylous
C. An increased volume of serous fluid
D. An inflammatory process affecting the appearance of a serous fluid

Body fluids/Apply knowledge of fundamental biological characteristics/Pleural fluid/1

23. Which of the following laboratory results is characteristic of a transudative fluid?
A. SG = 1.018
B. Total protein = 3.2 g/dL
C. LD fluid/serum ratio = 0.25
D. Total protein fluid/serum ratio = 0.65

Body fluids/Evaluate laboratory data to recognize health and disease states/Exudates/2

24. Which observation is *least* useful in distinguishing a hemorrhagic fluid from a traumatic tap?
A. Clearing of fluid as it is aspirated
B. Presence of xanthochromia
C. The formation of a clot
D. Diminished RBC count in successive aliquots

Body fluids/Correlate laboratory data with physiological processes/Serous fluids/2

25. Which of the following laboratory results on a serous fluid is most likely to be caused by a traumatic tap?
A. An RBC count of 8000/μL
B. A WBC count of 6000/μL
C. A hematocrit of 35%
D. A neutrophil count of 45%

Body fluids/Correlate laboratory data with physiological processes/Serous fluid/2

26. Which of the following conditions is commonly associated with an exudative effusion?
A. Congestive heart failure
B. Malignancy
C. Nephrotic syndrome
D. Cirrhosis

Body fluids/Correlate clinical and laboratory data/Transudate/2

Answers to Questions 21–26

21. **B** The serous fluids include pleural, pericardial, and peritoneal fluid. They form from ultrafiltration of plasma through serous membranes. These are lined with specialized epithelium called mesothelium. They make up about 5% of the cells in serous fluid and may be difficult to differentiate from malignant cells. Pleural fluid volume is normally less than 10 mL. The volume of pericardial fluid is normally 10–50 mL and peritoneal fluid 30–50 mL. X-rays can detect an increase in serous fluids of 300 mL or more. Normal serous fluids are clear and range in color from straw to amber.

22. **C** Effusions are classified as either transudates, exudates, or chylous. Transudates result from abnormal hemodynamics, and exudates and chylous fluids from local disease. A pleural fluid that is purulent is called an empyemic fluid. Such a fluid has a WBC count of 10,000/μL or greater.

23. **C** Transudative fluids are distinguished from exudative fluids by the physical appearance, SG, total protein, LD, cholesterol, and bilirubin. Exudative fluids have a fluid:serum LD ratio greater than 0.6 caused by release of the enzyme from inflammatory or malignant cells. Exudative fluids have a total protein greater than 3.0 g/dL, SG greater than 1.015, fluid:serum total protein ratio greater than 0.6, cholesterol greater than 60 mg/dL (fluid:serum ratio >0.3) and fluid:serum bilirubin ratio greater than 0.6. Exudates are caused by infection, infarction, malignancy, rheumatoid diseases, and trauma.

24. **C** Xanthochromia indicates either an exudative process or prior traumatic tap. Hemorrhagic pleural fluids usually have RBC counts greater than 100,000/μL and are usually caused by lung neoplasms. Clearing of fluid or diminished RBC counts in successive tubes favors a diagnosis of a traumatic tap. A clot may form from a traumatic tap, but not from a subarachnoid hemorrhage. However, clots can form from other causes and are usually absent unless there is extensive trauma during sample collection.

25. **A** Normal fluids have a WBC count less than 1000/μL, but counts between 1000 and 2500/μL may be seen in both exudates or transudates. All WBC types are present, but no type should account for more than 50% of the leukocyte count. An RBC count below 10,000/μL is usually caused by a traumatic tap. A fluid hematocrit similar to blood is caused by a hemothorax.

26. **B** Transudative fluids are caused by circulatory problems, usually decreased oncotic pressure or increased hydrostatic pressure. In contrast, exudative effusions are caused by inflammatory processes and cellular infiltration as seen in malignancy.

27. An exudative pleural fluid can be caused by:
A. Malignancy, commonly lung or breast cancer
B. Pulmonary infarction or infection
C. SLE or rheumatoid arthritis (RA)
D. All of the above

Body fluids/Correlate clinical and laboratory data/Exudates/2

28. Which of the following conditions is most often associated with a pleural fluid glucose below 30 mg/dL?
A. Diabetes mellitus
B. Pancreatitis
C. RA
D. Bacterial pneumonia

Body fluids/Correlate clinical and laboratory data/Pleural fluid/2

29. In which condition is the pleural fluid pH likely to be above 7.3?
A. Bacterial pneumonia with parapneumonic exudate
B. Rheumatoid pleuritis
C. Esophageal rupture
D. Pneumothorax

Body fluids/Correlate clinical and laboratory data/Pleural fluid/2

30. Which of the following hematology values best frames the upper reference limits for peritoneal fluid?

	WBC Count	Percentage of PMNs	RBC Count
A.	300/μL	25%	100,000/μL
B.	10,000/μL	50%	500,000/μL
C.	50,000/μL	50%	500,000/μL
D.	100,000/μL	75%	1,000,000/μL

Body fluids/Apply knowledge of fundamental biological characteristics/Serous fluids/2

31. Which of the following characteristics is higher for synovial fluid than for the serous fluids?
A. SG
B. Glucose
C. Total protein
D. Viscosity

Body fluids/Apply knowledge of fundamental biological characteristics/Synovial fluid/1

Answers to Questions 27–31

27. **D** The conditions above are all characterized by inflammation with increases in protein, WBCs, and lactate dehydrogenase. In addition, exudates are caused by tuberculosis, pancreatitis, and lymphoma. Lymphatic obstruction is often associated with lymphoma and causes a chylous exudate.

28. **C** Normal pleural fluid has the same glucose concentration as plasma. Hyperglycemia is the only condition that is associated with a high pleural fluid glucose. Low glucose levels (<60 mg/dL) may be seen in infection, malignancy, and rheumatic diseases. However, glucose levels are lowest (often below 30 mg/dL) and are a constant finding when rheumatoid disease affects the lungs. Pancreatitis causes an exudative peritoneal and pleural effusion with an elevated peritoneal fluid amylase (without a low glucose).

29. **D** The pH of pleural fluid is approximately 7.64, and values below 7.30 are usually associated with a poorer prognosis and usually require drainage. Esophageal rupture produces the lowest pH with values in the range of 6.0–6.3. In addition, pleural fluid pH is low in rheumatoid disease involving the lungs and pleura, some malignancies, and SLE. Low pH and glucose in pleural fluid are seen in lung abscess and exudative bacterial pneumonia (termed *parapneumonic effusion*). Pneumothorax results from air entering the pleural space and does not produce a low pH.

30. **A** Peritoneal fluid normally has a WBC count of less than 300/μL. Neutrophils should account for no more than 25% of the WBCs. A majority of PMNs indicates bacterial infection of the peritoneum. Lymphocytosis suggests malignancy, tuberculosis, cirrhosis, and lymphatic leakage. Peritoneal fluid amylase is elevated in most cases of acute pancreatitis. Peritonitis is suspected when the fluid LD is greater than 40% of the serum level. Normal pleural fluid has a WBC count usually below 1000/μL. Exudative fluids usually have a WBC count above 10,000/μL, but values tend to overlap noninflammatory fluids. The PMNs should comprise 50% of the WBCs or less, and the RBC count should be less than 100,000/μL.

31. **D** Synovial fluid has approximately the same SG and glucose as plasma and the serous fluids but is far more viscous due to a high content of mucoprotein (hyaluronate) secreted by the synovium. Viscosity is estimated by pulling the fluid from the tip of a syringe. Normal fluid gives a string longer than 4 cm. Low viscosity indicates inflammation. The total protein of synovial fluid is usually lower than serous fluids, the upper reference limit being 2.0 g/dL.

32. In which type of arthritis is the synovial WBC count likely to be greater than 50,000/μL?
A. Septic arthritis
B. Osteoarthritis
C. RA
D. Hemorrhagic arthritis

Body fluids/Correlate clinical and laboratory data/Synovial fluid/2

33. What type of cell is a "ragocyte"?
A. Cartilage cell seen in inflammatory arthritis
B. A PMN with inclusions formed by immune complexes
C. A plasma cell seen in RA
D. A macrophage containing large inclusions

Body fluids/Apply knowledge of fundamental biological characteristics/Morphology/1

34. Which of the following crystals is the cause of gout?
A. Uric acid or monosodium urate
B. Calcium pyrophosphate or apatite
C. Calcium oxalate
D. Cholesterol

Body fluids/Apply knowledge of fundamental biological characteristics/Synovial fluid/1

35. Which crystal causes "pseudogout"?
A. Oxalic acid
B. Calcium pyrophosphate
C. Calcium oxalate
D. Cholesterol

Body fluids/Apply knowledge of fundamental biological characteristics/Synovial fluid/1

36. A synovial fluid sample is examined using a polarizing microscope with a red compensating filter. Crystals are seen that are yellow when the long axis of the crystal is parallel to the slow vibrating light. When the long axis of the crystal is perpendicular to the slow vibrating light the crystals appear blue. What type of crystal is present?
A. Calcium oxalate
B. Calcium pyrophosphate
C. Uric acid
D. Cholesterol

Body fluids/Apply principles of special procedures/Synovial fluid/2

37. In which condition is the synovial fluid glucose most likely to be within normal limits?
A. Septic arthritis
B. Inflammatory arthritis
C. Hemorrhagic arthritis
D. Gout

Body fluids/Correlate clinical and laboratory data/Synovial fluid/2

Answers to Questions 32–37

32. A The WBC count is elevated in all types of arthritis, but is greatest (50,000–100,000/μL) in septic arthritis. Neutrophils comprise less than 25% of WBCs in normal and noninflammatory arthritis, but are above 50% in inflammatory and septic arthritis. Fluids are diluted in saline because acetic acid causes a mucin clot to form.

33. B Ragocytes are PMNs containing dark granules composed of immunoglobulins, but they may be seen in gout and septic arthritis as well as RA. LE cells may be seen in fluid from patients with SLE, and Reiter's cells, macrophages with ingested globular inclusions, are seen in Reiter's syndrome and other inflammatory diseases.

34. A Although all of the crystals mentioned can cause crystal-induced arthritis, uric acid and sodium urate crystals cause gout and are seen in about 90% of gout patients.

35. B Calcium pyrophosphate crystals occur as needles or small rhombic plates and can be confused with uric acid. They rotate plane polarized light but not as strongly as uric acid. Synovial fluid should never be collected in tubes containing powdered ethylenediaminetetraacetic acid (EDTA) because it may form crystals that can be mistaken for *in vivo* crystals.

36. C Synovial fluid is collected in sodium heparin because other anticoagulants may cause crystal artifacts. Polarized microscopy with a red compensating filter differentiates uric acid and pseudogout crystals. When the long axis of uric acid needles is parallel to the slow vibrating light, the crystals appear yellow. When the long axis is perpendicular to the slow vibrating light, the crystals appear blue. Calcium pyrophosphate gives the reverse effect.

37. C Synovial fluid glucose is normally less than 10 mg/dL below the serum glucose and should be collected after an 8-hour fast to ensure that the fluid and plasma are equilibrated. In septic arthritis, the glucose level is often more than 40 mg/dL below the serum level and about 25–40 mg/dL lower in inflammatory arthritis, which includes gout. Osteoarthritis and hemorrhagic arthritis are not usually associated with low joint fluid glucose.

38. Which statement about synovial fluid in RA is true?
  A. Synovial/serum IgG is usually 1:2 or higher.
  B. Total hemolytic complement is elevated.
  C. Ninety percent of RA cases test positive for rheumatoid factor in synovial fluid.
  D. Demonstration of rheumatoid factor in joint fluid is diagnostic for RA.

Body fluids/Correlate clinical and laboratory data/Synovial fluid/2

39. Which of the following organisms accounts for the majority of septic arthritis cases in young and middle age adults?
  A. *H. influenzae*
  B. *Neisseria gonorrhoeae*
  C. *Staphylococcus aureus*
  D. *Borrelia burgdorferi*

Body fluids/Apply knowledge of fundamental biological characteristics/Synovial fluid/2

40. Which of the following hematology values best frames the upper reference limits for synovial fluid?

	WBC Count	Percentage of PMNs	RBC Count
A.	200/μL	25%	2,000/μL
B.	5,000/μL	50%	10,000/μL
C.	10,000/μL	50%	50,000/μL
D.	20,000/μL	5%	500,000/μL

Body fluids/Apply knowledge of fundamental biological characteristics/Synovial fluid/2

Answers to Questions 38–40

38. **A** Rheumatoid factor can be present in both serum and synovial fluids from patients with RA, SLE, and other inflammatory diseases. Rheumatoid factor is present in synovial fluid of approximately 60% of patients with RA. Normally, IgG in synovial fluid is about 10% of the serum IgG level. CH_{50} levels in serum and synovium are more differential. Both are increased in Reiter's syndrome but are often low in SLE; synovial CH_{50} is decreased and serum CH_{50} is normal (or increased) in RA.

39. **B** Synovial fluid is normally sterile, and all of the organisms listed may cause septic arthritis. *N. gonorrhoeae* is responsible for about 75% of septic arthritis cases occurring in young and middle-aged adults. *Staphylococcus* spp is responsible for the majority of cases involving the elderly. *Haemophilus* spp, *Staphylococcus* spp, and *Streptococcus* spp are the most common causes of arthritis in children.

40. **A** The WBC count of normal joint fluid is 200/μL or less. Values above 5000/μL cause the fluid to be purulent and occur in septic arthritis, RA, and gout. WBC counts greater than 50,000 μL indicate septic arthritis. The majority of WBCs are monocytes, which usually account for 50%–65%. Neutrophils and lymphocytes should account for no more than 25% each. An increase in RBCs occurs in cases of infectious and hemorrhagic arthritis or results from a traumatic tap. Hemorrhagic fluid will appear turbid, red to brown, and often clotted. Inflammatory arthritis can allow fibrinogen to enter the fluid and thus clot. Fluid from a hemophiliac will not clot in spite of its bloody appearance.

Amniotic, Gastrointestinal, and Seminal Fluids

1. Which of the following statements about amniotic fluid bilirubin measured by scanning spectrophotometry is true?
   A. The 410-nm peak is due to hemoglobin and the 450-nm peak to bilirubin.
   B. Baseline correction is not required if a scanning spectrophotometer is used.
   C. Chloroform extraction is necessary only when meconium is present.
   D. In normal amniotic fluid bilirubin increases with gestational age.

   Body fluids/Apply principles of special procedures/Amniotic fluid/2

2. Which of the following statements regarding pregnancy testing is true?
   A. β Subunits of human chorionic gonadotropin (HCG), thyroid-stimulating hormone (TSH), and follicle-stimulating hormone (FSH) are very similar.
   B. Antibodies against the β subunit of HCG cross-react with luteinizing hormone (LH).
   C. A false-positive result may occur in patients with heterophile antibodies.
   D. Serum should not be used for pregnancy tests because proteins interfere.

   Body fluids/Apply principles of basic laboratory procedures/Pregnancy test/2

Answers to Questions 1–2

1. **A** Amniotic fluid bilirubin reflects the extent of fetal RBC destruction in cases of hemolytic disease of the newborn (HDN). It is measured by scanning the fluid from 350 to 600 nm, then drawing a baseline using the points at 365 nm and 550 nm. The delta absorbance (ΔA) of hemoglobin at 410 nm and bilirubin at 450 nm are determined by subtracting the absorbance of the baseline from the respective peaks. Samples that are not grossly hemolyzed can be corrected for oxyhemoglobin by subtracting 5% of the ΔA at 410 nm from the ΔA at 450 nm. When hemolysis is severe or meconium is present the bilirubin must be extracted in chloroform before measuring absorbance. Bilirubin normally decreases with increasing gestational age because fetal urine contributes more to amniotic fluid volume as the fetus matures. The bilirubin concentration must be correlated with gestational age in order to correctly evaluate the severity of HDN.

2. **C** The α subunit of HCG is very similar to the α subunit of TSH and FSH and identical to LH. Although the β subunits of HCG and LH are very similar, antibodies can be made to the β subunit of HCG that do not crossreact with LH or other pituitary hormones. Most enzyme immunoassay (EIA) methods utilize two monoclonal antibodies against different sites of the HCG molecule. One antibody is specific for the carboxy terminal end of the β chain, and the other reacts with the α chain resulting in a positive test only when intact HCG is present. Because monoclonal antibodies are derived from mouse hybridomas, rare false-positives may occur in patients who have antimouse Ig antibodies. Although the test can detect lower levels of HCG, 25 mIU/mL is the positive cutoff point for pregnancy. Serum is preferred over urine because serum levels are more consistently above the cutoff point than random urine in early pregnancy.

3. Which assay result is often approximately 25% below the expected level in pregnancies associated with Down syndrome?
A. Serum unconjugated estriol
B. Lecithin/sphingomyelin (L/S) ratio
C. Amniotic fluid bilirubin assay
D. Urinary chorionic gonadotropin

Body Fluids/Correlate laboratory data with physiological processes/Estriol/2

4. Which is the test of choice for determining fetal lung maturity?
A. Human placental lactogen
B. L/S ratio
C. Amniotic fluid bilirubin
D. Urinary estriol

Body Fluids/Correlate laboratory data with physiological processes/L/S/ratio/2

5. Which test best correlates with the severity of HDN?
A. Rh antibody titer of the mother
B. L/S ratio
C. Amniotic fluid bilirubin
D. Urinary estradiol

Body Fluids/Correlate clinical and laboratory data/Amniotic fluid/2

6. Which of the following statements about AFP is correct?
A. Maternal serum may be used to screen for open neural tube defects.
B. Levels above 4 ng/mL are considered positive.
C. Elevated levels in amniotic fluid are specific for spina bifida.
D. AFP levels increase in pregnancies associated with Down syndrome.

Body Fluids/Apply principles of special procedures/Alpha fetoprotein/2

Answers to Questions 3–6

3. **A** Estriol is produced by the placenta as well as the fetal and maternal adrenal glands and liver. Free estriol produced by the placenta is rapidly conjugated by the maternal liver. Maternal serum unconjugated (free) estriol is almost all derived from the fetus and is a direct reflection of current fetal placental function. Serum unconjugated estriol (uE_3) measured during the second trimester is used along with serum AFP and HCG as the triple marker screening test for Down syndrome. α-Fetoprotein (AFP) and uE_3 are decreased by approximately 25%, and HCG is increased by approximately 2.5 times in some Down syndrome pregnances. Each test as a detection rate of 25% or less when used alone, but when all three assays are combined with maternal age the detection rate is approximately 65%.

4. **B** Respiratory distress syndrome develops when surfactants are insufficient to prevent collapse of the infant's alveoli during expiration. Tests measuring pulmonary phospholipid surfactants are the most specific and sensitive indicators of respiratory distress syndrome. An L/S ratio greater than 2:1 (in some laboratories 2.5:1) is the most widely accepted measure of fetal lung maturity.

5. **C** Amniotic fluid bilirubin is the best index of the severity of HDN and is measured by scanning spectrophotometry from 550–365 nm. When hemoglobin produces a positive slope at 410 nm the bilirubin should be extracted with chloroform prior to scanning. Extraction methods give the best correlation with RBC destruction.

6. **A** Maternal serum AFP increases and amniotic fluid AFP decreases with gestational age. Because serum levels are dependent upon gestational age, upper reference limits depend upon the last menstrual period dating. AFP levels are reported as multiples of the median in order to permit interlaboratory comparison. When serum levels are high, ultrasound is used to determine fetal age and rule out twins. Increased fetal AFP levels (>2.5 MOM) may result from many diseases in addition to open neural tube defects such as spina bifida. These include anencephaly, ventral wall defects, congenital hypothyroidism, and Turner's syndrome. Decreased levels (<0.75 MOM) may be seen in aproximately 25% of Down syndrome pregnancies.

7. Which of the following statements accurately describes HCG levels in pregnancy?
   A. Levels of HCG rise throughout pregnancy.
   B. In ectopic pregnancy serum HCG doubling time is below expected levels.
   C. Molar pregnancies are associated with lower levels than expected for the time of gestation.
   D. HCG returns to nonpregnant levels within 2 days following delivery, stillbirth, or abortion.

Body fluids/Correlate clinical and laboratory data/Chorionic gonadotropin/2

8. Which of the following statements regarding the L/S ratio is true?
   A. A ratio of 2:1 or greater usually indicates adequate pulmonary surfactant to prevent respiratory distress syndrome (RDS).
   B. A ratio of 1.5:1 indicates fetal lung maturity in pregnancies associated with diabetes mellitus.
   C. Sphingomyelin levels increase during the third trimester causing the L/S ratio to fall slightly during the last 2 weeks of gestation.
   D. A phosphatidylglycerol (PG) spot indicates the presence of meconium in the amniotic fluid.

Body fluids/Correlate clinical and laboratory data/L/S ratio/2

9. Which of the following conditions is most likely to cause a falsely low L/S ratio?
   A. The presence of PG in amniotic fluid
   B. Freezing the specimen for one month at $-20°C$
   C. Centrifugation at $1000 \times g$ for 10 minutes
   D. Maternal diabetes mellitus

Body fluids/Apply knowledge to recognize sources of error/Amniotic fluid/2

10. Amniotic fluid samples for cytogenetic studies are usually collected at:
    A. 12–16 weeks' gestation
    B. 17–21 weeks' gestation
    C. 22–26 weeks' gestation
    D. 27–31 weeks' gestation

Body fluids/Apply knowledge of standard operating procedures/Specimen collection and handling/1

Answers to Questions 7–10

7. **B** In normal pregnancy HCG levels rise exponentially following implantation and peak at weeks 9–12, reaching in excess of 100,000 mIU/mL. Levels fall after the first trimester to about 20,000 mIU/mL and then remain at about that level through term. The HCG doubling time averages 2.2 days. In ectopic pregnancy the expected increase between consecutive days is below normal. Hydatiform moles are associated with greatly elevated levels of HCG. Serum HCG can take up to 4 weeks to return to nonpregnant (<25 mIU/mL) or baseline (<5 mIU/mL) levels following delivery, stillbirth, or abortion.

8. **A** Pulmonary surfactants are mainly disaturated lecithins produced by type II granular pneumocytes. The L/S ratio increases toward the end of the third trimester due to increased production of lecithin. The concentration of sphingomyelin remains constant throughout gestation and serves as an internal reference. Meconium contains less lecithin than amniotic fluid and will usually decrease the L/S ratio; however, meconium produces a spot that can be misinterpreted as lecithin, leading to a falsely increased L/S ratio. Sufficient PG to produce a spot is seen only when the L/S ratio is 2:1 or higher. PG is not present in either blood or meconium and, therefore, its presence indicates fetal lung maturity. In diabetes the fetal lungs may mature more slowly than normal, and infants may develop RDS when the L/S ratio is 2:1 or slightly higher. For this reason, an L/S of 3:1 more closely correlates with fetal lung maturity when testing amniotic fluid from diabetic mothers.

9. **C** Pulmonary surfactants are largely present in the form of lamellar bodies and can be lost by centrifuging the amniotic fluid at high g force. Centrifuge speed should be the minimum required to spin down cells ($450 g$ for 10 minutes at $4°C$). Samples that cannot be measured immediately should be refrigerated or frozen. Samples are stable for up to 3 days at $2°–8°C$ and for months when frozen at $-20°C$ or lower. Meconium and blood may also introduce errors when measuring the L/S ratio. Blood has an L/S ratio of approximately 2:1 and will falsely raise the L/S ratio when fetal lungs are immature and depress the L/S ratio when fetal lungs are mature.

10. **A** Amniocentesis for cytogenetic studies is performed between 12 and 16 weeks' gestation in order to complete cell culture and karyotyping before week 20. For legal and ethical reasons, therapeutic abortions are performed prior to week 20.

11. Most cases of Down syndrome are the result of:
    A. Nondisjunction of an E chromosome (E trisomy)
    B. Nondisjunction of chromosome 21 (G trisomy)
    C. A 14–21 chromosome translocation
    D. Deletion of the long arm of G21

    Body fluids/Apply knowledge of fundamental biological characteristics/Cytogenetics/1

12. In Turner's syndrome the modal chromosome count and number of Barr bodies are:

	Chromosomes	Barr Bodies
A.	45	0
B.	46	1
C.	46	2
D.	47	2

    Body fluids/Correlate clinical and laboratory data/Cytogenetics/2

13. Genetic mosaicism results from:
    A. Balanced translocation during meiosis
    B. Nondisjunction during meiosis
    C. Nondisjunction during mitosis in the early embryo
    D. Translocation during development of the blastocyst

    Body fluids/Apply knowledge of fundamental biological characteristics/Cytogenetics/1

14. What is the term for sperm when the anterior portion of the headpiece is smaller than normal?
    A. Azoospermia
    B. Microcephaly
    C. Acrosomal deficiency
    D. Necrozoospermia

    Body fluids/Apply knowledge of fundamental biological characteristics/Seminal fluid/1

15. The most common cause of male infertility is:
    A. Mumps
    B. Klinefelter's syndrome
    C. Varicocele
    D. Malignancy

    Body fluids/Correlate clinical and laboratory data/Seminal fluid/2

16. Which of the following sperm counts would be classified as oligozoospermia?
    A. 40 million per mL
    B. 65 million per mL
    C. 100 million per mL
    D. All of the above

    Body fluids/Evaluate laboratory data to recognize health and disease states/Seminal fluid/2

Answers to Questions 11–16

11. **B** Down syndrome results from the presence of an extra chromosome 21. Although it can be caused by 14–21 translocation or isochromosome formation, most cases arise from nondisjunction. Down syndrome is also associated with low amniotic fluid AFP levels; unexplained low levels indicate the need for cytogenetic testing. A triple marker study consisting of serum AFP, HCG, and uE_3 is the most sensitive screening test for Down syndrome. AFP and estriol levels are approximately 25% lower and HCG 2.5-fold higher in Down syndrome pregnancies.

12. **A** Turner's syndrome is caused by nondisjunction of a sex chromosome during meiosis, producing an offspring with an XO genotype. This results in aneuploidy with a modal chromosome count of 45 (45,X). Patients with Turner's syndrome are phenotypically female but fail to develop sexually at puberty. They are often color-blind and short, and may have other metabolic and anatomic abnormalities.

13. **C** Mosaicism refers to the presence of more than a single cell line causing a bimodal chromosome count. It results from nondisjunction in the early embryo.

14. **C** Spermatozoa have a well-defined headpiece consisting of the acrosome and nucleus. A thin filament, the neckpiece, connects the head and tail. The tail is divided into the midpiece, mainpiece, and endpiece. The midpiece is the thick anterior end of approximately 6 μ containing a 9 + 2 longitudinal arrangement of microtubules (two central microtubules surrounded by nine doublets so that a cross section appears like a pinwheel). This is called the axoneme and is surrounded by nine radial fibers. The longest portion of the tail (40–45 μ) is the mainpiece. It is thinner than the midpiece and lacks the outer radial fibers. The distal portion, called the endpiece, is approximately 5 μ. It contains the axoneme but is unsheathed.

15. **C** Varicocele is the hardening of veins that drain the testes. This causes blood from the adrenal vein to flow into the spermatic vein. Adrenal corticosteroids retard the development of spermatozoa. Mumps, Klinefelter's syndrome, and malignancy cause testicular failure, accounting for about 10% of infertility cases in men.

16. **A** The reference range for spermatozoa is 60–150 $\times 10^6$/mL. Counts below 20×10^6/mL are termed azoospermia. This often results from obstruction of the ejaculatory duct or testicular failure.

17. Which morphological abnormality of sperm is most often associated with varicocele?
A. Tapering of the head
B. Cytoplasmic droplet below the neckpiece
C. Lengthened neckpiece
D. Acrosomal deficiency

Body fluids/Correlate clinical and laboratory data/Seminal fluid/2

18. Which of the following stains is used to determine sperm viability?
A. Eosin
B. Hematoxylin
C. Papanicolaou
D. Methylene blue

Body fluids/Apply principles of special procedures/Seminal fluid/1

19. In which of the following conditions is the fasting serum gastrin level usually within normal limits?
A. Pernicious anemia
B. Duodenal ulcers
C. Zollinger-Ellison (Z-E) syndrome
D. Atrophic gastritis

Body fluids/Correlate clinical and laboratory data/Gastric function/2

20. In which condition is the highest level of serum gastrin usually seen?
A. Atrophic gastritis
B. Pernicious anemia
C. Z-E syndrome
D. Cancer of the stomach

Body fluids/Correlate clinical and laboratory data/Gastric function/2

21. In determining free HCl, the gastric fluid is titrated to pH:
A. 6.5
B. 4.5
C. 3.5
D. 2.0

Body fluids/Apply principles of special procedures/Gastric pH/1

22. In which condition is the BAO:PAO ratio consistently greater than 0.6?
A. Duodenal ulcers
B. Achlorhydria
C. Z-E syndrome
D. Stomach cancer

Body fluids/Correlate clinical and laboratory data/Gastric pH/2

Answers to Questions 17–22

17. **A** Acrosomal deficiency, nuclear abnormalities, and lengthened neckpiece are the most common morphologic abnormalities of spermatozoa. Tapering of the head is a nuclear abnormality. Sperm morphology should be evaluated by classifying 200 mature sperm by strict criteria, the most commonly used of which defines the normal sperm head as having a length of 4.0–5.0 μ, a width of 2.5–3.5 μ, a L:W ratio of 1.5–1.75, and an acrosomal area of 40%–70%. Using strict criteria, there is a high likelihood of infertility when the number of normal forms is below 15%.

18. **A** Eosin is excluded by living sperm and is used to determine the percentage of living cells. Papanicolaou, Giemsa's, and hematoxylin stains are used to evaluate sperm morphology, but Wright's stain is not recommended.

19. **B** Gastrin is produced by specialized epithelium of the stomach and stimulates secretion of HCl by parietal cells. Secretion is controlled by negative feedback causing levels to be very high in conditions associated with achlorhydria and gastrin-secreting tumors. In duodenal ulcers, increased gastric acidity occurs and fasting serum gastrin levels are normal. However, postprandial gastrin levels may be elevated in these patients because they do not respond to the negative feedback signal caused by HCl release.

20. **C** Z-E syndrome results from a gastrin-secreting tumor, gastrinoma, usually originating in the pancreas. It is characterized by very high levels of gastrin and excessive basal gastric acidity. In Z-E syndrome the basal acid output (BAO) divided by the peak acid output (PAO) is greater than 0.6 and the serum gastrin is greater than 1000 pg/mL.

21. **C** Free HCl in gastric residue is completely titrated at pH 3.5. When gastric fluid is titrated to pH 7.0, other acids including proteins and salts of chloride are also titrated. Total acidity is titrated to pH 7.0 with 0.1 N NaOH using a pH meter or phenol red.

22. **C** The BAO:PAO ratio is normally less than 0.2. Patients with achlorhydria and gastric carcinoma have absent and diminished HCl production, respectively, and ratios are less than 0.2. In achlorhydria the fasting gastric pH is often greater than 6.0, and this is considered diagnostic. Patients with gastric ulcers may also have a ratio less than 0.2 or between 0.2 and 0.4. In duodenal ulcers the ratio is usually between 0.2 and 0.6. The ratio is greater than 0.6 only in Z-E syndrome.

23. Which of the following tests would be normal in pancreatic insufficiency?
   A. Secretin stimulation
   B. D-Xylose absorption
   C. Twenty-four-hour fecal fat
   D. β Carotene absorption

   Body fluids/Correlate clinical and laboratory data/Pancreatic function/2

24. Which of the following is commonly associated with occult blood?
   A. Malignancy
   B. Benign peptic ulcers
   C. Hookworm infestation
   D. All of the above

   Body fluids/Correlate clinical and laboratory data/Occult blood/2

25. Which statement regarding fecal trypsin screening is true?
   A. Deficiency of trypsin causes clearing of an x-ray film.
   B. It is useful in screening adults for steatorrhea.
   C. Fecal trypsin deficiency in newborns is associated with cystic fibrosis.
   D. Stool is diluted in phosphate buffer at pH 7.0.

   Body fluids/Correlate clinical and laboratory data/Fecal trypsin/2

Answers to Questions 23–25

23. **B** The xylose absorption test differentiates pancreatic insufficiency from malabsorption syndrome (both cause deficient fat absorption). Xylose is absorbed by the small intestine without the aid of pancreatic enzymes. It is not metabolized and is excreted into urine. Low levels indicate gastrointestinal malabsorption.

24. **D** Blood in feces is a very sensitive indicator of gastrointestinal bleeding and is an excellent screening test to detect asymptomatic ulcers and malignancy of the gastrointestinal tract. However, the test is nonspecific, and contamination with vaginal blood is a frequent source of error.

25. **C** In cystic fibrosis obstruction of pancreatic ducts causes deficient delivery of trypsin into the small intestine. This can be detected by the inability of feces to hydrolyze the gelatin of an x-ray film. However, this test is not useful in screening adults because trypsin inhibitors are present in the stool. The pH optimum for trypsin is between 7.8 and 8.0; samples are diluted in barbital, TRIS(hydroxymethyl)aminomethane, or other alkaline buffer.

Body Fluids Problem Solving

1. Given the following dry reagent strip urinalysis results, select the most appropriate course of action:

   pH = 8.0; protein = 1+; glucose = neg; ketone = neg; blood = neg; nitrite = neg; bilirubin = neg
   A. Report the results assuming acceptable quality control.
   B. Check pH with a pH meter before reporting.
   C. Perform a turbidimetric protein test and report instead of the dipstick protein.
   D. Request a new specimen.

   Body fluids/Evaluate laboratory data to recognize problems/Urinalysis/3

2. Given the following urinalysis results, select the most appropriate course of action:

   pH = 8.0; protein = tr; glucose = neg; ketone = sm; blood = neg; nitrite = neg; 0–2 RBCs/HPF; 20–50 WBCs/HPF; bacteria = lg; $CaCO_3$ crystals = sm
   A. Call for a new specimen because urine was contaminated *in vitro*.
   B. Recheck pH because calcium carbonate ($CaCO_3$) does not occur at alkaline pH.
   C. No indication of error is present; results indicate a UTI.
   D. Report all results except bacteria because the nitrite test was negative.

   Body fluids/Evaluate laboratory data to recognize inconsistent results/Urinalysis/3

3. **SITUATION:** A 6-mL pediatric urine sample is processed for routine urinalysis in the usual manner. The sediment is prepared by centrifuging all of the urine remaining after performing the biochemical tests. The following results are obtained:

   SG = 1.015; protein = 2+; blood = lg; 5–10 RBCs/HPF; 5–10 WBCs/HPF

   Select the most appropriate course of action.
   A. Report these results; blood and protein correlate with microscopic results.
   B. Report biochemical results only; request a new sample for the microscopic examination.
   C. Request a new sample and report as quantity not sufficient (QNS).
   D. Recentrifuge the supernatant and repeat the microscopic examination.

   Body fluids/Apply knowledge to recognize sources of error/Urinalysis/3

Answers to Questions 1–3

1. **C** Highly buffered alkaline urine may cause a false-positive dry reagent strip protein test by titrating the acid buffer on the reagent pad. The turbidimetric test with SSA is not subject to positive interference by highly buffered alkaline urine.

2. **C** A positive nitrite requires infection with a nitrate-reducing organism, dietary nitrate, and incubation of urine in the bladder. The test is positive in about 70% of UTI cases. Alkaline pH, bacteriuria, and leukocytes point to UTI.

3. **B** This discrepancy between the blood reaction and RBC count resulted from spinning less than 12 mL of urine. When volume is below 12 mL, the sample should be diluted with saline to 12 mL before concentrating. Results are multiplied by the dilution (12 mL/mL urine) to give the correct range.

4. Given the data for creatinine clearance below, select the most appropriate course of action:

 Volume = 2.8 L/day; surface area = 1.73 m²; urine creatinine = 100 mg/dL; serum creatinine = 1.2 mg/dL
 A. Report a creatinine clearance of 162 mL/min.
 B. Repeat the urine creatinine; results point to a dilution error.
 C. Request a new 24-hour urine sample.
 D. Request the patient's age and sex.

 Body fluids/Evaluate laboratory data to recognize problems/Creatinine clearance/3

5. Given the urinalysis results below, select the most appropriate course of action:

 pH = 6.5; protein = neg; glucose = neg; ketone = tr; blood = neg; bilirubin = neg; mucus = sm; ammonium urate crystals = lg
 A. Recheck urine pH.
 B. Report these results assuming acceptable quality control.
 C. Repeat the dry reagent strip tests to confirm the ketone result.
 D. Request a new sample and repeat the urinalysis.

 Body fluids/Evaluate laboratory data to recognize problems/Urinalysis/3

6. Given the following urinalysis results, select the most appropriate course of action:

 Color = amber; transparency = clear; pH = 6.0; protein = neg; glucose = neg; ketone = neg; blood = neg; bilirubin = neg; bilirubin granules = sm
 A. Perform a tablet test for bilirubin before reporting.
 B. Request a new sample.
 C. Recheck the pH.
 D. Perform a test for urinary urobilinogen.

 Body fluids/Evaluate laboratory data to determine possible inconsistent results/Urinalysis/3

7. A 5-hour urinary D-xylose test on a 7-year-old boy who was given 0.5 g of D-xylose per pound is 15%. The 2-hour timed blood D-xylose is 15 mg/dL (lower reference limit 30 mg/dL). Select the most appropriate action:
 A. Request that a β carotene absorption test be performed.
 B. Repeat the urinary result because it is borderline.
 C. Request a retest using a 25-g dose of D-xylose.
 D. Request a retest using only a 1-hour timed blood sample.

 Body fluids/Apply principles of special procedures/D-Xylose absorption/3

8. A biochemical profile gives the following results:

 Creatinine = 1.4 mg/dL; BUN = 35 mg/dL; K = 5.5 mmol/L

All other results are normal and all tests are in control. Urine from the patient has an osmolality of 975 mOsm/kg. Select the most appropriate course of action:
 A. Check for hemolysis.
 B. Repeat the BUN and report only if normal.
 C. Repeat the serum creatinine and report only if elevated.
 D. Report these results.

Body fluids/Evaluate laboratory data to recognize problems/Renal function/3

Answers to Questions 4–8

4. **C** A calculated clearance in excess of 140 mL/min is greater than the upper physiological limit. The high volume per day suggests addition of H_2O to the sample. The result should be considered invalid.

5. **A** Ammonium urate crystals occur at alkaline pH only. The pH should be checked, and if below 7.0, the crystals should be reviewed in order to identify correctly. The trace ketone does not require confirmation provided that the quality control of the reagent strips is acceptable.

6. **A** Bilirubin crystals cannot occur in urine without bilirubin. The tablet test is more sensitive than the dry reagent test and will confirm the presence of bilirubin. If negative, the crystals should be reviewed before reporting. Abnormal crystals occur only in acid or neutral urine.

7. **D** Urinary xylose excretion is less reliable in children under the age of 10, and peak blood levels occur sooner than in adults. A 60-minute blood sample should have been used. A serum D-xylose level greater than 30 mg/dL at 1 hour is considered normal.

8. **D** Patients with prerenal failure usually have a BUN:creatinine ratio greater than 20:1. Reduced renal blood flow causes increased urea reabsorption and high urine osmolality. Patients are usually hypertensive and show fluid retention and hyperkalemia.

9. An elevated amylase is obtained on a stat serum collected at 8 PM. A δ-check flag for amylase occurs because of a normal result from 8 AM. Amylase is also ordered on a 6 PM urine sample. Select the most appropriate course of action:
   A. Repeat the stat amylase; report only if the δ-check limit is not exceeded.
   B. Repeat both the AM and PM amylase and report only if they agree.
   C. Request a new specimen; do not report results of the stat sample.
   D. Review amylase on the 6 PM urine sample; if elevated, report the stat amylase.

   Body fluids/Select routine laboratory procedures to verify test results/Amylase/3

10. A 2 PM urinalysis has a trace glucose by the dry reagent strip test. A fasting blood glucose drawn 8 hours earlier is 100 mg/dL. No other results are abnormal. Select the most appropriate course of action.
    A. Repeat the urine glucose and report if positive.
    B. Perform a test for reducing sugars and report the result.
    C. Perform a quantitative urine glucose; report as trace if greater than 100 mg/dL.
    D. Request a new urine specimen.

    Body fluids/Evaluate laboratory data to determine possible inconsistent results/Glucose/3

11. Following a transfusion reaction, urine from a patient gives positive tests for blood and protein. The SG is 1.015. No RBCs or WBCs are seen in the microscopic examination. These results:
    A. Indicate renal injury induced by transfusion reaction
    B. Support the finding of an extravascular transfusion reaction
    C. Support the finding of an intravascular transfusion reaction
    D. Rule out a transfusion reaction caused by RBC incompatibility

    Body fluids/Correlate clinical and laboratory data/Urinalysis/3

12. A urine sample taken after a suspected transfusion reaction has a positive test for blood, but intact RBCs are not seen on microscopic examination. Which one test result would rule out an intravascular hemolytic transfusion reaction?
    A. Negative urine urobilinogen
    B. Serum unconjugated bilirubin below 1.0 mg/dL
    C. Serum potassium below 6.0 mmol/L
    D. Normal plasma haptoglobin

    Body Fluids/Select routine laboratory procedures to verify test results/Transfusion reaction/3

13. Given the following urinalysis results, select the most appropriate course of action:

pH = 5.0; protein = neg; glucose = 1%; ketone = mod; blood = neg; bilirubin = neg; SSA protein = 1%
A. Report the SSA protein result instead of the dry reagent strip result.
B. Call for a list of medications administered to the patient.
C. Perform a quantitative urinary albumin.
D. Perform a test for microalbuminuria.

Body fluids/Evaluate laboratory data to determine possible inconsistent results/Urinalysis/3

Answers to Questions 9–13

9. **D** Amylase often peaks 6–12 hours after an episode of acute pancreatitis and may cause a δ-check flag in the absence of laboratory error. Urinary amylase parallels serum amylase; a positive urine test at 6 PM makes sample collection error unlikely.

10. **A** The urine glucose is determined by the blood glucose at the time the urine is formed. The postprandial glucose (2 PM) level exceeded the renal threshold resulting in trace glycosuria. Tests for reducing sugars are not used to confirm a positive urine glucose test.

11. **C** RBCs usually remain intact at an SG of 1.015. The absence of RBCs, WBCs, and casts points to hemoglobinuria caused by intravascular hemolysis rather than glomerular injury. A positive protein reaction will occur if sufficient hemoglobin is present.

12. **D** The plasma free hemoglobin will be increased immediately after a hemolytic transfusion reaction, and the haptoglobin will be decreased. The hemoglobin will be eliminated by the kidneys, but the haptoglobin will remain low or undetectable for 2–3 days. Normal urine urobilinogen and serum unconjugated bilirubin help in ruling out extravascular hemolysis. Pretransfusion potassium is needed to evaluate the contribution of hemolysis to the posttransfusion result.

13. **B** The combination of glucose- and ketone-positive urine points to a patient with insulin-dependent diabetes. A false-positive SSA test is likely if tolbutamide (Orinase) has been administered.

14. A 24-hour urine sample from an adult submitted for catecholamines gives a result of 140 μg/day (upper reference limit 150 μg/day). The 24-hour urine creatinine level is 0.6 g/day. Select the best course of action:
    A. Check the urine pH to verify that it is less than 2.0.
    B. Report the result in μg catecholamines per mg creatinine.
    C. Request a new 24-hour urine sample.
    D. Measure the VMA and report the catecholamine result only if elevated.

    Body fluids/Evaluate to recognize problems/Catecholamines/3

15. Urinalysis results from a 35-year-old woman are:

    SG = 1.015; pH = 7.5; protein = tr; glucose = sm; ketone = neg; blood = neg; leukocyte esterase = mod; 5–10 RBCs/HPF; 25–50 WBCs/HPF

    Select the most appropriate course of action:
    A. Recheck the blood reaction; if negative look for budding yeast.
    B. Repeat the WBC count.
    C. Report all results except blood.
    D. Request a list of medications.

    Body fluids/Evaluate laboratory data to recognize sources of error/Urinalysis/3

16. A routine urinalysis gives the following results:

    pH = 6.5; protein = neg; glucose = tr; ketone = neg; blood = neg; 5–10 blood casts/LPF; mucus = sm; amorphous crystals = lg

    These results are most likely explained by:
    A. False-negative blood reaction
    B. False-negative protein reaction
    C. Pseudocasts of urate mistaken for true casts
    D. Mucus mistaken for casts

    Body fluids/Evaluate laboratory data to determine possible inconsistent results/Urinalysis/3

17. A toluidine blue chamber count on CSF gives the following values:

CSF Counts	Peripheral Blood Counts
WBCs 10 × 10⁶/L	WBCs 5 × 10⁹/L
RBCs 1000 × 10⁶/L	RBCs 5 × 10¹²/L

    After correcting the WBC count in CSF, one should next:
    A. Report the WBC count as 9 × 10⁶/L without additional testing.
    B. Report the WBC count and number of PMNs identified by the chamber count.
    C. Perform a differential on a direct smear of the CSF.
    D. Concentrate CSF using a cytocentrifuge and perform a differential.

    Body fluids/Apply knowledge of standard operating procedures/Cerebrospinal fluid/3

18. A blood-tainted pleural fluid is submitted for culture. Which test result would be most conclusive in classifying the fluid as an exudate?

Test	Result
A. LD fluid/serum	0.65
B. Total protein	3.2 g/dL
C. RBC count	10,000/μL
D. WBC count	1500/μL

    Body fluids/Correlate clinical and laboratory data/Pleural fluid/3

Answers to Questions 14–18

14. **C** Urine creatinine of less than 0.8 g/day indicates incomplete sample collection. The patient's daily catecholamine excretion would be misinterpreted from this result.

15. **A** A nonhemolyzed trace may have been overlooked and the blood test should be repeated. A false-negative (e.g., megadoses of vitamin C) rarely occurs. Yeast cells often accompany pyuria and glycosuria and are easily mistaken for RBCs.

16. **C** At pH 6.5 amorphous crystals are most often urate. These form yellow- or reddish-brown refractile deposits sometimes resembling blood or granular casts. The number of casts reported could not have occurred with negative protein and blood tests.

17. **D** A differential is performed using CSF concentrate regardless of the WBC count. A toluidine blue chamber count of PMNs is not sufficiently sensitive to detect neutrophilic pleocytosis.

18. **A** A traumatic tap makes classification of fluids difficult on the basis of cell counts and protein. The values reported for protein, RBCs, and WBCs can occur in either an exudate or bloody transudate, but the LD ratio is significant.

19. Results of a fetal lung maturity (FLM) study from a patient with diabetes mellitus are:

L/S = 2.0; PG = pos; creatinine = 2.5 mg/dL

Given these results one should:

A. Report the result and recommend repeating the L/S ratio in 24 hours.
B. Perform scanning spectrophotometry on the fluid to determine if blood is present.
C. Repeat the L/S ratio after 4 hours and report those results.
D. Report results as invalid.

Body fluids/Correlate laboratory data to verify test results/L/S ratio/3

20. A quantitative serum HCG is ordered on a male patient. One should:

A. Perform the test and report the result.
B. Request that the order be cancelled.
C. Perform the test and report the result if negative.
D. Perform the test and report the result only if greater than 25 IU/L.

Body fluids/Apply knowledge of standard operating procedures/Human chorionic gonadotropin/3

Answers to Questions 19–20

19. **A** In patients with diabetes, lung maturity may be delayed and an L/S ratio of 2:1 may be associated with respiratory distress syndrome. A positive PG spot correlates with an L/S ratio of 2:1 or higher and rules out a falsely increased result caused by blood contamination. The best course of action is to wait an additional 24 hours and perform another L/S ratio on a fresh sample of amniotic fluid because an L/S ratio of 3:1 would indicate a high probability of fetal lung maturity.

20. **A** HCG may be produced in men by tumors of trophoblastic origin, such as teratoma and seminoma, and is an important marker for nontrophoblastic tumors as well.

BIBLIOGRAPHY

1. Brunzel, NA: Fundamentals of Urine and Body Fluid Analysis. WB Saunders, Philadelphia, 1994.
2. Burtis, CA and Ashwood, ER (eds): Tietz Textbook of Clinical Chemistry. WB Saunders, Philadelphia, 1994.
3. Haber, MH: Urinary Sediment: A Textbook Atlas. ASCP Press, Chicago, 1981.
4. Henry, JB (ed): Clinical Diagnosis and Management by Laboratory Methods. WB Saunders, Philadelphia, 1996.
5. Kaplan, LA and Pesce, AJ (eds): Clinical Chemistry Theory Analysis and Correlation. CV Mosby, St. Louis, 1996.
6. Kjeldsberg, CR and Knight, JA: Body Fluids. ASCP Press, Chicago, 1993.
7. Strasinger, SK: Urinalysis and Body Fluids. FA Davis, Philadelphia, 1994.

CHAPTER SIX

Microbiology

UNIT 1

Specimen Collection, Media, and Methods

1. The aseptic collection of blood cultures requires that the skin be cleansed with:
   A. 2% iodine and then 70% alcohol
   B. 80%–95% alcohol and then 2% iodine or an iodophor
   C. 70% alcohol and then 95% alcohol
   D. 95% alcohol only

   Microbiology/Apply knowledge of standard operating procedures/Specimen collection/1

2. When cleansing the skin with alcohol and then iodine for the collection of a blood culture, the iodine (or iodophor) should remain intact on the skin for at least:
   A. 10 seconds
   B. 30 seconds
   C. 60 seconds
   D. 5 minutes

   Microbiology/Apply knowledge of standard operating procedures/Specimen collection and handling/1

3. What is the purpose of adding 0.025%–0.050% sodium polyanethol sulfonate (SPS) to nutrient broth media for the collection of blood cultures?
   A. Inhibits phagocytosis and complement
   B. Promotes formation of a blood clot
   C. Enhances growth of anaerobes
   D. Functions as a preservative

   Microbiology/Apply knowledge of standard operating procedures/Media/1

4. A flexible calcium alginate nasopharyngeal swab is the collection device of choice for recovery of which organism from the nasopharynx?
   A. *Staphylococcus aureus*
   B. *Streptococcus pneumoniae*
   C. *Corynebacterium diphtheriae*
   D. *Bacteroides fragilis*

Microbiology/Apply knowledge of standard operating procedure/Specimen collection and handling/1

Answers to Questions 1–4

1. **B** In order to attain asepsis of the skin, 90%–95% alcohol followed by 2% iodine is used for obtaining blood cultures.

2. **C** The iodine should remain on the skin for 1 minute because instant antisepsis does not occur when cleansing the skin for a blood culture.

3. **A** SPS is used in most commercial blood culture products because it functions as an anticoagulant and prevents phagocytosis and complement activation. In addition, SPS neutralizes aminoglycoside antibiotics. Addition of SPS may inhibit some *Neisseria* and *Peptostreptococcus,* but this can be reversed with 1.2% gelatin.

4. **C** *C. diphtheriae* must be recovered from the deep layers of the pseudomembrane that forms in the nasopharyngeal area. A flexible calcium alginate nasopharyngeal swab is the best choice for collecting a specimen from the posterior nares and pharynx.

281

5. Semisolid transport media such as Amies, Stuart, or Cary-Blair are suitable for the transport of swabs for culture of most pathogens *except:*
 A. *Neisseria gonorrhoeae*
 B. *Enterobacteriaceae*
 C. *Campylobacter fetus*
 D. *S. pneumoniae*

Microbiology/Select methods/Reagents/Media/ Specimen collection and handling/2

6. Select the method of choice for recovery of anaerobic bacteria from a deep abscess.
 A. Cotton fiber swab of the abscess area
 B. Skin snip of the surface tissue
 C. Needle aspirate after surface decontamination
 D. Swab of the scalpel used for debridement

Microbiology/Apply knowledge of standard operating procedure/Specimen collection and handling/2

7. Select the primary and differential media of choice for recovery of most fecal pathogens.
 A. MacConkey, blood, birdseed, and *Campilobacter* (*Campy*) agars
 B. Hektoen, MacConkey, *Campy*, colistin-nalidixic acid (CNA) agars
 C. CNA and Christensen urea agars and thioglycollate media
 D. Blood, *Campy*, Mueller-Hinton agars, and thioglycollate media

Microbiology/Select methods/Reagents/Media/Stool culture/2

8. Select the media of choice for recovery of *Vibrio cholerae* from a stool specimen.
 A. MacConkey agar and thioglycollate media
 B. Thiosulfate-citrate-bile-sucrose (TCBS) agar and alkaline peptone water (APW) broth
 C. Blood agar and selenite-F (SEL) broth
 D. CNA agar

Microbiology/Select methods/Reagents/Media/Stool culture/2

9. CNA is used primarily for the recovery of:
 A. *Neisseria* species
 B. *Enterobacteriaceae*
 C. *P. aeruginosa*
 D. *S. aureus*

Microbiology/Select methods/Reagents/Media/ Gram-positive cocci/2

10. In the United States most blood agar plates are prepared with 5% or 10% red blood cells (RBCs) obtained from:
 A. Sheep
 B. Horses

 C. Humans
 D. Dogs

Microbiology/Select methods/Reagents/Media/ Culture/1

Answers to Questions 5–10

5. A Specimens for culture of *N. gonorrhoeae* are best if plated immediately or transported in a medium containing activated charcoal to absorb inhibitory substances that hinder their recovery.

6. C Anaerobic specimens are easily contaminated with organisms present on the skin or mucosal surfaces, when a swab is used. Needle aspiration of an abscess following surface decontamination provides the least exposure to ambient oxygen.

7. B Hektoen agar selectively isolates pathogenic coliforms, especially *Salmonella* and *Shigella*. MacConkey agar differentiates lactose fermenters from nonfermenters. CNA agar contains antibiotics that prohibit growth of gram-negative coliforms but not gram-positive cocci. Campy agar contains the antibiotics cephalothin, trimethoprim, vancomycin, polymyxin B, and amphotericin B to prevent growth of *Enterobacteriaceae*, *Pseudomonas* spp and fungi.

8. B TCBS agar is used to grow *V. cholera*, which appear as yellow colonies due to the use of both citrate and sucrose. APW is used as an enrichment broth and should be subcultured to TCBS agar for further evaluation of *Vibrio* colonies.

9. D CNA agar inhibits the growth of gram-negative bacteria and is used to isolate gram-positive cocci from specimens. This medium is especially useful for stool and wound cultures because these may contain large numbers of gram-negative rods.

10. A Sheep RBCs are used in blood agar plates because they are readily available and less inhibitory than cells of other species. The type of hemolysis is determined by the source of RBCs. Sheep RBCs are chosen because of the characteristic clear hemolysis produced by β-hemolytic *Streptococcus*, *Staphylococcus*, and other pathogens producing β hemolysins. Sheep blood does not support the growth of *Haemophilus haemolyticus*, eliminating the possibility of confusing it with β-hemolytic *Streptococcus* in throat cultures.

11. All of the following are appropriate when attempting to isolate *N. gonorrhoeae* from a genital specimen *except:*
    A. Transport the genital swab in charcoal transport medium.
    B. Plate the specimen on Modified Thayer-Martin (MTM) medium.
    C. Plate the specimen on New York City or Martin-Lewis agar.
    D. Culture specimens in ambient oxygen at 37°C.

    Microbiology/Select methods/Reagents/Media/ Culture/1

12. Chocolate agar and modified Thayer-Martin agar are used for the recovery of:
    A. *Haemophilus* spp and *Neisseria* spp, respectively
    B. *Haemophilus* spp and *N. gonorrhoeae*, respectively
    C. *Neisseria* spp and *Streptococcus* spp, respectively
    D. *Streptococcus* spp and *Staphylococcus* spp, respectively

    Microbiology/Select methods/Reagents/Media/ Stool culture/2

13. Cycloserine-cefoxitin-fructose agar (CCFA) is used for the recovery of:
    A. *Yersinia enterocolitica*
    B. *Yersinia intermedia*
    C. *Clostridium perfringens*
    D. *Clostridium difficile*

    Microbiology/Select methods/Reagents/Media/Stool culture/1

14. Deoxycholate agar (DCA) is useful for the isolation of:
    A. *Enterobacteriaceae*
    B. *Enterococcus* spp
    C. *Staphylococcus* spp
    D. *Neisseria* spp

    Microbiology/Select methods/Reagents/Media/Stool culture/1

15. Xylose lysine deoxycholate (XLD) agar is a highly selective medium used for the recovery of which bacteria?
    A. *Staphylococcus* spp from normal flora
    B. *Yersinia* spp that do not grow on Hektoen agar
    C. *Enterobacteriaceae* from gastrointestinal specimens
    D. *Streptococcus* spp from stool cultures

    Microbiology/Select methods/Reagents/Media/ Stool culture/1

Answers to Questions 11–15

11. **D** MTM, New York City, and Martin-Lewis agars contain blood factors needed to support the growth of *N. gonorrhoeae,* as well as antibiotics that prevent growth of normal genital flora. Cultures must be incubated in 3%–7% CO_2 at 35°C. Cultures should be held a minimum of 48 hours before being considered negative.

12. **B** Chocolate agar provides X factor (hemin) and V factor (NAD) required for the growth of *Haemophilus* spp. MTM is a chocolate agar containing the antibiotics vancomycin, colistin, nystatin, and trimethoprim. These permit isolation of *N. gonorrhoeae* in specimens containing large numbers of gram-negative bacteria, including commensal *Neisseria* species.

13. **D** CCFA is used for recovery of *C. difficile* from stool cultures. Cycloserine and cefoxitin inhibit growth of gram-negative coliforms in the stool specimen. *C. difficile* ferments fructose, forming acid that, in the presence of neutral red, causes the colonies to become yellow.

14. **A** DCA inhibits gram-positive organisms. *N. gonorrhoeae* and *Neisseria meningitidis* are too fastidious to grow on DCA. Citrate and deoxycholate salts inhibit growth of gram-positive bacteria. The media contains lactose and neutral red allowing differentiation of lactose fermenters (pink colonies) from nonfermenters (colorless).

15. **C** XLD agar is selective for gram-negative coliforms due to a high concentration (0.25%) of deoxycholate, which inhibits gram-positive bacteria. In addition, XLD is differential for *Shigella* and *Salmonella* spp. The medium contains xylose, lactose, and sucrose, which are fermented by most normal intestinal coliforms producing yellow colonies. *Shigella* does not ferment the sugars and produces red (or clear) colonies. *Salmonella* spp ferment xylose; however, they also decarboxylate lysine in the medium causing production of ammonia. Therefore, *Salmonella* first appear yellow but become red. Some *Salmonella* produce hydrogen sulfide (H_2S) from sodium thiosulfate and, therefore, appear as red colonies with black centers.

16. A sheep blood agar plate is used as a primary isolation medium when all of the following organisms are to be recovered from a wound specimen *except:*
- A. β-Hemolytic *Streptococcus* and coagulase-positive *Staphylococcus*
- B. *Haemophilus influenzae* and *Haemophilus parainfluenzae*
- C. *Proteus* spp and *Escherichia coli*
- D. *Pseudomonas* spp and *Acinetobacter* spp

Microbiology/Select methods/Reagents/Media/ Wound culture/2

17. Prereduced and vitamin K_1-supplemented blood agar plates are recommended isolation media for:
- A. *Mycobacterium marinum* and *Mycobacterium avium-intercellulare*
- B. *Bacteroides*, *Peptostreptococcus*, and *Clostridium* spp
- C. *Proteus* spp
- D. *Enterococcus* spp

Microbiology/Select methods/Reagents/Media/ Anaerobes/2

18. Which procedure is appropriate for culture of genital specimens in order to recover *Chlamydia* spp?
- A. Inoculate cycloheximide-treated McCoy cells.
- B. Plate onto blood and chocolate agar.
- C. Inoculate into thioglycollate (THIO) broth.
- D. Plate onto modified Thayer-Martin agar within 24 hours.

Microbiology/Select methods/Reagents/Media/ Virus culture/1

19. Specimens for virus culture should be transported in media containing:
- A. Antibiotics and 5% sheep blood
- B. Saline and 5% sheep blood
- C. 22% bovine albumin
- D. Antibiotics and nutrient

Microbiology/Select methods/Reagents/Media/ Virus culture/1

20. Cerebrospinal fluid (CSF) should be cultured immediately, but if delayed the specimen should be:
- A. Refrigerated at 4°–6°C
- B. Frozen at −20°C
- C. Stored at room temperature for not longer than 24 hours

D. Incubated at 37°C and cultured as soon as possible

Microbiology/Apply knowledge of standard operating procedure/Specimen collection and transport/1

Answers to Questions 16–20

16. **B** Both gram-positive cocci and gram-negative bacilli will grow on blood agar plates, but the medium is used in conjunction with a selective medium such as CNA agar for gram-positive cocci and MacConkey agar for gram-negative bacilli. *H. influenzae* requires X and V factors, and *H. parainfluenzae* requires V factor; the primary isolation medium for *Haemophilus* is chocolate agar.

17. **B** Anaerobic culture medium can be prereduced before sterilization by boiling, saturation of oxygen-free gas, and addition of cysteine or other thiol compound. The final oxidation reduction potential (Eh) of the medium should be approximately −150 mV to minimize the effects of exposure of organisms to oxygen during inoculation.

18. **A** *Chlamydia* are strict intracellular organisms and must be cultured using living cells. Direct smears can also be made at the time of culture. Staining cells with iodine may reveal the characteristic reddish-brown inclusions sometimes seen in *Chlamydia* infections. Fluorescein-conjugated monoclonal antibodies may be used to identify the organisms in infected cells.

19. **D** Media for transporting specimens for virus culture include Hanks balanced salt solution with bovine albumin, Stuart transport media, and Leibovitz-Emory media. Media used for transporting specimens for virus culture are similar to those for bacteria with the addition of a nutrient such as fetal calf serum or albumin and antibiotics. Specimens should be refrigerated after being placed in the transport media until the culture media can be inoculated.

20. **D** Fastidious organisms such as *Neisseria* and *Haemophilus* frequently isolated from CSF of patients with bacterial meningitis are preserved by placing the fluid in 3%–7% CO_2 at 35°–37°C (or at room temperature for no longer than 30 minutes), if the specimen cannot be cultured immediately.

21. The most sensitive method for the detection of β-lactamase in bacteria is by the use of:
    A. Chromogenic cephalosporin
    B. Penicillin
    C. Oxidase
    D. Chloramphenicol acetyltransferase

    Microbiology/Select methods/Reagents/Media/Sensitivity testing/2

22. The breakpoint of an antimicrobial drug refers to:
    A. The amount needed to cause bacteriostasis
    B. A minimum inhibitory concentration of 16 μg/mL or greater
    C. A minimum inhibitory concentration of 64 μg/mL or greater
    D. The level of drug that is achievable in serum

    Microbiology/Apply principle of theory and practice related to laboratory operations/Sensitivity testing/2

23. Which of the following variables may change the results of an MIC?
    A. Inoculum size
    B. Incubation time
    C. Growth rate of the bacteria
    D. All of the above

    Microbiology/Apply knowledge to identify sources of error/Sensitivity testing/2

24. According to the Kirby-Bauer standard antimicrobial susceptibility testing method, what should be done when interpreting the zone size of a motile, swarming organism such as a *Proteus* species?
    A. The swarming area should be ignored.
    B. The results of the disk diffusion method are invalid.
    C. The swarming area should be measured as the growth boundary.
    D. The isolate should be retested after diluting to a 0.05 McFarland standard.

    Microbiology/Apply knowledge of standard operating procedures/Sensitivity testing/2

25. Which class of antibiotics is used for the treatment of serious gram-negative infections as well as infections with *Mycobacterium tuberculosis*?
    A. Cephalosporins
    B. Penicillins
    C. Tetracyclines
    D. Aminoglycosides

Microbiology/Apply knowledge of fundamental biological characteristics/Antibiotics/1

Answers to Questions 21–25

21. **A** β-Lactamase production by bacteria that are resistant to penicillin and cephalosporin is detected using one of these drugs as a substrate. Penicillin is hydrolyzed by β-lactamase into acidic products that can be detected as a color change by a pH indicator. In the iodometric method, a disk containing a penicillin-starch substrate turns blue when a drop of iodine is added. A loop of β-lactamase-positive organisms applied to the center of the blue spot will reduce the iodine to iodide causing the area to clear. The most sensitive method of detection is based upon the ability of the organism to hydrolyze the β-lactam ring of a chromogenic cephalosporin.

22. **D** The breakpoint refers to an antimicrobial concentration in the serum associated with optimal therapy using the customary dosing schedule. An organism is susceptible if the minimum inhibitory concentration (MIC) is at or below the breakpoint.

23. **D** *In vitro* testing of drugs is reliable if the method is standardized. In addition to the first three variables, the type of media and the stability of antibiotics will affect the results of MIC testing and must be carefully controlled.

24. **A** A thin film of growth appearing in the zone area of inhibition around the susceptibility disk should be ignored when swarming *Proteus* or other organism is encountered. Discontinuous, poor growth or tiny colonies near the end of the zone are also ignored.

25. **D** The aminoglycoside antibiotics are bactericidal agents that act by inhibiting protein synthesis. They show a low incidence of bacterial resistance but must be monitored carefully because at high doses they can cause ototoxicity and nephrotoxicity. The group includes amikacin, gentamicin, tobramycin, kanamycin, streptomycin, and spectinomycin. These drugs are usually administered intravenously or intramuscularly because they are poorly absorbed from the gastrointestinal tract.

Enterobacteriaceae

1. Biochemically, the *Enterobacteriaceae* are gram-negative rods that:
   A. Ferment glucose, reduce nitrate to nitrite, and are oxidase-negative
   B. Ferment glucose, produce indophenol oxidase, and form gas
   C. Ferment lactose, reduce nitrite to nitrogen gas
   D. Ferment lactose, produce indophenol oxidase

   Microbiology/Apply knowledge of fundamental biological characteristics/Biochemical/Gram-negative bacilli/1

2. The ortho-nitrophenyl-β-galactopyranoside (ONPG) test is most useful when differentiating:
   A. *Salmonella* spp from *Pseudomonas* spp
   B. *Shigella* spp from some strains of *E. coli*
   C. *Klebsiella* spp from *Enterobacter* spp
   D. *Proteus vulgaris* from *Salmonella* spp

   Microbiology/Apply principles of basic laboratory procedures/Biochemical/2

3. The Voges-Proskauer (VP) test detects which end product of glucose fermentation?
   A. Acetoin
   B. Nitrite
   C. Acetic acid
   D. Hydrogen sulfide

   Microbiology/Apply principles of basic laboratory procedures/Biochemical/1

4. At which pH does the methyl red (MR) test become positive?
   A. 7.0
   B. 6.5
   C. 6.0
   D. 4.5

   Microbiology/Apply principles of basic laboratory procedures/Biochemical/1

5. A positive Simmons citrate test is seen as a:
   A. Blue color in the medium after 24 hours' incubation at 35°C
   B. Red color in the medium after 18 hours' incubation at 35°C
   C. Yellow color in the medium after 24 hours' incubation at 35°C
   D. Green color in the medium after 18 hours' incubation at 35°C

   Microbiology/Apply principles of basic laboratory procedures/Biochemical/1

Answers to Questions 1–5

1. **A** The family *Enterobacteriaceae* consists of more than 100 species and represents the most commonly encountered isolates in clinical specimens. All *Enterobacteriaceae* ferment glucose and are oxidase-negative and nonsporulating. Most *Enterobacteriaceae* are motile, but the genera *Shigella* and *Klebsiellae* are not.

2. **B** The ONPG test detects β-galactosidase activity and is most useful in distinguishing late lactose fermenters from lactose nonfermenters. Some strains of *E. coli* are slow lactose fermenters and may be confused with *Shigella* spp, which do not ferment lactose. *E. coli* are ONPG-positive while *Shigella* spp are ONPG-negative.

3. **A** Acetoin or carbinol, an end product of glucose fermentation, is converted to diacetyl after the addition of the VP reagents (α-naphthol and 40% potassium hydroxide [KOH]). Diacetyl is seen as a red- to pink-colored complex.

4. **D** Both MR and VP tests detect acid production from the fermentation of glucose. However, a positive MR test denotes a more complete catabolism of glucose to highly acidic end products such as formate and acetate than occurs with organisms that are VP-positive only (e.g., *Klebsiella pneumoniae*).

5. **A** The Simmons citrate test determines if an organism can utilize citrate as the sole source of carbon. The medium turns blue indicating the presence of alkaline products such as carbonate. Tubes are incubated a minimum of 24 hours at 35°C with a loose cap before reading.

6. In the test for urease production, ammonia reacts to form which product?
A. Ammonium citrate
B. Ammonium carbonate
C. Ammonium oxalate
D. Ammonium nitrate

Microbiology/Apply principles of basic laboratory procedures/Biochemical/1

7. Which of the following reagents is added to detect the production of indole?
A. *p*-Dimethylaminobenzaldehyde
B. Bromcresol purple
C. Methyl red (MR)
D. Cytochrome oxidase

Microbiology/Apply principles of basic laboratory procedures/Biochemical/1

8. Decarboxylation of the amino acids lysine, ornithine, and arginine results in the formation of:
A. Ammonia
B. Urea
C. CO_2
D. Amines

Microbiology/Apply principles of basic laboratory procedures/Biochemical/1

9. Lysine iron agar (LIA) showing a purple slant and a blackened butt indicates:
A. *E. coli*
B. *Citrobacter* spp
C. *Salmonella* spp
D. *Proteus* spp

Microbiology/Evaluate laboratory data to make identifications/Gram-negative bacilli/2

10. Putrescine is an alkaline amine product of which bacterial enzyme?
A. Arginine decarboxylase
B. Phenylalanine deaminase
C. Ornithine decarboxylase
D. Lysine decarboxylase

Microbiology/Apply principles of basic laboratory procedures/Biochemical/1

11. Which genera are positive for phenylalanine deaminase?
A. *Enterobacter, Escherichia,* and *Salmonella*
B. *Morganella, Providencia,* and *Proteus*
C. *Klebsiella* and *Enterobacter*
D. *Proteus, Escherichia,* and *Shigella*

Microbiology/Evaluate laboratory data to make identifications/Gram-negative bacilli/2

12. Kligler iron agar (KIA) differs from triple sugar iron agar (TSI) in the:
A. Ratio of lactose to glucose
B. The ability to detect H_2S production
C. The use of sucrose in the medium
D. The color reaction denoting production of acid

Microbiology/Apply principles of basic laboratory procedures/Methods/Reagents/Media/Gram-negative bacilli/2

Answers to Questions 6–12

6. **B** The test for urease production is based upon the ability of the colonies to hydrolyze urea in Stuart broth or Christensen's agar to form CO_2 and ammonia. These products form ammonium carbonate resulting in alkalinization. This turns the pH indicator (phenol red) pink at pH 8.0.

7. **A** The indole test detects the conversion of tryptophan (present in the media) to indole by the enzyme tryptophanase. Indole is detected by the reaction with the aldehyde group of *p*-dimethylaminobenzaldehyde (the active reagent in Kovacs and Ehrlich reagents) in acid, formimg a red complex.

8. **D** Specific decarboxylases split dibasic amino acids (lysine, arginine, and ornithine) forming alkaline amines. These products turn the pH indicators in the medium (cresol red and bromcresol purple) from yellow to purple.

9. **C** LIA is used as an aid for the identification of *Salmonella* species. It contains phenylalanine, lysine, glucose, thiosulfate, ferric ammonium citrate, and bromcresol purple. *Salmonella* produce H_2S from thiosulfate. This reduces ferric ammonium citrate forming ferrous sulfate causing the butt to blacken. *Salmonella* also decarboxylates lysine to produce alkaline amines giving the slant its purple color and differentiating it from *Citrobacter* spp, which are lysine decarboxylase-negative.

10. **C** Putrescine is the amine product of the decarboxylation of ornithine.

11. **B** Phenylalanine deaminase oxidatively deaminates phenylalanine forming phenylpyruvic acid. When a solution of ferric chloride is added the iron reacts with phenylpyruvic acid, forming a green colored complex. Phenylalanine deaminase is found in the genera *Morganella, Providencia,* and *Proteus,* and is an excellent test to determine if an organism belongs to this group. Rarely, isolates of *Enterobacter* may be phenylalanine deaminase-positive as well.

12. **C** Both KIA and TSI contain tenfold more lactose than glucose, peptone, and phenol red to detect acid production (turns yellow) and sodium thiosulfate and ferrous ammonium sulfate to detect H_2S production. However, TSI contains sucrose and KIA does not. Organisms fermenting either sucrose or lactose will turn the slant of the agar tube yellow. Therefore, some organisms, (e.g., many species of *Cedecea, Citrobacter, Edwardsiella,* and *Serratia*) will produce a yellow slant on TSI but a red slant on KIA.

13. The malonate test is most useful in differentiating which members of the *Enterobacteriaceae?*
  A. *Shigella*
  B. *Proteus*
  C. *Salmonella* subgroups 2, 3 (the former *Arizona*)
  D. *Serratia*

Microbiology/Evaluate laboratory data to make identifications/Gram-negative bacilli/2

14. Which genera of the *Enterobacteriaceae* are known to cause diarrhea and are considered enteric pathogens?
  A. *Enterobacter, Klebsiella, Providencia,* and *Proteus*
  B. *Escherichia, Salmonella, Shigella,* and *Yersinia*
  C. *Pseudomonas, Moraxella, Acinetobacter,* and *Aeromonas*
  D. *Enterobacter, Citrobacter,* and *Morganella*

Microbiology/Apply knowledge of fundamental biological characteristics/Gram-negative bacilli/1

15. An isolate of *E. coli* recovered from the stool of a patient with severe bloody diarrhea should be tested for which sugar before sending to a reference laboratory for serotyping?
  A. Sorbitol (fermentation)
  B. Mannitol (oxidation)
  C. Raffinose (fermentation)
  D. Sucrose (fermentation)

Microbiology/Evaluate laboratory data to recognize health and disease states/Gram-negative bacilli/3

16. Care must be taken when identifying biochemical isolates of *Shigella* because serological cross-reactions occur with:
  A. *E. coli*
  B. *Salmonella* spp
  C. *Pseudomonas* spp
  D. *Proteus* spp

Microbiology/Apply knowledge of fundamental biological characteristics/Gram-negative bacilli/2

17. Which species of *Shigella* is most commonly associated with diarrheal disease in the United States?
  A. *S. dysenteriae*
  B. *S. flexneri*
  C. *S. boydii*
  D. *S. sonnei*

Microbiology/Apply knowledge of fundamental biological characteristics/Gram-negative bacilli/2

18. Which of the following tests best differentiate *Shigella* species from *E. coli?*
  A. Hydrogen sulfide, VP, citrate, and urea
  B. Lactose, indole, ONPG, and motility
  C. Hydrogen sulfide, MR, citrate, and urea
  D. Gas, citrate, and VP

Microbiology/Evaluate laboratory data to make identifications/Gram-negative bacilli/2

Answers to Questions 13–18

13. **C** The malonate test determines whether an organism can utilize sodium malonate as the sole source of carbon. Malonate is broken down forming alkaline metabolites that raise the pH of the broth above 7.6. This causes bromthymol blue to turn from green to deep blue (Prussian blue). *E. coli, Shigella,* and most *Salmonella* are malonate-negative while *Enterobacter* and *Salmonella* (formerly *Arizona*) subgroups 2, 3a, and 3b are positive. *Proteus* and *Providencia* as well as *Serratia* and *Yersinia* are also malonate-negative.

14. **B** *Escherichia, Salmonella, Shigella,* and *Yersinia* are responsible for the majority of enteric diarrhea cases attributable to the *Enterobacteriaceae* family.

15. **A** An isolate of *E. coli* recovered from a stool culture in hemorrhagic colitis can be definitely identified only by serotyping. The isolate is identified as *E. coli* by the usual biochemical reactions. The strain of *E. coli* responsible for hemorrhagic colitis is O157:H7, and is usually negative for sorbitol fermentation. Colonies of this strain of *E. coli* will appear colorless on MacConkey agar with sorbitol added.

16. **A** Serological confirmation of *Shigella* isolates is based upon O antigen typing. If a suspected *Shigella* spp is serologically typed with polyvalent sera before it has been correctly identified biochemically, a false-positive confirmation may occur with an isolate that is *E. coli* (i.e., anaerogenic nongas-producing, lactose-negative or delayed, and nonmotile strains). These strains were formerly known as the Alkalescens-Dispar serotype.

17. **D** The *Shigella* spp are lactose nonfermenters that for the most part are biochemically inert and are classified into serogroups A, B, C, D as a result of their biochemical similarity. *S. sonnei* is the species most often isolated from diarrhea cases in the United States. It is more active biochemically than the other species due to ornithine decarboxylase and β-galactosidase activity. These enzymes, found in most strains of *S. sonnei* distinguish it from other *Shigella* species.

18. **B** *E. coli,* positive for lactose, indole, and ONPG, are usually motile. *Shigella* species do not ferment lactose or produce indole, lack β-galactosidase, and are nonmotile.

19. Which genera of *Enterobacteriaceae* are usually nonmotile at 36°C?
  A. *Shigella, Klebsiella,* and *Yersinia*
  B. *Escherichia, Edwardsiella,* and *Enterobacter*
  C. *Proteus, Providencia,* and *Salmonella*
  D. *Serratia, Morganella,* and *Hafnia*

Microbiology/Apply knowledge of fundamental biological characteristics/Gram-negative bacilli/2

20. Fever, abdominal cramping, watery stools, and fluid and electrolyte loss preceded by bloody stools 2–3 days before is characteristic of Shigellosis but may also result from infection with:
  A. *Campylobacter* spp
  B. *Salmonella* spp
  C. *Proteus* spp
  D. *Yersinia* spp

Microbiology/Apply knowledge of fundamental biological characteristics/Gram-negative bacilli/2

21. Cold enrichment of feces (incubation at 4°C) in phosphate-buffered saline prior to subculture onto enteric media enhances the recovery of:
  A. Enterotoxigenic *E. coli*
  B. *Salmonella paratyphi*
  C. *Hafnia alvei*
  D. *Y. enterocolitica*

Microbiology/Apply principles of special procedures/Gram-negative bacilli/2

22. Which group of tests, along with colonial morphology on primary media, aids most in the rapid identification of the *Enterobacteriaceae?*
  A. MR and VP, urea and blood agar plate
  B. Phenylanine deaminase, urea and CDC agar plate
  C. Bacitracin, β-lactamase, and MacConkey agar plate
  D. Indole, oxidase, MacConkey, and blood agar plates

Microbiology/Select methods/Reagents/Media/Gram-negative bacilli/2

23. A *routine,* complete stool culture procedure should include media for the isolation of *E. coli* O157:H7 as well as:
  A. *Salmonella, Shigella, Yersinia, Campylobacter,* and *S. aureus*
  B. *V. cholerae, Brucella,* and *Yersinia* spp
  C. *S. aureus,* group B *Streptococcus,* and group D *Streptococcus*
  D. *C. difficile, C. perfringens,* and *Yersinia* spp

Microbiology/Select methods/Reagents/Media/Gram-negative bacilli/2

24. Which group of tests best identifies the *Morganella* and *Proteus* genera?
  A. Motility, urease, and phenylalanine deaminase

  B. Malonate, glucose fermentation, and deoxyribonuclease (DNase)
  C. Indole, oxidase, MR, and VP
  D. Indole, citrate, and urease

Microbiology/Evaluate laboratory data to make identifications/Gram-negative bacilli/2

Answers to Questions 19–24

19. **A** *Shigella* spp and *Klebsiella* spp are for the most part nonmotile. *Yersinia* can be motile at 22°C but is nonmotile at 36°C. Other members of *Enterobacteriaceae* that have been isolated from human specimens and are usually nonmotile include *Leminorella, Rahnella,* and *Tatumella.*

20. **A** *Shigella* spp and *Campylobacter* spp are both causes of diarrhea, abdominal pain, fever, and sometimes vomiting. Blood is present in stools of patients infected with *Shigella* due to invasion and penetration of the bowel. Young children may also exhibit bloody stools when infected with *Campylobacter.*

21. **D** Cold enrichment is especially useful when specimens contain large numbers of normal flora that are sensitive to prolonged exposure to near-freezing temperature. In addition to *Yersinia,* the technique has been used to enhance recovery of *Listeria monocytogenes* from specimens containing other bacteria.

22. **D** The *Enterobacteriaceae* are all oxidase-negative. Because *E. coli* and *Proteus* spp comprise a majority of the organisms recovered from clinical specimens, they can be initially identified through rapid testing without additional overnight testing. *E. coli* display a positive indole test, and the colonial morphology on MacConkey agar is distinctive, showing flat, pink (lactose-positive) colonies with a ring of bile precipitation. *Proteus* spp swarm on blood agar and are indole-negative.

23. **A** *V. cholerae* and *C. difficile* are usually not included in a routine stool culture. If *Vibrio* spp are suspected, a special request should be included. Although MacConkey agar will support the growth of *Vibrio* spp, normal enteric flora will overgrow and occlude these organisms. *C. difficile* culture requires special media (CCFA) that inhibit other anaerobic flora and facultative anaerobic flora, and should be requested specifically if symptoms warrant. MacConkey agar with sorbitol will allow the *E. coli* O157:H7 to be recovered. *Yersinia* spp can be detected on a regular MacConkey agar plate.

24. **A** *Morganella* and *Proteus* spp are motile, produce urease, and deaminate phenylalanine.

25. Which group of tests best differentiates *Enterobacter aerogenes* from *Edwardsiella tarda*?
A. Motility, citrate, and urease
B. Hydrogen sulfide (H_2S) production, sucrose fermentation, indole, and VP
C. Lysine decarboxylase, urease, and arginine dihydrolase
D. Motility, H_2S production, and DNase

Microbiology/Evaluate laboratory data to make identifications/Gram-negative bacilli/2

26. *Enterobacter sakazakii* can best be differentiated from *Enterobacter cloacae* by its:
A. Yellow pigmentation and negative sorbitol fermentation
B. Pink pigmentation and positive arginine dihydrolase
C. Yellow pigmentation and positive urease
D. H_2S production on TSI

Microbiology/Evaluate laboratory data to make identifications/Gram-negative bacilli/2

27. Members of the genus *Cedecea* are best differentiated from *Serratia* spp by which test result?
A. Positive motility
B. Positive urease
C. Positive phenylalanine deaminase
D. Negative DNase

Microbiology/Evaluate laboratory data to make identifications/Gram-negative bacilli/2

28. Which of the following organisms is often confused with the *Salmonella* species biochemically and on plated media?
A. *E. coli*
B. *Citrobacter freundii*
C. *E. cloacae*
D. *Shigella dysenteriae*

Microbiology/Apply knowledge of fundamental biological characteristics/Gram-negative bacilli/2

29. A gram-negative rod is recovered from a catheterized urine sample from a nursing home patient. The lactose-negative isolate tested positive for indole, urease, KCN, ornithine decarboxylase, and phenylalanine deaminase and negative for H_2S. The most probable identification is:
A. *Ewardsiella* spp
B. *Morganella* spp
C. *Ewingella* spp
D. *Shigella* spp

Microbiology/Evaluate laboratory data to make identifications/Gram-negative bacilli/3

30. Which single test best separates *Klebsiella oxytoca* from *K. pneumoniae*?
A. Urease
B. Sucrose
C. Citrate
D. Indole

Microbiology/Evaluate laboratory data to make identifications/Gram-negative bacilli/2

Answers to Questions 25–30

25. B

Test	*E. aerogenes* (% positive)	*E. tarda* (% positive)
H_2S	0	100
Sucrose	>90	0
Indole	<20	100
VP	100	0
Citrate	95	0

26. A *E. sakazakii* is called a yellow-pigmented *E. cloacae* and is best differentiated from *E. cloacae* by sorbitol fermentation (95% positive for *E. cloacae* and 0% for *E. sakazakii*). In addition *E. cloacae* is usually positive for urease and malonate (65% and 75%, respectively) and *E. sakazakii* is usually negative (1% and <20%, respectively). Both species are usually motile and arginine dihydrolase-positive.

27. D DNase is not produced by *Cedecea* spp but is produced (along with proteinases) by *Serratia* spp. Other key differential tests include lipase (positive for *Cedecea*, negative for *Serratia*) and gelatin hydrolysis (negative for *Cedecea*, positive for *Serratia*).

28. B Biochemical differentiation is essential because *Citrobacter* isolates may give a false-positive agglutination test with *Salmonella* grouping sera. *C. freundii* strains, like *Salmonella* spp, are usually H_2S producers and may be confused with *Salmonella* spp unless the proper biochemical tests are utilized. *C. freundii* and *Salmonella* spp are adonitol-, indole-, and malonate-negative. However, *C. freundii* is KCN-positive, and *Salmonella* spp are KCN-negative.

29. B *Morganella* are biochemically similar to *Proteus* spp, both being lactose-negative, motile, and positive for phenylalanine deaminase and urease. However, *Morganella* can be differentiated from *Proteus* spp based upon H_2S, indole, ornithine decarboxylase, and xylose fermentation. *Ewingella* spp are usually positive (70%) for lactose fermentation, while the other three genera are lactose-negative.

30. D *K. oxytoca* and *K. pneumoniae* are almost identical biochemically, except for the ability to produce indole. Both organisms are usually positive for urease, sucrose, and citrate. However, *K. oxytoca* is indole-positive and *K. pneumoniae* is indole-negative.

31. Which of the following organisms, found in normal fecal flora, may be mistaken biochemically for the genus *Yersinia?*
A. *Klebsiella* spp
B. *Proteus* spp
C. *E. coli*
D. *Enterobacter* spp

Microbiology/Apply knowledge of fundamental biological characteristics/Gram-negative bacilli/2

32. Why might it be necessary for both pink (lactose-positive) and colorless (lactose-negative) colonies from an initial stool culture on MacConkey agar to be subcultured and tested further for possible pathogens?
A. Most *Shigella* strains are lactose-positive.
B. Most *Salmonella* strains are maltose-negative.
C. Most *Proteus* spp are lactose-negative.
D. Pathogenic *E. coli* can be lactose-positive or lactose-negative.

Microbiology/Evaluate laboratory data to make identifications/Gram-negative bacilli/2

33. Which agar that is used for routine stool cultures is the medium of choice for the isolation of *Yersinia* strains from stool specimens?
A. *Salmonella-Shigella* agar
B. Hektoen enteric agar
C. MacConkey agar
D. CNA agar

Microbiology/Select methods/Reagents/Media/Gram-negative bacilli/2

34. Which organism is sometimes mistaken for *Salmonella* and will agglutinate in *Salmonella* polyvalent antiserum?
A. *C. freundii* strains
B. *Proteus mirabilis* strains
C. *S. sonnei* strains
D. *Alkalencens-dispar* group

Microbiology/Apply knowledge of fundamental biological characteristics/Gram-negative bacilli/2

35. A bloody stool from a 26-year-old woman with 3 days of severe diarrhea showed the following results at 48 hours after being plated on the following media:

MacConkey agar: little normal flora with many non lactose-fermenting colonies
Hektoen enteric agar: many blue-green colonies
Campylobacter blood agar and *C. difficile* agar: no growth
Clear colonies (from MacConkey) tested negative for oxidase, indole, urea, motility and H₂S
The most likely identification is:

A. *Shigella* spp
B. *Salmonella* spp
C. *Proteus* spp
D. *E. coli*

Microbiology/Evaluate laboratory data to make identifications/Gram-negative bacilli/2

Answers to Questions 31–35

31. **B** *Proteus* spp are urease-positive as are approximately 70% of *Y. enterocolitica* isolates. Both organisms are lactose-negative and motile. However, *Yersinia* is motile at 22°C and not at 35°C (demonstrated using motility media).

32. **D** Possible pathogenic strains of *E. coli* should be picked from MacConkey agar and subcultured onto MacConkey agar with sorbitol. After subculture, these strains can be serotyped or sent to a reference laboratory. Most *E. coli* normal flora ferment D-sorbitol and appear pink to red on MacConkey-sorbitol agar. The *E. coli* strain O157:H7 causes the enteric disease hemorrhagic colitis. It ferments D-sorbitol slowly or not at all and appears as colorless colonies on MacConkey-sorbitol agar.

33. **C** Cefsulodin-irgasan-novobiocin (CIN) medium is the best agar for the isolation of *Yersinia* strains because it inhibits growth of other coliforms, but it is not used routinely in clinical laboratories. *Yersinia* spp grow well on MacConkey agar incubated at 37°C, but the colonies are much smaller than the other *Enterobacteriaceae;* therefore, 25°C is the temperature recommended for isolation. Some serotypes of *Yersinia* may be inhibited on more selective media, such as *Salmonella-Shigella* or Hektoen. CNA agar inhibits the growth of gram-negatives.

34. **A** *C. freundii* and *Salmonella* spp are H₂S-positive, indole, VP, and phenylalanine deaminase-negative. Biochemical characteristics that help to differentiate *C. freundii* from *Salmonella* include lactose fermentation (50% of *C. freundii* are lactose-positive while 100% of *Salmonella* are lactose-negative) and urease production (70% of *Citrobacter* are positive and >99% of *Salmonella* are negative).

35. **A** *Shigella* is the most likely organism biochemically. *E. coli* are usually indole- and motility-positive, and *Proteus* are motility- and urea-positive. Most *Salmonella* are H₂S-positive. *Shigella* and *Campylobacter* cause bloody diarrhea because they invade the epithelial cells of the large bowel; however, *Campylobacter* spp do not grow on MacConkey agar and they are oxidase-positive.

36. Which of the following organisms are generally positive for β-galactosidase?
A. *Salmonella* spp
B. *Shigella* spp
C. *Proteus* spp
D. *E. coli*

Microbiology/Evaluate laboratory data to make identifications/Gram-negative bacilli/2

37. In the Kauffmann-White schema, the combined antigens used for serological identification of the *Salmonella* spp are:
A. O antigens
B. H antigens
C. Vi and H antigens
D. O, Vi, and H antigens

Microbiology/Apply knowledge of fundamental biological characteristics/Gram-negative bacilli/1

38. The drugs of choice for treatment of infections with *Enterobacteriaceae* are:
A. Aminoglycosides, trimethoprim-sulfamethexazole, third-generation cephalosporins
B. Ampicillin and naladixic acid
C. Streptomycin and isoniazid
D. Chloramphenicol, ampicillin, and colistin

Microbiology/Apply knowledge of fundamental biological characteristics/Gram-negative bacilli/2

39. The Shiga-like toxin (verotoxin) is produced mainly by which *Enterobacteriaceae*?
A. *K. pneumoniae*
B. *E. coli*
C. *Salmonella typhimurium*
D. *E. cloacae*

Microbiology/Apply knowledge of fundamental biological characteristics/Gram-negative bacilli/2

40. Infections caused by *Yersinia pestis* are rare in the United States. Those cases that do occur are most frequently located in which region?
A. New Mexico, Arizona, and California
B. Alaska, Oregon, and Utah
C. North and South Carolina and Virginia
D. Ohio, Michigan, and Indiana

Microbiology/Apply knowledge of fundamental biological characteristics/Gram-negative bacilli/2

Answers to Questions 36–40

36. **D** *Enterobacteriaceae* are grouped according to their ability to ferment lactose, a β-galactoside. *Salmonella, Shigella, Proteus, Providencia,* and *Morganella* are usually lactose nonfermenters. Others including certain strains of *E. coli, S. sonnei, Hafnia alvei, Serratia marcescens,* and some *Yersinia* appear to be lactose nonfermenters because they lack the permease enzyme that actively transports lactose across the cell membrane. However, true lactose nonfermenters do not possess β-galactosidase. The test for β-galactosidase uses the substrate *o*-nitrophenyl-β-galactopyranoside. At an alkaline pH, β-galactosidase hydrolyses the substrate forming *o*-nitrophenol, which turns the medium yellow.

37. **D** The Kaufmann-White schema groups the *Salmonellae* on the basis of the somatic O (heat-stable) antigens and subdivides them into serotypes based on their flagellar H (heat-labile) antigens. The Vi (or K) antigen is a capsular polysaccharide that may be removed by heating. There are over 2200 serotypes of the *Salmonellae*.

38. **A** The drugs of choice for the *Enterobacteriaceae* vary and several genera display patterns of resistance that aid in their identification. *K. pneumoniae* and *Citrobacter diversus* are resistant to ampicillin and carbenicillin; most *Enterobacter* spp and *Hafnia* are resistant to ampicillin and cephalothin. *Proteus, Morganella,* and *Serratia* are resistant to colistin. *Providencia* and *Serratia* are resistant to multiple drugs. Several genera are resistent to chloramphenicol and most are resistant to penicillin.

39. **B** Strains of *E. coli* that produce one or both of the Shiga-like toxins (SLT I and SLT II) can cause a bloody diarrhea (hemorrhagic colitis). In the United States, *E. coli* strain O157:H7 is the serotype most often associated with hemorrhagic colitis.

40. **A** Approximately 15 cases of *Y. pestis* infection are confirmed in the United States annually. Most originate in the Southwest. It is necessary to be aware of this regional occurrence because untreated cases are associated with a mortality rate of approximately 60%. *Y. pestis* is not fastidious and grows well on blood agar. It is inactive biochemically, which helps to differentiate it from other *Enterobacteriaceae*.

41. A leg culture from a nursing home patient grew gram-negative rods on MacConkey agar as pink to dark pink oxidase-negative colonies. Given the following results, which is the most likely organism?

TSI = A/A	Indole = Neg
MR = Neg	VP = +
Citrate = +	H_2S = Neg
Urea = +	Motility = Neg

Antibiotic susceptibility: resistant to carbenicillin and ampicillin

A. *S. marcescens*
B. *P. vulgaris*
C. *E. cloacae*
D. *K. pneumoniae*

Microbiology/Evaluate laboratory data to make identifications/Gram-negative bacilli/3

42. Four blood cultures were taken over a 24-hour period from a 20-year-old woman with severe diarrhea. The cultures grew motile (room temperature), gram-negative rods. A urine specimen obtained by catheterization also showed gram-negative rods, 100,000 col/mL. Given the following results, which is the most likely organism?

TSI = A/A gas	Indole = +
VP = Neg	MR = +
H_2S = Neg	Citrate = Neg
Urea = Neg	Lysine decarboxylase = +
Phenylalanine deaminase = Neg	

A. *P. vulgaris*
B. *Salmonella typhi*
C. *Y. enterocolitica*
D. *E. coli*

Microbiology/Evaluate laboratory data to make identifications/Gram-negative bacilli/3

43. A stool culture from a 30-year-old man suffering from bloody mucoid diarrhea gave the following results on differential enteric media:

MacConkey agar = clear colonies; XLD agar = clear colonies; Hektoen agar = green colonies; *Salmonella-Shigella* agar = small, clear colonies

Which tests are most appropriate for identification of this enteric pathogen?

A. TSI, motility, indole, urea, *Shigella* typing with polyvalent sera
B. TSI, motility, indole, lysine, *Salmonella* typing with polyvalent sera
C. TSI, indole, MR, VP, citrate
D. TSI, indole, MR, and urea

Microbiology/Evaluate laboratory data to make identifications/Gram-negative bacilli/3

44. A leg-wound culture from a hospitalized 70-year-old diabetic man grew motile, lactose-negative colonies on MacConkey agar. Given the following biochemical reactions at 24 hours, what is the most probable organism?

H_2S (TSI) = Neg	Indole = Neg
MR = Neg	VP = +
Phenylalanine deaminase = Neg	DNase = +
Citrate = +	Urea = Neg
Ornithine and lysine decarboxylase = +	
Arginine decarboxylase = Neg	
Gelatin = +	

A. *P. vulgaris*
B. *S. marcescens*
C. *P. mirabilis*
D. *E. cloacae*

Microbiology/Evaluate laboratory data to make identifications/Gram-negative bacilli/3

Answers to Questions 41–44

41. D *K. pneumoniae* and *E. cloacae* display similar IMViC (indole, MR, VP, and citrate) reactions (00++) and TSI results. However, approximately 65% of *E. cloacae* strains are urea-positive compared to 98% of *K. pneumoniae*. *Enterobacter* spp are motile and *Klebsiella* are nonmotile. The antibiotic pattern of resistance to carbenicillin and ampicillin is characteristic for *Klebsiella*.

42. D Typically, the IMViC reactions for the organisms listed are:

E. coli	(++00)
S. typhi	(0+00)
Y. enterocolitica	(V+00)
P. vulgaris	(++00)

Note: Indole reaction is variable (V) for *Y. enterocolitica*.

43. A The most likely organism is a species of *Shigella*. Typically, *Salmonella* spp produce H_2S-positive colonies that display black centers on the differential media (except MacConkey agar). The biochemical tests above are necessary to differentiate *Shigella* from *E. coli* because some *E. coli* strains cross-react with *Shigella* typing sera. *Shigella* spp are one of the most common causes of bacterial diarrhea; group D (*S. sonnei*) and group B (*S. flexneri*) are the most often isolated species.

44. B *S. marcescens* has been implicated in numerous nosocomial infections and is recognized as an important pathogen with invasive properties. Gelatin hydrolysis and DNase are positive for both the *Proteus* spp and *Serratia*, but the negative urea and phenylalanine deaminase is differential. *E. cloacae* does not produce DNase, gelatinase, or lysine decarboxylase.

45. Three blood cultures taken from a 30-year-old cancer patient receiving chemotherapy and admitted with a urinary tract infection grew lactose-negative, motile, gram-negative rods prior to antibiotic therapy. Given the following biochemical reactions, which is the most likely organism?

H_2S (TSI) = +	Indole = +
MR = +	VP = Neg
Phenylalanine deaminase = +	DNase = +
Citrate = Neg	Urea = +
Gelatin hydrolysis = +	Ornithine de- carboxylase = Neg

A. *P. vulgaris*
B. *P. mirabilis*
C. *S. marcescens*
D. *K. pneumoniae*

Microbiology/Evaluate laboratory data to make identifications/Gram-negative bacilli/3

Answer to Question 45

45. **A** Although *P. mirabilis* is more frequently recovered from patients with urinary tract infections, *P. vulgaris* is commonly recovered from immunosuppressed patients. *P. mirabilis* is indole-negative and ornithine decarboxylase-positive but otherwise is very similar to *P. vulgaris*.

Nonfermentative Bacilli

1. What are the most appropriate screening tests to presumptively differentiate and identify the nonfermentative gram-negative bacilli (NFB) from the *Enterobacteriaceae?*
   A. Catalase, decarboxylation of arginine, growth on blood agar
   B. Motility, urease, morphology on blood agar
   C. Oxidase, TSI, nitrate reduction, growth on MacConkey agar
   D. Oxidase, indole, and growth on blood agar

   Microbiology/Evaluate laboratory data to make identifications/NFB/2

2. Presumptive tests used for identification of the *Pseudomonas* spp are:
   A. Oxidase, oxidation-fermentation (OF) glucose (open), OF glucose (sealed), motility, pigment production
   B. Growth on blood agar plate (BAP) and eosin-methylene blue (EMB) agars, lysine decarboxylation, catalase
   C. Growth on MacConkey, EMB, and XLD agars and motility
   D. Growth on mannitol salt agar and flagellar stain

   Microbiology/Evaluate laboratory data to make identifications/NFB/2

3. Which tests are most appropriate to differentiate between *P. aeruginosa* and *Pseudomonas putida?*
   A. Oxidase, motility, pyoverdin
   B. Oxidase, motility, lactose
   C. Oxidase, ONPG, DNase
   D. Mannitol, nitrate reduction, growth at 42°C

   Microbiology/Evaluate laboratory data to make identifications/NFB/2

4. Which test group best differentiates *Acinetobacter* spp from *P. aeruginosa?*
   A. Oxidase, motility, 42°C growth
   B. MacConkey growth, 37°C growth, catalase
   C. Blood agar growth, oxidase, catalase
   D. Oxidase, TSI, MacConkey growth

   Microbiology/Evaluate laboratory data to make identifications/NFB/2

Answers to Questions 1–4

1. **C** Nonfermentative bacilli will grow on the slant of TSI or KIA, but they do not acidify the butt (glucose fermentation) as do the *Enterobacteriaceae.* Nonfermentative bacilli can be cytochrome oxidase–positive or –negative, but all the *Enterobacteriaceae* are oxidase-negative. The *Enterobacteriaceae* grow well on MacConkey agar and reduce nitrate to nitrite, but the NFB grow poorly or not at all and most do not reduce nitrate. Nearly 70% of the NFB recovered from clinical specimens are:

   Strains of *P. aeruginosa*
   Acinetobacter baumannii (*A. anitratus*)
   Stenotrophomonas (*Xanthomonas*) *maltophilia*

2. **A** The use of OF tubes helps to determine the presumption of a nonfermentative bacillus (glucose oxidation–positive and glucose fermentation–negative). The positive cytochrome oxidase test and pigment production indicate a possible *Pseudomonas* spp. Several NFB produce pigments that aid in species identification: *P. aeruginosa* produces yellow pyoverdins (fluorescein) and/or pyocyanin (blue aqua pigment). The characteristic grapelike odor of aminoacetophenone as well as growth at 42°C are characteristics of *P. aeruginosa.*

3. **D** Both organisms are oxidase-positive, motile, and produce pyoverdin. Both are negative for ONPG and DNase. The differentiating tests are:

	P. aeruginosa	*P. putida*
Mannitol	+	0
Reduce NO$_3$ → NO$_2$	+	0
42°C growth	+	0

4. **A** *Acinetobacter* are nonmotile rods that appear as coccobacillary forms from clinical specimens. All are oxidase-negative and catalase-positive. *Acinetobacter* will grow at 30°C and 35°C, but not at 42°C.

5. In addition to motility, which test best differentiates *Acinetobacter* spp and *Alcaligenes* spp?
A. TSI
B. Oxidase
C. Catalase
D. Flagellar stain

Microbiology/Select methods/Reagents/Media/ NFB/Identification/2

6. The most noted differences between *P. aeruginosa* and *S. (X.) maltophilia* are:
A. Oxidase, catalase, and TSI
B. Oxidase, catalase, and ONPG
C. Oxidase, 42°C growth, and polar tuft of flagella
D. Catalase, TSI, and pigment

Microbiology/Evaluate laboratory data to make identifications/NFB/2

7. Which *Pseudomonas* is usually associated with a lung infection related to cystic fibrosis?
A. *P. fluorescens*
B. *P. aeruginosa*
C. *P. putida*
D. *Burkholderia (P.) pseudomallei*

Microbiology/Apply knowledge of fundamental biological characteristics/NFB/2

8. A nonfermenter recovered from an eye wound is oxidase-positive, motile with polar monotrichous flagella, and grows at 42°C. Colonies are dry, wrinkled or smooth, and buff to light brown in color, and are difficult to remove from the agar. In which DNA homology group should this organism be placed?
A. *Pseudomonas stutzeri*
B. *P. fluorescens*
C. *Pseudomonas alcaligenes*
D. *Pseudomonas diminuta*

Microbiology/Apply knowledge of fundamental biological characteristics/NFB/2

9. Which organism is associated with immunodeficiency syndromes and melioidosis (a glanderslike disease in Southeast Asia and northern Australia)?
A. *P. aeruginosa*
B. *P. stutzeri*
C. *P. putida*
D. *B. (P.) pseudomallei*

Microbiology/Apply knowledge of fundamental biological characteristics/NFB/2

10. Which biochemical tests are needed to differentiate *Burkholderia (P.) cepacia* from *S. (X.) maltophilia?*
A. Pigment on blood agar, oxidase, DNase
B. Pigment on MacConkey agar, flagellar stain, motility
C. Glucose, maltose, lysine decarboxylase
D. TSI, motility, oxidase

Microbiology/Evaluate laboratory data to make identifications/NFB/2

Answers to Questions 5–10

5. **B** The two genera, *Acinetobacter* and *Alcaligenes*, are very similar. Both use oxidation for the metabolism of carbohydrate, with some strains being nonsaccharolytic. Both grow well on MacConkey agar. However, *Acinetobacter* is nonmotile and oxidase-negative. *Alcaligenes* is motile by peritrichous flagella and oxidase-positive.

6. **C** The two genera, *Pseudomonas* and *Stenotrophomonas* (*Xanthomonas*), are motile and grow well on MacConkey agar. However, *P. aeruginosa* is oxidase-positive and grows at 42°C but is motile only by polar monotrichous flagella. *S. (X.) maltophilia* is oxidase-negative, does not grow at 42°C, and is motile by a polar tuft of flagella.

7. **B** *P. aeruginosa* is often recovered from the respiratory secretion of cystic fibrosis patients. If the patient is chronically infected with the mucoid strain of *P. aeruginosa*, the biochemical identification is very difficult. The mucoid strain results from production of large amounts of alginate, a polysaccharide that surrounds the cell.

8. **A** *P. stutzeri* produces dry, wrinkled colonies that are tough and adhere to the media as well as smooth colonies. *B. (P.) pseudomallei* produces similar colony types but is distinguished by biochemical tests and susceptibility to the polymixins. The colonies of *P. stutzeri* are buff to light brown due to the relatively high concentration of cytochromes.

9. **D** *B. (P.) pseudomallei* produces wrinkled colonies resembling *P. stutzeri*. Infections are usually asymptomatic and can be diagnosed only by serological methods. The organism exists in soil and water in an area of latitude 20° north and south of the equator (mainly in Thailand and Vietnam). Thousands of U.S. military personnel were infected during the 1960s and 1970s. The disease may reactivate many years after exposure and has been called the "Vietnamese time bomb."

10. **A** Both organisms produce yellowish pigment and have polar tuft flagella, but the oxidase and DNase tests are differential.

	B. (P.) cepacia	*S. (X.) maltophilia*
Pigment on BAP	Green-yellow	Lavender-green
Oxidase	+	0
DNase	0	+
Motility	+	+
Glucose OF (open)	+	+
Maltose OF (open)	+	+
Lysine decarboxylase	+	+

11. The following results were obtained from a pure culture of gram-negative rods recovered from the pulmonary secretions of a 10-year-old cystic fibrosis patient with pneumonia:

Oxidase = + Motility = +
Glucose OF (open) = + Gelatin = +
Pigment = Red Arginine dihydrolase = +
  (nonfluorescent)
Growth at 42°C = + Flagella = + (polar
   monotrichous)

Which is the most likely organism?
A. *B. (P.) pseudomallei*
B. *P. stutzeri*
C. *B. (P.) cepacia*
D. *P. aeruginosa*

Microbiology/Evaluate laboratory data to make identifications/NFB/3

12. *Alcaligenes faecalis* (formerly *A. odorans*) is distinguished from *Bordetella bronchiseptica* with which test?
A. Urea (rapid)
B. Oxidase
C. Growth on MacConkey agar
D. Motility

Microbiology/Evaluate laboratory data to make identifications/NFB/2

13. *Flavobacterium* spp are easily distinguished from *Acinetobacter* spp by which of the following two tests?
A. Oxidase, growth on MacConkey agar
B. Oxidase and OF (glucose)
C. TSI and urea hydrolysis
D. TSI and VP

Microbiology/Evaluate laboratory data to make identifications/NFB/2

14. A gram-negative coccobacillus was recovered on chocolate agar from CSF of an immunosuppressed patient. The organism was nonmotile and positive for indophenol oxidase but failed to grow on MacConkey agar. The organism was highly susceptible to penicillin. The most probable identification is:
A. *Acinetobacter* spp
B. *P. aeruginosa*
C. *P. stutzeri*
D. *Moraxella lacunata*

Microbiology/Evaluate laboratory data to make identifications/NFB/2

15. Cetrimide agar is used as a selective isolation agar for which organism?
A. *Acinetobacter* spp
B. *P. aeruginosa*
C. *Moraxella* spp
D. *S. (X.) maltophilia*

Microbiology/Select methods/Reagents/Media/ NFB/Identification/2

Answers to Questions 11–15

11. **D** The oxidase test and red pigment (pyorubin), as well as growth at 42°C, distinguish *P. aeruginosa* from the other pseudomonads listed, particularly *B. cepacia*, which is also associated with cystic fibrosis.

12. **A** *Alcaligenes* and *Bordetella* are genera belonging to the *Alcaligenaceae* family. The two organisms are very similar biochemically, but *B. bronchiseptica* is urea-positive. Both organisms are oxidase-positive, grow on MacConkey agar, and are motile by peritrichous flagella. *B. bronchiseptica* grows well on MacConkey, but other species of *Bordetella* are fastidious gram-negative rods.

13. **A** *Flavobacterium* spp and *Acinetobacter* spp often produce a yellow pigment on blood or chocolate agar and are nonmotile. *Acinetobacter* spp are oxidase-negative, grow on MacConkey agar, and are coccobacillary on the Gram stain smear. In contrast, *Flavobacterium* spp are oxidase-positive, do not grow on MacConkey agar, and are typically rod-shaped. *Flavobacterium meningosepticum* is highly pathogenic for premature infants.

14. **D** *Moraxella* spp are oxidase-positive and nonmotile, which distinguish them from *Acinetobacter* spp and most *Pseudomonas* spp. *Moraxella* spp are highly sensitive to penicillin, but *Acinetobacter* spp and *Pseudomonas* spp are penicillin-resistant. *M. lacunata* is implicated in infections involving immunosuppressed patients.

15. **B** Cetrimide (acetyl trimethyl ammonium bromide) agar is used for the isolation and identification of *P. aeruginosa*. With the exception of *P. fluorescens*, the other pseudomonads are inhibited along with related nonfermentative bacteria.

16. A specimen from a 15-year-old female burn patient was cultured after debridement, and the following results were obtained:

Oxidase = +

Catalase = +

Ornithine decarboxylase = Neg

Arginine dihydrolase = +

Penicillin = Resistant

Colistin (Polymixin B) = Susceptible

Lysine decarboxylase = Neg

Motility = +

Glucose = + for oxidation (open tube)

Maltose = Neg for oxidation (open tube)

Aminoglycosides = Susceptible

These results indicate which of the following organisms?
A. *A. (calcoaceticus) baumannii*
B. *M. lacunata*
C. *P. aeruginosa*
D. *Acinetobacter lwoffii*

Microbiology/Evaluate laboratory data to make identifications/NFB/ 3

17. A yellow pigment-producing organism that is oxidase-positive, nonmotile, and does not grow on MacConkey agar is:
A. *A. (calcoaceticus) baumannii*
B. *A. lwoffii*
C. *B. (P.) cepacia*
D. *F. meningosepticum*

Microbiology/Evaluate laboratory data to make identifications/NFB/2

18. Which reagent(s) is(are) used to develop the red color indicative of a positive reaction in the nitrate reduction test?
A. Sulfanilic acid and α-naphthylamine
B. Ehrlich and Kovacs reagents
C. *o*-Nitrophenyl-β-D-galactopyranoside
D. Kovac's reagent

Microbiology/Apply knowledge of biochemical reactions/bacteria/1

19. A culture from an intra-abdominal abscess produced orange-tan colonies on blood agar that gave the following results:

Oxidase = +

KIA = Alk/Alk (H$_2$S) +

DNase = +

Ornithine decarboxylase = +

Nitrate reduction = +

Motility = + (single polar flagellum)

Growth at 42°C = Neg

The most likely identification is:
A. *Shewanella (Pseudomonas) putrefaciens*
B. *Acinetobacter* spp
C. *P. aeruginosa*
D. *Flavobacterium* spp

Microbiology/Evaluate laboratory data to make identifications/NFB/3

20. *Flavobacterium* spp and *B. (P.) cepacia* are easily differentiated by which test?
A. Motility
B. OF glucose
C. Oxidase
D. Cetrimide agar

Microbiology/Evaluate laboratory data to make identifications/NFB/2

Answers to Questions 16–20

16. **C** *P. aeruginosa* is a cause of a significant number of burn wound infections; these organisms can exist in distilled water and underchlorinated water. *Acinetobacter* spp are oxidase-negative and *Moraxella* spp are highly susceptible to penicillin, ruling them out as possible causes.

17. **D** All species of *Acinetobacter* are oxidase-negative and grow on MacConkey agar. *Flavobacterium* spp produce yellow pigment like *Acinetobacter* but are oxidase-positive and do not grow on MacConkey agar. *B. (P.) cepacia* also produces a yellow pigment but is motile.

18. **A** In the nitrate test, nitrites formed by bacterial reduction of nitrates will diazotize sulfanilic acid. The diazonium compound complexes with α-naphthylamine, forming a red product. Media containing nitrates are used for the identification of nonfermenters. When testing nonfermenters, it is wise to confirm a negative reaction using zinc dust. The diazonium compound detects nitrite only, and the organism may have reduced the nitrates to nitrogen, ammonia, nitrous oxide, or hydroxylamine. Zinc ions reduce residual nitrates in the media to nitrites. A red color produced after addition of zinc indicates the presence of residual nitrates confirming a true negative reaction. If a red or pink color does not occur after adding zinc, then the organism reduced the nitrate to a product other than nitrite, and the test is considered positive.

19. **A** *S. putrefaciens* produces abundant H$_2$S on KIA or TSI (alkaline butt distinguishes it from other dextrose-negative nonfermentative bacilli).

20. **A** *B. (P.) cepacia* (93%) are weakly oxidase-positive and motile. *Flavobacterium* spp are oxidase-positive but are nonmotile.

Miscellaneous and Fastidious Gram-Negative Rods

1. A visitor to South America who returned with diarrhea is suspected to be infected with *V. cholerae*. Select the best media for recovery and identification of this organism.
   A. MacConkey agar
   B. Blood agar
   C. TCBS agar
   D. XLD agar

   Microbiology/Select methods/Reagents/Media/ Bacteria/Identification/2

2. A curved gram-negative rod producing oxidase-positive colonies on blood agar was recovered from a stool culture. Given the following results, what is the most likely identification?

   Lysine = +   Arginine = Neg Indole = +
   KIA = Alk/Acid VP = Neg   Lactose = Neg
   Urease = ±   String test = Neg TCBS agar =
                                    Green colonies

   A. *V. cholerae*
   B. *Vibrio parahaemolyticus*
   C. *Shigella* spp
   D. *Salmonella* spp

   Microbiology/Evaluate laboratory data to make identifications/Bacteria/3

3. A gram-negative S-shaped rod recovered from selective media for *Campylobacter* species gave the following results:

   Catalase = +   Oxidase = +
   Motility = +   Hippurate hydrolysis = +
   Growth at 42°C = Pos   Naladixic acid = Susceptible
   Pigment = Neg   Grape odor = Neg
   Cephalothin = Resistant

   The most likely identification is:
   A. *P. aeruginosa*
   B. *Campylobacter jejuni*

   C. *C. fetus*
   D. *P. putida*

   Microbiology/Evaluate laboratory data to make identifications/Bacteria/3

Answers to Questions 1–3

1. **C** The growth of yellow colonies on TCBS agar (citrate utilization and acid from sucrose) is diagnostic for *V. cholerae*. On blood agar, *V. cholerae* of the *El Tor* biotype appear as large, translucent, β-hemolytic colonies, and will agglutinate chicken erythrocytes.

2. **B** *V. parahaemolyticus* appear as green colonies on TCBS agar, while *V. cholerae* appear as yellow colonies on TCBS. *V. cholerae* is the only *Vibrio* species that will cause a positive string test. In the test, a loopful of bacterial colonies is suspended in sodium deoxycholate, 0.5%, on a glass slide. After 60 seconds, the inoculating loop is lifted out of the suspension. *V. cholerae* forms a long string resembling a string of pearls. *Salmonella* spp and *Shigella* spp are oxidase-negative.

3. **B** The only *Campylobacter* spp to hydrolyze hippurate are *C. jejuni* and subsp *doylei*. However, some strains of *P. aeruginosa* will grow on agar selective for the *Campylobacter* at 42°C. *C. fetus* will not grow at 42°C but will grow at 25°C and 37°C.

4. Which atmospheric condition is needed to recover *Campylobacter* spp from specimens inoculated onto a Campy-selective agar at 35°–37°C and 42°C?
   A. 5% O_2, 10% CO_2, and 85% N_2
   B. 20% O_2, 10% CO_2, and 70% N_2
   C. 20% O_2, 20% CO_2, and 60% N_2
   D. 20% O_2, 5% CO_2, and 75% N_2

   Microbiology/Apply knowledge of fundamental biological characteristics/Bacteria/2

5. Which group of tests best differentiates *Helicobacter pylori* from *C. jejuni*?
   A. Catalase, oxidase, and Gram stain
   B. Catalase, oxidase, and nalidixic acid sensitivity
   C. Catalase, oxidase, and cephalothin sensitivity
   D. Urease, nitrate, and hippurate hydrolysis

   Microbiology/Select methods/Reagents/Media/ Bacteria/Identification/2

6. Which of the following tests should be done first in order to differentiate *Aeromonas* spp from the *Enterobacteriaceae*?
   A. Urease
   B. OF glucose
   C. Oxidase
   D. Catalase

   Microbiology/Select methods/Reagents/Media/ Bacteria/Identification/2

7. Which is the best rapid test to differentiate *Plesiomonas shigelloides* from a *Shigella* species on selective enteric agar?
   A. Oxidase
   B. Indole
   C. TSI
   D. Urease

   Microbiology/Select methods/Reagents/Media/ Bacteria/Identification/2

8. Which are the best two tests to differentiate *A. hydrophilia* from *P. shigelloides*?
   A. Oxidase and motility
   B. DNase and VP
   C. Indole and lysine decarboxylase
   D. Growth on MacConkey and blood agar

   Microbiology/Select methods/Reagents/Media/ Bacteria/Identification/2

Answers to Questions 4–8

4. **A** *Campylobacter* spp are best recovered in a microaerophilic atmosphere (reduced O_2). The use of a CO_2 incubator or candle jar is not recommended because the amount of O_2 and CO_2 do not permit any but the most aerotolerant *Campylobacter* to survive. Cultures for *Campylobacter* should be incubated for 48–72 hours before reporting no growth.

5. **D** *H. pylori* is found in specimens from gastric secretions and biopsies and has been implicated as a cause of gastric ulcers. It is found only in the mucus-secreting epithelial cells of the stomach. Both *H. pylori* and *C. jejuni* are catalase- and oxidase-positive. However, *Helicobacter* spp are urease-positive, which differentiates them from *Campylobacter* spp.

	H. pylori	*C. jejuni*
Nitrate reduction	0	+
Hippurate hydrolysis	0	+
Urease	+	0
Cephalothin sensitivity	S	R
Nalixidic acid sensitivity	R	S

6. **C** *Aeromonas hydrophilia* and other *Aeromonas* spp have been implicated in acute diarrheal disease as well as cellulitis and wound infections. Infections usually follow exposure to contaminated soil, water, or food. *Aeromonas* growing on enteric media are differentiated from the *Enterobacteriaceae* by demonstrating that colonies are oxidase-positive. The *Aeromonas* are sometimes overlooked as pathogens because most strains grow on selective enteric agar as lactose fermenters.

7. **A** *P. shigelloides* is a lactose nonfermenter that will resemble *Shigella* spp on MacConkey agar. Both are TSI Alk/Acid and urease-negative. *Plesiomonas* produces indole and *Shigella* usually causes delayed production of indole. However, *Plesiomonas* is oxidase-positive while *Shigella* spp are oxidase-negative.

8. **B** Both of these bacteria cause diarrhea, grow well on enteric agar, and may be confused with *Enterobacteriaceae*. Both organisms are oxidase–, motility–, indole–, and lysine decarboxylase– positive. The following reactions are differential:

	A. hydrophilia	*P. shigelloides*
β-Hemolysis on sheep blood agar	+	0
DNase	+	0
VP	+	0

9. Which genus (in which most species are oxidase- and catalase-positive) of small gram-negative coccobacilli is associated mainly with animals but may cause endocarditis, bacteremia, wound, and dental infections in humans?
A. *Actinobacillus*
B. *Pseudomonas*
C. *Campylobacter*
D. *Vibrio*

Microbiology/Apply fundamental biological characteristics/Bacteria/2

10. Which of the following tests may be used to differentiate *Cardiobacterium hominis* from *Actinobacillus* spp?
A. Gram stain
B. Indole
C. Anaerobic incubation
D. Oxidase

Microbiology/Select methods/Reagents/Media/ Bacteria/Identification/2

11. A mixture of slender gram-negative rods and coccobacilli with rounded ends was recovered from blood cultures following root canal surgery. Given the following results after 48 hours, what is the most likely organism?

Catalase = Neg	Ornithine
Urease = Neg	decarboxylase = +
Oxidase = +	Lysine decarboxylase = +
Indole = Neg	X and V requirement = Neg
Carbohydrates =	Growth on blood and
Neg (no acid	chocolate agar = + (with
produced)	pitting of agar)
	Growth on MacConkey agar
	= Neg

A. *Eikenella corrodens*
B. *Actinobacillus* sp
C. *C. hominis*
D. *Proteus* sp

Microbiology/Evaluate laboratory data to make identifications/Bacteria/3

12. *Kingella kingae* can best be differentiated from *E. corrodens* using which media?
A. Sheep blood agar
B. Chocolate agar
C. MacConkey agar
D. XLD agar

Microbiology/Select methods/Reagents/Media/ Bacteria/Identification/2

13. *K. kingae* is usually associated with which type of infection?
A. Middle ear
B. Endocarditis

C. Meningitis
D. Urogenital

Microbiology/Apply fundamental biological characteristics/Bacteria/1

Answers to Questions 9–13

9. **A** *Actinobacillus* spp (formerly CDC groups HB-3 and HB-4) share many biochemical characteristics of the *Haemophilus* spp. Infections most often associated with this gram-negative coccobacillus are subacute bacterial endocarditis and periodontal disease (its main habitat is in the mouth). The most common human isolate is *Actinobacillus actinomycetemcomitans*, which grows slowly on chocolate agar. It is positive for catalase, nitrate reduction, and glucose fermentation. It does not grow on MacConkey agar and is negative for oxidase, urease, indole, X, and V requirements.

10. **B** *C. hominis* is a gram-negative coccobacillus biochemically similar to *Actinobacillus* spp. Like *Actinobacillus*, it is a cause of endocarditis. However, *Cardiobacterium* spp are positive for cytochrome oxidase and negative for nitrate reduction, while most *Actinobacillus* are negative for oxidase and positive for nitrate reduction. *C. hominis* will grow on blood agar after 48–72 hours in 5% CO_2 at 35°C, but *Actinobacillus* requires chocolate agar.

11. **A** *E. corrodens* is a part of the normal flora of the upper respiratory tract and the mouth. It is often seen after trauma to the head, neck; dental infections; and human bite wounds. It requires blood for growth. The organism causes a pitting of the agar where colonies are located. The smell of bleach may be apparent when the plates are uncovered for examination. *Actinobacillus* spp and *C. hominis* both utilize several carbohydrates, and *Proteus* spp are oxidase-negative.

12. **A** Both *K. kingae* and *E. corrodens* are gram-negative rods that are oxidase-positive and catalase-negative. Both grow well on blood and chocolate agars and cause pitting of the media, and neither grow on MacConkey or XLD agar. However, *K. kingae* strains produce a narrow zone of β-hemolysis on blood agar (sheep) similar to group B *Streptococcus*.

13. **B** *Kingella* spp are gram-negative coccobacilli or plump-looking rods. They are part of the normal flora of the upper respiratory and urogenital tracts of humans. Infection is seen primarily with patients having underlying heart disease, poor oral hygiene, or iatrogenic mucosal ulcerations (e.g., radiation therapy) where the organism is recovered from blood cultures.

14. Cultures obtained from a dog bite wound produced yellow, tan, and slightly pink colonies on blood and chocolate agar with a margin of fingerlike projections appearing as a film around the colonies. Given the following results at 24 hours, which is the most likely organism?

Oxidase = +; Catalase = +; growth on MacConkey agar = neg; motility = neg
A. *Actinobacillus* spp
B. *Eikenella* spp
C. *Capnocytophaga* spp
D. *Pseudomonas* spp

Microbiology/Evaluate laboratory data to make identifications/Bacteria/3

15. Smooth gray colonies showing no hemolysis are recovered from an infected cat scratch on blood and chocolate agar but fail to grow on MacConkey agar. The organisms are gram-negative pleomorphic rods that are both catalase- and oxidase-positive and strongly indole-positive. The most likely organism is:
A. *Capnocytophaga* spp
B. *Pasteurella* spp
C. *Proteus* spp
D. *Pseudomonas* spp

Microbiology/Evaluate laboratory data to make identifications/Bacteria/3

16. Which media should be used to recover *Bordetella pertussis* from a nasopharyngeal specimen?
A. Chocolate agar
B. Blood agar
C. MacConkey agar
D. Bordet-Gengou agar

Microbiology/Select methods/Reagents/Media/ Bacteria/Identification/2

17. Which media is recommended for the recovery of *Brucella* spp from blood and bone marrow specimens?
A. Biphasic Castenada bottles with *Brucella* broth
B. Blood culture bottles with *Brucella* broth
C. Bordet-Gengou agar plates and THIO broth
D. Blood culture bottles with THIO broth

Microbiology/Select methods/Reagents/Media/ Bacteria/Identification/2

Answers to Questions 14–17

14. **C** *Capnocytophaga gingivalis, C. sputigena,* and *C. ochracea* are part of the normal oropharyngeal flora of humans; however, *C. canimorsus* and *C. cynodegmi* (formerly CDC groups DF-2 and DF-2-like bacteria) are associated with infections resulting from dog bite wounds.

15. **B** *Pasteurella multocida* (*P. canis*) is part of the normal mouth flora of cats and dogs and is frequently recovered from wounds inflicted by them. It produces large amounts of indole and therefore an odor resembling colonies of *E. coli*. *Pseudomonas* spp are also catalase- and oxidase-positive but can be ruled out because they grow on MacConkey agar and do not produce indole.

16. **D** *B. pertussis* is an oxidase-positive, nonmotile gram-negative coccobacillus and appears as small, round colonies resembling droplets of mercury. It is fastidious and does not grow on chocolate or MacConkey agar. However, *B. pertussis* will adapt to blood agar, growing within 3–6 days. This organism is the cause of whooping cough, which has declined with the policy of mandatory diphtheria, tetanus, pertussis (DPT) immunization of infants in the United States. The DPT vaccine contains diphtheria and tetanus toxoids and killed whole-cell *B. pertussis*.

17. **A** Although blood agar will support the growth of *Brucella* spp, Castenada bottles are the media of choice. Castenada bottles contain a slant of enriched agar medium that is partially submerged and surrounded by an enriched broth medium. As the specimen is injected into the bottles and mixed, the agar slant is simultaneously coated with the blood (or bone marrow). *Brucella* is the cause of undulant fever and is responsible for many cases of fever of unknown origin. *Brucella* spp are facultative intracellular organisms and grow very slowly, usually requiring 4–6 weeks for recovery. *Brucella melitensis* is the most often recovered species.

18. In addition to CO_2 requirements and biochemical characteristics, *B. melitensis* and *Brucella abortus* are differentiated by growth on media containing which two dyes?
A. Basic fuchsin and thionin
B. Methylene blue and crystal violet
C. Carbol fuchsin and iodine
D. Safranin and methylene blue

Microbiology/Select methods/Reagents/Media/ Bacteria/Identification/2

19. Which of the following amino acids are required for growth of *Francisella tularensis*?
A. Leucine and ornithine
B. Arginine and lysine
C. Cysteine and cystine
D. Histidine and tryptophan

Microbiology/Apply fundamental biological characteristics/Bacteria/1

20. Which media is best for recovery of *Legionella pneumophila* from clinical specimens?
A. Chocolate agar
B. Bordet-Gengou agar
C. New yeast extract agar
D. Buffered charcoal-yeast extract (CYE) agar

Microbiology/Select methods/Reagents/Media/ Bacteria/Identification/1

21. *H. influenzae*, which requires X and V factors for growth, can be differentiated from subspecies *Haemophilus aegyptius* by which two tests?
A. Indole and xylose
B. Glucose and urease
C. Oxidase and catalase
D. Indole and oxidase

Microbiology/Select methods/Reagents/Media/ Bacteria/Identification/2

22. *Haemophilus* species that require the V factor (NAD) are easily recovered on which agar plate?
A. Blood agar made with sheep red cells
B. Blood agar made with horse red cells
C. Chocolate agar
D. Xylose agar

Microbiology/Select methods/Reagents/Media/ Bacteria/Identification/2

23. Which of the following products is responsible for satellite growth of *Haemophilus* spp around colonies of *Staphylococcus* and *Neisseria* spp on sheep blood agar?
A. NAD
B. Hemin
C. Indole
D. Oxidase

Microbiology/Apply fundamental biological characteristics/Bacteria/1

Answers to Questions 18–23

18. **A** *B. abortus* can be differentiated from *B. melitensis* by the reactions shown at the bottom of the page:

19. **C** *F. tularensis* is a fastidious gram-negative rod that is best recovered from lymph node aspirates and tissue biopsies. It is oxidase-negative, nonmotile, and inert biochemically. Cysteine blood agar is the medium of choice, but *F. tularensis* will grow on commercially prepared chocolate agar because it contains X factor and is supplemented with a growth enrichment (IsoVitaleX) that contains cysteine. *F. tularensis* may not grow well on MacConkey agar.

20. **D** *L. pneumophilia* should be recovered on buffered CYE agar. This agar is nonselective but can be made more selective for *Legionella* spp by addition of the antibiotics cefamandole, polymyxin B, and anisomycin. Any small, glistening, convex colonies on buffered CYE agar after 2–3 days of incubation that do not grow on L-cysteine–deficient buffered CYE agar or routine nonselective media should be further tested by the direct fluorescent antibody test (DFA) for confirmation of *L. pneumophila*.

21. **A** *H. influenzae* and subspecies *H. aegyptius* are both glucose, urease, oxidase, and catalase-positive. *H. influenzae* (biotype II) is positive for both indole and xylose, while *H. aegyptius* is negative for both tests. Biotype II encompasses 40%–70% of *H. influenzae* strains recovered from clinical specimens. *H. influenzae* subspecies *aegyptius* is responsible for epidemics of conjunctivitis in children.

22. **C** The V factor, NAD, must first be released from RBCs before it can be assimilated by *Haemophilus* spp. Chocolate agar is made by heating blood agar in order to lyse RBCs. The released NAD is directly available to those *Haemophilus* species requiring it. Chocolate agar also contains the X factor (hemin). All *Haemophilus* except *H. ducreyi* and *H. aphrophilus* require V factor, while X factor is required by *H. influenzae*, *H. haemolyticus*, and *H. ducreyi*.

23. **A** Colonies growing on sheep blood agar secreting NAD (V factor) or producing β-hemolysins (which lyse the sheep RBCs releasing NAD) allow pinpoint-size colonies of *Haemophilus* spp to grow around them. Sheep blood agar alone does not support the growth of *Haemophilus* spp, which require V factor due to the presence of V factor-inactivating enzymes that are present in the agar.

	H$_2$S	Urease	CO$_2$ Requirement	Basic Fuchsin	Thionin (20 mg)
B. melitensis	0	V	0	+	+
B. abortus	+	+	+/V	+	0

24. Which of the following plates should be used in order to identify *H. haemolyticus* and *Haemophilus parahaemolyticus*?
A. Sheep blood agar and chocolate agar
B. Horse blood agar and Mueller-Hinton agar with X and V strips
C. Brain-heart infusion agar with sheep red cells added
D. Chocolate agar and Mueller-Hinton agar with X factor added

Microbiology/Select methods/Reagents/Media/ Bacteria/Identification/2

25. The majority of *H. influenzae* infections are caused by which of the following capsular serotypes?
A. a
B. b
C. c
D. d

Microbiology/Correlate clinical and laboratory data/Bacteria/Haemophilus/2

26. Which *Haemophilus* species is generally associated with endocarditis?
A. *H. influenzae*
B. *H. ducreyi*
C. *H. aphrophilus*
D. *H. haemolyticus*

Microbiology/Correlate clinical and laboratory data/Bacteria/Haemophilus/2

27. Which *Haemophilus* species is difficult to isolate and recover from genital ulcers and swollen lymph nodes?
A. *H. aphrophilus*
B. *H. ducreyi*
C. *H. haemolyticus*
D. *H. parahaemolyticus*

Microbiology/Correlate clinical and laboratory data/Bacteria/Haemophilus/2

28. Which of the following is a characteristic of strains of *H. influenzae* that are resistant to ampicillin?
A. Production of β-lactamase enzymes
B. Hydrolysis of chloramphenicol
C. Hydrolysis of urea
D. All of the above

Microbiology/Apply fundamental biological characteristics/Bacteria/1

Answers to Questions 24–28

24. B Production of β-hemolysis is used to distinguish these two species from other *Haemophilus* with the same X and V requirements. Horse blood agar furnishes X factor and, when supplemented with yeast extract, supports the growth of *Haemophilus* spp. Sheep blood agar is not used because it contains growth inhibitors of some *Haemophilus* spp. The chart below summarizes the characteristics of the *Haemophilus* spp.

25. B The majority of *H. influenzae* infections occur in children under 5 years old, and are caused by capsular serotype b, one of six serotypes designated a through f. This strain appears to contain a virulence factor making it resistant to phagocytosis and intracellular killing by neutrophils. Serotyping of *Haemophilus* is performed by mixing colonies with agglutinating antibodies available as commercial agglutination kits.

26. C *H. aphrophilus* does not require either X or V factor for growth and is differentiated from the other *Haemophilus* species by its ability to produce acid from lactose and a positive δ-aminolevulinic acid (ALA) test. *H. influenzae* and *H. haemolyticus* are incapable of synthesizing protoporphyrin from δ-ALA and are negative for this test.

27. B *H. ducreyi* requires exogenous X factor and causes genital lesions referred to as "soft chancres." The media used for recovery is commercial chocolate agar or gonococcus base media containing 1%–2% hemoglobin, 5% fetal calf serum, and 1% IsoVitaleX enrichment. The plates must be incubated in a 3%–5% CO_2 environment for 2–3 days. Most specimens are recovered from heterosexuals, and outbreaks in the United States are traced to female prostitutes.

28. A Roughly 20% of *H. influenzae* strains produce β-lactamase, which hydrolyses and inactivates the β-lactam ring of ampicillin (and penicillin).

	H. influenzae	*H. parainfluenzae*	*H. haemolyticus*	*H. parahaemolyticus*	*H. aphrophilus*	*H. aegyptius*	*H. ducreyi*
X factor	+	0	+	0	0	+	+
V factor	+	+	+	+	0	+	0
Hemolysis	0	0	+	+	0	0	0

29. A small, gram-negative coccobacillus recovered from CSF of a 2-year-old gave the following results:

Indole = +   Glucose = + (acid)
X requirement = +   V requirement = +
Urease = +   Lactose = Neg
Sucrose = Neg   Hemolysis = Neg

Which is the most likely identification?
A. *H. parainfluenzae*
B. *H. influenzae*
C. *H. ducreyi*
D. *H. aphrophilus*

Microbiology/Evaluate laboratory data to make identifications/Bacteria/3

30. The δ-ALA test (for porphyrins) is a confirmatory procedure for which test used for identification of *Haemophilus* species?
A. X factor requirement
B. V factor requirement
C. Urease production
D. Indole production

Microbiology/Apply knowledge to recognize sources of error/Bacteria/Identification/3

Answers to Questions 29–30

29. **B** Although several biotypes of *H. parainfluenzae* produce indole and urease, *H. parainfluenzae* does not require X factor for growth. *H. ducreyi* requires X factor but not V factor. *H. aphrophilus* does not require either X factor or V factor for growth.

30. **A** The X factor requirement for growth is the cause of many inaccuracies when identifying *Haemophilus* spp requiring this factor. False-negative results have been attributed to the presence of small amounts of hemin present in the basal media, or X factor carryover from colonies transferred from primary media containing blood. The δ-ALA test determines the ability of an organism to synthesize protoporphyrin intermediates in the biosynthetic pathway to hemin from the precursor compound δ-aminolevulinic acid. *Haemophilus* species that need exogenous X factor to grow are unable to synthesize protoporphyrin from δ-ALA and are negative for the δ-ALA test. These include *H. influenzae, H. haemolyticus, H. aegyptius,* and *H. ducreyi.*

Gram-Positive and Gram-Negative Cocci

1. The test(s) used most often to separate the *Micrococcaceae* family from the *Streptococcaceae* family is (are) the:
   A. Bacitracin
   B. Catalase
   C. Hemolysis pattern
   D. All of the above

   Microbiology/Select methods/Reagents/Media/ Bacteria/Identification/1

2. *Micrococcus* and *Staphylococcus* species are differentiated by which test(s)?
   A. Fermentation of glucose (OF tube)
   B. Catalase test
   C. Gram stain
   D. All of the above

   Microbiology/Select methods/Reagents/Media/ Bacteria/Identification/1

3. Lysostaphin is used to differentiate a *Staphylococcus* from which other genus?
   A. *Streptococcus*
   B. *Stomatococcus*
   C. *Micrococcus*
   D. *Planococcus*

   Microbiology/Select methods/Reagents/Media/ Bacteria/Identification/2

Answers to Questions 1–3

1. **B** The catalase test (utilizing a 3% hydrogen peroxide (H_2O_2) solution stored in a brown bottle under refrigeration) is positive for the four genera belonging to the *Micrococcaceae* family: *Planococcus, Micrococcus, Stomatococcus,* and *Staphylococcus.* Members of the *Streptococcaceae* family are negative. *Planococcus* spp are associated with marine life and not human infections. *Stomatococcus* spp are implicated in endocarditis following cardiac catheterization; they are weakly catalase-positive and produce white or transparent, sticky colonies on agar, which help to differentiate them from *Staphylococcus.*

2. **A** Both micrococci and staphylococci are catalase-positive and gram-positive cocci. On direct smears they both appear as pairs, short chains (resembling *Streptococcus* spp), or clusters. However, the micrococci fail to produce acid from glucose under anaerobic conditions. The OF tube reactions are:

	Staphylococcus spp	*Micrococcus* spp
Open tube (oxidation)	+	+
Closed tube (fermentation)	+	0

3. **C** Lysostaphin is an endopeptidase that cleaves the glycine-rich pentapeptide crossbridges in the staphylococcal cell wall peptidoglycan. The susceptibility of the staphylococci to lysostaphin is used to differentiate them from the micrococci. Staphylococci are susceptible and show a 10–16 mm zone of inhibition, while micrococci are not inhibited.

4. Which of the following tests is used routinely to identify *S. aureus?*
A. Slide coagulase test
B. Tube coagulase test
C. Latex agglutination
D. All of the above

Microbiology/Select methods/Reagents/Media/ Bacteria/Identification/2

5. Which of the following enzymes contribute to the virulence of *S. aureus?*
A. Urease and lecithinase
B. Hyaluronidase and β-lactamase
C. Lecithinase and catalase
D. All of the above

Microbiology/Apply knowledge of fundamental biological characteristics/Bacteria/1

6. Toxic shock syndrome is attributed to infection with:
A. *Staphylococcus epidermidis*
B. *Staphylococcus hominis*
C. *S. aureus*
D. *Staphylococcus saprophyticus*

Microbiology/Correlate clinical and laboratory data/Bacteria/Staphylococcus/2

7. Which *Staphylococcus* species, in addition to *S. aureus*, also produces coagulase?
A. *S. intermedius*
B. *S. saprophyticus*
C. *S. hominis*
D. All of the above

Microbiology/Correlate clinical and laboratory data/Bacteria/Staphylococcus/2

8. *S. epidermidis* (coagulase-negative) is recovered from which of the following sources?
A. Prosthetic heart valves
B. Intravenous catheters
C. Urinary tract
D. All of the above

Microbiology/Correlate clinical and laboratory data/Bacteria/Staphylococcus/2

9. Slime production is associated with which *Staphylococcus* species?
A. *S. aureus*
B. *S. epidermidis*
C. *S. intermedius*
D. *S. saprophyticus*

Microbiology/Apply knowledge of fundamental biological characteristics/Bacteria/1

Answers to Questions 4–9

4. **D** The slide coagulase test using rabbit plasma with ethylenediaminetetraacetic acid (EDTA) detects bound coagulase or "clumping factor" on the surface of the cell wall, which reacts with the fibrinogen in the plasma. This test is not positive for all strains of *S. aureus,* and a negative result must be confirmed by the tube method for detecting "free coagulase" or extracellular coagulase. The tube test is usually positive within 4 hours at 35°C; however, a negative result must then be incubated at room temperature for the remainder of 18–24 hours. Some strains produce coagulase slowly or produce fibrinolysin, which dissolves the clot, at 35°C. Latex agglutination procedures utilize fibrinogen and IgG-coated latex beads that detect protein A on the staphylococcal cell wall.

5. **B** In addition to coagulase, the virulence of *S. aureus* is attributed to hyaluronidase, which damages the intercellular matrix (basement membrane) of tissues. β-Lactamase-producing strains are able to inactivate penicillin and ampicillin making the organism resistant to these antibiotics. Lecithinase is not produced by *S. aureus,* and urease is not a virulence factor.

6. **C** *S. aureus* is the organism most often recovered from female patients. These strains produce toxic shock syndrome toxin 1 (TSST-1). Toxic shock syndrome is attributed to the use of certain highly absorbent tampons by menstruating females. The toxin is also recovered from sites other than the genital area and produces fever and life-threatening systemic damage as well as shock.

7. **A** *S. intermedius* infects mammals and certain birds, but not usually humans. Cases involving humans result from animal bites and are most often seen in persons who work closely with animals.

8. **D** *S. epidermidis* represents 50%–80% of all coagulase-negative *Staphylococci* spp recovered from numerous clinical specimens. It is of special concern in nosocomial infections due to its high resistance to antibiotics.

9. **B** *S. epidermidis* produces an extracellular slime that enhances the adhesion of these organisms to indwelling plastic catheters. The slime production is considered a virulence factor and is associated with prostheses infections.

10. Strains of *Staphylococcus* species resistant to the β-lactam antibiotics by standardized disk diffusion and broth microdilution susceptibility methods are called:
A. Heteroresistant
B. Bacteriophage group 52A
C. Cross-resistant
D. Plasmid altered

Microbiology/Apply knowledge of fundamental biological characteristics/Bacteria/1

11. *S. saprophyticus* is best differentiated from *S. epidermidis* by resistance to:
A. 5 μg of lysostaphin
B. 5 μg of novobiocin
C. 10 units of penicillin
D. 0.04 units of bacitracin

Microbiology/Correlate clinical and laboratory data/Bacteria/Staphylococcus/2

12. The following results were observed by using a tube coagulase test:

Coagulase at 4 hours = +   Coagulase at 18 hours = Neg
Novobiocin = sensitive   Hemolysis on blood
   (16-mm zone)   agar = β
DNase = +   Mannitol salt plate
                                   = + (acid
                                   production)

What is the most probable identification?
A. *S. saprophyticus*
B. *S. epidermidis*
C. *S. aureus*
D. *S. hominis*

Microbiology/Evaluate laboratory data to make identifications/Bacteria/3

13. *S. aureus* recovered from a wound culture gave the following antibiotic sensitivity pattern by the standardized Kirby-Bauer method (S = sensitive; R = resistant):

Penicillin = R   Ampicillin = S
                                   (moderate)
Cephalothin = R   Cefoxitin = R
Vancomycin = S (moderate)   Methicillin = R

Which is the drug of choice for treating this infection?
A. Penicillin
B. Ampicillin
C. Cephalothin
D. Vancomycin

Microbiology/Correlate clinical and laboratory data/Bacteria/Staphylococcus/2

14. Which of the following tests should be used to differentiate *S. aureus* from *S. intermedius*?
A. Acetoin
B. Catalase

C. Slide coagulase test
D. Urease

Microbiology/Select methods/Reagents/Media/ Bacteria/Identification/2

Answers to Questions 10–14

10. **A** Methicillin-resistant *S. aureus* (MRSA) and methicillin-resistant *S. epidermidis* (MRSE) are termed *heteroresistant*. This refers to two subpopulations in a culture, one that is susceptible and the other resistant to antibiotic(s). The resistant population grows more slowly than the susceptible one and can be overlooked. Therefore, the more resistant subpopulation should be promoted growthwise by using a neutral pH (7.0–7.4), cooler incubation temperature (30°–35°C), addition of 2%–4% NaCl, and incubation up to 48 hours.

11. **B** *S. saprophyticus* is coagulase-negative and resistant to 5 μg of novobiocin. Using the standardized Kirby-Bauer sensitivity procedure, a 6–12 mm zone of growth inhibition is considered resistant. Susceptible strains will measure 16–27 mm (inhibition) zones.

12. **C** *S. aureus* can produce fibrinolysins that dissolve the clot formed by the coagulase enzyme. The tube method calls for an incubation of 4 hours at 35°–37°C and 18–24 hours at room temperature. Both must be negative to interpret the result as coagulase-negative. This organism is coagulase-positive and, therefore, identified as *S. aureus.*

13. **D** Vanomycin, along with rifampin, is used for strains of *S. aureus* that are resistant to the β-lactams. MRSA strains pose problems when reading the zone sizes for these strains. Their heteroresistance results in a film of growth consisting of very small colonies formed within the defined inhibition zone surrounding the antibiotic disk. Initially, this appears as a mixed culture or contaminant.

14. **A** The production of acetoin by *S. aureus* from glucose or pyruvate differentiates it from *S. intermedius*, which is also coagulase-positive. This test is also called the VP test. Acetoin production is detected by addition of 40% KOH and 1% α-napthol to the VP test broth after 48 hours of incubation. A distinct pink color within 10 minutes denotes a positive test.

15. A gram-positive coccus recovered from a wound ulcer from a 31-year-old diabetic patient showed pale yellow, creamy, β-hemolytic colonies on blood agar. Given the following test results, what is the most likely identification?

Catalase = +; glucose OF: positive open tube, negative sealed tube; mannitol salt = neg; slide coagulase = neg
A. *S. aureus*
B. *S. epidermidis*
C. *Micrococcus* spp
D. *Streptococcus* spp

Microbiology/Evaluate laboratory data to make identifications/Bacteria/3

16. Urine cultured from the catheter of an 18-year-old female patient produced greater than 100,000 col/mL on a CNA plate. Colonies were catalase-positive, coagulase-negative by the latex agglutination slide method as well as the tube coagulase test. The best single test for identification is:
A. Lactose fermentation
B. Urease
C. Catalase
D. Novobiocin susceptibility

Microbiology/Select methods/Reagents/Media/Bacteria/Identification/3

17. A *Staphylococcus* sp recovered from a wound (cellulitis) was negative for the slide coagulase test (clumping factor) and negative for novobiocin resistance. The next test(s) needed for identification is (are):
A. Tube coagulase test
B. β-Hemolysis on blood agar
C. Mannitol salt agar plate
D. All of the above

Microbiology/Select methods/Reagents/Media/Bacteria/Identification/3

18. Furazolidone (furoxone) susceptibility is a test used to differentiate:
A. *Staphylococcus* spp from *Micrococcus* spp
B. *Streptococcus* spp from *Staphylococcus* spp
C. *Staphylococcus* spp from *Pseudomonas* spp
D. *Streptococcus* spp from *Micrococcus* spp

Microbiology/Select methods/Reagents/Media/Bacteria/Identification/2

19. Bacitracin resistance (0.04 units) is used to differentiate:
A. *Micrococcus* spp from *Staphylococcus* spp
B. *Staphylococcus* spp from *Neisseriae* spp
C. *Planococcus* spp from *Micrococcus* spp
D. All of the above

Microbiology/Select methods/Reagents/Media/Bacteria/Identification/2

20. Which of the following tests will rapidly differentiate micrococci from staphylococci?
A. Catalase
B. Coagulase
C. Modified oxidase
D. Novobiocin susceptibility

Microbiology/Select methods/Reagents/Media/Bacteria/Identification/2

Answers to Questions 15–20

15. **C** *Micrococcus* spp utilize glucose oxidatively, but not under anaerobic conditions (sealed tube). *Staphylococcus* spp utilize glucose oxidatively and anaerobically. The catalase differentiates the *Micrococcaceae* family (positive) from the *Streptococcaceae* family (negative).

16. **D** *S. epidermidis* and *S. saprophyticus* are the two possibilities because they are both catalase-positive, coagulase-negative, urease positive, and ferment lactose. Novobiocin susceptibility is the test of choice for differentiating these two species. *S. epidermidis* is sensitive, but *S. saprophyticus* is resistant to 5 μg of novobiocin.

17. **D** *S. aureus* is novobiocin-sensitive and cannot be ruled out by a negative clumping factor test. Most *S. aureus* produce β-hemolysis on sheep blood agar plates and are mannitol salt-positive (produce acid and are not inhibited by the high salt concentration). The tube test should be performed because the slide test was negative.

18. **A** Staphylococci are susceptible to furazolidone, giving zones of inhibition that are 15 mm or greater. *Micrococcus* spp are resistant to furazolidone, giving zones of 6–9 mm. The test is performed as a disk susceptibility procedure using a blood agar plate.

19. **A** A bacitracin disk (0.04 units) is used to identify group A β-hemolytic streptococci, but it will also differentiate catalase-positive organisms. A zone of 10 mm or greater is considered susceptible. The *Staphylococcus* species are resistant and grow up to the disk, while *Micrococcus* species are sensitive.

20. **C** The modified oxidase test is used to rapidly identify catalase-positive gram-positive cocci as a *Micrococcus* spp (positive) or *Staphylococcus* spp (negative). Filter paper disks that are saturated with oxidase reagent (tetramethyl-*p*-phenylenediamine in dimethylsulfoxide) are used. A colony of the isolate is rubbed onto the paper. Oxidase-positive organisms produce a purple color within 30 seconds.

21. *Streptococcus* species exhibit which of the following properties?
- A. Aerobic, oxidase, and catalase-positive
- B. Facultative anaerobe, oxidase-negative, catalase-negative
- C. Facultative anaerobe, β-hemolytic, catalase-positive
- D. May be α- , β- , or γ-hemolytic, catalase-positive

Microbiology/Apply knowledge of fundamental biological characteristics/Streptococci/1

22. Which group of streptococci is associated with erythrogenic toxin production?
- A. Group A
- B. Group B
- C. Group C
- D. Group G

Microbiology/Apply knowledge of fundamental biological characteristics/Bacteria/1

23. A fourfold rise in titer of which antibodies is the best indicator of a recent infection with group A β-hemolytic streptococci?
- A. Anti-streptolysin O
- B. Anti-streptolysin S
- C. Anti-A
- D. Anti-B

Microbiology/Select methods/Reagents/Media/ Bacteria/Identification/1

24. Bacitracin A disks (0.04 units) are used for the presumptive identification of which group of β-hemolytic streptococcus?
- A. Group A
- B. Group B
- C. Group C
- D. Group F

Microbiology/Select methods/Reagents/Media/ Bacteria/Identification/1

25. Trimethoprim-sulfamethoxazole (SXT) disks are used along with bacitracin disks to differentiate which streptococci?
- A. α-Hemolytic streptococci
- B. β-Hemolytic streptococci
- C. γ-Hemolytic streptococci
- D. All of the above

Microbiology/Select methods/Reagents/Media/ Bacteria/Identification/1

26. β-Hemolytic streptococci, not of group A or B, usually exhibit which of the following reactions?

	Bacitracin	Trimethoprim-sulfamethoxazole
A.	Susceptible	Resistant
B.	Resistant	Resistant
C.	Resistant	Susceptible
D.	Susceptible	Indeterminant

Microbiology/Correlate clinical and laboratory data/Bacteria/Streptococci/2

Answers to Questions 21–26

21. **B** *Streptococcus* species are facultative anaerobes that grow aerobically as well, and are oxidase- and catalase-negative. In order to demonstrate streptolysin O on blood agar, it is best to stab the agar to create anaerobiosis because streptolysin O is oxygen labile.

22. **A** Group A β-hemolytic streptococci are the cause of scarlet fever, and some strains produce toxins (pyrogenic exotoxins A, B, and C) which cause a scarlatiniform rash.

23. **A** The antistreptolysin O (ASO) titer is used to indicate a recent infection with group A β-hemolytic streptococci. Streptolysin O may also be produced by some strains of groups C and G streptococci.

24. **A** The bacitracin disk test is used in conjunction with other confirmatory tests for the β-hemolytic streptococci. In addition to group A, groups C, F, and G are also β-hemolytic and will give a positive test for bacitracin (a zone of inhibition of any size). Therefore, a positive test does not confirm the presence of group A β-hemolytic streptococci.

25. **B** β-Hemolytic streptococci are the only streptococci that should be tested. *S. pneumoniae*, which is α-hemolytic, is susceptible to small concentrations of bacitracin, as are other α-hemolytic streptococci. SXT is inhibitory to most streptococci *except Streptococcus pyogenes and Streptococcus agalactiae.* For this reason, SXT is used in a commercially available streptococcal selective agar (SSA) as a primary plating agar for the detection of group A streptococci.

26. **C** Streptococci that are not group A or B may be either resistant or susceptible to bacitracin, but are usually susceptible to SXT.

β-Hemolytic Streptococci	Bacitracin	Trimethoprim-Sulfamethoxazole
Group A	S	R
Group B	R	R
Non-A, non-B groups	S or R	S

27. A false-positive CAMP test for the presumptive identification of group B streptococci may occur if the plate is incubated in a:
A. Candle jar or CO_2 incubator
B. Ambient air incubator
C. 35°C incubator
D. 37°C incubator

Microbiology/Apply knowledge to identify sources of error/Identification/Streptococci/3

28. Which test is used to differentiate the viridans streptococci from the group D streptococci and enterococci?
A. Bacitracin disk test
B. CAMP test
C. Hippurate hydrolysis test
D. Bile esculin test

Microbiology/Select methods/Reagents/Media/ Bacteria/Identification/2

29. The bile solubility test causes the lysis of:
A. *Streptococcus bovis* colonies on a blood agar plate
B. *S. pneumoniae* colonies on a blood agar plate
C. Group A streptococci in broth culture
D. Group B streptococci in broth culture

Microbiology/Apply knowledge to identify sources of error/Identification/Streptococci/1

30. *S. pneumoniae* and the viridans streptococcus type can be differentiated by which test?
A. Optochin disk test, 5 μg/mL or less
B. Bacitracin disk test, 0.04 units
C. CAMP test
D. Bile esculin test

Microbiology/Select methods/Reagents/Media/ Bacteria/Identification/2

31. The salt tolerance test (6.5% salt broth) is used to presumptively identify:
A. *S. pneumoniae*
B. *S. bovis*
C. *Streptococcus equinus*
D. *Enterococcus faecalis*

Microbiology/Select methods/Reagents/Media/ Bacteria/Identification/2

32. In addition to *Enterococcus faecalis*, which other streptococci will grow in 6.5% salt broth?
A. Group A streptococci
B. Group B streptococci
C. *S. pneumoniae*
D. Group D streptococci (nonenterococci)

Microbiology/Correlate clinical and laboratory data/Bacteria/Streptococci/2

Answers to Questions 27–32

27. A The CAMP (hemolytic phenomenon first described by Christie, Atkins, and Munch-Petersen in 1944) test refers to a hemolytic interaction that is seen on a blood agar plate between the β-hemolysins produced by most strains of *S. aureus* and an extracellular protein produced by both hemolytic and nonhemolytic isolates of group B streptococci. When performing a CAMP test the plate must be placed in an ambient air incubator at 35°–37°C. Group A streptococci may be CAMP-positive if the plate is incubated in a candle jar, high CO_2 atmosphere, or anaerobically.

28. D The bile esculin test differentiates those bacteria that can hydrolyze esculin and also grow in the presence of 4% bile salts or 40% bile. The bile esculin slant is inoculated on the surface and incubated for 24–48 hours in a non-CO_2 incubator. Group D streptococci (enterococci and nonenterococci) are positive causing blackening of half or more of the slant within 48 hours. Viridans streptococci are negative (will not grow or hydrolyze esculin).

29. B The bile solubility test can be performed directly by dropping 2% sodium deoxycholate onto a few well-isolated colonies of *S. pneumoniae*. The bile salts speed up the autolysis observed in pneumococci cultures. The colonies lyse and disappear when incubated at 35°C for 30 minutes, leaving a partially hemolyzed area on the plate. The same phenomenon can be seen using a broth culture; addition of 10% deoxycholate to broth containing *S. pneumoniae* results in visible clearing of the suspension after incubation at 35°C for 3 hours.

30. A Optochin at a concentration of 5 μg/mL or less will inhibit the growth of *S. pneumoniae,* but *not* viridans streptococci. However, optochin at a concentration in excess of 5 μg/mL will inhibit other viridans streptococci as well. A zone of inhibition of 14 mm or more around the 6-mm disk is considered a presumptive identification of *S. pneumoniae*. A questionable zone size should be confirmed by performing a bile solubility test.

31. D *Enterococcus faecalis* will grow in 6.5% salt and the nonenterococci (*S. bovis* and *S. equinus*) will not. This test distinguishes the enterococci group from *S. bovis* and *S. equinus* (nonenterococci group). Both groups will grow on bile esculin agar.

32. B Approximately 80% of group B streptococci are capable of growing in 6.5% salt broth; however, they do not hydrolyze esculin or grow in media containing 4% bile salts.

33. The quellung test is used to identify which
Streptococcus species?
A. *S. pyogenes*
B. *S. agalactiae*
C. *S. sanguis*
D. *S. pneumoniae*

*Microbiology/Apply knowledge of fundamental
biological characteristics/Streptococci/1*

34. The L-pyrrolidonyl-β-napthylamide (PYR) hydrolysis
test is a presumptive test for which streptococci?
A. Group A and D (enterococcus) streptococci
B. Group A and B β-hemolytic streptococci
C. Nongroup A or B β-hemolytic streptococci
D. *S. pneumoniae* and group D streptococci
   (nonenterococcus)

*Microbiology/Apply knowledge of fundamental
biological characteristics/Streptococci/1*

35. A pure culture of β-hemolytic streptococci
recovered from a leg wound ulcer gave the
following reactions:

CAMP test = Neg	Hippurate hydrolysis = Neg
Bile esculin = Neg	6.5% salt = Neg
PYR = Neg	Bacitracin = R
Optochin = R	SXT = S

The most likely identification is:
A. Group A streptococci
B. Group B streptococci
C. *Enterococcus faecalis*
D. Nongroup A, nongroup B, nongroup D
   streptococci

*Microbiology/Evaluate laboratory data to make
identifications/Bacteria/3*

36. β-Hemolytic streptococci, greater than 50,000
col/mL, were isolated from a urinary tract catheter.
Given the following reactions, what is the most
likely identification?

CAMP test = Neg	Hippurate hydrolysis = ±
Bile solubility = Neg	6.5% salt = +
PYR = +	Bile esculin = +
SXT = R	Bacitracin = R
Optochin = R	

A. Group A streptococci
B. Group B streptococci
C. *Enterococcus faecalis*
D. Nongroup A, nongroup B, nongroup D strepto-
   cocci

*Microbiology/Evaluate laboratory data to make
identifications/Bacteria/3*

37. Nutritionally variant streptococci (NVS) require
specific thiol compounds, cysteine, or the active
form of vitamin B_6. Which of the following tests
supplies these requirements?
A. CAMP test
B. Bacitracin susceptibility test

C. Bile solubility test
D. Staphylococcal cross-streak test

*Microbiology/Apply knowledge of fundamental
biological characteristics/Streptococci/1*

Answers to Questions 33–37

33. D A precipitin reaction seen microscopically with
methylene blue stain (microprecipitin reaction)
occurs between the carbohydrate of the capsule of
S. pneumoniae and anticapsular antibody. The
antibody may be type-specific or polyvalent.
Binding of antibodies to the bacteria causes the
capsule to swell, identifying the organisms as *S.
pneumoniae*.

34. A The PYR hydrolysis test is highly specific for
group A streptococci and group D enterococci.
The test detects the pyrrolidonylarylamidase
enzyme, which hydrolyses PYR.

35. D The β-hemolytic streptococci, not of groups A,
B, or D, are sensitive to SXT and may be either
sensitive or resistant to bacitracin. Groups A and B
are both resistant to SXT. Group A and
Enterococcus faecalis are PYR-positive.
Enterococcus faecalis is also positive for bile
esculin and 6.5 % salt broth.

36. C Group A streptococci are sensitive to bacitracin
and negative for bile esculin and 6.5% salt broth.
Group B streptococci will grow in 6.5% salt broth
but are negative for bile esculin and PYR. The
nongroup A, B, or D streptococci will not grow in
6.5% salt broth and are sensitive to SXT. Some
group D streptococci will hydrolyze hippurate.
Enterococcus faecalis is positive for bile esculin,
6.5% salt broth, and PYR.

37. D The staphylococcal streak, across the NVS
inoculum, provides the nutrients needed. Very
small colonies of NVS can be seen growing
adjacent to the staphylococcal streak on the blood
agar plate in a manner similar to the satellite phenomenon of *Haemophilus* spp around *S. aureus*.

38. Many α-hemolytic streptococci recovered from a wound were found to be penicillin-resistant. Given the following results, what is the most likely identification?

Bile esculin = +   Bile solubility   6.5% salt
                    = Neg   = +

Hippurate   PYR = +   SXT = R
  hydrolysis = +

A. *E. faecalis*
B. *S. pneumoniae*
C. *S. bovis*
D. Group B streptococci

Microbiology/Evaluate laboratory data to make identifications/Bacteria/3

39. Which two tests best differentiate *S. bovis* (group D streptococcus, nonenterococcus) from *Streptococcus salivarius*?
A. Bile esculin and 6.5% salt broth
B. Starch hydrolysis and acid production from mannitol
C. Bacitracin and PYR
D. Trimethoprim-sulfamethoxazole susceptibility and PYR

Microbiology/Select methods/Reagents/Media/Bacteria/Identification/2

40. Two blood cultures on a newborn grew β-hemolytic streptococci with the following reactions:

CAMP test = +   Hippurate hydrolysis = +
Bile solubility = Neg   6.5% salt = +
Bacitracin = R   Bile esculin = Neg
PYR = Neg   Trimethoprim-
                           sulfamethoxazole = R

Which is the most likely identification?
A. Group A streptococci
B. Group B streptococci
C. Group D streptococci
D. Nongroup A, nongroup B, nongroup D streptococci

Microbiology/Evaluate laboratory data to make identifications/Bacteria/3

41. MTM medium is used primarily for the selective recovery of which organism from genital specimens?
A. *N. gonorrhoeae*
B. *Neisseria lactamica*
C. *Neisseria sicca*
D. *Neisseria flavescens*

Microbiology/Select methods/Reagents/Media/Bacteria/Identification/1

42. Variation in colony types seen with fresh isolates of *N. gonorrhoeae* and sometimes with *N. meningitidis* are the result of:
A. Multiple nutritional requirements
B. Pili on the cell surface
C. Use of a transparent medium
D. All of the above

Microbiology/Apply knowledge of fundamental biological characteristics/Neisseria/2

Answers to Questions 38–42

38. **A** *E. faecalis* is highly resistant to penicillin and ampicillin, as well as some of the aminoglycoside antibiotics. Pneumococci, group B streptococci, and *S. bovis* are PYR-negative.

39. **B** *S. bovis* and *S. salivarius* are physiologically and biochemically similar. They are both PYR and 6.5% salt broth-negative and bile esculin-positive, but only *S. bovis* is positive for mannitol and starch reactions. See chart below.

40. **B** Group B streptococci (*S. agalactiae*) is resistant to both bacitracin and SXT. Unlike group A and group D streptococci, the group B streptococci are negative for PYR. With some exceptions, group B streptococci will grow in 6.5% salt broth.

41. **A** Both *N. gonorrhoeae* and *N. meningitidis* grow selectively on MTM due to the addition of vancomycin and colistin, which inhibit gram-positive and gram-negative bacteria, respectively. Trimethoprim is added to inhibit swarming of *Proteus* spp because a rectal swab may be used for culture. Nystatin and amphotericin B are used to prevent growth of yeasts and molds from vaginal specimens.

42. **D** Upon subculture from a primary plate, various sizes and appearances of gonococci are the result of multiple nutritional requirements, such as arginine-hypoxanthine-uracil (AHU)-requiring strains. Colony size and coloration (or light reflection) are the basis of Kellogg's scheme (types T1 through T5). Types T1 and T2 have pili on the surface and T3, T4, and T5 do not. Transparent media are not used routinely, but opaque and transparent colonial differences of the gonococci can be seen when using it.

	Bacitracin	**PYR**	**Bile Esculin**	**6.5% Salt**	**Mannitol**	**Starch**
S. bovis	R	0	+	0	+	+
S. salivarius	R	0	+	0	0	0

43. Gram-negative diplococci recovered from an MTM plate and giving a positive oxidase test can be presumptively identified as:
A. *N. gonorrhoeae*
B. *N. meningitidis*
C. *N. lactamica*
D. All of the above

Microbiology/Evaluate laboratory data to make identifications/Bacteria/2

44. The Superoxol test is used as a rapid presumptive test for:
A. *N. gonorrhoeae*
B. *N. meningitidis*
C. *N. lactamica*
D. *Moraxella (Branhamella) catarrhalis*

Microbiology/Apply knowledge of fundamental biological characteristics/Neisseria/1

45. Nonpathogenic *Moraxella* spp capable of growing on selective media for *Neisseria* can be differentiated from *Neisseria* spp by which test?
A. Catalase test
B. 10-unit penicillin disk
C. Oxidase test
D. Superoxol test

Microbiology/Select methods/Reagents/Media/ Bacteria/Identification/2

46. A Gram stain of a urethral discharge from a man showing extracellular and intracellular gram-negative diplococci within segmented neutrophils is a presumptive identification for:
A. *N. gonorrhoeae*
B. *N. meningitidis*
C. *M. (B.) catarrhalis*
D. All of the above

Microbiology/Evaluate laboratory data to make identifications/Bacteria/3

47. The β-galactosidase test aids in the identification of which *Neisseria* species?
A. *N. lactamica*
B. *N. meningitidis*
C. *N. gonorrhoeae*
D. *N. flavescens*

Microbiology/Apply knowledge of fundamental biological characteristics/Neisseria/1

48. Cystine tryptic digest (CTA) media used for identification of *Neisseria* spp should be inoculated and cultured in:
A. A CO_2 incubator at 35°C for 24 hours
B. A CO_2 incubator at 42°C for up to 72 hours
C. A non-CO_2 incubator at 35°C for up to 72 hours
D. An anaerobic incubator at 35°C for up to 72 hours

Microbiology/Apply knowledge of basic laboratory procedures/Gram-negative cocci/1

Answers to Questions 43–48

43. **D** All of the listed *Neisseria* spp grow on MTM and are oxidase-positive. *N. lactamica* is a nonpathogenic component of normal throat flora resembling *N. meningitidis,* but it grows well on selective MTM agar. Presumptive identification of *N. meningitidis* or *N. gonorrhoeae* is stated only if the source of the specimen (i.e., urogenital or CSF) is given. The identification must be confirmed by further testing such as carbohydrate utilization tests or rapid latex slide agglutination tests.

44. **A** *N. gonorrhoeae* colonies recovered from selective MTM media give an immediate positive reaction (bubbling) when 30% H_2O_2 is added. The catalase test uses 3% H_2O_2. This is a presumptive test for *N. gonorrhoeae; N. meningitidis* and *N. lactamica* give a weak or delayed bubbling reaction. *M. (B.) catarrhalis* is catalase-positive, superoxol-negative, and has a variable growth pattern on MTM.

45. **B** *Moraxella* spp are oxidase- and catalase-positive, as are the gonococci. *Neisseria* spp and *M. (B.) catarrhalis* will keep their typical coccal morphology after overnight incubation on blood agar with a 10-unit penicillin disk (CO_2 incubation). Other *Moraxella* species will form long filaments or long spindle-shaped cells when grown near a 10-unit penicillin disk.

46. **A** A Gram stain of urethral discharge (in men only) showing typical gonococcal cells in PMNs should be reported "presumptive *N. gonorrhoeae,* confirmation to follow." With female patients, the normal vaginal flora contain gram-negative cocci and diplococci resembling gonococci and, therefore, no presumptive identification should be reported for *N. gonorrhoeae* from the vaginal Gram stain smear.

47. **A** *N. lactamica* utilizes lactose by producing the enzyme β-galactosidase. All other *Neisseria* spp that grow on MTM media are lactose-negative.

48. **C** CTA agar with 1% carbohydrate and phenol red pH indicator added is used for the identification of *Neisseria* species. CTA carbohydrates must be placed in an ambient air incubator because a high CO_2 concentration may reduce the pH causing a false-positive (acid) result. The utilization of carbohydrates by some fastidious gonococcal strains may take up to 72 hours in order to produce a color change in the pH indicator.

49. Culture on MTM media of a vaginal swab produced several colonies of gram-negative diplococci that were catalase- and oxidase-positive and superoxol-negative. Given the following carbohydrate reactions, select the most likely identification.

Glucose = +; sucrose = Neg; lactose = +; maltose = +; fructose = Neg
A. *N. gonorrhoeae*
B. *N. sicca*
C. *N. flavescens*
D. *N. lactamica*

Microbiology/Evaluate laboratory data to make identifications/Bacteria/3

50. A sputum from a patient with pneumonia produced many colonies of gram-negative diplococci on a chocolate plate that were also present in fewer numbers on MTM after 48 hours. Given the results below, what is the most likely identification?

Catalase = +   Oxidase = +
DNase = +   Tributyrin hydrolysis = +
Glucose = Neg   Sucrose = Neg
Lactose = Neg   Maltose = Neg
Fructose = Neg
A. *M. (B.) catarrhalis*
B. *N. flavescens*
C. *N. sicca*
D. *Neisseria elongata*

Microbiology/Apply knowledge of fundamental biological characteristics/GPB/1

Answers to Questions 49–50

49. **D** *N. lactamica* is part of the normal vaginal and throat flora and is the only *Neisseria* species that grows on MTM that utilizes lactose. Other saprophytic *Neisseria* spp may utilize lactose but do not grow on MTM media.

50. **A** *M. (B.) catarrhalis* is part of the normal upper respiratory flora, but is implicated in lower respiratory infections including pneumonia. It produces stunted growth on MTM and is DNase-positive, characteristics differentiating it from the other saprophytic *Neisseria* species.

Aerobic Gram-Positive Rods, Spirochetes, Mycoplasmas and Ureaplasmas, and Chlamydia

1. A large gram-positive spore-forming rod growing on blood agar as large, raised, β-hemolytic colonies that spread and appear as frosted green-gray glass is most likely a:
   A. *Pseudomonas* spp
   B. *Bacillus* spp
   C. *Corynebacterium* spp
   D. *Listeria* spp

   Microbiology/Apply knowledge of fundamental biological characteristics/GPB/2

2. *Bacillus anthracis* and *Bacillus cereus* can best be differentiated by which tests?
   A. Motility and β-hemolysis on a blood agar plate
   B. Oxidase and β-hemolysis on a blood agar plate
   C. Lecithinase and glucose
   D. Lecithinase and catalase

   Microbiology/Select methods/Reagents/Media/ Bacteria/Identification/2

3. Which is the specimen of choice for proof of food poisoning by *B. cereus?*
   A. Sputum
   B. Blood
   C. Stool
   D. Food

   Microbiology/Apply knowledge of fundamental biological characteristics/GPB/2

Answers to Questions 1–3

1. **B** The only spore former listed is the *Bacillus* spp, which grow as large, spreading colonies on blood agar plates. *Pseudomonas* spp are gram-negative rods; *Corynebacterium* spp appear as small, very dry colonies on BAP; *Listeria* spp appear as very small β-hemolytic colonies on BAP resembling *Streptococcus* species.

2. **A** Both species of *Bacillus* are catalase- and lecithinase-positive and produce acid from glucose. *B. cereus* is β-hemolytic and motile, but *B. anthracis* is neither. See chart below.

3. **D** The best specimen is the suspected food itself. Stool cultures are not useful because *B. cereus* is part of the normal fecal flora. The suspected food can be the source of food poisoning by *B. cereus* if 100,000 or greater organisms per gram of infected food are demonstrated.

	β-Hemolysis	Motility	Oxidase	Catalase	Lecithinase	Glucose
B. cereus	+	+	0	+	+	+
B. anthracis	0	0	0	+	+	+

4. A suspected *B. anthracis* culture obtained from a wound specimen produced colonies that had many outgrowths (Medusa-head appearance), but were not β-hemolytic on sheep blood agar. Which test should be performed next?
A. Penicillin (10-unit) susceptibility test
B. Lecithinase test
C. Glucose test
D. Motility test

Microbiology/Select course of action/GPB/3

5. Which of the following tests should be performed for initial differentiation of *Listeria monocytogenes* from group B streptococci?
A. Gram stain, motility at room temperature, catalase
B. Gram stain, CAMP test, H₂S/TSI
C. Oxidase, CAMP test, glucose
D. Oxidase, bacitracin

Microbiology/Select methods/Reagents/Media/GPB/2

6. Culture of a finger wound specimen from a meat packer produced short gram-positive bacilli on a blood agar plate with no hemolysis. Given the following test results at 48 hours, what is the most likely identification?

Catalase = neg; H₂S/TSI = +; motility (wet prep) = neg; motility (media) = neg (bottle brush growth in stab culture)
A. *B. cereus*
B. *L. monocytogenes*
C. *Erysipelothrix rhusiopathiae*
D. *Bacillus subtilis*

Microbiology/Evaluate laboratory data to make identifications/Bacteria/3

7. A non-spore-forming, slender gram-positive rod forming palisades and chains was recovered from a vaginal culture and grew well on tomato juice agar. The most likely identification is:
A. *Lactobacillus* spp
B. *Bacillus* spp
C. *Neisseria* spp
D. *Streptococcus* spp

Microbiology/Evaluate laboratory data to make identifications/Bacteria/2

8. A *Corynebacterium* species recovered from a throat culture is considered a pathogen when it produces:
A. A pseudomembrane of the oropharynx
B. An exotoxin
C. Gray-black colonies with a brown halo on Tinsdale agar

D. All of the above

Microbiology/Apply knowledge of fundamental biological characteristics/GPB/2

Answers to Questions 4–8

4. **A** The best differentiating test to perform on a suspected *B. anthracis* culture is the 10-unit penicillin disk test. *B. anthracis* is susceptible but other *Bacillus* spp are not. Organisms suspected to be *B. anthracis* should be sent to a reference laboratory for final confirmation. All tests should be performed in a biological safety hood, and personnel should wear protective clothing to reduce risk from possible production of aerosols.

5. **A** *Streptococcus* spp are catalase-negative and *L. monocytogenes* is catalase-positive. *L. monocytogenes* appears on the Gram stain smear as gram-positive short, thin, diphtheroidal shapes, while streptococci usually appear as short gram-positive chains. The reactions shown in the chart below differentiate *L. monocytogenes* from the group B streptococci.

6. **C** *E. rhusiopathiae* is catalase-negative, while the other three organisms are catalase-positive. *E. rhusiopathiae* are seen primarily as skin infections on the fingers of meat and poultry workers. Colonies growing on blood agar are small and transparent, may be either smooth or rough, and are often surrounded by a green tinge. *E. rhusiopathiae* is characterized by H₂S production in the butt of a TSI slant which differentiates it from other catalase-negative, gram-positive rods.

7. **A** *Lactobacillus* spp produce both long, slender rods or short coccobacilli that form chains. It is part of the normal flora of the vagina (is not considered a pathogen) and is sometimes confused with the streptococci.

8. **D** *Corynebacterium* species recovered from a throat culture are usually considered part of the normal throat flora. *C. diphtheriae* is an exception and should be suspected when one of the conditions described occurs. In this event, direct inoculation on Loeffler serum medium or tellurite medium and the following biochemical tests should be performed to confirm the identification of *C. diphtheriae*.

Gelatin hydrolysis (−)	Catalase (+)
Motility (+)	Urease (+)
Acid from glucose (+)	Carbohydrate fermentation (+)

	Catalase	Motility	CAMP	H₂S	Bile Esculin
L. monocytogenes	+	+	+	0	+
Group B streptococci	0	0	+	0	0

9. A presumptive diagnosis of *Gardnerella vaginalis* can be made using which of the following findings?
A. Oxidase and catalase tests
B. Pleomorphic bacilli heavily colonized on vaginal epithelium
C. Hippurate hydrolysis test
D. All of the above

Microbiology/Select methods/Reagents/Media/ GPB/2

10. A gram-positive branching filamentous organism recovered from a sputum specimen was found to be positive with a modified acid-fast stain method. What is the most likely presumptive identification?
A. *Bacillus* spp
B. *Nocardia* spp
C. *Corynebacterium* spp
D. *Listeria* spp

Microbiology/Evaluate laboratory data to make identifications/Bacteria/2

11. Routine laboratory testing for *Treponema pallidum* involves:
A. Culturing
B. Serological analysis
C. Acid-fast staining
D. Gram staining

Microbiology/Select methods/Reagents/Media/ Spirochetes/1

12. Spirochetes often detected in the hematology laboratory, even before the physician suspects the infection are:
A. *Borrelia* spp
B. *Treponema* spp
C. *Campylobacter* spp
D. *Leptospira* spp

Microbiology/Apply knowledge of fundamental biological characteristics/Spirochetes/1

13. Which of the following organisms is the cause of Lyme disease?
A. *T. pallidum*
B. *N. meningitidis*
C. *Babesia microti*
D. *Borrelia burgdorferi*

Microbiology/Apply knowledge of fundamental biological characteristics/Spirochetes/1

14. The diagnostic method most commonly used for the identification of Lyme disease is:
A. Serology
B. Culture
C. Gram stain
D. Acid-fast stain

Microbiology/Select methods/Reagents/Media/ Spirochetes/1

Answers to Questions 9–14

9. **D** A Gram stain smear from vaginal secretion showing many squamous epithelial cells loaded with pleomorphic gram-variable (positive and negative) bacilli is considered presumptive for *G. vaginalis*. Other important findings are:

β-Hemolysis on BAP = +   Catalase = Neg
Oxidase = Neg   Hippurate hydrolysis = +

10. **B** *Nocardia* spp should be suspected if colonies that are partially acid-fast by the traditional method are positive with the modified acid-fast method using Kinyoun stain and 1% sulfuric acid as the decolorizing agent. The other organisms above are acid-fast-stain-negative.

11. **B** Serological tests of the patient's serum for evidence of syphilis is routinely performed, but culturing is not because research animals must be used for inoculation of the suspected spirochete. *T. pallidum* does not stain by either the Gram or acid-fast technique. Darkfield microscopy for *direct* visualization or *indirect* immunofluorescence using fluorescein-conjugated antihuman globulin (the fluorescent treponemal antibody-absorption test, FTA-ABS) may be used to identify syphilis.

12. **A** *Borrelia* spp are often seen on Wright's-stained smears of peripheral blood as helical bacteria with 3–10 loose coils. They are gram-negative but stain well with Giemsa stain.

13. **D** Lyme disease may result in acute arthritis and meningitis and is caused by *B. burgdorferi*. This spirochete is carried by the deer tick belonging to the *Ixodes* genus (*I. dammini* in the Eastern and Northcentral United States and *I. pacificus* in the Northwest United States). The life cycle of the tick involves small rodents such as the white-footed mouse and the white-tailed deer.

14. **A** Serological analysis using immunofluorescence or an enzyme immunoassay is the method of choice for diagnosis of Lyme disease. Titers of IgM remain high throughout the infection. *B. burgdorferi* can be cultured directly from lesions, and darkfield microscopy can be used for detection of spirochetes in blood cultures after 2–3 weeks of incubation at 34°–37°C.

15. Primary atypical pneumonia is caused by:
A. *S. pneumoniae*
B. *Mycoplasma pneumoniae*
C. *K. pneumoniae*
D. *Mycobacterium tuberculosis*

Microbiology/Apply knowledge of fundamental biological characteristics/1

16. Which organism typically produces "fried egg" colonies on agar within 1–5 days of culture from a genital specimen?
A. *Mycoplasma hominis*
B. *B. burgdorferi*
C. *Leptospira interrogans*
D. *T. pallidum*

Microbiology/Apply knowledge of fundamental biological characteristics/1

17. The manganous chloride-urea test is used for the identification of which organism?
A. *M. pneumoniae*
B. *U. urealyticum*
C. *B. cereus*
D. *B. burgdorferi*

Microbiology/Select methods/reagents/media/Mycoplasma/1

18. A gram-positive (gram-variable), beaded organism with delicate branching was recovered from the sputum of a 20-year-old patient with leukemia. The specimen produced orange, glabrous, waxy colonies on Middlebrook agar that showed partial acid-fast staining with the modified Kinyoun stain. What is the most likely identification?
A. *Rhodococcus* spp
B. *Actinomadura* spp
C. *Streptomyces* spp
D. *Nocardia* spp

Microbiology/Evaluate laboratory data to make identifications/Bacteria/3

19. A direct smear from a nasopharyngeal swab stained with Loeffler methylene blue stain showed various letter shapes and deep blue, metachromatic granules. The most likely identification is:
A. *Corynebacterium* spp
B. *Nocardia* spp
C. *Listeria* spp
D. *Gardnerella* spp

Microbiology/Evaluate laboratory data to make identifications/Bacteria/3

20. Which of the following is the best rapid, noncultural test to perform when *G. vaginalis* is suspected in a patient with vaginosis?
A. 10% KOH test
B. 3% H_2O_2 test
C. 30% H_2O_2 test
D. All of the above

Microbiology/Select methods/Reagents/Media/Gardnerella/2

Answers to Questions 15–20

15. **B** A common cause of respiratory tract illness, *M. pneumoniae*, generally causes a self-limited infection (3–10 days) and usually does not require antibiotic therapy. *M. pneumoniae* can be cultured from the upper and lower respiratory tract onto specially enriched (diphasic) media but is most frequently diagnosed by the change in antibody titer from acute to convalescent serum using enzyme immunoassay, cold agglutinins, or other serological methods.

16. **A** Genital mycoplasmas (*M. hominis* and *Ureaplasma urealyticum*) are grown on specific agars. *M. hominis* is grown on "M" agar containing arginine and phenol red. Colonies of mycoplasma are 50–300 μm in diameter and display a "fried egg" appearance with red holes. *U. urealyticum* is isolated from genital specimens on "U" agar (containing urea and phenol red), then subcultured to A7/A8 agar. Colonies of *Ureaplasma* are small and golden brown on A7/A8 agar.

17. **B** *U. urealyticum* is the only human mycoplasma that hydrolyses urea. The manganous chloride-urea test utilizes manganous chloride ($MnCl_2$) in the presence of urea. Urease produced by the organism hydrolyses the urea to ammonia. This reacts with $MnCl_2$ forming manganese oxide, which is insoluble and forms a dark brown precipitate around the colonies. The reaction is observed under a dissecting microscope and is a rapid test for the identification of *U. urealyticum*.

18. **D** All of the listed organisms produce mycelium (aerial or substrate) causing them to appear branched when gram-stained, but only the *Nocardia* spp are modified acid-fast stain-positive. *Nocardia* is an opportunistic pathogen, and cultures typically have a musty basement odor.

19. **A** *Corynebacterium* spp are part of the normal upper respiratory tract flora. Organisms display typical pleomorphic shapes often resembling letters such as Y or L, and metachromatic granules. Identification of *C. diphtheriae*, however, requires selective culture media and biochemical testing.

20. **A** The "whiff" test is used for a presumptive diagnosis of an infection with *G. vaginalis*. A fishlike odor is noted after the addition of 1 drop of 10% KOH to the vaginal washings. This odor results from the high concentration of amines found in women with vaginosis caused by *G. vaginalis*.

Anaerobic Bacteria

1. Obligate anaerobes, facultative anaerobes, and microaerophiles are terms referring to bacteria requiring:
   A. Increased nitrogen
   B. Decreased CO_2
   C. Increased O_2
   D. Decreased O_2

   Microbiology/Apply principles of fundamental biological characteristics/Anaerobes/1

2. Which of the following most affects the oxidation-reduction potential (Eh or redox potential) of media for anaerobic bacteria?
   A. O_2
   B. Nitrogen
   C. pH
   D. Glucose

   Microbiology/Apply principles of fundamental biological characteristics/Anaerobes/1

3. Which of the following is the medium of choice for the selective recovery of gram-negative anaerobes?
   A. Kanamycin-vancomycin (KV) agar
   B. Phenylethyl alcohol (PEA) agar
   C. CCFA
   D. THIO broth

   Microbiology/Select methods/Reagents/Media/Anaerobes/2

4. Anaerobic bacteria are routinely isolated from all of the following types of infections *except:*
   A. Lung abscesses
   B. Brain abscesses
   C. Dental infections
   D. Urinary tract infections

   Microbiology/Apply principles of fundamental biological characteristics/Anaerobes/1

Answers to Questions 1–4

1. **D** The anaerobic bacteria are subdivided according to their requirement for O_2. Obligate anaerobes are killed by exposure to atmospheric O_2 for 10 minutes or longer. Facultative anaerobes grow under aerobic or anaerobic conditions. Microaerophilic organisms will not grow in an aerobic incubator on solid media, and only minimally under anaerobic conditions. However, they will grow in minimal oxygen (5% O_2). Superoxide dismutase (SOD) is produced by many anaerobes, which catalyzes the conversion of superoxide radicals to less toxic H_2O_2 and molecular O_2.

2. **C** The Eh is most affected by pH and is expressed at pH 7.0. In cultivating anaerobic bacteria, reducing agents such as thioglycollate and L-cysteine are added to anaerobic transport and culture media in order to maintain a low Eh. Certain anaerobes will not grow in the media above a specific critical Eh level.

3. **A** KV allows the growth of *Bacteroides* spp, *Prevotella* spp, and *Fusobacterium* spp, and inhibits most facultative anaerobic gram-negative rods and gram-positive bacteria (both aerobic and anaerobic). PEA inhibits facultative gram-negative bacteria but will support gram-positive aerobes and anaerobes and gram-negative obligate anaerobes. CCFA is selective for *C. difficile* from stool, while THIO broth supports gram-positive and gram-negative aerobes and anaerobes.

4. **D** The incidence of anaerobic bacteria recovered from the urine is approximately 1% of isolates. The other three types of infection are associated with a 60%–93% incidence of anaerobic recovery. Urine is not cultured routinely under anaerobic conditions unless obtained surgically (e.g., suprapubic aspiration).

5. Methods other than packaged microsystems used to identify anaerobes include:
   A. Antimicrobial susceptibility testing
   B. Gas-liquid chromatography (GLC)
   C. Special staining
   D. Enzyme immunoassay

   Microbiology/Select methods/Reagents/Media/ Anaerobes/1

6. Which broth is used for the cultivation of anaerobic bacteria in order to detect volatile fatty acids as an aid to identification?
   A. Prereduced peptone-yeast extract-glucose (PYG)
   B. THIO broth
   C. Gram-negative (GN) broth
   D. SEL broth

   Microbiology/Select methods/Reagents/Media/ Anaerobes/1

7. A gram-positive spore-forming bacilli growing on sheep-blood agar anaerobically produces a double zone of β-hemolysis and is positive for lecithinase. What is the presumptive identification?
   A. *Bacteroides ureolyticus*
   B. *B. fragilis*
   C. *C. perfringens*
   D. *C. difficile*

   Microbiology/Evaluate laboratory data to make identifications/Bacteria/2

8. Egg yolk agar is used to detect which enzyme produced by *Clostridium* species?
   A. Lecithinase
   B. β-Lactamase
   C. Catalase
   D. Oxidase

   Microbiology/Apply principles of fundamental biological characteristics/Anaerobes/1

9. Which of the following organisms will display lipase activity on egg yolk agar?
   A. *Clostridium botulinum*
   B. *Clostridium sporogenes*
   C. *Clostridium novyi* (A)
   D. All of the above

   Microbiology/Evaluate laboratory data to make identifications/Bacteria/2

10. Which spore type and location is found on *Clostridium tetani?*
   A. Round, terminal spores
   B. Round, subterminal spores
   C. Ovoid, subterminal spores
   D. Ovoid, terminal spores

   Microbiology/Apply principles of fundamental biological characteristics/Anaerobes/1

Answers to Questions 5–10

5. **B** Anaerobic bacteria can be identified by analysis of metabolic products using gas-liquid chromatography. Results are evaluated along with Gram staining characteristics, spore formation, and cellular morphology in order to make the identification.

6. **A** Peptone yeast and chopped meat with carbohydrates support the growth of anaerobic bacteria. The end products from the metabolism of the peptone and carbohydrates are volatile fatty acids that help to identify the bacteria. After incubation the broth is centrifuged and the supernatant injected into a gas-liquid chromatograph. Peaks for acetic, butyric, or formic acid, for example, can be identified by comparison to the elution time of volatile organic acid standards.

7. **C** *C. perfringens* produces a double zone of β-hemolysis on blood agar, which makes identification relatively easy. The inner zone of complete hemolysis is caused by a θ-toxin and the outer zone of incomplete hemolysis is caused by an α-toxin (lecithinase activity). The *Bacteroides* spp are gram-negative bacilli, and *C. difficile* is lecithinase-negative and does not produce a double zone of β-hemolysis.

8. **A** Egg yolk agar (modified McClung or neomycin egg yolk agar) is used to determine the presence of lecithinase activity, which causes an insoluble, opaque, whitish precipitate within the agar. Lipase activity is indicated by an iridescent sheen or pearly layer on the surface of the agar.

9. **D** Lipase is produced by some *Clostridium* spp and is seen as an iridescent pearly layer on the surface of the colonies that extends onto the surface of the egg yolk agar medium surrounding them. *C. perfringens*, the most frequently isolated *Clostridium* species, is negative for lipase production.

10. **A** Spore appearance and location, along with Gram stain morphology, aids in distinguishing the *Clostridium* spp. Round, terminal spores are demonstrated when *C. tetani* is grown in chopped meat with glucose broth. Recognition of spores is particularly important because *C. tetani* sometimes appears as gram-negative.

11. Gram-positive bacilli recovered from two blood cultures from a 60-year-old diabetic patient gave the following results:

    Spores seen = Neg   Hemolysis = + (double zone)
    Motility = Neg   Lecithinase = +
    Volatile acids by GLC (PYG) = acetic acid (A) and butyric acid (B)

    What is the most likely identification?
    A. *C. tetani*
    B. *C. perfringens*
    C. *C. novyi* (B)
    D. *C. sporogenes*

    Microbiology/Evaluate laboratory data to make identifications/Bacteria/3

12. Which mechanism is responsible for botulism in infants caused by *C. botulinum*?
    A. Ingestion of spores in food or liquid
    B. Ingestion of preformed toxin in food
    C. Virulence of the organism
    D. Lipase activity of the organism

    Microbiology/Apply principles of fundamental biological characteristics/Anaerobes/2

13. The classic form of foodborne botulism is characterized by the ingestion of:
    A. Spores in food
    B. Preformed toxin in food
    C. Toxin H
    D. All of the above

    Microbiology/Apply principles of fundamental biological characteristics/Anaerobes/2

14. Which test is performed in order to confirm an infection with *C. botulinum*?
    A. Toxin neutralization
    B. Spore forming test
    C. Lipase test
    D. Gelatin hydrolysis test

    Microbiology/Select methods/Reagents/Media/Anaerobes/2

15. Which *Clostridium* spp causes pseudomembranous colitis or antibiotic-associated colitis?
    A. *Clostridium ramosum*
    B. *C. difficile*
    C. *C. perfringens*
    D. *C. sporogenes*

Microbiology/Apply principles of fundamental biological characteristics/Anaerobes/2

Answers to Questions 11–15

11. **B** Spores are generally not demonstrated from clinical specimens containing *C. perfringens*, which is the only species above producing a double zone of hemolysis. The reactions in the chart below distinguish the four species listed.

12. **A** Infant botulism is the most frequent form occurring in the United States. Epidemiological studies have demonstrated that infant botulism results from the ingestion of spores via breast-feeding or exposure to honey. Preformed toxin has not been detected in food or liquids taken by the infants. *C. botulinum* multiplies in the gut of the infant and produces the neurotoxin *in situ*.

13. **B** Foodborne botulism in adults and children is caused by ingestion of the preformed toxin (botulinum toxins A, B, E, and F) in food. The neurotoxins of *C. botulinum* are protoplastic proteins made during the growing phase and released during lysis of the organisms. Confirmation of botulism is made by demonstration of the toxin in serum, gastric, or stool specimens.

14. **A** *C. botulinum* and *C. sporogenes* have similar characteristics biochemically, and definitive identification of *C. botulinum* is made by the mouse neutralization test for its neurotoxins in serum or feces.

	Spore Type	Motility	Lipase	GLC Products
C. botulinum	Subterminal	+	+	A, (P)*, B, (IB)[†], IV[‡]
C. sporogenes	Subterminal	+	+	A, (P), B, (IB), IV

*( ) = variable
[†]Isobutyric acid
[‡]Isovaleric acid

15. **B** *C. difficile* is also implicated in hospital-acquired diarrhea and colitis. Clinical testing for *C. difficile* includes culture and cytotoxin testing by latex agglutination. The cytotoxin assay requires that specimens be shipped to a reference laboratory on dry ice or kept at 4°–6°C if done in-house.

	Spores	Motility	Lecithinase	Double-Zone Hemolysis	GLC Products
C. tetani	Terminal*	+	0	0	A,B
C. perfringens	Subterminal	0	+	+	A,B
C. novyi (B)	Subterminal	+	+	0	A,B,P[†]
C. sporogenes	Subterminal	+	0	0	A,B

*Usually lacking
[†]Proprionic acid

16. Identification of *C. tetani* is based upon:
A. Gram stain of the wound site
B. Anaerobic culture of the wound site
C. Blood culture results
D. Clinical findings

Microbiology/Apply principles of fundamental biological characteristics/Anaerobes/2

17. Obligate anaerobic gram-negative bacilli that do not form spores grow well in 20% bile and are resistant to penicillin 2-unit disks are most likely:
A. *Porphyromonas* spp
B. *Bacteroides* spp
C. *Fusobacterium* spp
D. *Prevotella* spp

Microbiology/Evaluate laboratory data to make identifications/Bacteria/2

18. Which *Bacteroides* spp is noted for "pitting" of the agar and is sensitive to penicillin 2-unit disks?
A. *Bacteroides vulgatus*
B. *Bacteroides ovatus*
C. *Bacteroides thetaiotaomicron*
D. *Bacteroides ureolyticus*

Microbiology/Evaluate laboratory data to make identifications/Bacteria/2

19. Which gram-negative bacilli produce black pigment and brick red fluorescence when exposed to an ultraviolet light source?
A. *Porphyromonas* spp and *Prevotella* spp
B. *Fusobacterium* spp and *Actinomyces* spp
C. *Bacteroides* spp and *Fusobacterius* spp
D. All of the above

Microbiology/Evaluate laboratory data to make identifications/Bacteria/2

20. The following characteristics of an obligate anaerobic gram-negative bacilli best describe which of the genera below?

Gram stain: long slender rods with pointed ends
Colonial appearance: dry bread crumbs or "fried egg" appearance
Penicillin 2-unit disk test = susceptible

A. *Bacteriodes* spp
B. *Fusobacterium* spp
C. *Prevotella* spp
D. *Porphyromonas* spp

Microbiology/Evaluate laboratory data to make identifications/Bacteria/3

21. All of the following genera are anaerobic cocci that stain gram-positive *except:*
A. *Peptococcus* spp
B. *Peptostreptococcus* spp
C. *Streptococcus* spp
D. *Veillonella* spp

Microbiology/Apply principles of fundamental biological characteristics/Anaerobes/2

22. The gram-positive non-spore-forming anaerobic rods most frequently recovered from blood cultures as a contaminant are:
A. *Proprionibacterium acnes*
B. *C. perfringens*
C. *S. intermedius*
D. *Veillonella parvula*

Microbiology/Apply knowledge of fundamental biological characteristics/Anaerobes/2

Answers to Questions 16–22

16. **D** The culture and Gram stain of the puncture wound site usually does not produce any evidence of *C. tetani*. The diagnosis is usually based upon clinical findings, which are characterized by spastic muscle contractions, lockjaw, and backward arching of the back due to muscle contraction.

17. **B** The *Bacteroides* group grows well in 20% bile and are resistant to penicillin 2-unit disks with the exception of *B. ureolyticus*. Most *Prevotella* are also resistant to penicillin 2-unit disks, but most *Fusobacterium* and *Porphyromonas* are sensitive.

18. **D** *B. ureolyticus* is the only species listed that is susceptible to penicillin and produces urease. The other organisms listed are resistant to penicillin.

19. **A** Pigmenting *Porphyromonas* spp and *Prevotella* spp also show hemolysis on sheep blood agar.

20. **B** *Fusobacterium* spp are usually spindle-shaped, slim rods while the other genera are small rods (variable length for *Bacteroides* spp and tiny coccoid rods for *Prevotella* and *Porphyromonas* spp). *Fusobacterium* spp and *Porphyromonas* spp are susceptible to penicillin 2-unit disks, while most *Bacteroides* spp and *Prevotella* spp are resistant.

21. **D** *Veillonella* spp are gram-negative cocci. All four genera are part of the normal human flora and are the most frequently isolated anaerobic cocci from blood cultures, abscesses, wounds, and body fluids. The *Streptococcus* spp are facultative anaerobes, but only *Streptococcus intermedius* is classified an obligate anaerobe.

22. **A** *P. acnes* is a nonspore former and is described as a diphtheroid-shaped rod. It is part of the normal skin, nasopharynx, genitourinary, and gastrointestinal tract flora but is implicated as an occasional cause of endocarditis.

23. Which *Clostridium* spp is most often recovered from a wound infection with gas gangrene?
A. *C. sporogenes*
B. *Clostridium sordellii*
C. *C. novyi*
D. *C. perfringens*

Microbiology/Apply knowledge of fundamental biological characteristics/Anaerobes/1

24. Gram stain of a smear taken from the periodontal pockets of a 30-year-old man with poor dental hygiene showed sulfur granules containing gram-positive rods (short diphtheroids and some unbranched filaments). Colonies on blood agar resembled "molar teeth" in formation. The most likely organism is:
A. *Actinomyces israelii*
B. *P. acnes*
C. *S. intermedius*
D. *Peptostreptococcus anaerobius*

Microbiology/Evaluate laboratory data to make identifications/Bacteria/3

25. Antimicrobial susceptibility testing of anaerobes is done by which of the following methods?
A. Broth disk elution
B. Disk agar diffusion
C. Microtube broth dilution
D. β-Lactamase testing

Microbiology/Apply knowledge of standard operating procedures/Anaerobes/1

Answers to Questions 23–25

23. **D** Wounds infected with clostridia are characterized by invasion and liquefactive necrosis of muscle tissue with gas formation. The most frequent isolate is *C. perfringens* followed by *C. novyi* and *C. septicum*.

24. **A** *A. israelii* is part of the normal flora of the mouth and tonsils but may cause upper or lower respiratory tract infection. The sulfur granules are granular microcolonies with a purulent exudate. Like *Nocardia*, *Actinomyces* produces unbranched mycelia and is sometimes (erroneously) considered a fungus. It has also been implicated in pelvic infection associated with intrauterine contraceptive devices (IUDs).

25. **C** The anaerobes are not suited for the broth disk elution or disk agar diffusion tests because of their slow rate of growth. Kirby-Bauer method reference charts are not designed to be used as a reference of susceptibility for anaerobes.

Mycobacteria

1. The best specimen for recovery of the mycobacteria from a sputum sample is:
   A. First morning specimen
   B. 10-hour evening specimen
   C. 12-hour pooled specimen
   D. 24-hour pooled specimen

   Microbiology/Apply knowledge of standard operating procedures/Mycobacteria/1

2. What concentration of sodium hydroxide (NaOH) is used to prepare a working decontamination solution for the processing of not normally sterile specimens for mycobacteria?
   A. 1% NaOH
   B. 4% NaOH
   C. 8% NaOH
   D. 12% NaOH

   Microbiology/Apply knowledge of standard operating procedures/Mycobacteria/1

3. Which is the most appropriate nonselective media for recovery of mycobacteria from a heavily contaminated specimen?
   A. Löwenstein-Jensen agar
   B. Middlebrook 7H10 agar
   C. Petragnani agar
   D. American Thoracic Society medium

   Microbiology/Select method/Reagents/Media/Mycobacteria/2

4. Mycobacteria stained by the Ziehl-Neelsen or Kinyoun methods with methylene blue counterstain are seen microscopically as:
   A. Bright red rods against a blue background
   B. Bright yellow rods against a yellow background
   C. Orange-red rods against a black background
   D. Bright blue rods against a pink background

   Microbiology/Apply knowledge of fundamental biological characteristics/Mycobacteria/1

Answers to Questions 1–4

1. **A** Contamination by fungi and other bacteria contribute to lower yields of mycobacteria in a 24-hour sample. The first morning specimen collected by expectoration or nebulization produces the highest concentration of mycobacteria in sputum.

2. **B** A strong decontamination solution (6% NaOH or greater) may kill or severely damage the mycobacteria. A 4% NaOH solution is mixed with an equal volume of N-acetyl-L-cysteine (NALC), a digestant or mucolytic agent, to yield a final working concentration of 2% NaOH. The time of exposure of the specimen to the digestion/decontamination solution must be monitored because overtreatment may result in fewer positive cultures.

3. **C** All four media contain malachite green as an inhibitory agent of nonmycobacteria, but Petragnani medium contains a higher concentration (0.052 g/dL) than Löwenstein-Jensen (0.025 g/dL), Middlebrook 7H10 (0.0025 g/dL), or American Thoracic Society medium (0.02 g/dL). The last is used for normally sterile specimens, such as cerebrospinal fluid and bone marrow.

4. **A** The carbolfuchsin (fuchsin with phenol) stains the mycobacteria red and does not decolorize after the acid-alcohol is added. The background and any other bacterial elements will decolorize and are counterstained blue by the methylene blue. A fluorescent staining procedure may be used as an alternative to acid-fast staining. Auramine fluorochrome produces bright yellow fluorescent mycobacteria and auramine-rhodamine causes an orange-red (gold) fluorescence against a dark background. A fluorescent microscope must be used, but with this method the smear can be scanned with a 25X objective instead of the 100X objective permitting more rapid identification of mycobacteria.

5. Acid-fast staining of a smear prepared from a digested sputum showed slender, slightly curved, beaded, red mycobacterial rods. Growth on Middlebrook 7H10 slants produced buff-colored microcolonies with a serpentine pattern after 14 days at 37°C. Niacin and nitrate reduction tests were positive. What is the most probable presumptive identification?
A. *M. tuberculosis*
B. *Mycobacterium ulcerans*
C. *Mycobacterium kansasii*
D. *M. avium* complex

Microbiology/Evaluate laboratory data to make identifications/Mycobacteria/3

6. Which organism, associated with tuberculosis in cattle, causes tuberculosis in humans, especially in regions where dairy farming is prevalent?
A. *M. avium* complex
B. *M. kansasii*
C. *M. marinum*
D. *Mycobacterium bovis*

Microbiology/Apply knowledge of fundamental biological characteristics/Mycobacteria/1

7. Which of the following organisms are used as controls for rapid-growers and slow-growers?
A. *Mycobacterium fortuitum* and *M. tuberculosis*
B. *M. avium* and *M. tuberculosis*
C. *Mycobacterium chelonei* and *M. fortuitum*
D. *M. kansasii* and *M. tuberculosis*

Microbiology/Apply knowledge of fundamental biological characteristics/Mycobacteria/2

8. Which of the following mycobacteria produces pigmented colonies in the dark (is a scotochromogen)?
A. *M. szulgai*
B. *M. kansasii*
C. *M. tuberculosis*
D. All of the above

Microbiology/Apply knowledge of fundamental biological characteristics/Mycobacteria/2

9. All of the following mycobacteria are associated with skin infections *except:*
A. *M. marinum*
B. *M. hemophilum*
C. *M. ulcerans*
D. *M. kansasii*

Microbiology/Apply knowledge of fundamental biological characteristics/Mycobacteria/

Answers to Questions 5–9

5. **A** *M. tuberculosis* is niacin accumulation-positive, while the other three species are niacin-negative. *M. ulcerans* is associated with skin infections (in the tropics), does not grow at 37°C (optimal temperature is 33°C), and is not recovered from sputum. A serpentine pattern of growth indicates production of cording factor, a virulence factor for *M. tuberculosis*.

6. **D** *M. bovis* is also called the bovine tubercle bacillus. A nonvirulent strain, bacillus Calmette-Guérin (BCG), is used as a tuberculosis vaccine throughout the world. Infections with *M. bovis* resemble infections caused by *M. tuberculosis* and are seen in circumstances where there is close contact between humans and cattle.

7. **A** Growth rates of mycobacteria are used along with biochemical tests as an aid to identification. *M. fortuitum* grows within 3–5 days at 37°C and is used as the control for rapid-growers. *M. tuberculosis* grows in 12–25 days at 37°C and is a control organism for slow-growers. In addition to *M. fortuitum*, *M. chelonei* is a rapid-grower (3–5 days at 28°–35°C). In addition to *M. tuberculosis*, *M. avium* and *M. kansasii* are slow-growers (10–21 days at 37°C).

8. **A** *M. tuberculosis* does not produce pigmentation in the dark or after exposure to light (photochromogen). A common tapwater scotochromogen is *Mycobacterium gordonae*. The pathogenic scotochromogens are *Mycobacterium szulgai*, *Mycobacterium scrofulaceum,* and *Mycobacterium xenopi*. *M. kansasii* is a photochromogen producing a yellow pigment following exposure to light and red β-carotene crystals after long incubation periods.

9. **D** *M. kansasii* is a photochromogen that causes chronic pulmonary disease (classic tuberculosis). The other three species cause cutaneous or subcutaneous disease. It is important to culture skin lesions at the correct temperature to facilitate growth.

	Optimum temperature	Growth at 37°C
M. marinum	30°–32°C	Poor
M. hemophilum	28°–32°C	Poor or no
M. ulcerans	33°C	No

10. All of the following *Mycobacterium* spp produce the enzyme required to convert niacin to niacin ribonucleotide *except:*
A. *M. kansasii*
B. *M. tuberculosis*
C. *M. avium* complex
D. *M. szulgai*

Microbiology/Apply knowledge of fundamental biological characteristics/Mycobacteria/2

11. The catalase test for mycobacteria differs from that used for other types of bacteria by using:
A. 1% H_2O_2 and 10% Tween 80
B. 3% H_2O_2 and phosphate buffer, pH 6.8
C. 10% H_2O_2 and 0.85% saline
D. 30% H_2O_2 and 10% Tween 80

Microbiology/Select method/Reagents/Media/Mycobacteria/2

12. Growth inhibition by thiophene-2-carboxylic hydrazide (T_2H) is used to differentiate *M. tuberculosis* from which other *Mycobacterium* sp?
A. *M. bovis*
B. *M. avium* complex
C. *M. kansasii*
D. *M. marinum*

Microbiology/Apply knowledge of fundamental biological characteristics/Mycobacteria/2

13. Which of the following mycobacteria is best differentiated by the rapid hydrolysis of Tween 80?
A. *M. fortuitum*
B. *M. chelonae*
C. *M. kansasii*
D. *M. gordonae*

Microbiology/Apply knowledge of fundamental biological characteristics/Mycobacteria/2

14. Mycobacteria isolated from the hot water system of a hospital grew at 42°C. Colonies on Löwenstein-Jensen medium were not pigmented after exposure to light and negative for niacin accumulation and nitrate reduction. The most likely identification is:
A. *M. xenopi*
B. *M. marinum*
C. *M. ulcerans*
D. *M. haemophilum*

Microbiology/Evaluate laboratory data to make identifications/Mycobacteria/3

Answers to Questions 10–14

10. **B** Niacin production is common to all mycobacteria. However, the niacin accumulates as a water-soluble metabolite in the culture medium when the organism cannot form niacin ribonucleotide. *M. tuberculosis, M. simiae,* and some strains of *M. marinum, M. chelonae,* and *M. bovis* lack the enzyme and therefore are termed niacin-positive because of the accumulation of niacin detected in the test medium.

11. **D** One milliliter of an equal mixture of 30% H_2O_2 (Superoxal) and Tween 80 (a strong detergent) is added to a 2-week-old subculture on Löwenstein-Jensen medium and placed upright for 5 minutes. Catalase activity is determined semiquantitatively by measuring the height of the column of bubbles produced above the culture surface.

12. **A** *M. bovis* and *M. tuberculosis* are very similar biochemically, and some strains of *M. bovis* also accumulate niacin. The T_2H test differentiates *M. tuberculosis* from *M. bovis*. *M. tuberculosis* is not inhibited by T_2H.

13. **C** The hydrolysis of Tween 80 is usually positive when testing the clinically insignificant mycobacteria. *M. fortuitum, M. chelonae,* and *M. gordonae* are saprophytic (and opportunistic) species, but *M. kansasii* is a pathogen. *M. kansasii* hydrolyses Tween 80 more rapidly than the other species (within 3–6 hours). A positive reaction is indicated by a change in the color of neutral red from yellow to pink.

14. **A** *M. xenopi* causes a pulmonary infection resembling *M. tuberculosis* and is frequently isolated from patients with an underlying disease such as alcoholism, AIDS, diabetes, and malignancy. It is often recovered from hot water taps and contaminated water systems and is a possible source of nosocomial infection. The other three species cause skin infections and grow on artificial media at a much lower temperature than *M. xenopi* (below 32°C).

15. A *Mycobacterium* species recovered from a patient with AIDS gave the following results:

Niacin = Neg T_2H = +
Tween 80   Nitrate reduction = Neg
    hydrolysis = Neg
Heat stable catalase (68°C) = ±
Nonphotochromogen

What is the most likely identification?
A. *M. gordonae*
B. *M. bovis*
C. *M. avium* complex
D. *M. kansasii*

Microbiology/Evaluate laboratory data to make identifications/Mycobacteria/3

16. The urease test is needed to differentiate *M. scrofulaceum* from which of the following mycobacteria?
A. *M. gordonae*
B. *M. kansasii*
C. *M. avium* complex
D. *M. bovis*

Microbiology/Apply knowledge of fundamental biological characteristics/Mycobacteria/2

17. A laboratory provides the following services for identification of mycobacteria:

Acid-fast staining of clinical specimens
Inoculation of cultures
Shipment of positive cultures to a reference laboratory for identification

According to the American Thoracic Society's definition for levels of service this laboratory is:
A. Level I
B. Level II
C. Level III
D. Level IV

Microbiology/Apply knowledge of laboratory operations/Mycobacteria/ 2

18. According to the College of American Pathologists (CAP) guidelines, which services for mycobacteria would be performed by a level II laboratory?
A. No procedures performed
B. Acid-fast staining, inoculation, and referral to a reference laboratory
C. Isolation and identification of *M. tuberculosis;* preliminary identification of other species
D. Definitive identification of all mycobacteria

Microbiology/Apply knowledge of laboratory operations/Mycobacteria/2

Answers to Questions 15–18

15. **C** With the exception of *M. tuberculosis, M. avium-intracellulare* (MAI) complex is the *Mycobacterium* species most often isolated from AIDS patients. It is biochemically inert, which is a distinguishing factor for identification. MAI complex is highly resistant to the antibiotics used to treat tuberculosis including multidrug therapy. Treatment with streptomycin, rifampin, ethionamide, ethambutol with cycloserine, or kanamycin has shown little success.

16. **A** Both pathogenic and saprophytic mycobacteria may produce urease, and urease production is used to differentiate several mycobacteria species. Biochemically, *M. scrofulaceum* is identical to *M. gordonae*, except for the urease reaction for which *M. scroflaceum* is positive and *M. gordonae* is negative. Urease reactions for the other pathogenic mycobacteria are:

M. tuberculosis = +   *M. kansasii* = +
M. bovis = +   *M. avium* complex = Neg

17. **A** The American Thoracic Society recognizes three levels of laboratory services for mycobacteria testing. Level I laboratories are those that grow mycobacteria and perform acid-fast stains but do not identify *M. tuberculosis* (they may or may not perform drug susceptibility tests on *M. tuberculosis*). Level II laboratories perform all of the functions of level I laboratories and also identify *M. tuberculosis*. Level III laboratories identify all mycobacteria species from clinical specimens and perform drug susceptibility tests on all species.

18. **B** The CAP lists four options for laboratories to follow in order to correlate the services provided with guidelines for inspection and accreditation. A laboratory's performance on CAP proficiency tests is evaluated by interlaboratory comparison to laboratories within these levels of performance.

19. Culture of a skin (hand) wound from a manager of a tropical fish store grew on Löwenstein-Jensen agar slants at 30°C in 10 days but did not grow on the same media at 37°C in 20 days. Given the results below, what is the most likely identification?

Photochromogen = +   Niacin = Neg
Urease = +   Heat stable catalase
                         (68°C) = Neg
Nitrate reduction = Neg   Tween 80 hydrolysis = +

A. *M. marinum*
B. *M. kansasii*
C. *M. avium* complex
D. *M. tuberculosis*

Microbiology/Evaluate laboratory data to make identifications/Mycobacteria/3

20. Which nonpathogenic *Mycobacterium* sp is isolated most often from clinical specimens and is called the "tapwater bacillus"?
A. *M. kansasii*
B. *M. avium* complex
C. *Mycobacterium leprae*
D. *M. gordonae*

Microbiology/Apply knowledge of laboratory operations/Mycobacteria/2

21. Which of the following drugs are first-line antibiotics used to treat classic tuberculosis for which susceptibility testing is performed by the disk diffusion method on 7H11 agar plates?
A. Ampicillin, penicillin, and carbenicillin
B. Ampicillin, penicillin, and methicillin
C. Vancomycin, methicillin, and carbenicillin
D. Isonicotinic acid hydrazide (INH), rifampin, ethambutol

Microbiology/Apply principles of special procedures/Mycobacteria/2

22. How long should *M. tuberculosis*-positive cultures be kept by the laboratory after identification and antibiotic susceptibility testing have been performed?
A. 1–2 months
B. 2–4 months
C. 5–6 months
D. 6–12 months

Microbiology/Apply knowledge of standard operating procedures/Mycobacteria/2

Answers to Questions 19–22

19. **A** *M. marinum* is typically recovered from cutaneous wounds resulting from infection when the skin is traumatized and comes into contact with inadequately chlorinated fresh water or salt water, such as in swimming pools or fish aquariums. The other three species are slow-growers at 37°C. *M. tuberculosis* and *M. avium* complex are nonphotochromogens. *M. avium* complex is urease-negative, *M. tuberculosis* is positive for niacin and nitrate, and *M. kansasii* is positive for nitrate and catalase.

20. **D** *M. gordonae* is a nonpathogen, scotochromogen, and rapid-grower (7 days at 37°C). Rarely it is implicated in opportunistic infections in patients with shunts, prosthetic heart values, or hepatoperitoneal disease. The other three species are pathogenic mycobacteria.

21. **D** Streptomycin and pyrazinamide are also included as first-line drugs. The first-line antibiotics, except for ethambutol, are bactericidal. Second-line antibiotics used to treat first-line drug-resistant tuberculosis include *p*-aminosalicylic acid, cycloserine, ethionamide, kanamycin, amikacin, viomycin, and capreomycin.

22. **D** Standard therapy using INH and rifampin for classic, uncomplicated pulmonary tuberculosis is 9 months. The patient may not respond to therapy, even when the organism is susceptible to the antibiotics *in vitro;* therefore, cultures must be kept for up to 1 year in order to facilitate testing of additional antibiotics should the infection become refractory to therapy.

23. According to the reporting standards of the American Lung Association (ALA), one or more acid-fast bacilli (AFB) per oil immersion field is reported as:
  A. Numerous or 3+.
  B. Few or 1+.
  C. Rare or 2+.
  D. Indeterminant; a new specimen should be requested.

Microbiology/Apply knowledge of standard operating procedures/Mycobacteria/1

24. Which of the following *Mycobacterium* spp would be most likely to grow on a MacConkey agar plate?
  A. *M. chelonae-fortuitum* complex
  B. *M. ulcerans*
  C. *M. marinum*
  D. MAI complex

Microbiology/Apply knowledge of fundamental biological characteristics/Mycobacteria/1

25. Rapid methods for identifying classic infection with *M. tuberculosis* include:
  A. GLC
  B. Nucleic acid probes
  C. Acid-fast smears
  D. All of the above

Microbiology/Apply principles of speial procedures/Mycobacteria/2

Answers to Questions 23–25

23. **A** Acid-fast smears are standardized by the ALA for reporting the number of AFB seen. The following criteria should be used to uniformly report results:

  1–2 AFB per smear → report negative and request another sample
  3–9 AFB per smear → report as rare (1+)
  10 or more per smear → report as few (2+)
  1 or more per oil immersion field → report as numerous (3+)

24. **A** Mycobacteria growing on MacConkey agar are usually nonpathogens. *M. chelonae* and *M. fortuitum* are both nonpathogenic rapid-growers that will grow on MacConkey agar (with no crystal violet) within 5 days. MAI complex is variable on MacConkey agar but takes much longer to grow. *M. marinum* and *M. ulcerans* will not grow on MacConkey agar.

25. **D** *M. tuberculosis* is a slow-grower with a prolonged culture time of 12–25 days and requires 3–6 weeks for definitive identification and antibiotic susceptibility testing. The acid-fast smear remains the number one rapid test for the detection of mycobacterial infection. A positive smear has a predictive value of 96% when all laboratory and clinical findings are considered. GLC is used to evaluate cell wall lipid patterns for identification. Nucleic acid probes consist of single strands of iodine 125 (^{125}I) labeled DNA complementary in base sequence to the rRNA of *M. tuberculosis*. Hybridization results in formation of double-stranded complexes, which are separated from the unhybridized probe DNA and then measured for radioactivity. DNA probes are available for rapid identification of *M. tuberculosis*, *M. bovis*, *M. avium* complex, and *M. gordonae*.

UNIT 9

Mycology

1. All of the following are examples of appropriate specimens for the recovery of fungi *except:*
   A. Tissue biopsy
   B. Cerebrospinal fluid
   C. Aspirate of exudate
   D. Swab

   Microbiology/Apply knowledge to identify sources of error/Mycology/1

2. For which clinical specimens is the KOH direct mount technique for examination of fungal elements used?
   A. Skin
   B. Cerebrospinal fluid
   C. Blood
   D. Bone marrow

   Microbiology/Apply principles of basic laboratory procedures/Mycology/1

3. The India ink stain is used as a presumptive test for the presence of which organism?
   A. *Aspergillus niger* in blood
   B. *Cryptococcus neoformans* in CSF
   C. *Histoplasma capsulatum* in CSF
   D. *Candida albicans* in blood or body fluids

   Microbiology/Correlate clinical and laboratory data/Mycology/2

4. Cutaneous disease involving skin, hair, and nails usually indicates an infection with a:
   A. Dimorphic fungus
   B. Dermatophyte
   C. Zygomycetes
   D. *Candida* species

   Microbiology/Correlate clinical and laboratory data/Mycology/2

Answers to Questions 1–4

1. **D** Specimens for fungal culture must be kept in a moist, sterile environment. Swabs that are dried out or submitted with insufficient material on them should be rejected. Generally, swabs are inadequate for the recovery of fungi because they are easily contaminated with surrounding skin flora.

2. **A** A solution of 10% KOH is used for contaminated specimens such as skin, nail scrapings, hair, and sputum to clear away background debris that may resemble fungal elements. Normally sterile specimens (CSF, blood, and bone marrow) do not require KOH for clearing.

3. **B** Meningitis caused by *C. neoformans* is diagnosed through culture, biochemical reactions, and the latex test for cryptococcal antigen. The India ink test is not diagnostic for cryptococcal meningitis because positive staining results are demonstrated in less than 50% of confirmed cases. A positive India ink test shows yeast cells in CSF with a surrounding clear area (the capsule) because the capsule of *C. neoformans* is not penetrated by ink particles.

4. **B** Superficial dermatophytes rarely invade the deeper tissues and are the cause of most cutaneous fungal infections. Fungal infections of the skin are most often caused by *Microsporum* spp, *Trichophyton* spp, and *Epidermophyton* spp, although *Candida* spp are sometimes implicated as the cause of nail infections.

5. What is the first step to be performed in the identification of an unknown yeast isolate?
  A. Gram stain smear
  B. India ink stain
  C. Catalase test
  D. Germ tube test

Microbiology/Select methods/Reagents/Media/Mycology/2

6. An isolate produced a constriction that was interpreted as a positive germ tube, but *C. albicans* was ruled out when confirmatory tests were performed. Which of the following fungi is the most likely identification?
  A. *Candida tropicalis*
  B. *Cryptococcus neoformans*
  C. *Candida glabrata*
  D. *Rhodotorula rubra*

Microbiology/Apply knowledge of fundamental biological characteristics/Mycology/2

7. Cornmeal agar with Tween 80 is used to identify which characteristic of an unknown yeast isolate?
  A. Hyphae (true and pseudo)
  B. Blastospores and arthrospores
  C. Chlamydospores
  D. All of the above

Microbiology/Apply knowledge of basic laboratory procedures/Mycology/1

8. Blastospores (blastoconidia) are the beginning of which structures?
  A. Arthrospores
  B. Germ tubes
  C. Pseudohyphae
  D. True hyphae

Microbiology/Apply knowledge of fundamental biological characteristics/Mycology/1

9. An isolate from CSF growing on cornmeal agar produces the following structures:

  Blastospores = +   Pseudohyphae = Neg
  Chlamydospores = Neg   Arthrospores = Neg

  Which tests should be performed next?
  A. Birdseed agar and urease
  B. Germ tube and glucose
  C. India ink and germ tube
  D. All of the above

Microbiology/Select methods/Reagents/Media/Mycology/2

10. Which of the following yeast enzymes is detected using birdseed (niger seed) agar?
  A. Phenol oxidase
  B. Catalase
  C. Urease
  D. Nitrate reductase

Microbiology/Apply knowledge of fundamental biological characteristics/Mycology/2

11. Which of the following yeasts is characteristically positive for germ tube production?
  A. *Candida tropicalis*
  B. *Candida pseudotropicalis*
  C. *Cryptococcus neoformans*
  D. *Candida albicans*

Microbiology/Apply knowledge of fundamental biological characteristics/Mycology/1

Answers to Questions 5–11

5. **D** The true germ tube (filamentous extension from a yeast cell) is approximately one-half the width and 3–4 times the length of the cell with no true hyphae constriction at the point of origin. *C. albicans* produce germ tubes (95%), and a positive test is considered a presumptive identification.

6. **A** *C. tropicalis* forms pseudohyphae that resemble true germ tubes by producing a constriction at the point of origin of the yeast cell. A germ tube represents a true hyphae without constriction, and therefore, the test should have been repeated along with carbohydrate tests before making a presumptive identification. The other three species of yeast listed do not form hyphae.

7. **D** Cornmeal agar with Tween 80 (polysorbate) reduces the surface tension and allows for enhanced formation of hyphae, blastospores, and chlamydospores.

8. **C** Pseudohyphae are the result of a pinching off process, blastoconidiation, with the growth of filaments with constrictions. Germ tubes are the beginning of true hyphae (no constrictions). Arthrospores are the result of a breaking off process of true septate hyphae resulting in square conidia.

9. **A** A yeast isolated from CSF producing blastospores is most likely to be *C. neoformans*, which is positive for urease and produces brown colonies on birdseed agar.

10. **A** Most isolates of *C. neoformans* produce phenol oxidase when grown on *Guizotia abyssinica* medium (birdseed medium) producing brown to black pigmented colonies. *C. neoformans* is the only *Cryptococcus* species that oxidizes *o*-diphenol to melanin, which is responsible for the color.

11. **D** *C. albicans* and *Candida stellatoidea*, a variant of *C. albicans*, are the only yeasts that produce germ tubes within 1–3 hours of incubation at 37°C. *C. tropicalis* produces pseudohyphae after incubation for 3 hours, which may be mistaken for germ tubes. A careful evaluation of the tube origin for constriction is required in order to avoid a false-positive interpretation.

12. Arthrospore (arthroconidia) production is used to differentiate which two yeast isolates?
   A. *Candida albicans* and *C. stellatoidea*
   B. *Trichosporon pullulans* and *Cryptococcus neoformans*
   C. *C. albicans* and *C. tropicalis*
   D. *Saccharomyces cerevisiae* and *Candida (Torulopsis) glabrata*

   Microbiology/Apply knowledge of fundamental biological characteristics/Mycology/2

13. The urease test, niger seed agar test, and the germ tube test are all used for the presumptive identification of:
   A. *R. rubra*
   B. *Cryptococcus neoformans*
   C. *T. pullulans*
   D. *Candida albicans*

   Microbiology/Apply knowledge of fundamental biological characteristics/Mycology/2

14. Which of the following yeasts produces only blastospores on cornmeal Tween 80 agar?
   A. *Candida* spp
   B. *Trichosporon* spp
   C. *Geotrichum* spp
   D. *Cryptococcus* spp

   Microbiology/Apply knowledge of fundamental biological characteristics/Mycology/2

15. Ascospores are formed by which yeast isolate?
   A. *S. cerevisiae*
   B. *Candida albicans*
   C. *Cryptococcus neoformans*
   D. All of the above

   Microbiology/Apply knowledge of fundamental biological characteristics/Mycology/2

16. A germ tube-negative, pink yeast isolate was recovered from the respiratory secretions and urine of a patient with AIDS. Given the following results, what is the most likely identification?

   Cornmeal Tween 80 Agar
   Blastospores = +   Pseudohyphae = +
   Arthrospores = Neg   Urease = +

   A. *C. albicans*
   B. *Rhodotorula* spp
   C. *Cryptococcus* spp
   D. *Trichosporon* spp

   Microbiology/Evaluate laboratory data to make identifications/Mycology/3

Answers to Questions 12–16

12. **B** *T. pullulans* and *C. neoformans* are both urease-positive, but *T. pullulans* produces arthrospores and *C. neoformans* does not. In addition to *Trichosporon* spp arthrospores are produced by *Geotrichum* spp.

13. **B** A germ tube negative isolate producing black colonies on niger seed agar and a positive urease test is a presumptive identification of *C. neoformans*. A positive germ tube test is a presumptive identification for *C. albicans*, as well as for *C. stellatoidea*. See the first chart below.

14. **D** *Cryptococcus* spp do not form either pseudohyphae or arthrospores. *Candida* spp produce blastospores or pseudohyphae. *Trichosporon* spp and *Geotrichum* spp produce pseudohyphae, blastospores, and arthrospores. See the second chart below.

15. **A** Sexual spore production is a characteristic of the *Ascomycotina*, which produce an ascus (saclike structure) after the union of two nuclei. The resulting spore is termed an ascospore. *S. cerevisiae* produces ascospores when grown on ascospore agar for 10 days at 25°C.

16. **B** *Rhodotorula* spp produce pink- to coral-colored colonies on Sabouraud agar and cornmeal agar. It is usually considered a contaminant but is an opportunistic pathogen and must be identified when found in specimens from immunosuppressed patients.

	C. neoformans	R. rubra	T. pullulans	C. albicans
Urease	+	+	+	0
Germ tube	0	0	0	+
Black colonies on niger seed agar	+	0	0	0

	Blastospores	Pseudohyphae	Arthrospores
Cryptococcus spp	+	0	0
Candida spp	+	+	0
Trichosporon spp	+	+	+
Geotrichum spp	+	+	+

17. Chlamydospore production is demonstrated by which *Candida* species?
A. *C. glabrata*
B. *Candida krusei*
C. *C. albicans*
D. *C. tropicalis*

Microbiology/Apply knowledge of fundamental biological characteristics/Mycology/1

18. Carbohydrate assimilation tests are used for the identification of yeast isolates by inoculating media:
A. Free of carbohydrates
B. Free of niger seed
C. Containing carbohydrates
D. Containing yeast extract

Microbiology/Apply principles of basic laboratory procedures/Mycology/1

19. Yeast recovered from the urine of a catheterized patient receiving chemotherapy for cancer gave the following results:

Cornmeal Tween 80 Agar

Germ tube = +   Blastospores = +
Pseudohyphae = +   Arthrospores = Neg
Chlamydospores = +

What further testing is necessary?
A. Carbohydrate assimilation and urease
B. Urease and niger seed
C. Nitrate reductase and carbohydrate fermentation
D. No further testing is needed for identification

Microbiology/Select course of action/Mycology/3

20. A blood agar plate inoculated with sputum from a patient with diabetes mellitus grew very few bacterial flora and a predominance of yeast. Given the following results, what is the most likely identification of the yeast isolate?

Cornmeal Tween 80 Agar

Germ tube = Neg   Pseudohyphae = +
Arthrospores = Neg   Blastoconidia = + (arranged
Chlamydospores =   along pseudohyphae)
   Neg
A. *C. tropicalis*
B. *C. pseudotropicalis*
C. *Trichosporon beigelii*
D. *Geotrichum condidum*

Microbiology/Evaluate laboratory data to make identifications/Mycology/3

21. Dimorphic molds are found in infected tissue in which form?
A. Mold phase
B. Yeast phase
C. Encapsulated
D. Latent

Microbiology/Apply knowledge of fundamental biological characteristics/Mycology/1

22. The mycelial form of which dimorphic mold produces thick-walled, rectangular or barrel-shaped alternate arthroconidia?
A. *Coccidioides immitis*
B. *Sporothrix schenckii*
C. *H. capsulatum*
D. *Blastomyces dermatitidis*

Microbiology/Apply knowledge of fundamental biological characteristics/Mycology/2

Answers to Questions 17–22

17. C Cornmeal Tween 80 agar supports the growth of *C. albicans* and formation of its distinctive thick-walled, terminal (at the tip of the pseudohyphae) chlamydospores. *C. stellatoidea* may also produce chlamydospores, but it is considered a variant of *C. albicans* and is not usually differentiated.

18. A The yeast isolate is inoculated directly into the molten agar base free of carbohydrates, or is poured as a suspension onto a yeast nitrogen agar base plate. Carbohydrate disks are then added to the surface of the agar and the plates incubated for 24–48 hours at 30°C. Growth around the disk indicates the ability of the yeast to utilize the carbohydrate(s) as a sole source of carbon.

19. D This isolate is *C. albicans*, which also produces some true hyphae along with pseudohyphae. A positive germ tube is a presumptive identification; no further testing is needed because no other yeast produces blastospores and chlamydospores along with pseudohyphae.

20. A *C. tropicalis* and *C. pseudotropicalis* differ in their arrangement of blastoconidia along the pseudohyphae. *C. pseudotropicalis* forms elongated blastoconidia arranged in parallel clusters that simulate logs in a stream. *Trichosporon* spp and *Geotrichum* spp form arthrospores.

21. B Dimorphic molds are in the yeast form in infected tissues because they are in the yeast form at 37°C. Specimens are cultured and incubated at both room temperature and 35°–37°C. To prove that a mold growing at room temperature (or 30°C) is a dimorphic fungus, conversion to the yeast form must be demonstrated via subculture and incubation at 37°C.

22. A The mold form of *C. immitis* shows barrel-shaped arthroconidia separated by empty cells (ghost cells) that cause an uneven staining effect when they are examined under a microscope. *Trichosporon* spp and *Geotrichum* spp show rectangular, evenly stained arthroconidia.

23. The yeast form of which dimorphic fungus appears as oval or elongated cigar shapes, some with multiple buds?
- A. *C. immitis*
- B. *S. schenckii*
- C. *H. capsulatum*
- D. *B. dermatitidis*

Microbiology/Apply knowledge of fundamental biological characteristics/Mycology/2

24. The mycelial form of *H. capsulatum* seen on agar resembles:
- A. *Sepedonium* spp
- B. *Penicillium* spp
- C. *Sporothrix* spp
- D. *Coccidioides* spp

Microbiology/Apply knowledge of fundamental biological characteristics/Mycology/2

25. The yeast form of which dimorphic mold shows a large parent yeast cell surrounded by smaller budding yeast cells?
- A. *Paracoccidioides brasiliensis*
- B. *S. schenkii*
- C. *C. immitis*
- D. *H. capsulatum*

Microbiology/Apply knowledge of fundamental biological characteristics/Mycology/2

26. Which group of molds can be ruled out when septate hyphae are observed in a culture?
- A. Dematiaceous
- B. Zyomycetes
- C. Dermatophytes
- D. Dimorphic molds

Microbiology/Apply knowledge of fundamental biological characteristics/Mycology/1

27. Tinea versicolor is a skin infection caused by:
- A. *Malassezia furfur*
- B. *Trichophyton rubrum*
- C. *Trichophyton schoenleinii*
- D. *Microsporum gypseum*

Microbiology/Apply knowledge of fundamental biological characteristics/Mycology/1

28. Which of the following structures is invaded by the genus *Trichophyton?*
- A. Hair
- B. Nails
- C. Skin
- D. All of the above

Microbiology/Apply knowledge of fundamental biological characteristics/Mycology/1

Answers to Questions 23–28

23. **B** *S. schenckii* is usually acquired by humans through thorns or splinters because it is commonly found on living or dead vegetation. It is called "rose gardener's disease" because gardeners, florists, and farmers are most often infected. *S. schenckii* is often recovered from exudates of unopened subcutaneous nodules or open draining lesions.

24. **A** *Sepedonium* spp are saprophytic molds that do not have a yeast phase and produce large spherical tuberculate macroconidia like *H. capsulatum*. Histoplasmosis is a chronic granulomatous infection primarily found in the lungs that invades the reticuloendothelial system. Infection occurs via spores released from decaying bird or chicken droppings which are inhaled when disturbed.

25. **A** *P. brasiliensis* yeast forms are sometimes seen as a "mariner's wheel" because multiple budding cells completely surround the periphery of the parent cell.

26. **B** Zygomycetes commonly recovered from clinical specimens are *Rizopus* spp and *Mucor* spp. Both display aseptate hyphae, while the other groups above display septate hyphae. Zygomycetes usually not encountered in clinical specimens are also aseptate and include *Absidia* spp, *Rhizomucor* spp, *Cincinella* spp, *Cunninghamella* spp, and *Syncephalastrum* spp.

27. **A** *M. furfur* has a worldwide distribution and causes a superficial, brownish, dry, scaly patch on the skin of light-skinned persons and lighter patches on persons with dark skin. *M. furfur* is not cultured because diagnosis can be made from microscopic examination of the skin scales. Skin scrapings prepared in KOH show oval or bottle-shaped cells that exhibit monopolar budding in the presence of a cell wall and also produce small hyphae.

28. **D** *Trichophyton* spp, *Microsporum* spp, and *Epidermophyton* spp are the organisms causing human dermatomycoses or cutaneous infections. *Trichophyton* spp infect hair and nails as well as skin. Infections with members of the genus *Microsporum* are confined to the hair and skin, while infections caused by the genus *Epidermophyton* are seen only on the skin and nails.

29. An organism cultured from the skin produces colonies displaying a cherry red color on Sabouraud dextrose agar after 3–4 weeks, and teardrop-shaped microconidia along the sides of the hyphae. The most likely identification is:
A. *T. rubrum*
B. *Trichophyton tonsurans*
C. *T. schoenleinii*
D. *Trichophyton violacium*

Microbiology/Apply knowledge of fundamental biological characteristics/Mycology/1

30. Which *Microsporum* species causes an epidemic form of tinea capitis in children?
A. *Microsporum canis*
B. *Microsporum audouinii*
C. *M. gypseum*
D. All of the above

Microbiology/Correlate clinical and laboratory data/Mycology/2

31. Microscopic examination of a fungus cultured from a patient with athlete's foot showed large, smooth-walled, club-shaped macroconidia appearing singly or in clusters of 2–3 from the tips of short conidiophores. The colonies did not produce microconidia. What is the most likely identification?
A. *Trichophyton* spp
B. *Alternaria* spp
C. *Epidermophyton* spp
D. *Microsporum* spp

Microbiology/Evaluate laboratory data to make identifications/Mycology/2

32. Which *Trichophyton* species causes the favus type of tinea capitis seen in the Scandinavian countries and in the Appalachian region of the United States?
A. *T. verrucosum*
B. *T. violaceum*
C. *T. tonsurans*
D. *T. schoenleinii*

Microbiology/Correlate clinical and laboratory data/Mycology/2

33. The Hair Baiting Test is used to differentiate which two species of *Trichophyton* that produce red colonies on Sabouraud agar plates?
A. *Trichophyton mentagrophytes* and *T. rubrum*
B. *T. tonsurans* and *T. schoenleinii*
C. *T. tonsurans* and *T. violaceum*
D. *T. verrucosum* and *T. rubrum*

Microbiology/Correlate clinical and laboratory data/Mycology/2

34. A mold that produces colonies with a dark brown, green-black, or black appearance of both the surface and reverse side is classified as a:
A. Dematiaceous mold
B. Dermatophyte
C. Hyaline mold
D. Dimorphic fungus

Microbiology/Apply knowledge of fundamental biological characteristics/Mycology/1

Answers to Questions 29–34

29. **A** Members of the genus *Microsporum* produce club-shaped microconidia and are usually pigmented white, buff, yellow, or brown. *Epidermophyton* does not display microconidia and produces yellow-green, or yellow-tan colonies. *T. rubrum* can be differentiated from the other members of the genus by its distinctive cherry red color. *Trichophyton mentagrophytes* may also produce a red pigment, but it is usually rose-colored or orange, or deep red. *T. tonsurans* produces white-tan to yellow suedelike colonies. *T. schoenleinii* produces white to cream-colored colonies, and *T. violaceum* produces port wine to deep violet colonies.

30. **B** *M. audouinii* and *T. tonsurans* may both cause epidemic tinea capitis in children. *M. audouinii* causes a chronic infection transmitted directly via infected hairs on caps, hats, combs, upholstery, and hair clippers. Infected hair shafts fluoresce yellow-green under a Wood's lamp. *M. audouinii* does not usually sporulate in culture and forms atypical vegetative forms such as antler and racquet hyphae and terminal chlamydospores. In contrast, *M. canis* produces spindle-shaped, thick-walled multicelled macroconidia, and *M. gypseum* produces ellipsoidal, multicellular macroconidia.

31. **C** *Epidermophyton* spp do not produce microconidia; this differentiates them from *Trichophyton* spp and *Microsporum* spp. *Alternaria* is not a dermatophyte. *Epidermophyton floccosum* is the most frequently isolated member of the genus and infects the skin, but not the hair or nails.

32. **D** *T. schoenleinii* is identified microscopically by its characteristic antler-shaped hyphae and chlamydospores in the absence of conidia.

33. **A** *T. mentagrophytes* may produce a deep red pigment seen through the reverse side of the agar plate that resembles the cherry red pigment produced by *T. rubrum*. However, *T. mentagrophytes* can be differentiated by its ability to invade the hair shaft. *T. rubrum* grows on the surface of the hair but does not penetrate the shaft.

34. **A** The dematiaceous molds are easily recognized and confirmed by observing dark yellow or brown septate hyphae upon microscopic examination.

35. A rapidly growing hyaline mold began as a white colony but soon developed a black "pepper" effect on the agar surface. The older colony produced a black matte making it resemble a dematiaceous mold. What is the most likely identification?
A. *Penicillium notatum*
B. *Aspergillus niger*
C. *Paecilomyces* spp
D. *Scopulariopsis* spp

Microbiology/Apply knowledge of fundamental biological characteristics/Mycology/1

36. Which dematiaceous mold forms flask-shaped phialides each with a flask-shaped collarette.
A. *Phialophora* spp
B. *Exophila* spp
C. *Wangiella* spp
D. All of the above

Microbiology/Apply knowledge of fundamental biological characteristics/Mycology/1

37. Which *Aspergillus* species, recovered from sputum or bronchial mucus, is the most common cause of pulmonary aspergillosis?
A. *A. niger*
B. *A. flavus*
C. *A. fumigatus*
D. All of the above

Microbiology/Correlate clinical and laboratory data/Mycology/2

38. A hyaline mold recovered from a patient with AIDS produced rose-colored colonies with lavender centers on Sabouraud dextrose agar. Microscopic examination showed multiseptate macroconidia appearing as sickles or canoes. What is the most likely identification?
A. *Fusarium* spp
B. *Wangiella* spp
C. *Exophiala* spp
D. *Phialophora* spp

Microbiology/Evaluate laboratory data to make identifications/Mycology/3

39. Material from a fungus-ball infection produced colonies with a green surface on Sabouraud agar in 5 days at 30°C. Microscopic examination showed club-shaped vesicles with sporulation only from the top half of the vesicle. This hyaline mold is most probably which *Aspergillus* spp?
A. *A. niger*
B. *A. fumigatus*
C. *A. flavus*
D. *A. terreus*

Microbiology/Evaluate laboratory data to make identifications/Mycology/3

40. A rapidly growing nonseptate mold produced colonies with a gray surface resembling cotton candy that covered the entire plate. Microscopic examination revealed sporangiophores arising between, not opposite, the rhizoids and producing pear-shaped sporangia. What is the most likely identification?
A. *Absidia* spp
B. *Penicillium* spp
C. *Rhizopus* spp
D. *Aspergillus* spp

Microbiology/Evaluate laboratory data to make identifications/Mycology/3

Answers to Qestions 35–40

35. **B** *A. niger* is the only species listed producing black conidia, which causes a "pepper" effect as the colony grows. The reverse side of the agar plate remains buff- or cream-colored, which differentiates it from the dematiaceous (dark) molds.

36. **A** *Phialophora, Exophila,* and *Wangiella* all produce phialides, but the last two genera form elongated, tubelike phialides without a collarette, as opposed to the flask-shaped phialides of *Phialophora,* which contain clusters of conidia at the tips.

37. **C** *A. fumigatus* is most often associated with compost piles and is found in the soil of potted plants. *A. niger* is the cause of cavitary fungus ball lesions of the lungs and nasal passages.

38. **A** *Fusarium* spp are usually a contaminant but are sometimes seen as a cause of mycotic eye, nail, or skin infection in debilitated patients. *Fusarium* sp is a hyaline *Hyphomycetes* and grows on Sabouraud agar plates at 30°C within 4 days. The other three organisms are members of the *Dematiaceae* family (dark molds).

39. **B** *A. fumigatus* is the most common cause of aspergillosis. It is characterized by sporulation only from the upper half or two-thirds of the vesicle. Colonies of *A. niger* are yellow with black pepper growth and produce phialides over the entire vesicle forming the classic "radiate" head. *A. flavus* colonies are yellow to yellow-green and produce phialides that cover the entire vesicle and point out in all directions. *A. terreus* produces brown colonies and phialides that also cover the entire vesicle.

40. **A** *Absidia* spp are similar to *Rhizopus* spp except for the location of rhizoids (rootlike hyphae). The rhizoids of *Rhizopus* spp are located at the point where the stolons and sporangiophores meet, while those of *Absidia* spp arise at a point on the stolon between the rhizoids. *Penicillium* spp and *Aspergillus* spp do not form rhizoids.

1. Classification of viruses is made by:
   A. Complement fixation serology
   B. Electron microscopy
   C. Nucleic acid composition
   D. Cellular inclusion bodies

   Microbiology/Apply knowledge of fundamental biological characteristics/Viruses/1

2. Which virus is the most common etiologic agent of viral respiratory diseases in infants and children?
   A. Respiratory syncytial virus (RSV)
   B. Measles virus
   C. Coxsackie A virus
   D. Coxsackie B virus

   Microbiology/Apply knowledge of fundamental biological characteristics/Viruses/1

3. The most common viral syndrome of pericarditis and myocarditis and pleurodynia (pain upon breathing) is caused by:
   A. Herpes simplex
   B. Respiratory syncytial virus
   C. Epstein-Barr virus
   D. Coxsackie B virus

   Microbiology/Apply knowledge of fundamental biological characteristics/Viruses/1

4. Which of the following viruses is implicated along with Epstein-Barr virus as a cause of infectious mononucleosis?
   A. Cytomegalovirus (CMV)
   B. Coxsackie A virus
   C. Coxsackie B virus
   D. Hepatitis B virus

   Microbiology/Apply knowledge of fundamental biological characteristics/Viruses/1

5. The most common causes of viral pneumonia in adults are:
   A. Influenza and adenovirus
   B. Hepatitis A and B viruses
   C. Coxsackie A and B viruses
   D. Herpes simplex and CMV

   Microbiology/Apply knowledge of fundamental biological characteristics/Viruses/1

Answers to Questions 1–5

1. **C** True viruses have nucleic acid that is either RNA or DNA, and this serves as the basis for initial classification. Members of these classes are further divided into groups that cause human disease based upon the mode of transmission, tissues invaded, diseases produced, and antigenic characteristics.

2. **A** RSV is the cause of croup, bronchitis, bronchiolitis, and interstitial pneumonia. Children under 1 year old who are hospitalized are the most susceptible group.

3. **D** Coxsackie A virus, coxsackie B virus, and the echoviruses are most commonly implicated in myocarditis and other syndromes, including acute cerebellar ataxia and hepatitis. Like poliovirus, infections are more common in the summer and fall and gain entry through the gastrointestinal tract.

4. **A** CMV infection in a previously healthy individual causes a self-limited mononucleosis syndrome. CMV is an opportunistic pathogen that may produce lifelong infections and can cause a variety of diseases including congenital and neonatal infection, hepatitis, pneumonia, and disseminated infection in immunocompromised patients.

5. **A** Influenza and adenoviruses are the main cause of respiratory infections including the common cold, tracheobronchitis, and pneumonia. Adenoviruses also cause conjunctivitis, keratitis, cystitis, and gastroenteritis.

6. Which virus belonging to the Reoviridae group causes gastroenteritis in infants and young children but an asymptomatic infection in adults?
A. Coxsackie B virus
B. Rotavirus
C. Respiratory syncytial virus
D. Rhabdovirus

Microbiology/Apply knowledge of fundamental biological characteristics/Viruses/1

7. A very small, single-stranded DNA virus that causes a febrile illness with a rash and is called the fifth childhood disease after rubeola, rubella, varicella, and roseola is:
A. Rotavirus
B. Adenovirus type 40
C. Coxsackie A virus
D. Parvovirus B19

Microbiology/Apply knowledge of fundamental biological characteristics/Viruses/1

8. Hepatitis B virus can be transmitted by:
A. Acupuncture
B. Tatoos
C. Sexual contact
D. All of the above

Microbiology/Apply knowledge of fundamental biological characteristics/Viruses/1

9. Which virus has been implicated in adult gastroenteritis resulting from ingestion of contaminated food (especially shellfish) and water?
A. Norwalk-like viruses
B. Rotavirus
C. Hepatitis C virus
D. Coronavirus

Microbiology/Apply knowledge of fundamental biological characteristics/Viruses/1

10. Which virus is associated with venereal and respiratory tract warts and produces lesions of skin and mucous membranes?
A. Polyomavirus
B. Poxvirus
C. Adenovirus
D. Papillomavirus

Microbiology/Apply knowledge of fundamental biological characteristics/Viruses/1

11. A clinical test used for the detection and identification of viral infections other than culture is:
A. Hemagglutination
B. Hemadsorption
C. Viral antigen detection
D. All of the above

Microbiology/Apply principles of basic laboratory procedures/Viruses/1

Answers to Questions 6–11

6. **B** Rotavirus has been implicated in both nosocomial infections and epidemic gastroenteritis. Children 3–24 months old are most commonly affected. Diarrhea begins after an incubation period of 3 days, lasts for 2–10 days, and is associated with vomiting and dehydration. In immunosuppressed children rotavirus causes a chronic infection.

7. **D** Parvovirus causes a fever and characteristic "slapped cheek" rash in young children. Adults are usually immune, but immunocompromised persons may exhibit an arthritis or anemia (the virus infects immature RBCs in the bone marrow).

8. **D** Although the most common mode of transmission of hepatitis B is via needle puncture, it may also be transmitted by other parenteral means including sexual transmission and contact with contaminated blood through broken skin or mucous membranes.

9. **A** Norwalk-like viruses are small RNA viruses that have been implicated in epidemics of community gastroenteritis as well as sporadic infections. Unlike rotavirus, which causes gastroenteritis in infants and young children, Norwalk-like viruses produce infection in all age groups.

10. **D** The human papillomaviruses (HPVs) cause genital warts. Several strains including HPV-6, HPV-11, HPV-16, and HPV-18 are associated with cervical and vaginal neoplasia. Because the virus cannot be cultured *in vitro*, diagnosis is usually made using DNA probes. A diagnostic characteristic of infected cells is koilocytosis, a perinuclear clearing in the squamous epithelium accompanied by nuclear atypica.

11. **D** In addition to serological tests for antibodies against the virus and DNA probes that identify viral DNA or RNA, the methods above aid in the rapid diagnosis of several viruses. Various species of animal RBCs are used for identification of viruses that contain receptors that agglutinate the RBCs. Some influenza A and parainfluenza viruses may be detected only by hemagglutination or hemadsorption. Testing for viral antigen in culture is used for detection of RSV, CMV, and varicella-zoster.

12. Which technique is most widely used for the confirmation of infection with human immunodeficiency virus (HIV-1)?
A. Western blot (immunoblot) assay
B. Enzyme-linked immunosorbent assay (ELISA)
C. Complement fixation
D. Polymerase chain reaction

Microbiology/Select methods/Reagents/Media/ Viruses/2

13. A 13-year-old boy was admitted to the hospital with a diagnosis of viral encephalitis. History revealed that the boy harbored wild racoons from a nearby woods. What is the best method to determine if the boy has contracted rabies?
A. Remove the brain stems from all of the racoons and examine for cytopathic effects.
B. Request immunofluorescent test for antibody on the saliva from all of the racoons.
C. Request immunofluorescent test for antigen in cutaneous nerves obtained by nuchal biopsy of the patient.
D. Isolate the virus from the saliva of both the animals and the patient.

Microbiology/Select methods/Reagents/Media/ Viruses/3

14. A 65-year-old woman was admitted to the hospital with acute respiratory distress, fever, myalgia, and headache. Influenza A or B was suspected after ruling out bacterial pneumonia. Which of the following methods could be used to confirm influenza infection?
A. Influenza virus culture in Madin-Darby canine kidney
B. Hemagglutination inhibition test for antibodies in the patient's serum
C. Direct examination of nasal epithelium for virus using fluorescent antibody stain
D. All of the above

Microbiology/Select methods/Reagents/Media/ Viruses/3

15. The most rapid definitive diagnosis of a genital herpes simplex (HSV-2) infection in a 20-year-old man is made by which method?
A. Direct immunofluorescence test for viral antigen in vesicle fluid
B. Titer of serum and seminal fluid for antibodies to herpes simplex
C. Detection of antiherpes simplex in seminal fluid
D. Cell culture of vesicle fluid

Microbiology/Select methods/Reagents/Media/ Viruses/2

Answers to Questions 12–15

12. **A** The Western blot assay is most often used to confirm a positive serological test of antibodies to HIV. A sample is confirmed positive if antibodies are demonstrated against two of the three major regions (env, pol, and gag).

13. **C** Using direct immunofluorescence, rabies antigen can be detected in the cutaneous nerves surrounding the hair follicles of the posterior region of the neck (nuchal biopsy) and in epithelial cells obtained by a corneal impression. Antibodies to rabies can be detected in the serum and CSF of infected persons within 8–10 days of illness; however, infection usually occurs several months before the onset of symptoms. Isolation of virus from the saliva of the patient may be accomplished by mouse inoculation or by inoculation of susceptible cell culture lines with subsequent detection by immunofluorescent antibodies.

14. **D** Influenza virus types A, B, and C may be grown and isolated in embryonated hen eggs or cell cultures using Madin-Darby canine kidney (MDCK), rhesus monkey, or cynomolgus monkey kidney cells. Cell culture using MDCK cells is the most rapid technique, permitting identification within 1–3 days. The hemagglutination inhibition test can be used to titer antibody to influenza virus and to distinguish virus subtypes, if specific antisera is available. Direct fluorescent and enzyme immunoassays using monoclonal antibodies to nucleoprotein antigens in infected nasal epithelium are used for rapid diagnosis of both influenza A and influenza B infection.

15. **A** Direct immunofluorescence testing of vesicle (lesion) fluid for virus using fluorescein-conjugated antibodies is the most rapid method for diagnosis of genital herpes infection. Immunofluorescence and immunoperoxidase methods are also used to distinguish HSV-1 and HSV-2. However, the most sensitive method is viral cell culture, which may yield a positive result within 24 hours when fluid contains a high concentration of virus. Vero cells or primary human embryonic cells are inoculated with vesicle fluid and examined for cytopathic effects (CPE), the most common of which are large "balloon" cells and multinucleated giant cells.

Parasitology

1. The *incorrect* match between organism and the appropriate diagnostic procedure is:
   A. *Onchocerca volvulus*—examination of skin snips
   B. *Cryptosporidium*—modified acid-fast stain
   C. *Echinococcus granulosus*—routine ova and parasite examination
   D. *Schistosoma haematobium*—examination of urine sediment

   Microbiology/Apply knowledge of diagnostic techniques/Parasitology/2

2. In a patient with diarrhea, occasionally *Entamoeba histolytica/E. dispar* (four nucleated cysts, no chromatoidal bars) are identified as being present; however, these cells which are misdiagnosed as protozoa are really:
   A. Macrophages
   B. Polymorphonuclear leukocytes
   C. Epithelial cells
   D. Eosinophils

   Microbiology/Apply knowledge of the morphology of artifacts/Parasitology/3

3. Charcot-Leyden crystals in stool may be associated with an immune response and are thought to be the breakdown products of:
   A. Neutrophils
   B. Eosinophils
   C. Monocytes
   D. Lymphocytes

   Microbiology/Apply knowledge of the morphology of artifacts/Parasitology/1

4. Parasitic organisms that are most often transmitted sexually include:
   A. *Entamoeba gingivalis*
   B. *Dientamoeba fragilis*
   C. *Trichomonas vaginalis*
   D. *Diphyllobothrium latum*

Microbiology/Apply knowledge of life cycles and epidemiology/Parasitology/1

Answers to Questions 1–4

1. **C** The appropriate procedure for the diagnosis of *E. granulosus* (hydatid disease) would involve the microscopic examination of hydatid fluid aspirated from a cyst. Immature scolices and/or hooklets would be found in the centrifuged fluid sediment and could be identified under the microscope.

2. **B** As polymorphonuclear leukocytes (PMNs) in stool begin to fragment and appear to have four nuclei, they will resemble *E. histolytica/E. dispar* cysts. However, *E. histolytica/E. dispar* cysts are rarely seen in cases of diarrhea. The species name *E. histolytica* is reserved for the true pathogen, whereas *E. dispar* is used for the non-pathogenic species. Unfortunately, morphologically they look identical. The only time *E. histolytica* could be identified morphologically would be from trophozoites containing ingested red blood cells (RBCs). Nonpathogenic *E. dispar* would not contain ingested RBCs. The correct way to report these organisms is *E. histolytica/E. dispar* (no trophozoites containing ingested RBCs) or *E. histolytica* (trophozoites seen that contain ingested RBCs). Physicians may treat based on patient symptoms.

3. **B** When eosinophils disintegrate, the granules reform into Charcot-Leyden crystals.

4. **C** *T. vaginalis* has been well documented to be a sexually transmitted flagellate.

5. The *incorrect* match between the organism and one method of acquiring the infection is:
   A. *Trypanosoma brucei rhodesiense*—bite of sand fleas
   B. *Giardia lamblia*—ingestion of water contaminated with cysts
   C. Hookworm—skin penetration of larvae from soil
   D. *Toxoplasma gondii*—ingestion of raw or rare meats

Microbiology/Apply knowledge of fundamental life cycles/Parasitology/1

6. Upon examination of stool material for *Isospora belli*, one would expect to see:
   A. Cysts containing sporozoites
   B. Precysts containing chromatoidal bars
   C. Oocysts that are acid fast
   D. Sporozoites that are hematoxylin-positive

Microbiology/Apply knowledge of life cycles and organism morphology/Parasitology/1

7. Which specimen is the *least* likely to provide recovery of *T. vaginalis*?
   A. Urine
   B. Urethral discharge
   C. Vaginal discharge
   D. Feces

Microbiology/Apply knowledge of pathogenesis and diagnostic procedures/Parasitology/2

8. Which of the following is the best technique to identify *D. fragilis* in stool?
   A. Formalin concentrate
   B. Trichrome-stained smear
   C. Modified acid fast–stained smear
   D. Giemsa's stain

Microbiology/Apply knowledge of diagnostic procedures/Parasitology/2

9. One of the following protozoan organisms has been implicated in waterborne and foodborne outbreaks within the United States. The suspect organism is:
   A. *Trichomonas hominis*
   B. *D. fragilis*
   C. *G. lamblia*
   D. *Balantidium coli*

Microbiology/Apply knowledge of life cycles and epidemiology/Parasitology/1

10. A Gram stain from a gum lesion showed what appeared to be amoebae. A trichrome smear showed amoebae with a single nucleus and partially digested PMNs. The correct identification is:
   A. *Trichomonas tenax*
   B. *E. histolytica/E. dispar*
   C. *E. gingivalis*
   D. *Entamoeba polecki*

Microbiology/Apply knowledge of organism morphology and body site/Parasitology/3

11. An *E. histolytica* trophozoite has the following characteristics:
   A. Central karyosome in the nucleus, ingested RBCs, and clear pseudopodia
   B. Ingested RBCs, clear pseudopodia, and uneven chromatin on the nuclear membrane
   C. Ingested RBCs, clear pseudopodia, and large glycogen vacuoles in cytoplasm
   D. Large, blotlike karyosome, ingested white blood cells (WBCs), and granular pseudopods

Answers to Questions 5–11

5. **A** East and West African trypanosomiasis (*T. b. rhodesiense* and *T. b. gambiense*) are caused when infective forms are introduced into the human body through the bite of the tsetse fly, not sand fleas.

6. **C** *I. belli* oocysts in various stages of maturity would be seen in the concentrate sediment or possibly the direct, wet preparation; these oocysts would stain positive with modified acid-fast stains.

7. **D** *T. vaginalis* is site specific. The organisms are found in the urogenital tract; thus, the intestinal tract is not the normal site for these organisms.

8. **B** Because there is no known cyst form, the best technique to recover and identify *D. fragilis* trophozoites would be the trichrome-stained smear.

9. **C** For a number of years, *G. lamblia* has been implicated in both waterborne and foodborne outbreaks from the ingestion of infective cysts within contaminated water and food.

10. **C** *E. gingivalis* is known to be an inhabitant of the mouth and is characterized by morphology that resembles *E. histolytica/E. dispar*. However, *E. gingivalis* tends to ingest PMNs, whereas *E. histolytica/E. dispar* does not.

11. **A** The trophozoite of *E. histolytica* has evenly arranged chromatin on the nuclear membrane; a central, compact karyosome in the nucleus; clear pseudopodia; and ingested RBCs in the cytoplasm.

12. A 12-year-old girl is brought to the emergency room with meningitis and a history of swimming in a warm-water spring. Motile amoebae that measure 10 μ in size are seen in the cerebrospinal fluid, and are most likely:
A. *Iodamoeba bütschlii* trophozoites
B. *Endolimax nana* trophozoites
C. *D. fragilis* trophozoites
D. *Naegleria fowleri* trophozoites

Microbiology/Apply knowledge of life cycle and epidemiology/Parasitology/3

13. Characteristics of the rhabditiform (noninfective) larvae of *Strongyloides stercoralis* include a:
A. Short buccal capsule and large genital primordium
B. Long buccal capsule and pointed tail
C. Short buccal capsule and small genital primordium
D. Small genital primordium and notch in tail

Microbiology/Apply knowledge of organism morphology and life cycle/Parasitology/2

14. Visceral larva migrans is associated with which of the following organisms?
A. *Toxocara*—serology
B. *Onchocerca*—skin snips
C. *Dracunculus*—skin biopsy
D. *Angiostrongylus*—cerebrospinal fluid (CSF) examination

Microbiology/Apply knowledge of life cycle and diagnostic procedures/Parasitology/2

15. The following organisms are linked with specific, relevant information. The *incorrect* combination is:
A. *S. stercoralis*—internal autoinfection
B. *E. granulosus*—hydatid examination
C. *Pneumocystis carinii*—more than 50% of population antibody-positive by age 4
D. *B. coli*—common within the United States

Microbiology/Apply knowledge of life cycle and epidemiology/Parasitology/2

16. Examination of 24-hour unpreserved urine specimen is sometimes helpful in the recovery of:
A. *T. vaginalis* trophozoites
B. *S. haematobium* eggs
C. *Enterobius vermicularis* eggs
D. *Strongyloides stercoralis* larvae

Microbiology/Apply knowledge of life cycle and diagnostic methods/Parasitology/1

17. The examination of sputum may be necessary to diagnose infection with:
A. *Paragonimus westermani*
B. *Trichinella spiralis*
C. *Wuchereria bancrofti*
D. *Fasciola hepatica*

Microbiology/Apply knowledge of life cycle and diagnostic methods/Parasitology/1

18. Two helminth eggs that may resemble one another are:
A. *D. latum* and *P. westermani*
B. *Opisthorchis sinensis* and *Fasciolopsis buski*
C. *Taenia saginata* and *Hymenolepis nana*
D. *Ascaris lumbricoides* and *Trichostrongylus*

Microbiology/Apply knowledge of organism morphology/Parasitology/2

Answers to Questions 12–18

12. **D** *N. fowleri* are free-living soil and water amoebae that cause primary amoebic meningoencephalitis, or PAM. The number of cases reported is few; however, the infection is very acute and almost always fatal.

13. **A** The rhabditiform larvae of *S. stercoralis* are characterized by the short buccal capsule (mouth) and large genital primordium, whereas hookworm larvae have a long buccal capsule and very small genital primordium.

14. **A** *Toxocara* spp are the cause of visceral larva migrans and occur when humans accidentally ingest the infective eggs of the dog or cat ascarid. The larvae migrate through the deep tissues, including the eye. The test of choice is the serology.

15. **D** *B. coli* is a ciliate that can cause watery diarrhea in humans; however, it is not commonly found within the United States. It is the largest of the intestinal protozoa and can be found in proficiency testing specimens. So, although it is not common, laboratories must still be able to identify these organisms.

16. **B** *S. haematobium* blood flukes reside in the veins over the bladder. When the eggs are passed from the body, they are often found in urine; egg viability can also be determined in unpreserved urine.

17. **A** *P. westermani* adult worms are found in the lung, and eggs may be coughed up in the sputum. Consequently, both sputum and stool (if the sputum containing the eggs are swallowed) are the recommended specimens for examination for the eggs.

18. **A** Both *D. latum* and *P. westermani* eggs are operculated and approximately the same size. The morphology is similar, although *D. latum* has a knob at the abopercular end, and *P. westermani* has a thickened abopercular end and shoulders into which the operculum fits.

19. Eating poorly cooked pork can lead to an infection with:
A. *Taenia solium* and *T. spiralis*
B. *T. saginata* and *H. nana*
C. *Trichuris trichiura* and *Hymenolepis diminuta*
D. *D. latum* and *A. lumbricoides*

Microbiology/Apply knowledge of organism life cycle/Parasitology/1

20. An operculated cestode egg that can be recovered from human feces is:
A. *Clonorchis sinensis*
B. *D. latum*
C. *P. westermani*
D. *Dipylidium caninum*

Microbiology/Apply knowledge of organism morphology/Parasitology/1

21. The adult tapeworm of *E. granulosus* is found in the intestine of:
A. Dogs
B. Sheep
C. Humans
D. Cattle

Microbiology/Apply knowledge of life cycle/ Parasitology/1

22. In infections with *T. solium,* humans can serve as the:
A. Definitive host
B. Intermediate host
C. Either the definitive or the intermediate host
D. None of the above

Microbiology/Apply knowledge of life cycle/ Parasitology/2

23. Humans acquire infections with *D. latum* adult worms by:
A. Ingestion of freshwater crabs
B. Skin penetration of cercariae
C. Ingestion of water chestnuts
D. Ingestion of raw freshwater fish

Microbiology/Apply knowledge of life cycle/ Parasitology/1

24. Humans can serve as both the intermediate and definitive host in infections caused by:
A. *E. vermicularis*
B. *H. nana*
C. *Schistosoma japonicum*
D. *A. lumbricoides*

Microbiology/Apply knowledge of life cycle/ Parasitology/1

25. *Babesia* is an organism that has been implicated in disease from both splenectomized and nonsplenectomized patients. Morphologically, the parasites resemble:
A. *Plasmodium falciparum* rings

B. *Leishmania donovani* amastigotes
C. *Trypanosoma cruzi* trypomastigotes
D. *P. carinii* cysts

Microbiology/Apply knowledge of parasite morphology/Parasitology/2

26. Organisms (and infections) that under normal conditions *cannot* be transmitted in the laboratory are:
A. *Cryptosporidium*—cryptosporidiosis
B. *T. solium*—cysticercosis
C. *A. lumbricoides*—ascariasis
D. *E. vermicularis*—pinworm infections

Microbiology/Apply knowledge of life cycles/Parasitology/2

Answers to Questions 19–26

19. **A** Both *T. solium* (pork tapeworm) and *T. spiralis* can be acquired from the ingestion of raw or poorly cooked pork.

20. **B** *D. latum* is the only operculated cestode egg that is found in humans; the infection is acquired from the ingestion of raw freshwater fish.

21. **A** Although the hydatid cysts are found in sheep or in humans (accidental intermediate host), the adult tapeworms of *E. granulosus* are found in the intestine of the dog.

22. **C** If humans ingest *T. solium* cysticerci in uncooked or rare pork, the adult tapeworm will mature within the intestine (human will serve as definitive host); if eggs from the adult tapeworm are ingested, then the cysticerci will develop in human tissues (accidental intermediate host), causing cysticercosis.

23. **D** The ingestion of raw freshwater fish containing the encysted larvae of *D. latum* will result in the development of an adult tapeworm within the human intestine.

24. **B** In infections with *H. nana,* humans serve as both intermediate and definitive hosts. When ingested, the oncosphere penetrates the intestinal mucosa, develops into the mature cysticercoid (human is intermediate host), and returns to the gut where the adult tapeworm matures (humans are definitive hosts).

25. **A** *Babesia* is an intracellular parasite that closely resembles the ring forms (early trophozoites) of *P. falciparum.* Often in babesiosis there are more rings per cell and the ring form is the only stage seen.

26. **C** *A. lumbricoides* eggs require a period of development in the soil before they are infective for humans. The other organisms listed can be transmitted within the laboratory or in the hospital setting.

27. *T. gondii* is characterized by:
- A. Possible congenital infection and ingestion of oocysts
- B. Cosmopolitan distribution and possible difficulties with interpretation of serologic results
- C. None of the above
- D. Both A and B

Microbiology/Apply knowledge of all areas of parasite biology, diagnostic procedures/Parasitology/3

28. Oocysts of *Cryptosporidium parvum* can be detected in stool specimens using:
- A. Modified Ziehl-Neelsen acid-fast stain
- B. Gram stain
- C. Methenamine silver stain
- D. Trichrome stain

Microbiology/Apply knowledge of diagnostic procedures, staining characteristics/Parasitology/1

29. Which microfilariae are usually *not* found circulating in the peripheral blood?
- A. *Brugia malayi*
- B. *Wuchereria bancrofti*
- C. *Onchocerca volvulus*
- D. *Loa loa*

Microbiology/Apply knowledge of diagnostic procedures, staining characteristics/Parasitology/1

30. Massive hemolysis, blackwater fever, and central nervous system involvement are most common with:
- A. *Plasmodium vivax*
- B. *P. falciparum*
- C. *Plasmodium ovale*
- D. *Plasmodium malariae*

Microbiology/Apply knowledge of disease pathogenesis/Parasitology/2

31. Organisms that should be considered in a nursery school outbreak of diarrhea include:
- A. *E. nana, G. lamblia,* and *Entamoeba coli*
- B. *G. lamblia, D. fragilis,* and *C. parvum*
- C. *C. parvum, T. vaginalis,* and *E. coli*
- D. *T. hominis, D. fragilis,* and *E. nana*

Microbiology/Apply knowledge of epidemiology/ Parasitology/2

32. The *incorrect* match between disease and symptoms is:
- A. Paragonimiasis—hemoptysis
- B. Cryptosporidiosis—watery diarrhea
- C. Toxoplasmosis in compromised host—central nervous system symptoms
- D. Enterobiasis—dysentery

Microbiology/Apply knowledge of life cycles/ Parasitology/2

33. The formalin-ether (ethyl acetate) concentration procedure for feces is used to demonstrate:

- A. Motility of helminth larvae
- B. Protozoan cysts and helminth eggs
- C. Formation of amoebic pseudopods
- D. Trophozoites

Microbiology/Apply knowledge of diagnostic procedures/Parasitology/2

Answers to Questions 27–33

27. D Infection with *T. gondii* is acquired through the ingestion of rare or raw meats, infective oocysts from cat feces, or as congenital transmission. The organism has a cosmopolitan distribution and although serologic testing is generally the test of choice, the results may be very difficult to interpret in certain situations (e.g., congenital infection and immunocompromised patients).

28. A The oocysts of *C. parvum* can be found and identified using microscopic examination of fecal smears stained with modified acid-fast stains. They appear as purple-red-pink round objects, measuring approximately 4–6 μ. Often the four sporozoites and residual body can be seen within the oocyst wall.

29. C The microfilariae of *O. volvulus* are normally found in the fluid right under the outer layer of skin. Therefore, the skin snip is the proper specimen to examine.

30. B The pathogenic sequelae of malarial infections with *P. falciparum* are the most severe of the four species. They can include massive hemolysis, blackwater fever, and multiple organ involvement, including the central nervous system (cerebral malaria).

31. B *G. lamblia, D. fragilis,* and *C. parvum* have been implicated in nursery school outbreaks. Among the many protozoa and coccidia found in the human, these three organisms have become the most likely parasites in this type of setting.

32. D Infections with *E. vermicularis* (the pinworm) may cause anal itching, sleeplessness, and possibly some vaginal irritation or discharge; however, dysentery (bloody diarrhea) has not been associated with this infection.

33. B The ova and parasite examination contains three components: the direct wet film (demonstrates protozoan trophozoite motility), the formalin-ethyl acetate concentration (demonstrates protozoan cysts, coccidian oocysts, and helminth eggs), and the trichrome or iron hematoxylin–stained smear (confirms protozoan cysts and trophozoites).

34. Cysts of *I. bütschlii* typically have:
   A. Chromatoidal bars with rounded ends
   B. A heavily vacuolated cytoplasm
   C. A large glycogen vacuole
   D. Many ingested bacteria and yeast cells

Microbiology/Apply knowledge of morphology/Parasitology/1

35. The miracidial hatching test helps to demonstrate the viability of eggs of:
   A. *Taenia* species
   B. *Schistosoma* species
   C. Hookworm species
   D. *Opisthorchis* species

Microbiology/Apply knowledge of diagnostic procedures/Parasitology/1

36. Organisms that should be considered in a waterborne outbreak of diarrheal disease include:
   A. *G. lamblia* and *C. parvum*
   B. *E. nana* and *E. histolytica*
   C. *Blastocystis hominis* and *T. vaginalis*
   D. *T. gondii* and *Schistosoma mansoni*

Microbiology/Apply knowledge of epidemiology/Parasitology/2

37. The use of the bronchoalveolar lavage (BAL) specimen has become much more widely used in:
   A. Any suspect patient with both toxoplasmosis and cryptosporidiosis
   B. Pediatric patients with pulmonary paragonimiasis
   C. AIDS patients with suspected *Pneumocystis* pneumonia
   D. Immunocompromised patients with disseminated strongyloidiasis

Microbiology/Apply knowledge of pathogenesis and diagnostic procedures/Parasitology/3

38. Primary infections with the microsporidia may originate in:
   A. The lung
   B. The nervous system
   C. The gastrointestinal tract
   D. Mucocutaneous lesions

Microbiology/Apply knowledge of life cycles/Parasitology/2

39. Eye infections with *Acanthamoeba* spp have most commonly been traced to:
   A. Use of soft contact lenses
   B. Use of hard contact lenses
   C. Use of contaminated lens care solutions
   D. Failure to remove lenses while swimming

Microbiology/Apply knowledge of epidemiology/Parasitology/2

40. Select the most sensitive recovery method for *Acanthamoeba* spp from lens care solutions or corneal biopsies.
   A. The trichrome staining method
   B. The use of monoclonal reagents for the detection of antibody
   C. The use of nonnutrient agar cultures seeded with *Escherichia coli*
   D. The Giemsa's stain method

Microbiology/Apply knowledge of diagnostic procedures/Parasitology/2

Answers to Questions 34–40

34. C The cyst of *I. bütschlii* is characterized by a large glycogen vacuole that is seen on the wet smear (stains brown with iodine) and on the permanent stained smear (vacuole will appear clear). Occasionally the vacuole will be so large that the organism will collapse on itself.

35. B The determination of egg viability is important in schistosomiasis; therefore, the miracidial hatching test is helpful in demonstrating the egg viability of *Schistosoma* species. Once the eggs are hatched, the living miracidium larvae will be visible in the water.

36. A Both *G. lamblia* and *C. parvum* have been implicated in waterborne outbreaks or diarrheal disease. These infections would result from the ingestion of *G. lamblia* cysts and/or *C. parvum* oocysts.

37. C With the advent of AIDS, the use of less invasive procedures for the diagnosis of *Pneumocystis* pneumonia, including the BAL method, has become much more common. These patients are often not able to tolerate an "open" procedure like the lung biopsy (more commonly used in non-AIDS patients).

38. C With the possible exception of direct inoculation infection in the eye, the microsporidia are thought to initially infect the gastrointestinal (GI) tract through ingestion of the infective spores; infections in other body sites are thought to disseminate from the GI tract.

39. C The majority of eye infections with *Acanthamoeba* spp have resulted from the use of contaminated eye care solutions, primarily the use of homemade saline. It is recommended that all solutions be discarded at the expiration date. Continued use may increase the risk of environmental contamination of the fluids.

40. C Currently, the most sensitive method for the recovery of *Acanthamoeba* spp from clinical specimens is the non-nutrient agar culture seeded with *E. coli*. The amoebae feed on the bacteria; both trophozoites and cysts can be recovered from the agar surface.

41. The microsporidia are protozoans that have been implicated in human disease primarily in:
A. Immunocompromised patients
B. Pediatric patients under the age of 5
C. Adult patients with congenital immuno-deficiencies
D. Patients who have been traveling in the tropics

Microbiology/Apply knowledge of pathogenesis and epidemiology/Parasitology/2

42. When staining *I. belli* oocysts with modified acid-fast stains, the important difference between these methods and the acid-fast stains used for acid-fast bacilli (AFB) is:
A. The staining time is much longer with regular AFB acid-fast stains.
B. The decolorizer is weaker than acid alcohol used for AFB decolorizing.
C. A counterstain must be used for the modified methods.
D. The stain is more concentrated when staining for AFB.

Microbiology/Apply knowledge of diagnostic procedures/Parasitology/2

43. The *incorrect* match between symptoms and disease is:
A. Dysentery and amoebiasis
B. Malabsorption syndrome and giardiasis
C. Cardiac involvement and chronic Chagas' disease
D. Myalgias and trichuriasis

Microbiology/Apply knowledge of life cycle and pathogenesis/Parasitology/2

44. The *incorrect* match between organism and characteristic is:
A. *Chilomastix mesnili* and Shepherd's crook and lemon shape
B. *P. malariae* and "band troph"
C. *H. nana* and striated shell
D. *W. bancrofti* and sheathed microfilariae

Microbiology/Apply knowledge of morphology/Parasitology/2

45. The *incorrect* match between method and method objective is:
A. Direct wet examination and detection of organism motility
B. Knott concentration and the recovery of operculated helminth eggs
C. Baermann concentration and the recovery of *Strongyloides*
D. Permanent stained fecal smear and confirmation of protozoa

Microbiology/Apply knowledge of diagnostic procedures/Parasitology/2

46. The *incorrect* match between organism and characteristic is:
A. *D. fragilis* and tetrad karyosome in the nucleus
B. *T. gondii* and diagnostic serology
C. *E. granulosus* and daughter cysts
D. *S. mansoni* and egg with terminal spine

Microbiology/Apply knowledge of morphology/Parasitology/2

Answers to Questions 41–46

41. **A** Although the microsporidia have been known as pathogens in many groups of animals, their involvement in humans has primarily been in immunocompromised patients, especially those with AIDS. Microsporidia can be found in different tissues, and currently there are eight genera implicated in human disease.

42. **B** The decolorizer in modified acid-fast stains (Kinyoun's cold method, modified hot method) is usually 1%–3% sulfuric acid, rather than the stronger acid alcohol used in the routine AFB stains.

43. **D** *T. trichiura* (whipworm) may cause diarrhea and occasionally dysentery in very heavy infections; however, the worms are confined to the intestine and myalgias are not seen in this helminth infection.

44. **C** *H. nana* has a thin eggshell containing a six-hooked embryo (oncosphere) and polar filaments that lie between the eggshell and the embryo. The striated eggshell is generally associated with *Taenia* spp eggs.

45. **B** The Knott concentration is designed to allow the recovery of microfilariae from a blood specimen. Dilute formalin (2%) is used; blood is introduced into the formalin, the red cells lyse, and the sediment can be examined as a wet preparation or permanent stained smear (Giemsa's or hematoxylin-based stain) for the presence of microfilariae.

46. **D** The egg of *S. mansoni* is characterized by a large lateral spine; *S. haematobium* has the characteristic terminal spine.

47. There are few procedures considered stat in parasitology. The most obvious situation would be:
   A. Ova and parasite examination for giardiasis
   B. Baermann concentration for strongyloidiasis
   C. Blood films for malaria
   D. Culture of amoebic keratitis

Microbiology/Apply knowledge of pathogenesis and diagnostic procedures/Parasitology/3

48. An immunosuppressed man has several episodes of pneumonia, intestinal pain, sepsis with gram-negative rods, and a history of military service in Southeast Asia 20 years earlier. The most likely cause is infection with:
   A. *T. cruzi*
   B. *S. stercoralis*
   C. *N. fowleri*
   D. *P. westermani*

Microbiology/Apply knowledge of pathogenesis and life cycles/Parasitology/3

49. In a non-AIDS patient, the recommended clinical specimen for recovery of *P. carinii* is the:
   A. Tracheobronchial apsirate
   B. BAL
   C. Bronchial brushings
   D. Open-lung biopsy

Microbiology/Apply knowledge of pathogenesis and life cycle/Parasitology/2

50. Eosinophilic meningoencephalitis is a form of larva migrans, causing fever, headache, stiff neck, and increased cells in the spinal fluid. It is generally a mild and self-limited infection and is caused by:
   A. *Necator americanus*
   B. *Angiostrongylus cantonensis*
   C. *Ancylostoma braziliense*
   D. *S. stercoralis*

Microbiology/Apply knowledge of pathogenesis and life cycle/Parasitology/2

51. "Cultures of parasites are different from bacterial cultures; no quality control is needed." This statement is:
   A. True, if two tubes of media are set up on each patient.
   B. True, if the media is checked every 24 hours.
   C. False, unless two different types of media are used.
   D. False, and organism and media controls need to be set up.

Microbiology/Apply knowledge of diagnostic procedures/Parasitology/2

52. Protozoan cysts were seen in a concentrate sediment and tentatively identified as *E. coli*. However, the organisms were barely visible on the permanent stained smear because:
   A. The organisms were actually not present in the concentrate sediment.

B. There were too few cysts to allow identification on the stained smear.
   C. *E. coli* cysts were present, but poorly fixed.
   D. The concentrate and permanent stained smear were not from the same patient.

Microbiology/Apply knowledge of fixatives and diagnostic procedures/Parasitology/3

53. When humans have hydatid disease, the causative agent and host classification are:
   A. *E. granulosus*—accidental intermediate host
   B. *E. granulosus*—definitive host
   C. *T. solium*—accidental intermediate host
   D. *T. solium*—definitive host

Microbiology/Apply knowledge of life cycles/Parasitology/3

Answers to Questions 47–53

47. **C** The request for blood films for malaria should always be considered a stat request. Any laboratory providing these services should be available 24 hours a day, 7 days a week. In cases of *P. falciparum* malaria, any delay in diagnosing the infection could be fatal for the patient.

48. **B** A latent infection with *S. stercoralis* acquired years before may cause severe symptoms in the immunosuppressed patient ("autoinfective" capability of life cycle and migratory route through the body).

49. **D** In a non-AIDS patient, the specimen of choice for the diagnosis of *P. carinii* pneumonia is the open lung biopsy. The lung is the site of the organisms and the optimal specimen for organism recovery.

50. **B** Eosinophilic meningoencephalitis is a form of larva migrans and is caused by *A. cantonensis*, the rat lungworm. This Pacific area infection is associated with CSF symptoms and sometimes eye involvement.

51. **D** Duplicate cultures should be set up, and specific American Type Culture Collection (ATCC) strains should be cultured along with the patient specimens to confirm that the culture system is operating properly. This approach is somewhat different from that used in diagnostic bacteriology and mycology.

52. **C** As *E. coli* cysts mature, the cyst wall becomes more impenetrable to fixatives. Consequently, the cysts may be visible in the concentrate sediment but appear very distorted or pale on the permanent stained smear.

53. **A** The cause of hydatid disease is *E. granulosus*, and the human is classified as the accidental intermediate host. Infection occurs when humans accidentally ingest the eggs of *E. granulosus* and the hydatid cyst(s) develop in the liver, lung, and other organs of the human instead of sheep (normal cycle).

54. A 45-year-old hunter developed fever, myalgia, and periorbital edema. He has a history of bear meat consumption. The most likely causative agent is:
A. *T. gondii*
B. *T. solium*
C. *H. nana*
D. *T. spiralis*

Microbiology/Apply knowledge of pathogenesis and life cycles/Parasitology/3

55. In a condition resulting from the accidental ingestion of eggs, the human becomes the interme-diate rather than the definitive host. The correct answer is:
A. Trichinosis
B. Cysticercosis
C. Ascariasis
D. Strongyloidiasis

Microbiology/Apply knowledge of pathogenesis and life cycles/Parasitology/3

56. A transplant patient on immunosuppressive drugs developed increasing shortness of breath and cyanosis. The most likely combination of disease and diagnostic procedure is:
A. Strongyloidiasis and trichrome stain
B. Pneumocystosis and silver stain
C. Toxoplasmosis and Gram stain
D. Paragonimiasis and wet preparation

Microbiology/Apply knowledge of pathogenesis and diagnostic procedures/Parasitology/3

57. After returning from a 2-year stay in India, the patient has eosinophilia, an enlarged left spermatic cord and bilateral inguinal lymphadenopathy. The most likely clinical specimen and organism match is:
A. Thin blood films and leishmania
B. Urine and concentration for *T. vaginalis*
C. Thin blood films and *Babesia*
D. Thick blood films and microfilariae

Microbiology/Apply knowledge of pathogenesis and diagnostic procedures/Parasitology/3

58. Patients with severe diarrhea should use "enteric precautions" to prevent nosocomial infections with:
A. *G. lamblia*
B. *A. lumbricoides*
C. *C. parvum*
D. *I. belli*

Microbiology/Apply knowledge of pathogenesis and life cycles/Parasitology/3

59. A 60-year-old Brazilian patient with cardiac irregu-larities and congestive heart failure suddenly dies. Examination of the myocardium revealed numerous amastigotes, an indication that the cause of death was most likely:
A. Leishmaniasis with *L. donovani*
B. Leishmaniasis with *Leishmania braziliense*
C. Trypanosomiasis with *Trypanosoma gambiense*

D. Trypanosomiasis with *T. cruzi*

Microbiology/Apply knowledge of pathogenesis and life cycles/Parasitology/3

60. When malaria smears are requested, what patient information should be obtained?
A. Diet, age, sex
B. Age, antimalarial medication, sex
C. Travel history, antimalarial medication, date of return to United States
D. Fever patterns, travel history, diet

Microbiology/Apply knowledge of pathogenesis and life cycle, and epidemiology/Parasitology/3

Answers to Questions 54–60

54. **D** Bear meat is another excellent source of *T. spiralis*. In this case, the patient had evidently consumed poorly cooked bear meat, thus ingesting the encysted larvae of *T. spiralis*.

55. **B** The accidental ingestion of *T. solium* eggs can result in the disease called cysticerosis. The cys-ticerci will develop in a number of different tissues, including the brain, and the human is the accidental intermediate host.

56. **B** The fact that the patient has received a trans-plant, is on immunosuppressive drugs, and has pulmonary symptoms suggests *Pneumocystis* pneumonia.

57. **D** Based on the history, the most relevant procedure to perform is the preparation and exam-ination of thick blood films for the recovery and identification of microfilariae. The symptoms suggest early filariasis.

58. **C** *C. parvum* oocysts (unlike those of *I. belli*) are immediately infective when passed in stool, and nosocomial infections have been well docu-mented with this coccidian.

59. **D** *T. cruzi,* the cause of Chagas' disease, has two forms within the human, the trypomastigote in the blood and the amastigote in the striated muscle (usually cardiac muscle and intestinal tract muscle).

60. **C** Travel history (areas of drug resistance), the date of return to the United States (primary versus relapse case), and history of antimalarial medication (severe illness, few organisms on smear) are very important questions to ask. Without this information, a malaria diagnosis can be missed or delayed with severe patient consequences.

61. In an outbreak of diarrheal disease traced to a municipal water supply, the most likely causative agents are:
A. *C. parvum* and *G. lamblia*
B. *G. lamblia* and *I. belli*
C. *I. belli* and *E. histolytica*
D. *E. histolytica* and *D. fragilis*

Microbiology/Apply knowledge of life cycles and epidemiology/Parasitology/2

62. Within the United States, sporadic minioutbreaks of diarrheal disease have been associated with the ingestion of strawberries, raspberries, fresh basil, and mesclun (baby lettuce leaves); the most likely causative agent is:
A. *D. fragilis*
B. *Cyclospora cayetanensis*
C. *S. mansoni*
D. *I. belli*

Microbiology/Apply knowledge of life cycles and epidemiology/Parasitology/2

63. Which of the following statements is true regarding onchocerciasis?
A. The adult worm is present in the blood.
B. The microfilariae are in the blood during the late evening hours.
C. The diagnostic test of choice is the skin snip.
D. The parasite resides in the deep lymphatics.

Microbiology/Apply knowledge of life cycles and diagnostic procedures/Parasitology/2

64. The most prevalent helminth to infect humans is:
A. *E. vermicularis,* the pinworm
B. *A. lumbricoides,* the large intestinal roundworm
C. *T. saginata,* the beef tapeworm
D. *S. mansoni,* one of the blood flukes

Microbiology/Apply knowledge of life cycles and epidemiology/Parasitology/1

65. A helminth egg is described as having terminal polar plugs. The most likely helminth is:
A. Hookworm
B. *T. trichiura*
C. *F. hepatica*
D. *D. caninum*

Microbiology/Apply knowledge of organism morphology/Parasitology/1

66. Ingestion of which of the following eggs will result in infection?
A. *S. stercoralis*
B. *S. japonicum*
C. *Toxocara canis*
D. *O. sinensis*

Microbiology/Apply knowledge of life cycles/Parasitology/2

67. *P. vivax* and *P. ovale* are similar because they:
A. Exhibit Schüffner's dots and have a true relapse in the life cycle
B. Have no malarial pigment and multiple rings
C. Commonly have appliqué forms in the red cells
D. Have true stippling, do not have a relapse stage, and infect old red cells

Microbiology/Apply knowledge of life cycles and morphology/Parasitology/2

Answers to Questions 61–67

61. **A** Both *C. parvum* oocysts and *G. lamblia* cysts can be transmitted through contaminated water. Such outbreaks have been well documented.

62. **B** The coccidian, *C. cayetanensis,* has been linked to mini-outbreaks of diarrheal disease. Epidemiological evidence strongly implicates various berries, basil, and mesclun as likely causes. These outbreaks are very sporadic and tend to occur primarily in March through May.

63. **C** The adult *O. volvulus* reside in subcutaneous nodules and the microfilariae are found in the fluids right under the outer layers of skin; thus the appropriate diagnostic test is the microscopic examination of skin snips for the presence of microfilariae.

64. **A** The pinworm, *E. vermicularis,* is the most common parasitic infection throughout the world, and the eggs are infective within just a few hours. Some have said, "You either had the infection as a child, have it now, or will have it again when you have children."

65. **B** The eggs of *T. trichiura* (the whipworm) have been described as being barrel-shaped with a thick shell and two polar plugs.

66. **C** The eggs of *T. canis* are infectious for humans and cause visceral larva migrans. These ascarid eggs of the dog can infect humans; the eggs hatch and the larvae wander through the deep tissues, occasionally the eye. In this case, the human becomes the accidental intermediate host.

67. **A** Both *P. vivax* and *P. ovale* infect young red cells, have true stippling (Schüffner's dots), contain malarial pigment, and have a true relapse stage in the life cycle.

68. The term *internal autoinfection* can be associated with the following parasites:
A. *C. parvum* and *G. lamblia*
B. *I. belli* and *S. stercoralis*
C. *C. parvum* and *S. stercoralis*
D. *G. lamblia* and *I. belli*

Microbiology/Apply knowledge of life cycles/Parasitology/2

69. Microsporidia have been identified as causing severe diarrhea, disseminated disease in other body sites, and ocular infections. Routes of infection have been identified as:
A. Ingestion
B. Inhalation
C. Direct contamination from the environment
D. Ingestion, inhalation, and direct contamination

Microbiology/Apply knowledge of life cycles/Parasitology/2

70. An immunocompromised patient continues to have diarrhea after repeated ova and parasites (O&P) examinations (sedimentation concentration, trichrome permanent stained smear) were reported as negative; organisms that might be responsible for the diarrhea include:
A. *C. parvum, G. lamblia,* and *I. belli*
B. *G. lamblia,* microsporidia, and *E. nana*
C. *T. solium* and *E. nana*
D. *C. parvum* and microsporidia

Microbiology/Apply knowledge of life cycles and diagnostic procedures/Parasitology/3

Answers to Questions 68–70

68. **C** Both *C. parvum* and *S. stercoralis* have an internal autoinfection capability in their life cycles. This means that the cycle and infection can continue, even after the patient has left the endemic area. In the case of *C. parvum*, the cycle continues in patients who are immunocompromised and unable to self-cure.

69. **D** Infectious routes for microsporidial infections have been confirmed as ingestion and inhalation of the spores; direct transfer of infectious spores from environmental surfaces to the eyes has also been reported.

70. **D** Routine O&P examinations will usually not allow the detection of *C. parvum* oocysts and microsporidial spores; special stains are required. Modified acid-fast stains for *C. parvum* and modified trichrome stains for the microsporidial spores are recommended.

Problem Solving in Microbiology and Parasitology

1. An emergency room physician ordered a culture and sensitivity on a catheterized urine specimen obtained from a 24-year-old female patient. A colony count was done and gave the following results after 24 hours:

   Blood agar plate = >100,000 col/mL of gram-positive cocci resembling staphylococci

MacConkey agar =	CNA plate =
No growth	Inhibited growth
Hemolysis = Neg	Catalase = Positive
Novobiocin = Resistant	

   This isolate is:
   A. *Staphylococcus saprophyticus*
   B. *Micrococcus luteus*
   C. *Staphylococcus aureus*
   D. *Streptococcus pyogenes*

   Microbiology/Select methods/Reagents/Media/Culture/3

2. An outbreak of *S. aureus* in the Nursery Department prompted the Infection Control Committee to proceed with an environmental screening procedure. The best screening media to use for this purpose would be:
   A. CNA agar
   B. THIO broth
   C. Mannitol salt agar
   D. PEA agar

   Microbiology/Select methods/Reagents/Media/Culture/3

3. A listless 12-month-old boy with a fever of 103°F was taken to the emergency room. He had been diagnosed with an ear infection 3 days earlier. A spinal tap was performed, but only one tube of CSF was obtained from the lumbar puncture. The single tube of CSF should be submitted *first* to which department?
   A. Chemistry
   B. Microbiology
   C. Hematology
   D. Cytology/Histology

   Microbiology/Select methods/Reagents/Media/Culture/3

Answers to Questions 1–3

1. **A** CNA inhibits most strains of *S. saprophyticus*. Therefore, blood agar should be used when culturing catheterized urine samples from young female patients. Most *S. saprophyticus* isolates are obtained from female patients 20–30 years old.

2. **C** The high concentration of NaCl (7.5%) in mannitol salt agar allows for the recovery of *S. aureus* from heavily contaminated specimens while inhibiting other organisms. Also, *S. aureus* ferments mannitol, thus allowing for easy detection of yellow-haloed colonies of *S. aureus* on red mannitol salt agar.

3. **B** Generally, tube 2 or 3 is submitted to the microbiology laboratory for culture and gram smear. To ensure recovery of any pathogens and correct diagnosis without other bacterial contamination, immediate centrifugation and inoculation to the appropriate media as well as a Gram stain smear should be performed prior to delivery of the specimen to the chemistry and hematology departments for testing.

4. A 65-year-old female outpatient was requested by her physician to submit a 24-hour urine specimen for protein and creatinine tests. He also requested testing for mycobacteria in the urine. Should the microbiology laboratory accept this 24-hour specimen for culture?
A. Yes, if the specimen is kept on ice.
B. Yes, if the specimen is for aerobic culture only.
C. No, the specimen must be kept at room temperature.
D. No, the specimen is unsuitable for the recovery of mycobacteria.

Microbiology/Select methods/Reagents/Media/ Culture/3

5. A lymph node biopsy obtained from a 30-year-old male patient was submitted to the microbiology laboratory for a culture and AFB smear for my-cobacteria. The specimen was fixed in formalin. This specimen should be:
A. Accepted for AFB smear and cultured
B. Rejected
C. Held at room temperature for 24 hours and then cultured
D. Cultured for anaerobes only

Microbiology/Select methods/Reagents/Media/ Culture/3

6. A 49-year-old man who traveled to Mexico City returned with a bad case of dysentery. Along with a fever, abdominal cramping and bloody, mucoidal, frequent stools, many WBCs were seen on the Gram stain smear. Stool culture gave the following results:

Gram stain: Lactose = +
  gram-negative rods
Indole = +   Lysine decarboxylase
                  = Neg
Urea = Neg   Motility = Neg

What is the most likely organism?
A. *Salmonella* spp
B. *P. mirabilis*
C. *E. coli*
D. *E coli* (EIEC)

Microbiology/Evaluate laboratory data to make identification/Gram-negative bacilli/3

7. An 80-year-old male patient was admitted to the hospital with a fever of 102°F. A sputum culture revealed many gram-negative rods on MacConkey agar and blood agar. The patient was diagnosed with pneumonia. The following biochemical results were obtained from the culture:

H_2S = Neg   Lactose = +
Urea = +   Citrate = +
Indole = +   VP = +   Motility = Neg
Resistance to ampicillin and carbenicillin

What is the most likely identification?
A. *K. oxytoca*
B. *P. mirabilis*
C. *E. coli*
D. *K. pneumoniae*

Microbiology/Evaluate laboratory data to make identification/Gram-negative bacilli/3

8. An immunocompromised 58-year-old female chemotherapy patient received two units of packed RBCs. The patient died 3 days later, and the report from the autopsy revealed that her death was due to septic shock. The blood bags were cultured and the following results were noted:

Growth of aerobic gram-negative rods on both MacConkey and blood agars
Lactose = Neg   Sucrose = +   Citrate = Neg
Indole = Neg   VP = Neg H_2S = Neg
Urea = +   Motility 22°C = +   Motility 37°C = Neg

What is the most likely identification?
A. *E. coli*
B. *Y. enterocolitica*
C. *Enterobacter cloacae*
D. *C. freundii*

Microbiology/Evaluate laboratory data to make identification/Gram-negative bacilli/3

Answers to Questions 4–8

4. **D** In general, a 24-hour urine is unsuitable for culture; a first morning specimen is best for the recovery of mycobacteria in the urine.

5. **B** Specimens submitted for culture and recovery of any bacteria should be submitted *without* fixatives.

6. **D** EIEC, or enteroinvasive *E. coli*, produces a dysentery similar to *Shigella*, with invasion and de-struction of the intestinal mucosal epithelium. Leukocytes are seen on the Gram stain smear. Adults who are travelers to foreign countries, espe-cially Mexico, are the group at greatest risk.

7. **A** *K. oxytoca* is similar to *K. pneumoniae* except the indole test is positive for *K. oxytoca*.

8. **B** *Y. enterocolitica* has been associated with fatal bacteremia and septic shock from contaminated blood transfusion products. The motility at room temperature is a clue to this identification.

9. A pediatric patient with severe bloody diarrhea who had been camping with his parents was admitted to the hospital with complications of hemolytic uremic syndrome (HUS). Several stool specimens were cultured with the following results noted:

Gram stain smear = many gram-negative rods with no WBCs seen

Blood agar = Normal flora   MacConkey agar = Normal flora

MacConkey agar with sorbitol = Many clear colonies (sorbitol negative)

Hektoen agar = Normal flora Campy agar = No growth

What is the most likely identification?
A. *Yersinia* spp
B. *E. coli* O157:H7
C. *Salmonella* spp
D. *Shigella* spp

Microbioloby/Evaluation laboratory data to make identification/Gram-negative bacilli/3

10. A 14-year-old emergency room patient had been to the doctor's office 2 days previously with abdominal pain, diarrhea, and a low-grade fever. He was diagnosed with pseudoappendicular syndrome. Cultures from the stool containing blood and WBCs showed the following results:

Aerobic gram-negative rods on MacConkey agar (clear colonies)

Campy agar = No growth

Lactose = Neg   Sucrose = +   Citrate = Neg
Indole = Neg   VP = Neg   H₂S = Neg
Motility 37°C   Motility 22°C Hektoen
  = Neg   = +   agar = NF

What is the most likely identification?
A. *Y. enterocolitica*
B. *Salmonella* spp
C. *Shigella* spp
D. *E. coli*

Microbiology/Evaluate laboratory data to make identification/Gram-negative nonfermenter/3

11. A sputum culture from a 13-year-old cystic fibrosis patient grew a predominance of short, gram-negative rods that tested oxidase-negative. On MacConkey, chocolate, and blood agar plates, the organism appeared to have a lavender-green pigment. Further testing showed:

Motility = +   DNase = +
Glucose = + (oxidative)   Maltose = + (oxidative)
Lysine decarboxylase = + Esculin hydrolysis = +

What is the most likely identification?
A. *S. (X.) maltophilia*
B. *A. baumanii*
C. *P. aeruginosa*
D. *B. cepacia*

Microbiology/Evaluate laboratory data to make identification/Gram-negative nonfermenter/3

12. A patient with a human bite wound on the right forearm arrived at the clinic for treatment. The wound was inflicted 36 hours earlier, and a culture was taken by the physician on duty. After 48 hours, the culture results were:

Gram-stain smear = Gram-negative straight, slender rods

Chocolate agar plate = "Pitting" of the agar by small, yellow, opaque colonies

Oxidase = +   Motility = Neg
Catalase = Neg   Glucose = +
Growth in increased CO₂ = +
Growth at 42°C = Neg

What is the most likely identification of this facultative anaerobe?
A. *P. aeruginosa*
B. *A. baumanii*
C. *K. kingae*
D. *Eikenella corrodens*

Microbiology/Evaluate laboratory data to make identification/Unusual gram-negative bacteria/3

Answers to Questions 9–12

9. **B** *E. coli* O157:H7 is usually the most common isolate from bloody stools of the enterohemorrhagic *E. coli* (EHEC) group, which results from undercooked beef. These strains are waterborne and foodborne, and the infections from *E. coli* O157:H7 are greatest during the summer months in temperate climates.

10. **A** *Y. enterocolitica* is responsible for diseases in younger persons. Blood and leukocytes can be present in stools. Patients (usually teens) exhibiting appendicitis-like symptoms with lactose-negative colonies growing on MacConkey agar (small colonies at 24 hours, but larger colonies at 48 hours if incubated at room temperature) should be tested for the growth of *Y. enterocolitica*.

11. **A** *S. (X.) maltophilia* is the third most frequently isolated nonfermentative gram-negative rod in the clinical laboratory. Cystic fibrosis patients are at greater risk for infections because of previous antimicrobial treatment and recurrent pneumonia, and because some strains may be colonizers.

12. **D** *E. corrodens* is part of the normal flora of the human mouth and typically "pits" the agar. This organism is capnophilic (needing increased CO₂).

13. A dog bite wound to the thumb of a 20-year-old male patient became infected. The culture grew a gram-negative, slender rod, which was a facultative anaerobe. The following results were noted:

Oxidase = +   Motility = Neg
Catalase = +   Capnophilic = +
"Gliding" on the agar was noted.

What is the most likely identification?
A. *P. aeruginosa*
B. *Capnocytophaga carnimorsus*
C. *A. baumannii*
D. *P. mirabilis*

Microbiology/Evaluate laboratory data to make identification/Unusual gram-negative bacteria/3

14. A patient exhibits fever, chills, abdominal cramps, diarrhea, vomiting, and bloody stools 10–12 hours after eating. Which organisms will most likely grow from this patient's stool culture?
A. *Salmonella* or *Yersinia* spp
B. *E. coli* O157:H7 or *Shigella* spp
C. *Staphylococcus aureus* or *C. perfringens*
D. *Salmonella* or *Staphylococcus* spp

Microbiology/Identification gram-negative bacteria/3

15. When testing for coagulase properties, staphylococci isolates from a 67-year-old male diabetic patient showed a positive tube test (free coagulase). The organism should be identified as:
A. *S. aureus*
B. *S. haemolyticus*
C. *S. saprophyticus*
D. *M. luteus*

Microbiology/Identification gram-positive cocci/2

16. An isolate of *S. aureus* was cultured from an ulcer obtained from the leg of a diabetic, 79-year-old female patient. The organism showed resistance to methicillin. Additionally, this isolate should be tested for resistance or susceptibility to:
A. Erythromycin
B. Gentamicin
C. Vancomycin
D. Kanamycin

Microbiology/Select antibiotic/Identification/3

17. An isolate, recovered from a vaginal culture obtained from a 25-year-old female patient who is 8 months pregnant is shown to be a gram-positive cocci, catalase-negative, and β-hemolytic on blood agar. Which tests are needed for further identification?
A. Optochin, bile solubility, PYR
B. Bacitracin, CAMP, PYR
C. Methicillin, PYR, trehalose
D. Coagulase, glucose, PYR

Microbiology/Evaluate data to make identification/Gram-positive cocci/3

18. Which organism is the most often recovered gram-positive cocci (catalase-negative) from a series of blood cultures obtained from individuals with endocarditis?
A. *S. agalactiae*
B. *C. perfringens*
C. *Enterococcus faecalis*
D. *Pediococcus* spp

Microbiology/Evaluate data to make identification/Gram-positive cocci/3

Answers to Questions 13–18

13. **B** *C. carnimorsus* is associated with septicemia or meningitis following dog bites. All *Capnocytophaga* strains are capnophilic, facultative anaerobic, gram-negative slender or filamentous rods with tapered ends.

14. **B** Both *E. coli* O157:H7 and *Shigella* spp are invasive and cause bloody stools.

15. **A** *S. aureus* is an opportunistic human pathogen. A wound or ulcer infected with *S. aureus* that is left untreated is especially detrimental to a diabetic patient.

16. **C** MRSA isolates are usually tested for susceptibility or resistance to vancomycin, a glycopeptide.

17. **B** Group B streptococci (*S. agalactiae*) are important pathogens and can cause serious neonatal infections. Women who are found to be heavily colonized vaginally with *S. agalactiae* pose a threat to the newborn, especially within the first few days after delivery. The infection acquired by the infant is associated with pneumonia.

18. **C** *Enterococcus* (*Streptococcus*) *faecalis* is the cause of up to 20% of the bacterial endocarditis cases and is the most commonly encountered species in this condition.

19. A presumptive diagnosis of gonorrhea can be made from an exudate from a 20-year-old emergency room patient, if which of the following criteria are present?
   A. Smear of urethral exudate (male only) shows typical gram-negative, intracellular diplococci; growth of oxidase-positive gram-negative diplococci on selective agar (modified Thayer-Martin).
   B. Smear from vaginal area shows gram-negative diplococci; growth of typical colonies on blood agar.
   C. Smear from rectum shows typical gram-negative diplococci; no growth on chocolate agar.
   D. Growth of gram-negative cocci on MacConkey agar and blood agar.

Microbiology/ Select/Reagents/Media/Gram-negative cocci identification/3

20. "Clue cells" are seen on a smear of vaginal discharge obtained from an 18-year-old female emergency room patient. This finding, along with a fishy odor (amine) after the addition of 10% KOH, suggests bacterial vaginosis caused by which organism?
   A. *Staphylococcus epidermides*
   B. *Streptococcus agalactiae*
   C. *G. vaginalis*
   D. *E. coli*

Microbiology/Evaluate laboratory data for identification/Gram-variable coccobacilli/3

21. A 1-month-old infant underwent a spinal tap to rule out bacterial meningitis. The CSF was cloudy, and the smear showed many pus cells and short gram-positive rods. After 18 hours, many colonies appeared on blood agar that resembled *Streptococcus* spp or *L. monocytogenes*. Which of the following preliminary tests should be performed on the colonies to best differentiate *L. monocytogenes* from *Streptococcus* spp?
   A. Hanging-drop motility (25°C) and catalase
   B. PYR and bacitracin
   C. Oxidase and glucose
   D. Coagulase and catalase

Microbiology/Select methods/Reagents/Media/ Culture/3

22. Acid-fast positive bacilli were recovered from the sputum of a 79-year-old man who had been treated for pneumonia. Which of the following test reactions after 3 weeks of incubation on Löwenstein-Jensen agar are consistent with *M. tuberculosis?*
   A. Niacin = +; nitrate reduction = +; photochromogenic = Neg
   B. Niacin = Neg; optochin = +; catalase = +
   C. PYR = +; urease = +; bacitracin = +
   D. Ampicillin = resistant; penicillin =Resistant

Microbiology/Evaluate laboratory data to make identification/Acid-fast bacilli/3

23. Which biochemical tests should be performed in order to identify colorless colonies growing on MacConkey agar (swarming colonies on blood agar) from a catheterized urine specimen?
   A. Indole, ornithine decarboxylase, and urease
   B. Glucose, oxidase, and lactose utilization
   C. Phenylalanine deaminase and bile solubility
   D. H₂S and catalase

Microbiology/Evaluate laboratory data to make identification/Gram-negative bacilli/3

24. A gram-negative nonfermenter was isolated from a culture taken from a burn patient. Which of the following is the best choice of tests to differentiate *P. aeruginosa* from *Acinetobacter* spp?
   A. Growth on MacConkey agar, catalase, growth at 37°C
   B. Oxidase, motility, growth at 42°C
   C. Growth on blood agar, oxidase, growth at 35°C
   D. String test and coagulase test

Microbiology/Select methods/Reagent/Media/ Identification nonfermentative gram-negatives/3

Answers to Questions 19–24

19. **A** *N. gonorrhoeae* can be presumptively identified from a male patient only from the Gram stain and growth on selective agar. In female patients, the normal flora from a urethral swab may appear to be *N. gonorrhoeae* (gram-negative diplococci), but may be part of the normal flora, such as *Veillonella* spp (an anaerobic gram-negative cocci resembling *N. gonorrhoeae*).

20. **C** *G. vaginalis*, a gram-negative or gram-variable pleomorphic coccobacilli, causes bacterial vaginosis but is also present as part of the normal vaginal flora of women of reproductive age with a normal vaginal examination. "Clue cells" are vaginal epithelial cells with gram-negative or gram-variable coccobacilli attached to them.

21. **A** *L. monocytogenes* is catalase-positive and displays a "tumbling" motility at room temperature. *Streptococcus* spp are catalase-negative and nonmotile.

22. **A** *M. tuberculosis* is niacin-positive and nonphotochromogenic. This organism takes up to 3 weeks to grow on selective agar.

23. **A** A swarmer on blood agar would most likely be a *Proteus* spp. A lactose nonfermenter and swarmer that is isolated often from urinary tract infections is *P. mirabilis*.

24. **B** *P. aeruginosa* has a distinctive grape odor. The best choice of tests is:

	42°C Growth	Oxidase	Motility
P. aeruginosa	+	+	+
Acinetobacter spp	Neg.	Neg.	Neg.

25. A *Haemophilus* spp, recovered from a throat culture obtained from a 59-year-old male patient undergoing chemotherapy required hemin (X factor) and NAD (V factor) for growth. This species also hemolyzed horse erythrocytes on blood agar. What is the most likely species?
A. *H. ducreyi*
B. *H. parahemolyticus*
C. *H. haemolyticus*
D. *H. aegyptius*

Microbiology/Evaluate laboratory data to make identification/Gram-negative coccobacilli/3

26. Large gram-positive bacilli (boxcar shaped) were recovered from a blood culture taken from a 70-year-old female diabetic patient. The following results were recorded:

Aerobic growth = Neg   Anaerobic growth = +
Spores = Neg   Motility = Neg
Lecithinase = +   Hemolysis = β
                          (double-zone)
GLC (volatile acids) = acetic acid and butyric acid

What is the most likely identification?
A. *C. perfringens*
B. *Fusobacterium* spp
C. *Bacteroides* spp
D. *C. sporogenes*

Microbiology/Evaluate laboratory data to make identification/Anaerobic gram-positive bacilli/3

27. Anaerobic gram-negative rods were recovered from the blood of a patient after gallbladder surgery. The bacteria grew well on agar containing 20% bile but was resistant to kanamycin and vancomycin. What is the most likely identification?
A. *C. perfringens*
B. *Bacteroides fragilis* group
C. *Prevotella* spp
D. *Porphyromonas* spp

Microbiology/Evaluate laboratory data to make identification/Anaerobic gram negataive bacilli/3

28. In Breakpoint Antimicrobial Drug Testing, interpretation of susceptible (S), intermediate (I), and resistant (R) refers to testing antibiotics by using:
A. The amount needed to cause bacteriostasis
B. Only the specific concentrations necessary to report S, I, or R
C. A minimum inhibitory concentration of 64 μg/mL
D. A dilution of drug that is one tube less than the toxic level

Microbiology/Select methods/Reagents/Media/Antibiotic testing/2

29. A CSF sample obtained from a 2-week-old infant with suspected bacterial meningitis grew gram-negative rods on blood and chocolate agars. The following results were noted:

MacConkey agar = No growth   ONPG = +
Glucose (open) OF = +   Urea = Neg
Glucose (closed) OF = Neg   Catalase = +
Indole = +   Oxidase = +
Motility = Neg   Pigment = Yellow
42°C growth = Neg

What is the correct identification?
A. *P. aeruginosa*
B. *F. meningosepticum*
C. *A. baumanii*
D. *E. coli*

Microbiology/Evaluate laboratory data for identification/Gram-negative rods/3

Answers to Questions 25–29

25. **C** *H. haemolyticus* requires both X and V factors for growth and lyses horse erythrocytes.

26. **A** *C. perfringens* is an anaerobic gram-positive rod that is often isolated from the tissue of patients with gas gangrene (myonecrosis). Spore production is not usually seen with this organism, which may also stain gram-negative.

27. **B** *B. fragilis* is the most often isolated gram-negative anaerobic bacillus. It is resistant to many antibiotics. A good screening agar is a 20% bile plate which does not support the growth of *Prevotella* spp or *Porphyromonas* spp.

28. **B** Breakpoint susceptibility testing is done by selecting only two appropriate drug concentrations for testing. If the results show growth at both concentrations, then resistance is indicated; growth only at the lower concentration signifies an intermediate result; no growth at either concentration is interpreted as susceptible.

29. **B** *F. meningosepticum* is a well-known cause of neonatal meningitis. It will grow well on chocolate agar producing yellow pigmented colonies.

30. During the summer break, several middle-aged elementary school teachers from the same school district attended a 3-day seminar in Chicago. Upon returning home, three female teachers from the group were hospitalized with pneumonia, flulike symptoms, and a nonproductive cough. Routine testing of sputum samples revealed normal flora. Further testing using buffered CYE agar with L-cysteine and α-ketoglutarate in 5% CO_2 produced growth of opaque colonies that stained faintly showing thin gram-negative rods. What is the most likely identification?
A. *L. pneumophila*
B. *H. influenzae*
C. *E. corrodens*
D. *S. pneumoniae*

Microbiology/Evaluate laboratory data for identification/Gram-negative rods/3

31. A vancomycin-resistant gram-positive coccobacillus resembling the streptococcus viridans group was isolated from the blood of a 42-year-old female patient undergoing a bone marrow transplant. The PYR and leucine aminopeptidase (LAP) tests were negative. The following results were noted:

Catalase = Neg   CAMP = Neg
Esculin hydrolysis = Neg   Gas from glucose = +
Hippurate hydrolysis = Neg 6.5% salt broth = Neg

What is the correct identification?
A. *Leuconostoc* spp
B. *Enterococcus* spp
C. *Staphylococcus* spp
D. *Micrococcus* spp

Microbiology/Evaluate laboratory data to make identification/Aerobic gram-positive coccobacilli/3

32. A catalase-negative, gram-positive coccus resembling staphylococcus (clusters on Gram-stained smear) was recovered from three different blood cultures obtained from a 60-year-old patient diagnosed with endocarditis. The following test results were noted:

PYR = Neg   LAP = Neg (V)
Esculin hydrolysis = Neg   6.5% Salt broth = Neg
Vancomycin = Sensitive   CAMP test = Neg

What is the correct identification?
A. *Leuconostoc* spp
B. *Gemella* spp
C. *Enterococcus* spp
D. *Micrococcus* spp

Microbiology/Evaluate laboratory data for identification/Gram-positive cocci/3

33. An immunocompromised patient with prior antibiotic treatment grew aerobic gram-positive cocci from several clinical specimens that were cultured. The organism was vancomycin-resistant and catalase-negative. Additional testing proved negative for enterococci. What other groups of organisms might be responsible?
A. *Leconostoc* spp and *Pediococcus* spp
B. *S. pyogenes* and *S. agalactiae*
C. *Micrococcus* spp and *Gemella* spp
D. *Clostridium* spp and *S. bovis*

Microbiology/Evaluate laboratory data for identification/Gram-positive cocci/3

34. A catalase-positive, gram-positive coccus (clusters under Gram stain) grew pale yellow, creamy colonies on 5% sheep blood agar. The specimen was recovered from pustules on the face of a 5-year-old girl with impetigo. The following test reactions indicate which organism?

Glucose = + (Fermentation) Oxidase = Neg
PYR = Neg   Bacitracin = Sensitive
Lysostaphin = Sensitive
A. *Micrococcus* spp
B. *Streptococcus* spp
C. *Enterococcus* spp
D. *Staphylococcus* spp

Microbiology/Evaluate laboratory data for identification/Gram-positive cocci/3

Answers to Questions 30–34

30. **A** *L. pneumophila* is the cause of pneumonia and can occur as part of an epidemic sporadically or nosocomically, or may be community acquired. The appearance of mottled, cut-glass colonies on buffered CYE agar under low power and the use of a direct immunofluorescence technique on sputum samples determine the presence of *L. pneumophila*. The most common environmental sites for recovery are shower heads, faucets, water tanks, and air-conditioning systems.

31. **A** *Leuconostoc* spp are vancomycin-resistant opportunistic pathogens and follow invasive procedures. They are often recovered from positive neonatal blood cultures resulting from colonization during delivery.

32. **B** *Gemella* spp are often recovered from patients with endocarditis and meningitis. On the Gram stain, they resemble staphylococci morphologically but are catalase-negative.

33. **A** *Leuconostoc* spp and *Pediococcus* spp are vancomycin-resistant, catalase-negative, gram-positive aerobic organisms recovered from immunosuppressed patients.

34. **D** *S. aureus* is a usual cause of skin infections and a common cause of cellulitis, impetigo, postsurgical wounds, and scalded skin syndrome in infants.

35. A 22-year-old pregnant woman (third trimester) entered the emergency room complaining of diarrhea, fever, and other flulike symptoms. Blood cultures were ordered along with a urine culture. After 24 hours, the urine culture was negative, but the blood cultures revealed a gram-positive short rod that grew aerobically on blood agar. The colonies were small and smooth, resembling a *Streptococcus* spp with a small narrow zone of β-hemolysis. The following test results indicate which organism?

Motility = +   Catalase = +
   (Wet mount = Tumbling)
Glucose = + (Acid)   Esculin hydrolysis = +
A. *L. monocytogenes*
B. *S. pneumoniae*
C. *S. agalactiae*
D. *Corynebacterium* spp

Microbiology/Evaluate laboratory data for identification/Gram-positive rod/3

36. Anaerobic gram-positive, spore-forming bacilli were recovered from the feces of a chemotherapy patient with severe diarrhea. The patient had undergone antibiotic therapy 1 week prior. The fecal culture produced growth only on the CCFA plate. No *aerobic* growth of normal flora was seen after 48 hours. The following results were noted:

Kanamycin =   Vancomycin =   Colistin =
  Sensitive   Sensitive   Resistant
Lecithinase = Neg Lipase = Neg   Nitrate = Neg
Indole = Neg   Urease = Neg   Catalase = Neg
Spores = +   CCFA agar = growth of yellow,
  "ground glass" colonies that fluoresce chartreuse
  (yellow-green)

What is the correct identification?
A. *C. perfringens*
B. *C. tetani*
C. *C. sordellii*
D. *C. difficile*

Microbiology/Evaluate laboratory data for identification/Anaerobic gram-positive rods/3

37. Anaerobic gram-positive diphtheroids (nonspore formers) were cultured from two separate blood culture bottles (at 5 days) obtained from a 25-year-old patient admitted to the hospital with dehydration, diarrhea, and other flulike symptoms. Four other blood culture bottles did not grow any organisms at 7 days and were discarded. The following results were obtained from the recovered anaerobe:

Indole = +   Nitrate = +
Catalase = +   Kanamycin = Sensitive
Vancomycin = Sensitive Colistin = Resistant
Major acid from PYG broth by GLC = Propionic acid

What is the correct identification?
A. *E. lentum*
B. *Propionibacterium acnes*

C. *Actinomyces* spp
D. *Peptostreptococcus* spp

Microbiology/Evaluate laboratory data for identification/Anaerobic gram-positive rods/3

38. Anaerobic gram-positive bacilli with subterminial spores were recovered from several blood cultures obtained from a patient diagnosed with a malignancy of the colon. The following results were recorded:

Indole = Neg   Growth on blood agar
                        = Swarming colonies
Urease = Neg   Lipase = Neg
Catalase = Neg   Lecithinase = Neg

What is the correct identification?
A. *C. septicum*
B. *C. perfringens*
C. *C. sordellii*
D. *P. acnes*

Microbiology/Evaluate laboratory data for identification/Anaerobic gram-positive rods/3

Answers to Questions 35–38

35. **A** Early detection in pregnant women is very important when dealing with *L. monocytogenes*. If it is not detected and treated, infection of the fetus, resulting in stillbirth, abortion, or premature birth may result. Detection can also be made post-partum by culturing the CSF, blood, amniotic fluid, and respiratory secretions of the neonate.

36. **D** The overgrowth of *C. difficile* in the bowel is the cause of antimicrobial-associated colitis. Culturing for *C. difficile* is the least specific but the most sensitive method to detect possible disease related to *C. difficile*. A characteristic "horse-stable" odor is noted on CCFA growing *C. difficile*.

37. **B** *P. acnes* is a diphtheroid (pleomorphic rod) that may appear to branch on the Gram stain smear. It is the most commonly isolated species found in blood cultures and is often considered a contaminant. Abundant propionic acid is produced by GLC.

38. **A** *C. septicum* is often recovered from patients with malignancies or other diseases of the colon, especially the cecum. The following chart defines the swarming *Clostidium* spp:

	Indole	**Urease**	**Spores**
C. septicum	Neg	Neg	Subterminal
C. tetani	−/+	Neg	Terminal
C. sordellii	+	+	Subterminal

39. Anaerobic gram-negative bacilli were recovered from fluid obtained from drainage of a postsurgical abdominal wound. The following test results were recorded:

Kanamycin = Resistant	Vancomycin = Resistant	Colistin = Resistant
Growth on 20% bile plate = +	Pigment = Neg	Indole = V (neg)
Nitrate = Neg	Urea = Neg	Lipase = Neg

What is the correct identification?
A. *Prevotella* spp
B. *Bacteroides fragilis* group
C. *Porphyromonas* spp
D. *Clostridium* spp

Microbiology/Evaluate laboratory data for identification/Anaerobic gram-negative rods/3

40. Anaerobic, nonpigmented, gram-negative rods were recovered from an anaerobic blood agar plate after 48 hours of incubation. The Gram stain smear showed thin bacilli with pointed ends. The colonies on blood agar had the appearance of dry, irregular, white breadcrumb-like morphology with greening of the agar. The following reactions were noted:

Kanamycin = Sensitive	Vancomycin = Resistant	Colistin = Sensitive
Growth on 20% bile agar = Neg	Nitrate = Neg	Indole = +
Catalase = Neg	Lipase = Neg	Urease = Neg

What is the correct identification?
A. *Fusobacterium nucleatum*
B. *Bacteroides fragilis*
C. *C. perfringens*
D. *Peptostreptococcus* spp

Microbiology/Evaluate laboratory data for identification/Anaerobic gram-negative rods/3

41. A 2-month-old infant in good health was scheduled for a checkup at the pediatrician's office. After arriving for the appointment, the mother noted white patches on the baby's tongue and in his mouth. The baby constantly used a pacifier. What is the most likely organism causing the white patches?
A. *Cryptococcus neoformans*
B. *Candida albicans*
C. *A. fumigatus*
D. None of the above

Microbiology/Evaluate laboratory data to make identification/Mycology/3

42. A 69-year-old male patient who was a cigarette smoker visited the doctor's office complaining of a cough and congestion of the lungs. Routine cultures of early morning sputum (× 3) for bacteria as well as for AFB revealed no pathogens. A fungal culture was also ordered that grew the following on Sabouraud dextrose agar after 3 days:

Hyphae = septate with dichotomous branching
Spores = produced by conidial heads with numerous conidia
Colonies = velvety or powdery, white at first, then turning dark greenish to gray (Reverse = white to tan)
Vesicle = holding phialides usually on upper two-thirds only

What is the most likely identification?
A. *Aspergillus niger*
B. *Absidia* spp
C. *Mucor* spp
D. *Aspergillus fumigatus*

Microbiology/Evaluate laboratory data to make identification/Mycology/3

Answers to Questions 39–42

39. **B** The *B. fragilis* group is a dominant part of the indigenous flora of the large bowel and is recovered most commonly from postoperative abdominal fluids. The *B. fragilis* group are more resistant to antibiotics and are not pigmented. *Prevotella* and *Porphyromonas* spp are pigmented.

40. **A** A slender gram-negative rod with pointed ends that does not grow on 20% bile agar rules out *B. fragilis* group and indicates *F. nucleatum.*

41. **B** *C. albicans* is the common cause of oral thrush involving the mucocutaneous membranes of the mouth. *C. albicans* is part of the normal flora of the skin, mucous membranes, and gastrointestinal tract.

42. **D** *A. fumigatus* is the cause of aspergillosis and involves the organism colonizing the mucous plugs in the lung. This is called allergic aspergillosis and is characterized by a high titer of IgE antibody to *Aspergillus*. Invasive aspergillosis seen in neutropenic patients exhibits sinusitis and is disseminated throughout the body.

43. A young male patient with a fungus of the feet visited the podiatrist for some relief for the itching. A culture was sent to the microbiology laboratory that grew after 8 days on Sabouraud dextrose agar. Colonies were powdery pink with concentric and radial folds, with the reverse side showing brownish-tan to red in color. Other observations were:

Hyphae = Septate   Macroconidia = Cigar-shaped, thin-walled with 1–6 cells
Urease = +   Microconidia = Round and clustered on branched conidiophores

Red pigment on cornmeal (1% dextrose) = 0
In vitro hair perforation = +

The most likely identification is:
A. *T. mentagrophytes*
B. *T. rubrum*
C. *C. albicans*
D. *A. niger*

Microbiology/Evaluate laboratory data to make identification/Mycology/3

44. A 79-year-old female nursing home patient was admitted to the hospital with a fever and central nervous system dysfunction. Routine blood work and blood cultures were ordered. After 48 hours, the blood cultures revealed a budding yeast. The following tests performed from Sabouraud dextrose agar (after 3 days of growth) showed:

Germ tube = 0   Birdseed agar = Brown
   growth
Urease = +   Pseudohyphae = 0
Blastospores = +   Chlamydospores = 0
Arthrospores = 0   Assimilation agar = +
                                 (dextrose, sucrose, maltose)

What is the most likely identification?
A. *C. albicans*
B. *Cryptococcus laurentii*
C. *Cryptococcus neoformans*
D. *Candida tropicalis*

Microbiology/Evaluate laboratory data for identification/Mycology/3

45. A dehydrated 25-year-old male patient was admitted to the hospital with symptoms similar to chronic fatigue syndrome. Serological testing proved negative for recent streptococcal infection, Epstein-Barr virus, and hepatitis. Which of the following viral serological tests should help with a possible diagnosis?
A. CMV
B. Echovirus

C. Respiratory syncytial virus
D. Measles virus

Microbiology/Select tests for identification/ Virology/3

46. A nursing student working in the emergency room accidentally stuck herself with a needle after removing it from an intravenous set taken from a suspected drug user. The best course of action, after reporting the incident to her supervisor is to:
A. Immediately test the student for hepatitis B virus.
B. Immediately test the patient and the student for HIV using an EIA or ELISA test.
C. Perform a Western blot assay on the student's serum.
D. Draw blood from the student only and freeze it for further testing.

Microbiology/Evaluate testing for viral testing/Virology/3

Answers to Questions 43–46

43. **A** *T. mentagrophytes*, a common cause of athletes foot, is sometimes confused with *T. rubrum*, the most common dermatophyte to infect humans. The differential tests are shown in the chart below.

44. **C** *C. neoformans* produces brown colonies on birdseed agar, is urease-positive, and produces only blastospores. Immunosuppressed patients are vulnerable to this organism.

45. **A** CMV infection in young adults causes a self-limited mononucleosis syndrome. CMV infections are common and usually self-limited, except in neonates and immunosuppressed patients, in whom they may cause a life-threatening infection.

46. **B** With the permission of the patient (state law may require him or her to sign a consent form) and counseling of the student nurse, the appropriate course of action is to test the patient for HIV using a screening test (EIA or ELISA). The student should also be baseline tested. If the test result is positive for the patient, the student will be administered the appropriate antiviral drug(s) immediately or within 2 hours of the incident. Confirmatory testing will be done on any positive HIV tests.

	Urease	**Hair Perforation**	**Red Pigment on Cornmeal (1% dextrose)**
T. mentagrophytes	+	+	0
T. rubrum	0 or W	0	+

47. A 30-year-old female patient complained of vaginal irritation and symptoms (fever, dysuria, and inguinal lymphadenopathy) associated with sexually transmitted diseases (STDs). Examination showed extensive lesions in the genital area. *Chlamydia* spp testing, *N. gonorrhoeae,* and *G. vaginalis* cultures were negative. Rapid plasma reagin (RPR) testing was also negative. What is the next line of testing?
A. Darkfield examination
B. Herpes simplex testing
C. *Trichomonas* spp testing
D. Group B streptococcal testing

Microbiology/Evaluate tesing for identification/ Virology/3

48. A patient is being seen in the emergency room for a low-grade fever, headache, and general malaise after returning from Africa on a photographic safari. The physician has requested blood for malaria; the laboratory would like to have patient information regarding:
A. Specific travel history and temperature every 4 hours
B. Liver function tests and prophylactic medication history
C. Transfusion history and temperature every 4 hours
D. Prophylactic medication history and specific travel history

Microbiology/Apply knowledge of life cycles, diagnostic techniques, and clinical presentation/ Parasitology/3

49. Examination of a modified acid-fast stained fecal smear reveals round structures measuring approximately 8–10 μm, some of which are stained and some of which are not. They do not appear to show any internal morphology. The patient is symptomatic with diarrhea, and the cause may be:
A. *Blastocystis hominis*
B. Polymorphonuclear leukocytes
C. *Cyclospora cayetanensis*
D. Large yeast cells

Microbiology/Apply knowledge of the morphology of artifacts, organism life cycles, and diagnostic methods/Parasitology/3

50. A patient has been diagnosed as having amebiasis but continues to be asymptomatic. The physician has asked for an explanation and recommendations regarding follow-up. Suggestions should include:
A. Consideration of *Entamoeba histolytica* versus *Entamoeba dispar*
B. A request for an additional three stools for culture
C. Initiating therapy, regardless of the patient's asymptomatic status
D. Performance of barium x-ray studies

Microbiology/Apply knowledge of the morphology of organisms and pathogenesis/Parasitology/3

Answers to Questions 47–50

47. **B** Herpes genitalis is an infection caused by HSV-2. Symptomatic primary herpes by HSV-2 is responsible for about 85% of herpes infections. HSV-1 (causing the other 15%) does not involve recurring infections of herpes. HSV-2 causes 99% of recurrent genital herpes.

48. **D** If the patient has malaria and has been taking prophylaxis (often sporadically), the number of parasites on the blood smear will be reduced and examination of routine thick and thin blood films should be more exhaustive. Also specific geographic travel history may help to determine whether chloroquine-resistant *Plasmodium falciparum* may be a factor.

49. **C** One of the newer coccidian parasites, *C. cayetanensis* has been implicated in cases of human diarrhea. The recommended stains are modified acid-fast stains, and the organisms are quite variable in their staining characteristics. The oocysts are immature when passed (no internal morphology) and they measure about 8–10 μm.

50. **A** It is now well established that *E. histolytica* is being used to designate pathogenic zymodemes (strains of former "*E. histolytica*" based on isoenzyme analysis patterns), while *E. dispar* is now being used to designate nonpathogenic zymodemes. However, unless trophozoites containing ingested red blood cells (*E. histolytica*) are seen, the two organisms cannot be differentiated on the basis of morphology. Based on this information, there are now two separate species, only one of which (*E. histolytica*) is pathogenic. Because this patient is asymptomatic, the organisms seen in the fecal smears are probably *E. dispar* (nonpathogen); the laboratory report should have said "*Entamoeba histolytica/E. dispar*"—unable to differentiate on the basis of morphology unless trophozoites are seen to contain ingested RBCs (*E. histolytica*).

51. Although a patient is strongly suspected of having giardiasis and is still symptomatic, three routine stool examinations (O&P exam) have been performed correctly and reported as negative. Biopsy confirmed the patient had giardiasis. Reasons for these findings may include:
A. The patient was coinfected with several bacterial species.
B. *Giardia lamblia* tends to adhere to the mucosal surface and more than three stool examinations may be required to confirm a suspected infection.
C. The organisms present did not stain with trichrome stain so the morphology is very atypical.
D. Special diagnostic procedures such as the Knott concentration and nutrient-free agar cultures should have been used.

Microbiology/Apply knowledge of life cycles, organism morphology, pathogenesis, and diagnostic procedures/Parasitology/3

52. A transplant patient is currently receiving steroids. The patient is now complaining of abdominal pain and has symptoms of pneumonia and positive blood cultures with gram-negative rods. The individual has been living in the United States for 20 years but grew up in Central America. The most likely parasite causing these symptoms is:
A. *Trypanosoma brucei rhodesiense*
B. *G. lamblia*
C. *Strongyloides stercoralis*
D. *Schistosoma japonicum*

Microbiology/Apply knowledge of fundamental life cycles, pathogenesis, and immunosuppressives/Parasitology/3

Answers to Questions 51–52

51. **B** It is well known that *G. lamblia* trophozoites adhere to the intestinal mucosal surface by means of the sucking disk. Although a patient may have giardiasis and be symptomatic, confirmation of the infection from stool examinations may require more than the routine three stools or may require the examination of duodenal contents.

52. **C** Although infection with *S. stercoralis* may have been acquired in Central America many years before, the patient may have remained asymptomatic while the infection was maintained at a low level in the body via the autoinfective portion of the life cycle. As the patient became more immunosuppressed (steroids), the life cycle began to reactivate with penetration of the larvae through the intestinal wall (abdominal pain), through the lungs (pneumonia), and the patient may present with evidence of sepsis (often with gram-negative bacteria carried with the larvae as they penetrate the intestinal wall). Patients who become immunosuppressed may see the life cycle of *Strongyloides* reactivated with serious illness resulting; this can occur many years after the initial infection and after the patient has left the endemic area.

BIBLIOGRAPHY

1. Baron, EJ, Peterson, LR, and Finegold, FM: Bailey and Scott's Diagnostic Microbiology. CV Mosby, St. Louis, 1994.
2. Garcia, LS, and Bruckner, DA: Diagnostic Medical Parasitology. ASM Press, Washington, DC, 1997.
3. Henry, JB (ed): Clinical Diagnosis and Management by Laboratory Methods. WB Saunders, Philadelphia, 1996.
4. Isenberg, HD (ed): Clinical Microbiology Procedures Handbook, Vols 1 and 2. American Society for Microbiology, Washington, DC, 1992
5. Koneman, EW, Allen, SD, Janda, WM, et al: Color Atlas and Textbook of Diagnostic Microbiology. JB Lippincott, Philadelphia, 1992.
6. Larone, DH: Medically Important Fungi: A Guide to Identification. ASM Press, Washington, DC, 1995.
7. Murray, PR, Baron, EJ, Pfaller, MA, et al: Manual of Clinical Microbiology. American Society for Microbiology, Washington, DC, 1995.
8. Summanen, P, Baron, EJ, Citron, DM, et al: Wadsworth Anaerobic Bacteriology Manual. Star, Belmont, CA, 1993.

CHAPTER SEVEN

Education and Management

1. A comparison of methods for the determination of alkaline phosphatase is categorized in which domain of educational objectives?
   A. Affective
   B. Psychomotor
   C. Cognitive
   D. Behavioral

   Education and management/Apply knowledge of educational methodology/1

2. Attitude, judgment, and interest refer to which domain of educational objectives?
   A. Cognitive
   B. Affective
   C. Psychomotor
   D. Competency

   Education and management/Apply knowledge of educational methodology/1

3. Criterion-referenced examinations are used in order to determine the:
   A. Competency of a student according to a prede-termined standard
   B. Validity of a test
   C. Status of one student compared to the whole group
   D. Accuracy of a test

   Education and management/Apply knowledge of educational testing/1

4. An instructor "curved" a blood bank exam given to medical technology students. The highest grade was an 85% and the lowest grade was a 60%. What type of test is this?

   A. Subjective
   B. Objective
   C. Norm-referenced
   D. Criterion-referenced

   Education and management/Apply knowledge of educational testing/2

Answers to Questions 1–4

1. **C** The cognitive domain of educational objectives deals with application, analysis, synthesis, and evaluation of information or knowledge learned to be utilized in problem solving.

2. **B** The affective domain of educational objectives includes those that emphasize values, attitudes, and interests that attach a worth to an activity, situation, or phenomenon.

3. **A** A criterion-referenced test is used to determine the mastery of predetermined competencies, while a norm-referenced test evaluates students by comparison to the group. Criterion-referenced ex-aminations use questions of known difficulty and can be calibrated against established criteria in order to evaluate the examinee's performance.

4. **C** This type of test compares the students to each other rather than grading the students on a set of standards or criterion that must be met.

5. A stated competency requirement for a medical technology student is to perform calibration, plot data, and evaluate the acceptability of controls. This competency requirement encompasses which educational objective?
A. Cognitive
B. Psychomotor
C. Affective
D. All of the above

Education and management/Apply knowledge of educational methodology/3

6. A chemistry test result from a chemotherapy patient was within normal limits on Tuesday. The same test was reported as abnormal on Monday ("flagged" high and approaching a critical value). The technologist performing the test noted a delta-check error and remembered that both controls ran much higher on Monday although they were within acceptable limits. The technologist's decision to follow-up this discrepancy before reporting the results is an example of which domain of behavioral objectives?
A. Cognitive
B. Affective
C. Psychomotor
D. Organizational

Education and management/Apply knowledge of educational methodology/3

7. In general, academic evaluation of students depends on the ability of the instructor to create a test that reflects the stated objectives of the course material as well as making the test:
A. Reliable and valid
B. Normally distributed and practical
C. Fair and short
D. Written and oral

Education and management/Apply knowledge of educational testing/1

8. When dealing with the instruction of complex instrumentation, a demonstration by the instructor is necessary and should include the following:
A. Detailed diagrams of the electrical system
B. A blueprint of the optical system
C. A step-by-step narrative with comparisons to a manual method
D. A quiz as soon as the demonstration is complete

Education and management/Apply knowledge of educational methodology/1

9. One method of learning is by giving a small group of students a topic to discuss or a problem to solve rather than a formal lecture by the instructor. Each participant is given a portion of the topic to discuss or solve. This method of learning is popular and used easily with which of the following approaches?

A. Case study
B. Manual demonstration
C. Implementing new equipment
D. Histogram evaluation

Education and management/Apply knowledge of educational methodology/2

Answers to Questions 5–9

5. **D** The student will perform the actual calibration (psychomotor skills), utilize the cognitive domain of analysis to plot the standards, construct a best-fit calibration line, and determine the concentration of the controls. The affective domain describes the student's ability to value the results as acceptable or to repeat the calibration, if an error is apparent.

6. **B** The technologist chose to investigate the situation in order to resolve a discrepancy. The responding, valuing, and characterization refer to the affective domain in dealing with the problem presented here. In doing so, a rule-based process is followed that includes evaluation of the specimen, instrument performance, potential sources of interference (such as the effects of drugs), and physiological variation before determining whether to report the result, repeat the test, or call for a new specimen.

7. **A** A test should be based on stated, measurable objectives and contain five attributes: reliability, validity, objectivity, fairness, and practicality.

8. **C** When a demonstration of a complex instrument is necessary, a small group of students should be assembled around the instrument to permit clear visibility. A diagram with the major functioning parts should be provided along with an assignment of a written summary or questions about the function, principle, testing done, and reagents needed.

9. **A** The case study approach allows a student to engage in problem solving and to utilize the input of all members of the group. This allows for interaction and use of higher cognitive levels in order to determine the cause of the patient's illness and various laboratory test results.

10. An instructor of clinical laboratory science was given the task of expanding the curriculum for the senior (baccalaureate degree) medical technology students. Which of the following courses should be included in the curriculum?
A. Cytology—cytogenetics
B. Histology—special stains
C. Computer (laboratory information systems [LIS])
D. Economics—budget analysis

Education and management/Education/Apply knowledge of entry level skills/1

11. McGregor's X-Y theory advocates managing employees by stressing:
A. Equal pay for equal work
B. A pyramid of attainable goals for satisfaction at work
C. Respect for the worker and acknowledgment of his/her ability to perform a task
D. Collective bargaining

Education and management/Apply knowledge of management theory/1

12. Maslow's theory of management is based upon:
A. The premise that all workers are unmotivated
B. A pyramid of goals for the satisfaction of employee needs
C. Use of detractors and perks to keep employees happy
D. The professional development of the employee

Education and management/Apply knowledge of management theory/1

13. Herzberg's theory relies on motivators that are part of the job design in order to instill job satisfaction. These same motivators can become dissatisfiers if they are lacking in a job. Herzberg's motivators are:
A. Opportunity for achievement and advancement
B. Performance evaluations every 24 months
C. Continuing education sessions requiring supervisory approval
D. Punitive actions taken when improvement diminishes

Education and management/Apply knowledge of management theory/1

14. Management by objective (MBO) is *least* effective for managing employees in which situation?
A. Employees must be creative in their work.
B. The laboratory is converting to a new computer system.
C. The laboratory is undergoing a renovation.
D. Employees jointly agree to institutional goals.

Education and management/Apply knowledge of management theory/2

15. The four essential functions of a manager are:
A. Staffing, decision making, cost analysis, evaluating
B. Directing, leading, forecasting, implementing
C. Planning, organizing, directing, controlling
D. Innovating, designing, coordinating, problem solving

Education and management/Apply knowledge of management theory/1

Answers to Questions 10–15

10. **C** The everchanging role of the medical technologist in a clinical laboratory prompts the curriculum committee to re-evaluate the courses required by the students on a yearly basis. The heart of the laboratory, the LIS, is one of the first important areas to which students are introduced when entering the professional clinical training portion of their degree.

11. **C** McGregor's theory deals with participatory management in which the employee is considered a valuable asset.

12. **B** Maslow's theory of managing people deals with six levels. As the basic needs of an employee are met, the next higher need is substituted. The needs, in ascending order, are physiological, safety, security, social, esteem and self-actualization. Unsatisfied needs are considered motivators.

13. **A** According to Frederick Herzberg, achievement, opportunity for advancement, recognition, challenging work, responsibility, and a chance for advancement and personal growth are motivators and should be included as part of a job design.

14. **A** MBO stresses teamwork and shared goals and objectives but stifles creativity.

15. **C** While managing may involve all of the functions listed, the four core processes for all managers are planning, organizing, directing, and controlling. Planning includes formulating of goals and objectives, organizing the tasks, and establishing schedules. Organizing includes establishing effective communication, relationships, job descriptions, and training. Directing involves oversight of the various steps and stages of the plan including coordination and leadership. Controlling involves evaluating resource utilization and outcomes, managing costs, and modifying the process to improve quality.

16. Which of the following questions is allowable during a pre-employment interview?
- A. How many times have you been pregnant?
- B. Have you been convicted of any felonies?
- C. Does your husband belong to any religious societies?
- D. Are you planning to use the hospital day care center?

Education and management/Labor law/3

17. Direct laboratory costs for tests include which of the following?
- A. Equipment maintenance
- B. Insurance
- C. Depreciation
- D. Overtime pay

Education and management/Laboratory economics/1

18. Which of the following accounts for the largest portion of the direct cost of a laboratory test?
- A. Reagents
- B. General supplies
- C. Technologist labor
- D. Instrument depreciation

Education and management/Laboratory economics/1

19. Using the surcharge/cost-plus method for determining test charges, determine the charge for an ova and parasite examination on fecal specimens, given the following information:

Collection, handling, clerical, and so forth = $2.00
Reference lab charge to lab = $20.00
Lab "markup" = 100%

- A. $22.00
- B. $32.00
- C. $42.00
- D. $122.00

Education and management/Laboratory economics/2

20. In deciding whether to adopt a new test on the laboratory's automated chemistry analyzer, which parameters are needed to determine the number of tests that must be performed to break even?
- A. Test turnaround time
- B. Cost of labor per hour
- C. Number of other tests performed per month
- D. Total fixed laboratory costs

Education and management/Laboratory economics/2

21. Which statement best represents the relationship between test volume and revenue or costs for batch-run tests?
- A. As volume increases the fixed cost per test also increases.
- B. As volume increases the revenue also increases.
- C. Revenue is approximately equal for both high and low volume tests.
- D. 90% of the revenue is generated by 5% of the tests offered.

Education and management/Laboratory economics/2

Answers to Questions 16–21

16. **B** Title VII of the Civil Rights Act of 1964 states that questions are permissible during interviews if they are related to legitimate occupational qualifications. Inquiries concerning convictions for drug use or theft are legitimate questions when hiring a laboratory night supervisor or other individuals who will utilize controlled substances.

17. **D** All costs that are specifically linked to a test (e.g., personnel, overtime, chemicals, supplies) are direct costs.

18. **C** Labor accounts for 60%–70% of the direct cost per test in most laboratories. The cost of labor, reagents, and supplies are direct costs, but instrument depreciation is not.

19. **C** The "markup" factor is used to establish part of the cost of a test in order to obtain the desired profit margin. Tests sent to reference laboratories or done in-house have the added cost that is referred to as the surcharge/cost-plus method of determining test charges.

20. **D** The formula for calculating the break-even point in test volume is:

No. tests = total fixed costs ÷ (average reimbursement − variable cost per test)

The total fixed costs are the expenses that are not expected to change as the workload increases (e.g., cost of the instrument). The variable cost per test includes any costs that increase as the workload increases (e.g., cost of reagents). The average reimbursement represents the expected revenue generated per billable test result.

21. **B** As volume increases, costs should decrease and revenues should increase. The large fixed costs such as instrumentation, labor, and management do not change with the size of the batch. As volume increases, reagent and consumable costs per test often become lower thus reducing the variable cost per test. In most laboratories, about 80% of the revenue is generated by the laboratory tests that comprise the top 20% of the test volume.

22. A hospital submits a bill for $200.00 to the patient's insurance company for the cost of outpatient laboratory tests. The laboratory services rendered by the hospital are paid according to an agreed fee schedule. The specific laboratory procedures are billed according to which system of coding?
A. Diagnosis-related group (DRG)
B. Current procedual terminolgy (CPT)
C. Medicare
D. Medicaid

Education and management/Laboratory economics/1

23. A hospital has a contract with a major medical insurer that reimburses the laboratory at a rate of $1.00 per insured life per year. This type of reimbursement is termed:
A. A prospective payment system
B. A preferred provider discount
C. Capitation
D. Diagnosis-related group

Education and management/Laboratory economics/2

24. According to federal and state regulations, a hospital's capital budget should include which of the following before projects costing $150,000 can be submitted for approval?
A. A time table of completion
B. A cost analysis
C. Salaries and wages for new employees
D. A certificate of need

Education and management/Laboratory economics/1

25. A rural hospital laboratory employs 8.25 FTEs (full-time equivalents). In order to budget for next year's salaries for these employees, the laboratory manager needs to submit which figures for the laboratory's projected annual budget?
A. Total (paid) hours
B. Productive (worked) hours
C. Total hours of full-time employees
D. Total hours of part-time employees

Education and management/Laboratory economics/1

26. A chemistry profile that includes electrolytes, glucose, blood urea nitrogen (BUN), and creatinine is ordered on an 80-year-old woman with symptoms of vomiting and dizziness. How should the laboratory submit the charge for these tests for reimbursement by Medicare?
A. Submit as one test.
B. Submit each test separately.
C. Submit Medicare-approved tests only.
D. Submit as four individual tests.

Education and management/Laboratory regulation and law/2

Answers to Questions 22–26

22. B The CPT code refers to Current Procedural Terminology. Codes are assigned to all medical procedures, which are grouped according to common disease characteristics. The insurance company or payer (e.g., Medicare) usually has agreed to a reimbursement amount per test or procedure. The American Medical Association publishes *Current Procedural Terminology*, or CPT, which is updated yearly.

23. C Capitation plans provide the laboratory with a fixed (known) revenue based upon a negotiated per capita fee for the members of the group. In order to profit the laboratory must manage its resources to provide covered laboratory tests to the group at a cost that does not equal or exceed its reimbursement. A prospective payment system is used by Medicare and Medicaid programs for outpatient reimbursements and is based upon projecting the cost of a laboratory test in a specific region. For inpatients the fees for laboratory tests are incorporated into the reimbursement covering the specific diagnosis-related group rather than the type or number of laboratory procedures performed.

24. D A certificate of need (CON) is an authorization to proceed with a needed project, such as a new obstetrics department or new wing to the laboratory. There are specific federal guidelines (most states also require them) to follow and the limit is set at $150,000. This is done to control duplication of services as well as oversupply of hospital beds.

25. A The total (paid) hours are the total number of hours for which employees are paid. This includes vacation time, sick time, and the actual time spent working in the laboratory. On the other hand, productive (worked) hours refers only to the actual hours worked, including overtime. A budget must include the total (paid) hours in order to give a clear picture of what is needed for the next year of wages and salaries.

26. A A chemistry profile that includes electrolytes, glucose, BUN, and creatinine is considered a billable procedure and has a single CPT code (currently this panel is called the Basic Metabolic Panel and is coded as CPT 80049). Splitting a profile into many individual tests for billing purposes may be prohibited by law. For example, a complete blood count (CBC) cannot be split into five parts with each component being charged separately.

27. According to the Clinical Laboratory Improvement Act of 1988 (CLIA '88), control of laboratory test reliability is accomplished by all of the following requirements *except:*
A. Documentation of quality control results and corrective actions
B. Participation in proficiency testing for all non-waivered tests
C. Professional certification of all testing personnel
D. Demonstration that all quantitative tests meet manufacturer's performance specifications

Education and management/Laboratory regulation and law/2

28. CLIA '88 specifies the minimum requirements for proficiency testing (PT) of analytes for which PT is required (excluding cytology) to be:
A. One challenge per analyte and one testing event per year
B. Ten challenges per analyte and five testing events per year
C. Five challenges per analyte and at least three testing events per year
D. Twelve challenges per analyte and one testing event per month

Education and management/Laboratory regulation and law/1

29. According to CLIA '88, satisfactory performance for ABO, Rh, and compatibility tests requires a score of:
A. 100%
B. 90%
C. 80%
D. 75%

Education and management/Laboratory regulation and law/1

30. In order to comply with CLIA '88 calibration materials must:
A. Be purchased by an authorized agency such as the College of Pathology
B. Have concentration values that cover the laboratory's reportable range
C. Be traceable to the National Calibration Board
D. Be identical in concentration to those sold by the reagent manufacturer

Education and management/Laboratory regulation and law/1

31. According to CLIA '88, calibration materials should be appropriate for the methodology and be:
A. Of bovine origin
B. Three times the normal range for the specific analyte
C. Traceable to a reference method and reference material of known value
D. Twice the laboratory's reference range for the analyte

Education and management/Laboratory regulation and law/1

32. Under CLIA '88, testing personnel with an associate degree and appropriate training in the clinical laboratory are authorized to perform:
A. Waivered tests only
B. Tests that are qualitative or waivered and some moderate-complexity tests
C. Waivered and moderate-complexity tests
D. Waivered, moderate-complexity, and high-complexity tests

Education and management/Laboratory regulation and law/1

Answers to Questions 27–32

27. **C** CLIA '88 requires all clinical laboratories to be certified, but the requirements differ for each of the three certification levels—waivered, moderate, or high complexity. For example, quality control must be practiced by all laboratories, but standards for testing personnel differ for all three levels and do not specify certification, only educational levels.

28. **C** Analytes for which proficiency testing is required are identified in section 493 subpart I of the CLIA rules. A minimum number of five challenges for each analyte and at least three testing events per year are required. The testing events are evenly spaced throughout the year. Unsatisfactory performance for the same analyte for two out of two events or two out of the three most recent events constitutes unsuccessful participation and may result in punitive action.

29. **A** Unsatisfactory performance occurs when any challenge for ABO, Rh, or compatibility testing is in error. For all other tests, a score below 80% is defined as unsatisfactory performance. Unsatisfactory performance for the same analyte for two out of two events or two out of the three most recent events constitutes unsuccessful participation.

30. **B** According to CLIA '88, the minimum requirement for calibration is every 6 months or more frequently if specified by the manufacturer. The calibrators must cover the reportable range of the method. A minimum of two levels of calibrant must be used (more if specified by the manufacturer).

31. **C** Calibrators must have an assigned concentration determined by assay using a reference method. The reference method should be calibrated using standards that are traceable to National Bureau of Standards material or acceptable primary standards.

32. **D** Testing personnel with an associate degree and approved laboratory training may perform high-complexity tests as well as waivered and moderate-complexity tests. However, the laboratory must be certified at all three levels.

33. Sexual harassment is a form of discrimination and therefore is prohibited by the:
  A. Occupational Safety and Health Administration (OSHA)
  B. Civil Rights Act of 1964 (Title VII)
  C. Right to Privacy Act of 1974
  D. Department of Health and Human Services

Education and management/Labor law/1

34. Which order of events should be followed at the conclusion of a laboratory worker's shift in order to prevent the spread of bloodborne pathogens?
  A. Remove gloves, disinfect area, wash hands, remove lab coat.
  B. Disinfect area, remove gloves, remove lab coat, wash hands.
  C. Disinfect area, remove gloves, wash hands, remove lab coat.
  D. Remove gloves, wash hands, remove lab coat, disinfect area.

Education and management/Laboratory safety and standard precautions/2

35. Records of a patient's laboratory test results may not be released without his or her consent to anyone outside the clinical laboratory *except* to the:
  A. American Red Cross
  B. Department of Health and Human Services
  C. Insurance carrier
  D. Physician who ordered the tests

Education and management/Laboratory regulation and law/2

36. Unethical behavior by a laboratory supervisor that results in a compromise of employee safety should be:
  A. Reported to a higher authority
  B. Directly confronted
  C. Reported to the EEOC
  D. All of the above

Education and management/Apply principles of laboratory management/Personnel/2

37. The most *common* deficiency cited during an onsite laboratory inspection by the College of American Pathologists (CAP) and the Joint Commission on Accreditation of Healthcare Organizations (JCAHO) is:
  A. Improper documentation
  B. Insufficient work space area
  C. Improper reagent storage
  D. Improper instrument calibration frequency

Education and management/Laboratory regulation and certification/2

38. Which of the following circumstances is considered a form a sexual harassment?
  A. Unwelcome sexual advances by a supervisor
  B. Requests for favors of a sexual nature from a fellow laboratory employee
  C. Physical conduct of a sexual nature from an employee working in another department
  D. All of the above

Education and management/Labor law/2

Answers to Questions 33–38

33. **B** The Civil Rights Act of 1964 prohibits by federal law discrimination in employment because of race, color, religion, or gender. The law established the Equal Employment Opportunity Commission (EEOC) to hear complaints of discrimination by employees and initiate legal action as appropriate.

34. **B** According to the OSHA Bloodborne Pathogens Rule of 1992, gloves and lab coats are to be removed after disinfection of the work area.

35. **D** The Privacy Act of 1974 prohibits the release of medical records without the patient's consent except to the patient's attending physician, attorney, or next of kin if deceased unless solicited by a valid subpoena.

36. **D** Direct confrontation is in order, followed by reporting the behavior to a higher authority at the clinical site. Major violations that are a threat to the safety of employees, patients, and the facility in general should be reported to the EEOC or OSHA, if the violations are not corrected in a timely fashion, and if all avenues of action have been exhausted.

37. **A** Improper documentation accounts for the majority of laboratory deficiencies while outdated or inadequate procedure manuals is the second most frequently cited deficiency.

38. **D** Sexual harassment is a form of discrimination and it is prohibited by the Civil Rights Act of 1964 (Title VII). The suggestion that a sexual favor must be performed to avoid punitive action or receive a favorable performance evaluation constitutes sexual harassment. Additionally, offensive language and behavior with sexual connotations are a form of sexual harassment.

39. The material safety data sheets (MSDS) for hazardous chemicals address which of the following conditions?
A. Physical characteristics of the chemical
B. Safe handling and storage of the chemical
C. Specific health hazards associated with the chemical
D. All of the above

Education and management/Laboratory regulation and safety/1

40. A new employee's performance is to be evaluated at the end of his or her probationary period, and must relate to:
A. The person's job description
B. Verbal instructions given
C. Wage and salary policies
D. Recruitment practices

Education and management/Apply principles of laboratory management/Personnel/1

Answers to Questions 39–40

39. **D** The MSDS documents describe the chemical and physical characteristics, safe handling and storage, and potential health hazards of reagents used in the laboratory. These documents must be located in an easily accessible place so that all employees have access to them. They should be reviewed at least once per year during safety inservice training.

40. **A** The information used for the employee's performance review should reflect the job description used at the time of hire. An employee should receive a written job description that states the responsibilities and activities of the position. Job performance criteria and the rating system used should be clearly stated and available to the employee.

BIBLIOGRAPHY

1. Erickson, RC and Wentling, TL: Measuring Student Growth: Techniques and Procedures for Occupational Education. Allyn and Bacon, Boston, 1977.
2. Snyder, JR and Senhauser, DA: Administration and Supervision in Laboratory Medicine. JB Lippincott, Philadelphia, 1989.
3. Umiker, WO: The Effective Laboratory Supervisor. Medical Economics, Oradell, NJ, 1982.
4. Regulations Implementing the Clinical Laboratory Improvement Amendments of 1988 (42 CFR Part 405). Federal Register. February 28, 1992:57(40).
5. Varnadoe, LA: Medical Laboratory Management and Supervision. FA Davis, Philadelphia, 1996.
6. Wallace, MA and Klosinski, DD: Clinical Laboratory Science Education and Management. WB Saunders, Philadelphia, 1998.

CHAPTER EIGHT

Photomicrographs and Color Plates

Refer to the photomicrographs and color plates that follow p. 383.

1. Plate 1 is a photomicrograph of an antinuclear antibody test using human fibroblasts, fluorescein isothiocyanate (FITC)–conjugated antihuman serum, and transmitted fluorescence microscopy. Which pattern of immunofluorescence is demonstrated in this 40× field?
   A. Homogenous
   B. Peripheral
   C. Nucleolar
   D. Speckled

   Immunology/Identify microscopic morphology/ Immunofluorescence/2

2. Plate 2 shows the electrophoresis of serum proteins on a high-resolution agarose gel at pH 8.6. Sample 1 (in lane 1) is a normal serum control. Which sample can be presumptively classified as a monoclonal gammopathy?
   A. Sample 2
   B. Sample 4
   C. Sample 6
   D. Sample 8

   Chemistry/Evaluate clinical and laboratory data/ Electrophoresis/3

Answers to Questions 1–2

1. **A** Using FITC-conjugated antihuman serum, diffuse apple green fluorescence seen over the entire nucleus characterizes the homogenous pattern. At a significant titer, this pattern occurs in a variety of systemic autoimmune diseases including systemic lupus erythematosus, rheumatoid arthritis, systemic sclerosis, and Sjögren's syndrome. The antibodies are directed against nucleoprotein; although they are mainly nonpathological, they are useful markers for active disease.

2. **C** A monoclonal gammopathy causes a band showing restricted electrophoretic mobility usually located in the γ or the β region. The band represents the accumulation of identical immunoglobulin molecules or fragments secreted by a malignant or benign clone of plasma cells. Confirmation of the band as immunoglobulin is required because other homogenous proteins (such as fibrinogen or carcinoembyronic antigen) can occur in the same regions.

3. Plate 3 shows a densitometric scan of a control serum for protein electrophoresis. The percentages of each fraction are shown below the scan. Given these results, what is the most appropriate initial corrective action?
A. Repeat the electrophoresis run using fresh control serum.
B. Report the results provided that the previous run was in control.
C. Move the fourth fraction mark to the right and redraw the scan.
D. Calculate the concentration of each fraction in grams per deciliter.

Chemistry/Identify sources of error/Densitometry/3

4. Plate 4 is an immunoelectrophoresis film. The patient's serum was added to the even-numbered wells and a normal control serum to the odd-numbered wells. Trough A contains antitotal immunoglobulin and troughs B through F contain monospecific antisera in the following order: B–anti-γ, C–anti-α, D–anti-μ, E–anti-λ, and F–anti-κ. Which monoclonal immunoglobulin can be identified in the patient's serum?
A. IgG κ
B. IgA λ
C. IgM λ
D. λ Light chain

Chemistry/Evaluate clinical and laboratory data/ Immunoelectrophoresis/2

5. Plate 5 is a densitometric scan of a serum protein electrophoresis sample. The relative and absolute concentration of each fraction and reference limits are shown below the scan. What is the correct classification of this densitometric pattern?
A. Polyclonal gammopathy associated with chronic inflammation
B. Nephrotic syndrome
C. Acute inflammation
D. Hepatic cirrhosis

Chemistry/Evaluate clinical and laboratory data/ electrophoresis/3

6. Plate 6 shows an agarose gel on which immunofixation electrophoresis (IFE) was performed at pH 8.6. The gel contains the same serum sample as number 6 shown in Plate 2. What is the heavy and light chain type of the monoclonal protein present in this sample?
A. IgA κ
B. IgG κ
C. IgG λ
D. IgM λ

Chemistry/Evaluate clinical and laboratory data/ Electrophoresis/3

Answers to Questions 3–6

3. **C** The fraction marker between the α_2- and β-fractions is marked improperly. High-resolution gels produce individual peaks for haptoglobin and α_2-macroglobulin, which partially splits the α_2- band into two subfractions. In addition, the β-band may contain three subfractions corresponding to β-lipoprotein, transferrin, and complement. In this scan, the valley between the α_2- subfractions was selected incorrectly as the boundary between the α_2- and β-fractions. This fraction marker should be placed at the next valley to the right and the scan redrawn to determine the area under the α_2- and β-fractions correctly.

4. **C** Restricted electrophoretic mobility characteristic of monoclonal protein is seen in three reactions: serum from well 1 with antitotal Ig, serum from well 5 with anti-μ, and serum from well 5 with anti-λ. The monoclonal immunoprecipitate is the same distance from the anode in all three cases. The dark staining ring around the wells containing the patient's serum is also characteristic of IgM monoclonal gammopathies and represents aggregated IgM that could not be washed out of the gel.

5. **C** This pattern is characterized by significant increases in the α_1- and α_2- fractions and a decrease in serum albumin concentration. This pattern is most often caused by increased production of acute phase reactants such as α_1-antitrypsin and haptoglobin that are associated with acute inflammation. This pattern is seen in myocardial infarction and other forms of acute tissue injury, the early stage of acute infection, and pregnancy.

6. **B** IFE is performed by placing the patient's sample in all six lanes and separating the proteins by electrophoresis. Following electrophoresis, the proteins in lane 1 are precipitated and fixed by overlaying sulfosalicylic acid onto the gel. Monospecific antiserum against each heavy or light chain is applied to the gel over the lanes as labeled and incubated to precipitate the immunoglobulins containing the corresponding chain. The gel is washed to remove unprecipitated proteins, then stained to visualize the precipitated bands. This IFE gel shows an insoluble immunoprecipitate restricted to a single band in lanes 2 and 5. The proteins in lane 2 reacted with anti-γ (anti-IgG), and the proteins in lane 5 reacted with anti-κ. Lane 5 also contains a small restricted band anodal to the IgG band. This band is not present in lane 2 (does not contain γ chains) and represents free κ light chains.

7. Plate 7 shows the electrophoresis of hemoglobin (Hgb) samples performed on agarose gel, pH 8.8. The control sample is located in lanes 2 and 10 and contains Hgb A, S, and C. Which sample(s) are from neonates?
   A. Samples 1 and 5
   B. Sample 3
   C. Sample 7
   D. Samples 8 and 9

   Chemistry/Evaluate clinical and laboratory data/ Hemoglobin electrophoresis/2

8. Plate 8 shows the electrophoresis of Hgb samples on acid agar gel, pH 6.0. The sample order is the same as for plate 7 with the A, S, C control hemolysate in lanes 2 and 10. Based upon the electrophoretic mobility of sample 7 as seen in both plate 7 and plate 8, what is the patient's Hgb phenotype?
   A. SS
   B. AS
   C. AD
   D. AG

   Chemistry/Evaluate clinical and laboratory data/ Hemoglobin electrophoresis/3

9. Plate 9 is a photomicrograph of a fungal slide culture stained with lactophenol cotton blue, 40×. Which of the following fungi is present?
   A. *Microsporum gypseum*
   B. *Microsporum canis*
   C. *Aspergillus niger*
   D. *Aspergillus fumigatus*

   Microbiology/Identify microscopic morphology/ Fungi/2

10. Plate 10 is a photomicrograph of a fungal slide culture stained with lactophenol cotton blue, 40×. Which of the following fungi is present?
    A. *M. gypseum*
    B. *M. canis*
    C. *Trichophyton schoenleinii*
    D. *Epidermophyton floccosum*

    Microbiology/Identify microscopic morphology/ Fungi/2

11. Plate 11 is a photomicrograph of a fungal slide culture stained with lactophenol cotton blue, 40×. The morphology is most consistent with which fungus?
    A. *Aspergillus* spp
    B. *Penicillium* spp
    C. *Scedosporium*
    D. *Fusarium*

    Microbiology/Identify microscopic morphology/ Mycology/2

Answers to Questions 7–11

7. **A** Neonates and infants up to 6 months old have Hgb F levels between 8% and 40%. The Hgb F level falls to below 2% in children over 2 years old. Hgb F is more acidic than Hgb S, and less acidic than Hgb A. Therefore, at an alkaline pH, Hgb F has a greater net negative charge than Hgb S but a lesser net negative charge than Hgb A, and migrates between Hgb A and Hgb S.

8. **A** Sample 7 demonstrates one major band on plate 7 in the Hgb S position. Because Hgb A is not present, there is no normal β-gene, and the patient can be classified as a homozygote for Hgb S, D, or G which migrate to the same position on agarose gel at a pH between 8.4 and 9.2. Hgb S can be differentiated from Hgbs D and G by performing electrophoresis on agar gel at pH 6.0–6.2. On agar at acid pH, Hgb C migrates furthest toward the anode. Hgb S migrates toward the anode, but not as far as Hgb C. Hgb F migrates furthest toward the cathode, while Hgbs A, D, G, and E migrate to the same position, slightly cathodal to the point of application. On plate 8, sample 7 shows a single large band that migrated toward the anode at the same position as the S band in the control sample.

9. **D** *A. fumigatus* produces hyaline, septate hyphae, and dome-shaped vesicles, the upper one-half to two-thirds of which are covered with a row of phialides producing long chains of conidia. *A. niger* produces spherical vesicles that are completely covered with phialides. The phialides produce jet black conidia that obscure the vesicle surface forming a radiated head. *M. gypseum* and *M. canis* produce septate macroconidia, not vesicles with phialides.

10. **A** *M. gypseum* produces enormous numbers of symmetric, rough macroconidia. These have thin walls with not more than six compartments and have rounded ends. *M. canis* produces spindle-shaped macroconidia with usually more than six compartments and pointed ends. *E. floccosum* forms macroconidia but not microconidia. The macroconidia are smooth and club-shaped with rounded ends. Each contains 2–6 cells and are found singly or in clusters. *T. schoenleinii* does not produce macroconidia or microconidia and is identified by its hyphae-forming characteristics. *T. schoenleinii* forms antler-like branching hyphae called *favic chandeliers*.

11. **A** This plate shows a fungus with thin, septate, branching hyphae. A conidiophore is present in the center that contains a double row of phialides producing round conidia. *Fusarium* sp produces canoe-shaped macroconidia. These are made by phialides attached to the hyphae in the absence of conidiophores. *Penicillium* spp produce conidia from a single row of phialides that resembles a brush or the skeleton of a hand. *Scedosporium* spp produce annellides on short conidiophores with oval conidia that are tapered at one end.

12. Plate 12 is a bronchoalveolar lavage sample concentrated by cytocentrifugation and stained with Wright's stain, 100×. The sample was obtained from a patient with AIDS who resides in the midwestern United States. Which infectious agent is present?
A. *Pneumocystis carinii*
B. *Mycobacterium avium-intracellulare*
C. *Histoplasmosis capsulatum*
D. *Cryptococcus neoformins*

Microbiology/Identify microscopic morphology/ Mycology/2

13. Plate 13 is a fecal specimen seen under 40× using brightfield microscopy. The plate shows the ovum of which parasite?
A. *Necator americanus*
B. *Trichuris trichiura*
C. *Ascaris lumbricoides*
D. *Enterobius vermicularis*

Microbiology/Identify microscopic morphology/ Parasites/2

14. Plate 14 is a fecal specimen unstained seen under 40× using brightfield microscopy. The plate shows the ovum of which parasite?
A. *N. americanus*
B. *T. trichiura*
C. *A. lumbricoides*
D. *E. vermicularis*

Microbiology/Identify microscopic morphology/ Parasites/2

15. Plate 15 is an iodine-stained fecal specimen seen under 40× using brightfield microscopy. The plate shows the ovum of which parasite?
A. Pinworm
B. Threadworm
C. Hookworm
D. Whipworm

Microbiology/Identify microscopic morphology/ Parasites/2

16. Plate 16 is a unstained fecal specimen seen under 40× using brightfield microscopy. The plate shows the ovum of which parasite?
A. *Clonorchis sinensis*
B. *Fasciola hepatica*
C. *Paragonimus westermani*
D. *Fasciolopsis buski*

Microbiology/Identify microscopic morphology/ Parasites/2

17. Plate 17 is an unstained fecal specimen seen under 40× using brightfield microscopy. The plate shows the ovum of which parasite?
A. *Fasciola hepatica*
B. *Paragonimus westermani*

C. *Metagonimus yokogawai*
D. *Opisthorchis viverrimi*

Microbiology/Identify microscopic morphology/ Parasites/2

Answers to Questions 12–17

12. **C** This plate shows abundant *Histoplasma capsulatum* (yeast phase) within the cytoplasm of both the macrophage and histiocyte. All of the organisms above may cause pulmonary pneumonia in immunodeficient patients. Small oval yeast cells, 2–5 μ in diameter, are seen.

13. **B** The ova of *T. trichiura* are brown and shaped like a football with mucus plugs at both ends. Ova have a thick wall and measure about 50 μ long by 20 μ wide. *Enterobius* ova are approximately the same size but have a clear (hyaline) shell, flat on one side with a visible larva within. *Necator* eggs are larger (approximately 65–75 μ long by 40 μ wide) and have a clear shell.

14. **C** *Ascaris* ova are large and oval usually measuring 50–75 μ long by 35–50 μ wide. They are often bile-stained and may have a thick shell with a coarse covering (corticated). This egg demonstrates a contracted embryo leaving space between the shell and the embryo at the opposing poles. This indicates that the egg is fertilized.

15. **C** Hookworm ova are approximately 60–75 μ in length and 35–40 μ in width. They have a thin outer shell usually containing an unembryonated or partly embryonated egg within. The ova of *Necator* and *Ancyclostoma* cannot be differentiated from one another. Threadworm (*Strongyloides*) produces similar ova, but these hatch in the intestine releasing the rhabditoid larvae that are found in the feces. Pinworm (*Enterobius*) ova are approximately the same size but are more elongated and flat on one side. Whipworm (*Trichuris*) ova are smaller and thick-walled with mucus plugs at both ends.

16. **A** *C. sinensis* produces small, bile-stained ova approximately 25–35 μ in length and 10–20 μ in width. Ova have a collar (shoulder) on both sides of the operculum and a knob at the end opposite the operculum. *Fasciola*, *Paragonimus*, and *Fasciolopsis* all produce large, yellow-brown operculated ova.

17. **B** *P. westermani* produces large, operculated ova measuring approximately 80–100 μ in length and 50–70 μ in width. They are yellow-brown and non-embryonated. *Metagonimus* and *Opisthorchis* ova are small ova resembling *Clonorchis*. *Fasciola* produces ova that are also yellow-brown, operculated, and unembryonated. The ova are larger than *Paragonimus* and lack the small shoulders adjacent to the operculum of *Paragonimus* ova.

18. Plate 18 is a peripheral blood film stained with Giemsa's stain, 100×. What condition is suspected from this field?
A. Macrocytic anemia
B. Agranulocytosis
C. Relapsing fever
D. Lead poisoning

Microbiology/Identify microscopic morphology/ Spirochete/2

19. Plate 19 shows an organism isolated from an eye wash of a patient with a cornea infection who had been wearing contact lenses for the past 2 years. What is the name of the causative agent?
A. *Naegleria* spp
B. *Acanthamoeba* spp
C. *Entamoeba histolytica*
D. *Trichomonas vaginalis*

Microbiology/Identify microscopic morphology/ Parasites/2

20. Plate 20 is a wright-stained peripheral blood film, 100×. Which malarial stage is present in the RBC in the center of the plate?
A. Ring trophozoite of *Plasmodium vivax*
B. Mature trophozoite of *Plasmodium malariae*
C. Macrogametocyte stage of *Plasmodium falciparum*
D. Mature gametocyte stage of *Plasmodium ovale*

Microbiology/Identify microscopic morphology/ Parasites/3

21. Plate 21 is a modified acid-fast stain with malachite green counterstain of a stool specimen, 100× magnification. The oocysts seen in this field are approximately 5 μ in diameter. Which organism is present?
A. *Isospora belli*
B. *Cryptosporidium parvum*
C. *Cyclospora* spp
D. *Sarcocystis* spp

Microbiology/Identify microscopic morphology/ Parasites/2

22. Plate 22 is a gram-stained CSF concentrated by centrifugation, 100×. Which organism is present?
A. *Neisseria meningitidis*
B. *Staphylococcus aureus*
C. *Streptococcus pneumonia*
D. *Listeria monocytogenes*

Microbiology/Identify microscopic morphology/ CSF/2

Answers to Questions 18–22

18. **C** This field shows long helical bacteria between red blood cells (RBCs) of normal size and color. These spirochetes are sometimes seen in the blood of patients suffering from the febrile septic phase of infection with *Borrelia* or *Leptospira* spp. The former are more commonly encountered in differential exams, especially in patients infected with *Borrelia recurrentis* and other species that cause relapsing fever. *Borrelia burgdorferi,* the causative agent of Lyme disease, is rarely seen in Wright's stained blood films and is usually diagnosed by enzyme-linked immunosorbent assay (ELISA) and other serological methods.

19. **B** This is a large trophozoite with spiculated cytoplasm characteristic of *Acanthamoeba*. Eye infections caused by this organism have been documented in contact lens wearers who do not properly disinfect lenses. *Acanthamoeba* spp are large trophozoites measuring 25–50 μ. They may also cause primary amoebic meningoencephalitis, although they are isolated less often than *Naegleria* in the cerebrospinal fluid (CSF) of patients with this disease.

20. **A** The infected RBC demonstrates enlarged amoeba-like cytoplasm and Schüffner's dots, which are characteristic of *P. vivax* and *ovale*. The parasite is at the ring-form trophozoite stage.

21. **B** All of the organisms above are coccidian parasites that cause diarrhea, especially in immunodeficient patients such as those with AIDS. *Cryptosporidium* produces the smallest oocysts (half the size of *Cyclospora,* which is the next smallest) and is visible in stools using either the acid-fast or immunofluorescent staining techniques. The oocysts are round, about 5 μ in diameter, and deep pink.

22. **C** This field shows abundant gram-positive diplococci with the lancet shape that is characteristic of *S. pneumoniae*. *Haemophilus* and group B *Streptococcus* are the most common causes of bacterial meningitis in infants. *Listeria* may cause bacterial meningitis in infants and elderly patients, while *S. pneumonia* is most often encountered in middle-aged adults and older patients. *Staphylococcus, Streptococcus,* and *Listeria* spp are gram-positive while *Neisseria* is gram-negative. *Listeria* is a small coccobacillus or rod. *Staphylococcus* is rarely isolated from CSF and appears as small grapelike cocci.

23. Plate 23 is a urinary sediment viewed under 40× magnification using a brightfield microscope. What is the object located in the center of the field?
A. *Schistosoma haematobium* ovum
B. Oval fat body
C. Glitter cell
D. Fecal contaminant

Body fluids/Identify microscopic morphology/Urine sediment/2

24. Plate 24 is a urinary sediment viewed under 40× magnification using a brightfield microscope. Which crystals are seen?
A. Uric acid
B. Calcium oxalate
C. Ammonium magnesium phosphate
D. Hippuric acid

Body fluids/Identify microscopic morphology/Urine sediment/2

25. Plate 25 is a urinary sediment viewed under 40× magnification using a brightfield microscope. Which crystals are seen?
A. Uric acid
B. Calcium oxalate
C. Ammonium magnesium phosphate
D. Hippuric acid

Body fluids/Identify microscopic morphology/Urine sediment/2

26. Plate 26 is a urinary sediment viewed under 40× magnification using a brightfield microscope. Which formed element is seen?
A. Hyaline cast
B. Broad cast
C. Waxy cast
D. Coarse granular cast

Body fluids/Identify microscopic morphology/Urine sediment/2

27. Plate 27 shows a urinary sediment viewed under 40× magnification using brightfield microscopy. This colorless crystal is presumptively identified as:
A. Calcium phosphate
B. Acetaminophen
C. Cystine
D. Hippuric acid

Body fluids/Identify microscopic morphology/Urine sediment/2

28. Plate 28 is a wright-stained cytocentrifuge preparation of pleural fluid, 100×. What is the correct classification of the largest mononuclear cell located in the center of the plate?
A. Histiocyte
B. Macrophage
C. Lymphoblast
D. Mesothelial cell

Body fluids/Identify microscopic morphology/ Pleural fluid/2

Answers to Questions 23–28

23. **B** Oval fat bodies are degenerated renal tubular epithelia that contain a high concentration of neutral fat, largely reabsorbed cholesterol droplets. These appear highly refractile under brightfield microscopy, and the fat globules produce a maltese cross effect under a polarizing microscope. Oval fat bodies occur in conditions associated with increased urinary lipoprotein excretion such as the nephrotic syndrome.

24. **A** Uric acid crystals are yellow to reddish brown in color and occur in acid or neutral urine. Common forms include whetstones and rhombic plates (as seen here), as well as thin needles and rosettes. Calcium oxalate crystals are usually colorless octahedrons. Ammonium magnesium phosphate crystals are long, colorless six-sided prisms, and hippuric acid crystals are colorless long, flat, hexagonal plates.

25. **C** Ammonium magnesium phosphate crystals (triple phosphate) occur in alkaline or neutral urine. They are long, colorless hexagonal prisms that often resemble a "coffin lid." They may also occur in a feathery form that resembles a fern leaf. Triple phosphate crystals may form calculi in the renal pelvis appearing on an x-ray as an outline of the calyces and referred to as "stag-horn" calculi.

26. **D** Coarse granular casts often form from degeneration of cellular casts. The finding of more than a rare granular cast is significant and helps to identify the kidney as the source of urinary protein and cells. Coarse and fine granular casts have the same significance as cellular casts and point to glomerular damage.

27. **C** Cystine crystals form in acid urine and appear as colorless uniform six-sided hexagonal plates in urinary sediment. Calcium phosphate crystals form in neutral to alkaline urine and appear as thin amorphous crystals resembling a sheet of ice or as flat needles that form a rosette. Acetaminophen crystals are cylinder-shaped with round edges. Hippuric acid crystals form long six-sided prisms in acid urine. Cystine crystals must be differentiated from uric acid on the basis of solubility, polarized microscopy, or biochemical testing. Cystine crystals are less anisotropic than uric acid. Cystine crystals are soluble in dilute hydrochloric acid (HCl), but uric acid is insoluble. Cystine causes a positive cyanide-nitroprusside test and uric acid does not.

28. **D** Mesothelial cells are specialized epithelium that line the serous membranes, and they may be seen in small numbers in normal pleural, pericardial, and ascites fluids. They are often seen in increased numbers when there is an inflammatory injury involving the serous membranes. They are large mononuclear or binucleate cells with an open chromatin pattern and abundant agranular cytoplasm. Mesothelial cells may transform into phagocytic cells and undergo morphologic changes that cause them to resemble malignant cells.

29. Plate 29 is a wright-stained smear of pleural fluid prepared by cytocentrifugation. The largest cell in this field (see arrow) is identified as a:
A. Signet ring macrophage
B. Reactive mesothelial cell
C. Foam cell
D. Metastatic cell from the breast

Body fluids/Identify microscopic morphology/ Pleural fluid/2

30. Plate 30 is from a wright-stained peripheral blood film, 100×. Which of the following best describes the cells in this plate?
A. Normal morphology
B. Macrocytic red blood cells
C. Hypersegmented neutrophil present
D. Reduced platelets

Hematology/Identify microscopic morphology/ RBCs/2

31. Plate 31 is a wright-stained peripheral blood film, 100×. What is the most appropriate classification of the red cell morphology seen in this field?
A. Microcytic, hypochromic
B. Microcytic, normochromic
C. Normocytic, normochromic
D. Macrocytic, normochromic

Hematology/Identify microscopic morphology/ RBCs/3

32. Plate 32 is a wright-stained peripheral blood film, 100×. What is the most appropriate classification of the white blood cells (WBCs) present in this field?
A. Reactive (atypical) lymphocytes
B. Large lymphoblasts exhibiting L2 morphology
C. The M4 subtype of acute granulocytic leukemia
D. Monocytes

Hematology/Identify microscopic morphology/ WBCs/3

33. Plate 33 is from a wright-stained peripheral blood film, 40×. Which of the following tests may be performed to enable an accurate diagnosis?
A. Leukocyte alkaline phosphatase (LAP) stain
B. Myeloid marker study by flow cytometry
C. Myeloperoxidase stain
D. Periodic acid-Schiff (PAS) stain

Hematology/Identify microscopic morphology/ WBCs/3

34. Plate 34 is from a wright-stained peripheral blood film, 40×. The cells seen are diagnostic of which condition?
A. Intravascular hemolytic anemia
B. Sickle cell disease
C. Myelofibrosis
D. Erythroleukemia

Hematology/Identify microscopic morphology/ RBCs/3

Answers to Questions 29–34

29. **A** Macrophages are frequently seen in serous fluids. They are present in increased numbers in exudative conditions. Signet ring forms result from compression of the nucleus against the cell wall usually caused by large vacuoles that form after phagocytosis of erythrocytes or fat.

30. **A** The size, shape, and central pallor of the red cells in this plate are normal. The morphology of the neutrophil is typical in appearance. Platelets of normal size and shape are present. On average, there should be less than three platelets per oil immersion (100×) field when thrombocytopenia is present.

31. **D** Many of the RBCs in this field are larger than the nucleus of the small lymphocyte indicating that they are macrocytic. Several of the RBCs are elliptical in shape and are classified as ovalocytes. The region of central pallor of most of the cells is normal. Macrocytic anemia (anemia with an increased mean cell volume [MCV]) is commonly seen in patients with chronic liver disease, vitamin B_{12} or folate deficiency, hypothyroidism, and alcoholism.

32. **A** These cells are lymphocytes characteristic of those found in viral infections such as infectious mononucleosis. In these conditions, the WBC count is increased (usually $15–25 \times 10^3/\mu L$), and lymphocytes account for the majority of the WBCs. Reactive lymphocytes are larger than normal. The cytoplasm is increased in volume and may be vacuolated, and the edges of the cell are often scalloped and basophilic. The nuclear chromatin pattern is open and reticular.

33. **A** This plate shows marked granulocytosis demonstrating cells at all stages of maturity and marked thrombocytosis. These characteristics suggest chronic granulocytic leukemia (CGL), but they also occur in the leukemoid response, which is a severe granulocytosis in response to infection, inflammation, tissue damage, or malignancy. The LAP test is performed to distinguish the two conditions. In CGL the LAP score is markedly reduced, usually 10 or below. In the leukemoid response (and leukoerythroblastosis) the LAP score is elevated (reference range 20–100). In addition to the LAP stain, cytogenetic evaluation is another important diagnostic marker for CGL. Ninety-five percent of patients with CGL display the Philadelphia (Ph[1]) chromosome in their granulocytes.

34. **B** This plate displays polychromasia, abundant target cells (leptocytes), and well-defined sickle cells (drepanocytes) characteristic of sickle cell disease. Sickle cells are elongated with pointed ends, and the Hgb is concentrated in the center of the cell. They may also be encountered in a few other hemoglobinopathies, such as Hgb SC disease but are rarely seen in patients with sickle cell trait.

35. Plate 35 is from a wright-stained peripheral blood film, 100×. Which description of the RBC morphology and platelets is correct?
   A. Microcytic, hypochromic with marked poikilocytosis and increased platelets
   B. Macrocytic, hypochromic with marked anisocytosis and normal platelets
   C. Normocytic, normochromic with mild poikilocytosis and increased platelets
   D. Microcytic, hypochromic, with mild anisocytosis and normal platelets

Hematology/Identify microscopic morphology/ RBCs/2

36. Plate 36 is a wright-stained peripheral blood film, 100×. The RBCs in this plate are characteristic of:
   A. Hemolytic anemia
   B. Myelofibrosis
   C. Hgb C disease
   D. Sideroblastic anemia

Hematology/Identify microscopic morphology/ RBCs/ 3

37. Plate 37 is a wright-stained peripheral blood film, 100×. The cells seen in this plate are associated with:
   A. Lead poisoning
   B. Aplastic anemia
   C. Iron deficiency anemia
   D. Intravascular hemolysis

Hematology/Identify microscopic morphology/ RBCs/3

38. Plate 38 is from a wright-stained peripheral blood film, 40×. Which of the following conditions is consistent with this RBC morphology?
   A. Erythroleukemia
   B. β Thalessemia major
   C. Folate deficiency anemia
   D. Autoimmune hemolytic anemia

Hematology/Identify microscopic morphology/ RBCs/3

39. Plate 39 is from a wright-stained smear of peripheral blood, 100× from a patient with a WBC count of 35 × 10^9/L. The patient is 60 years old with firm, enlarged lymph nodes and hepatosplenomegaly. These same cells comprise 50% of the bone marrow WBCs and are PAS-positive and myeloperoxidase and nonspecific esterase-negative. What is the most likely diagnosis?
   A. Epstein-Barr virus infection
   B. Infectious mononucleosis
   C. Chronic lymphocytic leukemia
   D. Waldenström's macroglobulinemia

Hematology/Evaluate clinical and laboratory data/ Leukemia/3

Answers to Questions 35–39

35. **A** These RBCs demonstrate extreme central pallor characteristic of cells that are microcytic and hypochromic. Target cells, ovalocytes, burr cells, and cell fragments are present. On average, when more than 20 platelets are seen per oil immersion field, the platelet count is elevated.

36. **B** The peripheral blood in myelofibrosis is leukoerythroblastic and is characterized by teardrop cells (dacrocytes), ovalocytes, nucleated RBCs, basophilic stippling, poikilocytosis, leukocytosis, and (often) micromegakaryocytes. Hgb C disease produces normocytic or slightly microcytic anemia with many target cells. Sideroblastic anemia produces both microcytic, hypochromic RBCs, and normocytic RBCs in the blood (dimorphic RBC morphology). Hemolytic anemias are usually normocytic, normochronic, or macrocytic with polychromasia, but morphology varies with the cause of hemolysis.

37. **A** Several RBCs in this plate show coarse basophilic stippling. Basophilic stippling results from unstable RNA within the cell and is associated with defects in Hgb synthesis. This is most often associated with lead poisoning, hemoglobinopathies, myelofibrosis, and megaloblastic anemias.

38. **B** This plate shows severe microcytic, hypochromic RBCs with numerous target cells and marked anisocytosis. A polychromatophilic normoblast is present. In addition, thalassemia is also associated with poikilocytes, Howell-Jolly bodies, ovalocytes, and siderocytes. Folate deficiency produces a macrocytic anemia, and autoimmune hemolytic anemia is usually normocytic, normochromic. The peripheral blood in erythroleukemia contains many nucleated RBC precursors demonstrating bizarre shapes.

39. **C** The WBCs in this plate (with the exception of one granulocyte) are small lymphocytes. Chronic lymphocytic leukemia is rare in patients under the age of 30. The peripheral blood demonstrates a predominance of small lymphocytes, usually 20–200 × 10^9/L, which comprise at least 40% of the bone marrow WBCs. Flow cytometry indicates these cells to be B cells in approximately 95% of cases. The bone marrow in Waldenström's macroglobulinemia is infiltrated by plasmacytoid lymphocytes, plasma cells, and mast cells, as well as small lymphocytes; however, a severe peripheral lymphocytosis is not seen. Lymphadenopathy and hepatosplenomegaly occur in infectious mononucleosis. The lymphocyte count is usually 15–25 × 10^9/L, but the cells are atypical, being characterized by reactive features. The bone marrow is usually hyperplastic but not infiltrated by small lymphocytes.

40. Plate 40 is from a wright-stained peripheral blood film, 40×. The RBC morphology is most consistent with which of the following anemias?
A. Folate deficiency
B. Iron deficiency
C. Hemolytic
D. Sideroblastic

Hematology/Identify microscopic morphology/ RBCs/3

41. Mr. Vacini, an Italian immigrant, has been hospitalized with tachycardia, a rapidly decreasing hematocrit, and blood in his urine. Twenty-four hours prior to admission he had taken his first dose of a sulfonamide prescribed for a urinary tract infection. Plate 41 is from a wright-stained smear of his peripheral blood, 100×. Which laboratory test would be helpful in establishing a diagnosis of Mr. Vacini's hematologic problem?
A. Heinz body preparation
B. Hgb H preparation
C. Iron stain
D. New methylene blue stain

Hematology/Identify microscopic morphology/ RBCs/3

42. Plate 42 is from a wright-stained smear of peripheral blood, 100×. The bone marrow aspirate of this patient demonstrated an abundance of cells with this morphology. Which of the following conditions is most likely to be associated with this sample?
A. Sézary syndrome
B. Hodgkin's disease
C. Burkitt's lymphoma
D. Multiple myeloma

Hematology/Identify microscopic morphology/ WBCs/3

43. Plate 43 is from a wright-stained peripheral blood film, 100×. The WBC appearing in this plate is most likely a:
A. Myeloblast
B. Promyelocyte
C. Myelocyte
D. Monoblast

Hematology/Identify microscopic morphology/ WBCs/2

Answers to Questions 40–43

40. **D** The RBC morphology of this field is characterized by the presence of both microcytic, hypochromic, and normocytic, normochromic cells. This dimorphic appearance is a characteristic of sideroblastic anemias. Folate deficiency causes a megaloblastic anemia causing a macrocytic, normochromic appearance. Iron deficiency is associated with a microcytic, hypochromic RBC morphology. Hemolytic anemias are often normocytic, normochromic.

41. **A** The RBC morphology seen in this plate shows both anisocytosis and poikilocytosis with prominent schistocytes that indicate a hemolytic anemia. The patient's ethnic background, clinical findings, and sulfonamide therapy point to a hemolytic episode of glucose-6-phosphate dehydrogenase (G-6-PD) deficiency as the cause. This can be substantiated by an assay of erythrocyte G-6-PD. The enzyme deficiency results in oxidative damage to RBCs causing formation of Heinz bodies (precipitated Hgb). Heinz bodies are demonstrated by staining with crystal violet and will be pitted from the RBCs by the spleen, resulting in RBC fragments sometimes called *bite* or *helmet* cells.

42. **D** The cell in the center of the plate is a plasma cell. Such cells have a dense, eccentric nucleus that is surrounded by a clear perinuclear area that represents the Golgi apparatus. The cytoplasm is basophilic and more abundant than is seen in small lymphocytes. Plasma cells are not normally seen in peripheral blood. They may be found in cases of viral and chronic infections and connective tissue diseases, as well as in myeloma and other plasma cell dyscrasias. The RBCs in this plate demonstrate rouleaux, which is a characteristic seen in multiple myeloma. The peripheral blood in Hodgkin's disease is characterized by neutrophilia and lymphopenia. Burkitt's lymphoma produces very large, intensely basophilic lymphoblasts (L3 morphology). Abnormal lymphocytes appearing in peripheral blood in Sézary syndrome are large with a convoluted nucleus of fine chromatin and almost no cytoplasm.

43. **A** Blasts are usually 15–20 μ in diameter with a large nucleus containing fine chromatin. The cytoplasm is usually agranular and basophilic. Lymphoblasts are differentiated from myeloblasts by cytochemical staining and flow cytometry. This blast contains uniform, unclumped chromatin, multiple nucleoli, the absence of azurophilic granules, and is from a patient with acute myelogenous leukemia, FAB M1. Lymphoblasts often display irregular clumping of the chromatin and azurophilic granules. They usually lack prominent nucleoli.

44. Plate 44 is a wright-stained peripheral blood film, 100×. The white blood cells in this field are peroxidase, chloroacetate esterase, and Sudan B–negative. The cells are positive for terminal deoxynucleotidyl transferase (Tdt) and PAS. On the basis of these findings, what is the most appropriate classification of these cells?
A. Lymphoblasts with L1 morphology
B. Lymphoblasts with L2 morphology
C. Lymphoblasts with L3 morphology
D. Chronic lymphocytic leukemia cells

Hematology/Identify microscopic morphology/ WBCs/3

45. Plate 45 is from a wright-stained peripheral blood film, 100×. Sixty percent of the WBCs are positive for naphthol AS-D chloroacetate esterase (specific esterase), and 70% are positive for α-naphthyl acetate esterase (nonspecific esterase). The WBCs in this plate are characteristic of which FAB subtype of acute nonlymphocytic leukemia?
A. M1
B. M2
C. M3
D. M4

Hematology/Identify microscopic morphology/ WBCs/3

46. Plate 46 is from a wright-stained peripheral blood film, 100×. The WBCs shown in this field are classified as:
A. Blasts
B. Prolymphocytes
C. Plasma cells
D. Myelocytes

Hematology/Identify microscopic morphology/ WBCs/3

47. Plate 47A shows cells from the same sample as plate 46 after peroxidase staining, 100×. Plate 47B is a normal peroxidase-stained peripheral blood film, 100×, which is used as a control. The blast cell shown in 47A is classified as:
A. Peroxidase-positive
B. Weakly peroxidase-positive
C. Peroxidase-negative
D. Invalid because of an improper control reaction

Hematology/Identify microscopic morphology/ Special stains/3

48. Plate 48 is from a wright-stained peripheral blood film, 100×. The WBC shown in the center of the field (see arrow) is classified as a:
A. Blast
B. Promyelocyte
C. Myelocyte
D. Prolymphocyte

Hematology/Identify microscopic morphology/ WBCs/2

Answers to Questions 44–48

44. **A** The cytochemistry of these cells is characteristic of lymphoblasts, and they exhibit morphology that is characteristic of the L1 subtype of acute lymphocytic leukemia. L1 cells have scarce cytoplasm that is moderately basophilic. The cells are small and uniform in size and shape. They either lack a nucleolus or have one or two small nucleoli. L2 cells are large and irregular in size and often contain one or more prominent nucleoli. L3 cells are large and uniform in size with deeply blue cytoplasm. The have multiple prominent nucleoli.

45. **D** These WBCs are large blasts containing a convoluted nucleus, large nucleoli, lacy nuclear chromatin, and abundant cytoplasm. These are characteristics of monoblasts. M1 is myeloblastic leukemia without maturation. M2 is myeloblastic leukemia with maturation. M3 is promyelocytic leukemia, and M4 is myelomonocytic leukemia. Acute myelomonocytic leukemia comprises 20%–30% of acute myelogenous leukemias in adults and usually occurs in persons over 50 years old. More than 30% of nucleated cells in the bone marrow are blasts and 20% or more of the nucleated bone marrow cells are monoblasts or monocytes.

46. **A** The nucleated cells shown in this photomicrograph have a large nucleus with open, unclumped chromatin and scant agranular blue cytoplasm. Chromatin is reticular and nucleoli are prominent. Although nuclear folding is present, Auer rods are not seen and, therefore, the origin of the blasts must be determined by cytochemical and immunological characteristics.

47. **A** The control slide shows peroxidase staining of the granules in three mature neutrophils and indicates that the stain is functioning properly. The cytoplasm of the blast in plate 47A is strongly positive for peroxidase, indicating that it is a myeloblast. When at least 3% of blasts stain positive, the test is considered positive. Acute myeloblastic leukemia (AML) with minimal differentiation, M0, is negative with peroxidase stain. M1 through M4 classes of AML are peroxidase-positive. M5 may be weakly positive, and myeloblasts in M6 are positive. Lymphoblasts, hairy cells, erythroid cells, megakaryocytes, and platelets are negative. Reactions for Sudan Black B parallel those of peroxidase.

48. **B** Promyelocytes are often larger than myeloblasts, and the cytoplasm is more abundant than in the myeloblast. The nuclear chromatin is open but usually is slightly condensed, and one or more nucleoli may be present. The cytoplasm is blue and contains large azurophilic (primary) granules, but no secondary granules. In contrast, the myelocyte has a round nucleus that is smaller, the chromatin is more condensed, and nucleoli are absent. The cytoplasm of the myelocyte is more orange-purple, and secondary granules predominate.

49. Plate 49 is a wright-stained peripheral blood film, 100×. What is the most appropriate classification of the WBCs seen in this field?
   A. Lymphoblasts
   B. Myeloblasts
   C. Promyelocytes
   D. Prolymphocytes

Hematology/Identify microscopic morphology/ WBCs/3

50. Plate 50 is a wright-stained peripheral blood film, 100×. Which description best characterizes the morphology of the neutrophil shown in this plate?
   A. Normal morphology
   B. Döhle bodies
   C. Toxic granulation
   D. Hypersegmentation

Hematology/Identify microscopic morphology/ WBCs/2

Answers to Questions 49–50

49. **B** The nucleated cells shown in this field are blasts. The large blast seen in the corner of the plate contains a prominent Auer rod. Auer rods are linear projections of azurophilic granules and are seen only in acute myelocytic leukemia. Auer rods are usually found in myeloblasts or promyelocytes and are most often seen in M1, M2, and M3 subtypes of AML.

50. **C** This neutrophil displays an abundance of large purple azurophilic granules characteristic of toxic granulation. The granules contain peroxidase and acid hydrolyases that result in increased basophilia. Toxic granulation is found in severe infections and inflammatory conditions and is often present in band cells and metamyelocytes, which are usually increased in these conditions. Döhle bodies and vacuolated neutrophils may be seen in association with toxic granulation.

BIBLIOGRAPHY

1. Harmening, D: Clinical Hematology and Fundamentals of Hemostasis. FA Davis, Philadelphia, 1996.
2. Henry, JB (ed): Clinical Diagnosis and Management by Laboratory Methods. WB Saunders, Philadelphia, 1996.
3. Garcia, LS, and Bruckner, DA: Diagnostic Medical Parasitology. ASM Press, Washington, DC, 1997.
4. Larone, DH: Medically Important Fungi: A Guide to Identification. ASM Press, Washington, DC, 1995.

COLOR PLATE SECTION

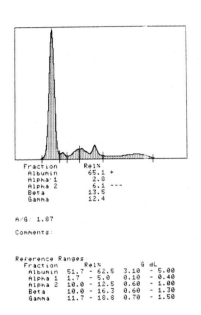

Plate - 1

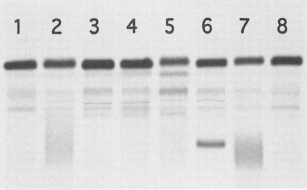

Plate - 2

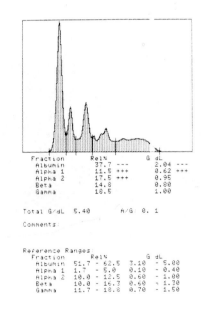

Fraction   Rel%
Albumin 65.1 +
Alpha 1   2.8
Alpha 2   6.1 ---
Beta   13.5
Gamma   12.4

A/G: 1.87

Comments:

Reference Ranges:
Fraction   Rel%   G dL
Albumin 51.7 - 62.5 3.10 - 5.00
Alpha 1   1.7 - 5.0 0.10 - 0.40
Alpha 2 10.0 - 12.5 0.60 - 1.00
Beta   10.0 - 16.3 0.60 - 1.30
Gamma   11.7 - 18.8 0.70 - 1.50

Plate - 3

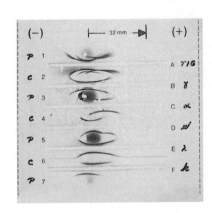

Plate - 4

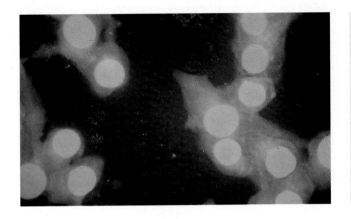

Fraction   Rel%   G dL
Albumin 37.7 ---   2.04 ---
Alpha 1 11.5 +++   0.62 +++
Alpha 2 17.5 +++   0.95
Beta   14.8   0.80
Gamma   18.5   1.00

Total G/dL 5.40   A/G: 0.1

Comments:

Reference Ranges:
Fraction   Rel%   G dL
Albumin 51.7 - 62.5 3.10 - 5.00
Alpha 1   1.7 - 5.0 0.10 - 0.40
Alpha 2 10.0 - 12.5 0.60 - 1.00
Beta   10.0 - 16.3 0.60 - 1.30
Gamma   11.7 - 18.8 0.70 - 1.50

Plate - 5

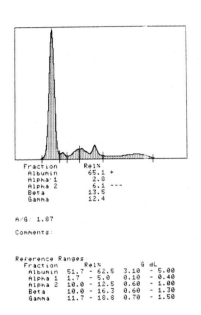

Plate - 6

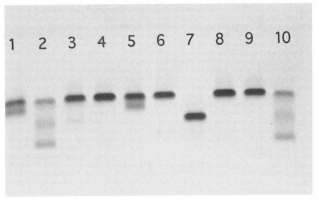

Plate - 7

COLOR PLATE SECTION

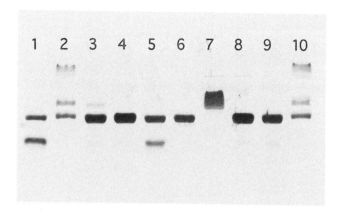

Plate - 8

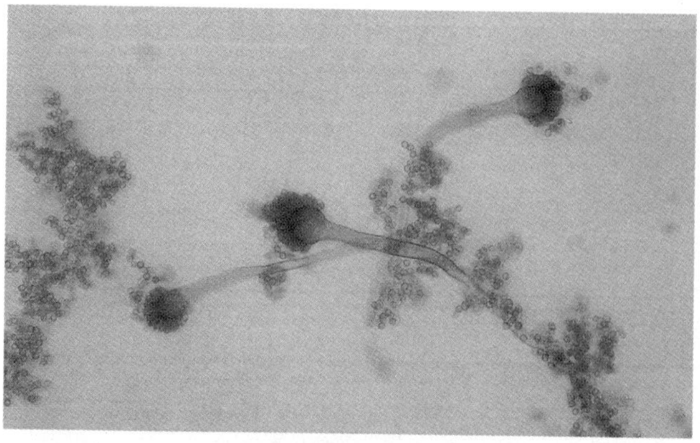

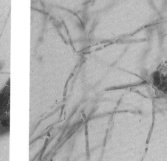

Plate - 9

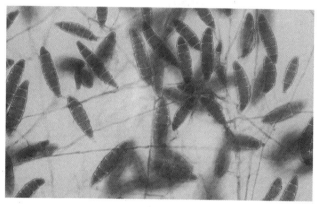

Plate - 10

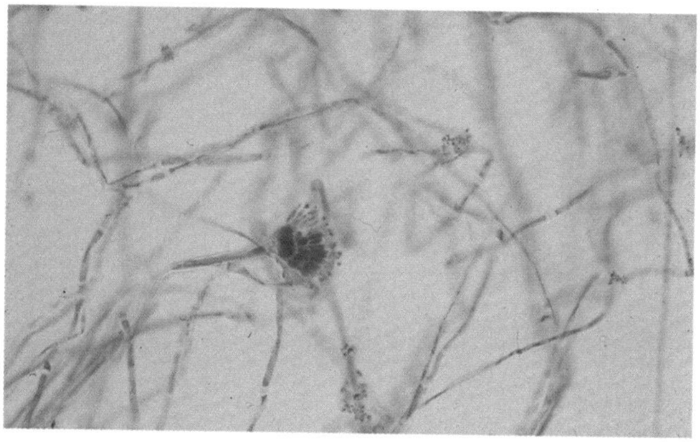

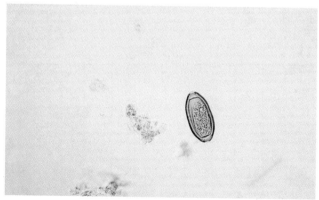

Plate - 11

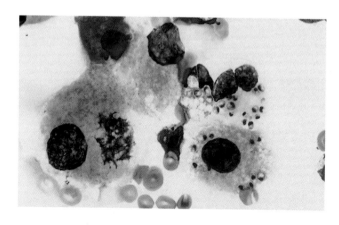

Plate - 12

Plate - 13

COLOR PLATE SECTION

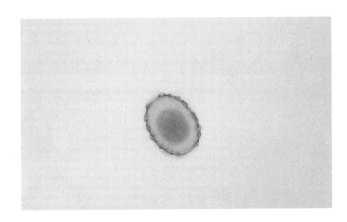

Plate - 14

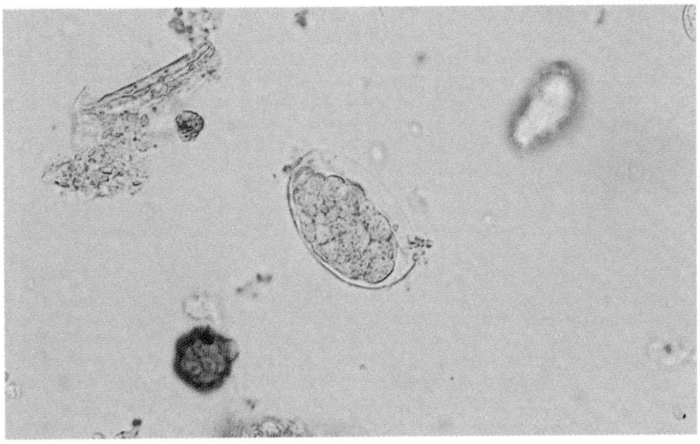

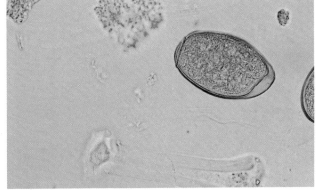

Plate - 15

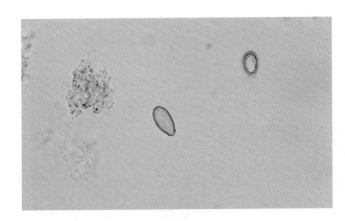

Plate - 16

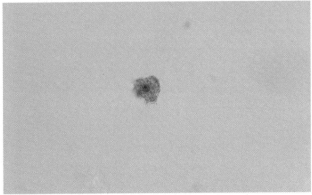

Plate - 17

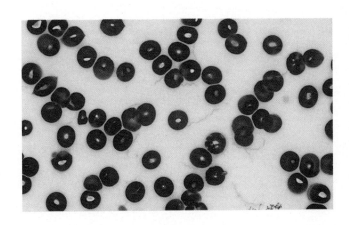

Plate - 18

Plate - 19

COLOR PLATE SECTION

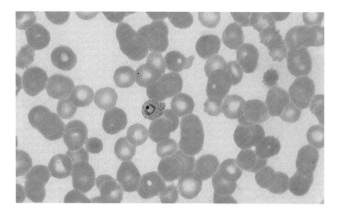

Plate - 20

Plate - 21

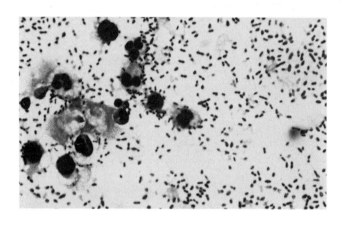

Plate - 22

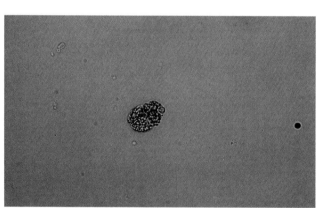

Plate - 23

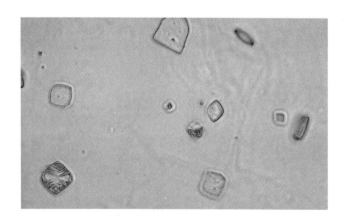

Plate - 24

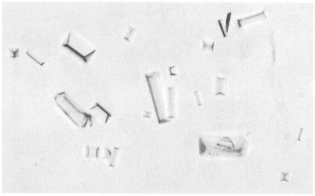

Plate - 25

COLOR PLATE SECTION

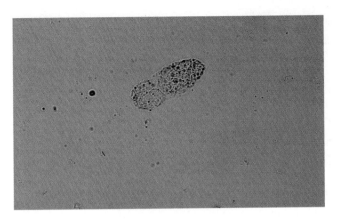

Plate - 26

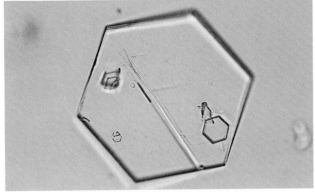

Plate - 27

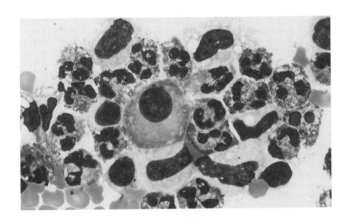

Plate - 28

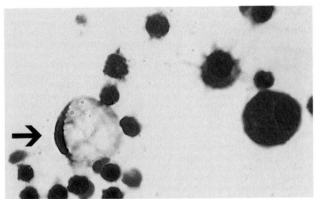

Plate - 29

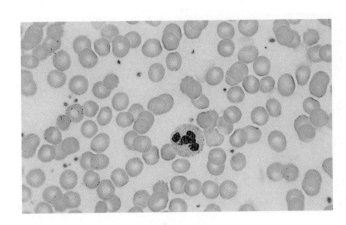

Plate - 30

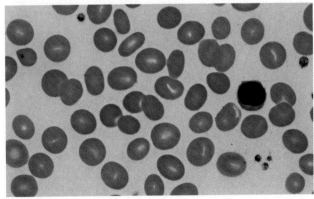

Plate - 31

COLOR PLATE SECTION

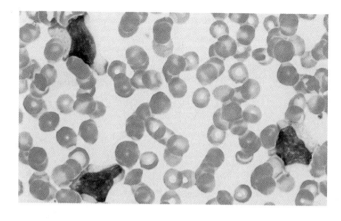

Plate - 32

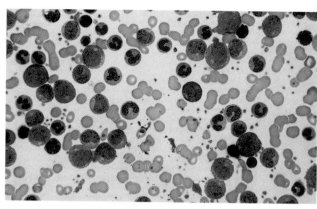

Plate - 33

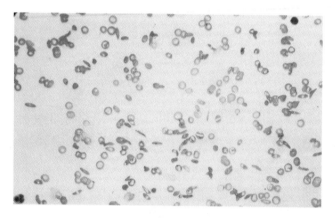

Plate - 34

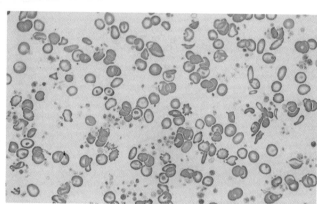

Plate - 35

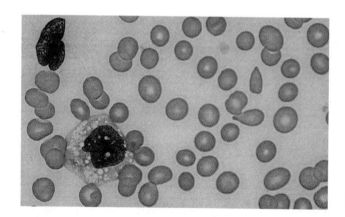

Plate - 36

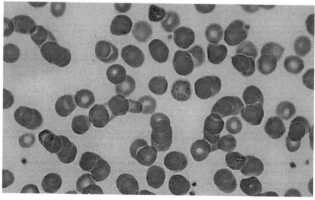

Plate - 37

COLOR PLATE SECTION

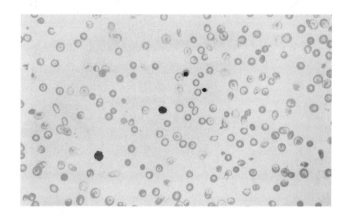

Plate - 38

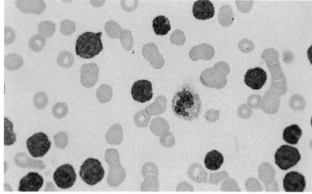

Plate - 39

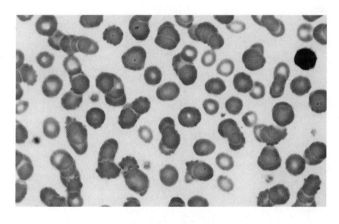

Plate - 40

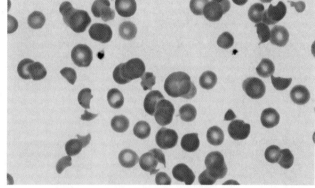

Plate - 41

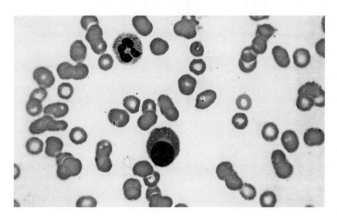

Plate - 42

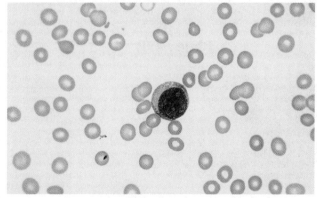

Plate - 43

COLOR PLATE SECTION

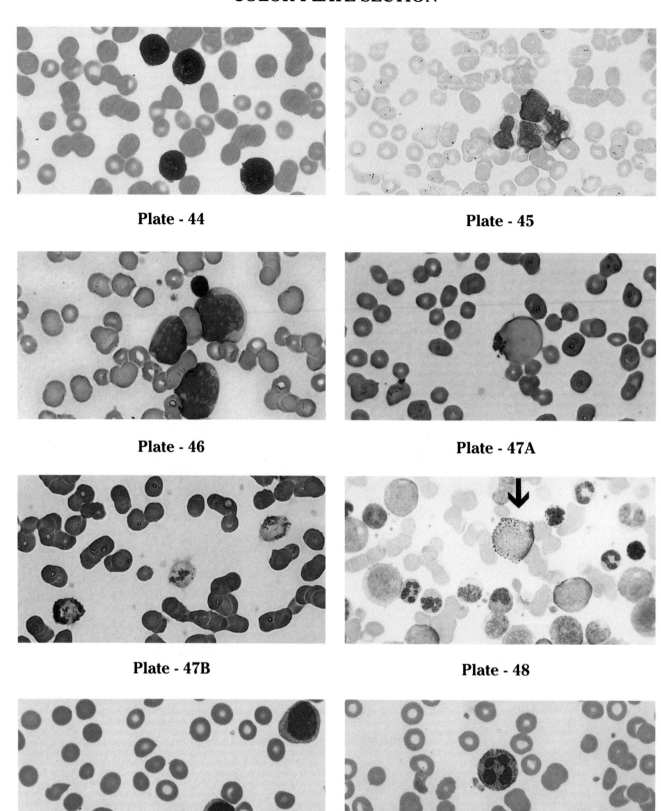

Plate - 44

Plate - 45

Plate - 46

Plate - 47A

Plate - 47B

Plate - 48

Plate - 49

Plate - 50

CHAPTER NINE

Sample Certification (Self-Assessment) Examination

Directions: Each question is followed by four answers, labeled A through D. Choose the best answer and write the corresponding letter in the space to the left of the question number. An answer key is provided on the page following the examination. Use the key to score your exam; a score below 70% correct on any section indicates the need for further study.

Chemistry

_____ 1. Which condition is a common cause of stray light?
A. Unstable source lamp voltage
B. Improper wavelength calibration
C. Dispersion from second-order spectra
D. Misaligned source lamp

_____ 2. The term RT/nF in the Nernst equation defines the:
A. Potential at the ion selective membrane
B. Slope of the electrode
C. Decomposition potential
D. Isopotential point of the electrode

_____ 3. Which of the following is a potential source of error in the hexokinase method?
A. Galactosemia
B. Hemolysis
C. Sample collected in fluoride
D. Ascorbic acid

_____ 4. Which condition is caused by deficient secretion of bilirubin into the bile canaliculi?
A. Gilbert's disease
B. Neonatal hyperbilirubinemia
C. Dubin-Johnson syndrome
D. Crigler-Najjar syndrome

_____ 5. Which of the following OGTT results at 2 hours would be classified as impaired glucose tolerance?

Two-Hour Serum Glucose
A. 105 mg/dL
B. 130 mg/dL
C. 150 mg/dL
D. 204 mg/dL

_____ 6. A patient's blood gas results are:
pH 7.50; PCO_2 55 mm Hg; HCO_3^- 40 mmol/L
These results indicate:
A. Respiratory acidosis
B. Metabolic alkalosis
C. Respiratory alkalosis
D. Metabolic acidosis

_____ 7. A blood sample is left on a phlebotomy tray for 4 hours before it is delivered to the laboratory. Which group of tests could be performed?
A. Glucose, Na, K, Cl, TCO_2
B. Uric acid, BUN, creatinine
C. Total and direct bilirubin
D. CK, ALT, ALP, ACP

_____ 8. A patient's blood urea nitrogen (BUN) is 60 mg/dL, and serum creatinine is 3.0 mg/dL. These results suggest:
A. Lab error measuring BUN
B. Renal failure
C. Prerenal failure
D. Patient was not fasting

_____ 9. Which condition produces the highest elevation of serum lactate dehydrogenase?
A. Pernicious anemia
B. Myocardial infarction (MI)
C. Acute hepatitis
D. Muscular dystrophy

_____ 10. Which substrate is used in the Bowers-McComb method for alkaline phosphatase?
A. p-Nitrophenylphosphate
B. β-Glycerophosphate
C. Phenylphosphate
D. α-Naphthylphosphate

_____ 11. Which of the following liver diseases produces the highest levels of transaminases?
A. Hepatic cirrhosis
B. Obstructive jaundice
C. Chronic hepatitis
D. Alcoholic hepatitis

_____ 12. Zollinger-Ellison syndrome is characterized by great (e.g., 20-fold) elevation of:
A. Gastrin
B. Cholecystokinin
C. Pepsin
D. Glucagon

_____ 13. Which of the following hormones is often decreased by approximately 25% in the serum of pregnant women who have a fetus with Down syndrome?
A. Estriol
B. Human chorionic gonadotropin (HCG)
C. Progesterone
D. Estradiol

_____ 14. SITUATION: A peak blood level for orally administered theophylline (therapeutic range 8–20 mg/L) measured at 8 AM is 5.0 mg/L. The preceding trough level was 4.6 mg/L. What is the most likely explanation of these results?
A. Laboratory made an error on peak measurement.
B. Specimen for peak level was collected from wrong patient.
C. Blood for peak level was drawn too soon.
D. Elimination rate has reached maximum.

_____ 15. Select the hormone that is associated with galactorrhea, pituitary adenoma, and amenorrhea.
A. Estradiol
B. Progesterone
C. Follicle-stimulating hormone
D. Prolactin

_____ 16. In the Oliver-Rosalki method the reverse reaction is used to measure creatine kinase activity. The enzyme(s) used in the coupling reactions are:
A. Hexokinase and glucose-6-phosphate dehydrogenase
B. Pyruvate kinase and lactate dehydrogenase
C. Luciferase
D. Adenylate kinase

_____ 17. The results given in the chart below are reported on an adult male patient being evaluated for chest pain. What is the most likely cause of these results?
A. The wrong sample was assayed for the first myoglobin.
B. The patient did not suffer an MI until after admission.
C. Hemolysis caused interference with the 3-hour and 6-hour myoglobin result.
D. The patient is suffering from unstable angina.

Time	Myoglobin (Cutoff = 100)	Troponin I (Cutoff = 1.5)	CK-MB (Cutoff = 10)
Admission	12 μg/L	3.1 μg/L	18 μg/L
3 hours postadmission	360 μg/L	3.8 μg/L	30 μg/L
6 hours postadmission	300 μg/L	4.0 μg/L	40 μg/L

Hematology

_____ **18.** Which of the following electrophoretic results is consistent with a diagnosis of sickle cell trait?
A. Hgb A: 40%   Hgb S: 35%   Hgb F: 5%
B. Hgb A: 60%   Hgb S: 38%   Hgb A_2: 2%
C. Hgb A: 0%   Hgb A_2: 5%   Hgb F: 95%
D. Hgb A: 80%   Hgb S: 10%   Hgb A_2: 10%

_____ **19.** Which ratio of anticoagulant to blood is correct for coagulation procedures?
A. 1:4
B. 1:5
C. 1:9
D. 1:10

_____ **20.** Which of the following is the preferable site for bone marrow aspiration and biopsy in an adult?
A. Iliac crest
B. Sternum
C. Tibia
D. Spinous processes of a vertebra

_____ **21.** An abnormal activated partial thromboplastin time (APTT) seen with a pathological circulating anticoagulant is:
A. Corrected with aged serum
B. Corrected with absorbed plasma
C. Corrected with normal plasma
D. Not corrected with any of the above

_____ **22.** A manual white blood cell (WBC) count gave a total of 36 cells counted in all 9 mm^2 of a Neubauer ruled hemacytometer. A 1:10 dilution was used; what is the WBC count?
A. 0.4×10^9/L
B. 2.5×10^9/L
C. 4.0×10^9/L
D. 8.0×10^9/L

_____ **23.** If a patient has a reticulocyte count of 7% and a hematocrit (Hct) of 20%, what is the corrected reticulocyte count?
A. 1.4%
B. 3.1%
C. 3.5%
D. 14%

_____ **24.** A decreased osmotic fragility test would be associated with which of the following conditions?
A. Sickle cell anemia
B. Hereditary spherocytosis
C. Hemolytic disease of the newborn
D. Acquired hemolytic anemia

_____ **25.** Given the following values, which set of red blood cell (RBC) indices suggests spherocytosis?
A. MCV 76 μm^3 MCH 19.9 pg   MCHC 28.5%
B. MCV 90 μm^3 MCH 30.5 pg   MCHC 32.5%
C. MCV 76 μm^3 MCH 36.5 pg   MCHC 39.0%
D. MCV 76 μm^3 MCH 29.0 pg   MCHC 34.8%

_____ **26.** Which anemia has red cell morphology similar to that seen in iron deficiency anemia?
A. Sickle cell anemia
B. Thalassemia syndrome
C. Pernicious anemia
D. Hereditary spherocytosis

_____ **27.** In myelofibrosis, the characteristic abnormal red cell morphology is that of:
A. Target cells
B. Schistocytes
C. Teardrop cells
D. Ovalocytes

_____ **28.** Which type of anemia is usually present in a patient with acute leukemia?
A. Microcytic, hyperchromic
B. Microcytic, hypochromic
C. Normocytic, normochromic
D. Macrocytic, normochromic

_____ **29.** **SITUATION:** The prothrombin time (PT) and APTT are corrected with aged serum, but not with absorbed plasma. What factor is deficient?
A. V
B. VII
C. X
D. XI

_____ **30.** Iron deficiency anemia may be distinguished from anemia of chronic infection by:
A. Serum iron level
B. Red cell morphology
C. Red cell indices
D. Total iron-binding capacity

_____ **31.** Which of the following are most characteristic of the red cell indices associated with megaloblastic anemias?
A. MCV 99 fL   MCH 28 pg   MCHC 31%
B. MCV 62 fL   MCH 27 pg   MCHC 30%
C. MCV 125 fL   MCH 36 pg   MCHC 34%
D. MCV 78 fL   MCH 23 pg   MCHC 30%

_____ **32.** **SITUATION:** The following laboratory values are seen:

WBCs 6.0×10^9/L	Hgb 6.0 g/dL
RBCs 1.90×10^{12}/L	Hct 18.5%
Platelets 130×10^9/L	Serum B_{12} and folic acid: normal

WBC Differential	Bone Marrow
6% PMNs	40% myeloblasts
40% lymphocytes	60% promegaloblasts
4% monocytes	40 megaloblastoid
50% blasts	NRBCs/100 WBC

These results are most characteristic of:
A. Pernicious anemia (PA)
B. Acute myeloblastic leukemia (M1)
C. Erythroleukemia (M6)
D. Myelomonocytic leukemia (M4)

_____ **33.** Disseminated intravascular coagulation (DIC) is most often associated with which of the following FAB designations of acute leukemia?
A. M1
B. M3
C. M4
D. M5

_____ **34.** When performing platelet aggregation studies, which set of platelet aggregation responses would most likely occur in a patient with Bernard-Soulier syndrome?
A. Normal platelet aggregation in response to collagen, adenosine diphosphate (ADP), and ristocetin
B. Normal platelet aggregation in response to collagen, ADP, and epinephrine; decreased in response to ristocetin
C. Normal platelet aggregation in response to epinephrine and ristocetin; decreased in response to collagen and ADP
D. Normal platelet aggregation in response to epinephrine, ristocetin, and collagen; decreased in response to ADP

_____ **35.** **SITUATION:** The following laboratory values are seen in the chart below:

Which test helps most to establish a diagnosis?
A. Leukocyte alkaline phosphatase (LAP) stain
B. Nonspecific esterase stain
C. Acid phosphatase
D. Sudan Black B stain

WBC Differential		
WBCs 76×10^9/L	55% PMNs	RBC morphology normocytic, normochromic
RBCs 4.20×10^{12}/L	15% bands	Occasional Döhle body
Platelets 398×10^9/L	12% lymphocytes	
Hgb 12.5 g/dL	7% monocytes	
Hct 26.7%	2% eosinophils	
	1% basophils	
	8% metamyelocytes	

Immunology

_____ **36.** What antibodies are represented by the peripheral or rim pattern of immunofluorescence in tests for antinuclear antibodies?
A. Antihistone antibodies
B. Anti-double-stranded DNA (anti-dsDNA) antibodies
C. Anti–extractable nuclear antigen (anti-ENA) including anti-Sm (anti-Smith) and anti-RNP (antiribonucleoprotein) antibodies

D. Anti-RNA (ribonucleic acid) antibodies

_____ **37.** Interpret the following quantitative rapid plasma reagin (RPR) test results:

RPR titer: weakly reactive 1:8; reactive 1:8–1:64
A. Excess antibody, prozone effect
B. Excess antigen, postzone effect
C. Equivalence of antigen and antibody
D. Impossible to interpret; testing error

_____ **38.** Which T helper-to-T suppressor ratio (T_h:T_s) is most likely in a patient with acquired immunodeficiency syndrome (AIDS)?
  A. 2:1
  B. 3:1
  C. 2:3
  D. 1:2

_____ **39.** Which hepatitis B marker is the best indicator of early acute infection?
  A. Hepatitis B surface antigen (HBsAg)
  B. HBeAg
  C. Antibody to hepatitis B core antigen (anti-HBc)
  D. Anti-HBs

_____ **40.** Which of the following diseases is most likely to cause a false-positive when testing for syphilis?
  A. Systemic lupus erythematosus (SLE)
  B. Idiopathic thrombocytopenic purpura
  C. Aplastic anemia
  D. Hypogammaglobulinemia

_____ **41.** Interpret the following results for Epstein-Barr virus (EBV) infection: IgG and IgM antibodies to viral capsid antigen (VCA): positive
  A. Infection in the past
  B. Infection with a mutual enhancer virus such as human immunodeficiency virus (HIV)
  C. Current infection
  D. Impossible to interpret; need more information

_____ **42.** What type of disorders would show a decrease in C3, C4, and CH_{50}?
  A. Autoimmune disorders such as SLE and rheumatoid arthritis (RA)
  B. Immunodeficiency disorders such as common variable immunodeficiency
  C. Tumors
  D. Bacterial, viral, fungal, or parasitic infections

_____ **43.** Blood products are tested for which virus before being transfused to newborns?
  A. EBV
  B. Human T-lymphotropic virus II (HTLV-II)
  C. Cytomegalovirus (CMV)
  D. Hepatitis D virus

_____ **44.** A 12-year-old female patient has symptoms of fatigue and presents with a localized lymphadenopathy. Laboratory tests reveal a peripheral blood lymphocytosis, a positive RPR, and a positive spot test for infectious mononucleosis. What test should be performed next?
  A. HIV test by enzyme-linked immunosorbent assay (ELISA)
  B. Venereal Disease Research Laboratory (VDRL)
  C. EBV specific antigen test
  D. Microhemagglutinin assay–_Treponema pallidum_ (MHA-TP)

_____ **45.** Which increase in antibody titer (dilution) best indicates an acute infection?
  A. From 1:2 to 1:8
  B. From 1:4 to 1:8
  C. From 1:16 to 1:256
  D. From 1:64 to 1:128

_____ **46.** Which of the following is used in rapid slide tests for detection of rheumatoid factors?
  A. Whole IgM molecules
  B. Fc portion of the IgG molecule
  C. Fab portion of the IgG molecule
  D. Fc portion of the IgM molecule

_____ **47.** Which major histocompatibility (MHC) class of antigens is necessary for antigen recognition by CD4-positive T cells?
  A. Class I
  B. Class II
  C. Class III
  D. No MHC molecule necessary for antigen recognition

_____ **48.** Interpret the results below for HIV infection.
  ELISA: positive; repeat ELISA: negative; Western blot: no bands
  A. Positive for HIV
  B. Negative for HIV
  C. Indeterminate
  D. Further testing needed

_____ **49.** Interpret the following description of an immunoelectrophoresis assay of urine:
  Heavy bowed arcs with anti-κ and anti-λ antisera when compared to the normal control.
  A. Normal
  B. Light chain disease
  C. Increased polyclonal Fab fragments
  D. Multiple myeloma

_____ **50.** What is the titer in tube 8 if tube 1 is undiluted and dilutions are doubled?
  A. 64
  B. 128
  C. 256
  D. 512

Blood Banking

_____ **51.** Which donor unit is selected for a recipient with anti-c?
A. $r'r$
B. R^oR^1
C. R^2r''
D. $r'r^y$

_____ **52.** Which of the following patients would be a candidate for Rh immune globulin (RhIg)?
A. B-positive mother; B-negative baby; first pregnancy; no anti-D in mother
B. O-negative mother; A-positive baby; second pregnancy; no anti-D in mother
C. A-negative mother; O-negative baby; fourth pregnancy; anti-D in mother
D. AB-negative mother; B-positive baby; second pregnancy; anti-D in mother

_____ **53.** Can crossmatching be performed on October 14, using a patient sample drawn on October 12?
A. Yes, a new sample would not be needed.
B. Yes, but only if the previous sample has no alloantibodies.
C. No, a new sample is needed because the 2-day limit has expired.
D. No, a new sample is needed for each testing.

_____ **54.** Interpret the following typing results:
Anti-A, 1+; anti-B, neg; A_1 cells, 1+; B cells, 4+
A. The patient is group A with autoantibodies.
B. The patient is group O with acquired A antigen.
C. The patient is group AB with excessive A_1.
D. The patient may be A_2 with anti-A_1.

_____ **55.** What should be done if all forward and reverse ABO results and the autocontrol are positive?
A. Wash the cells with warm saline; autoadsorb the serum at 4°C.
B. Retype the sample using a different lot number of reagents.
C. Use polyclonal typing reagents.
D. Report the sample as group AB.

_____ **56.** What antibodies could an R^1R^1 individual make if exposed to R^2R^2 blood?
A. Anti-e and anti-C
B. Anti-E and anti-c
C. Anti-E and anti-C
D. Anti-e and anti-c

_____ **57.** Which typing results characterize a secretor who is group O?
A. Anti-A + saliva + A cells = positive; anti-B + saliva + B cells = negative; anti-H + saliva + O cells = negative
B. Anti-A + saliva + A cells = positive; anti-B + saliva + B cells = positive; anti-H + saliva + O cells = positive
C. Anti-A + saliva + A cells = positive; anti-B + saliva + B cells = positive; anti-H + saliva + O cells = negative
D. Anti-A + saliva + A cells = negative; anti-B + saliva + B cells = negative; anti-H + saliva + O cells = negative

_____ **58.** What procedure would help to distinguish between an anti-e and anti-Fy^a in an antibody mixture?
A. Lower pH of test serum.
B. Run an enzyme panel.
C. Use a thiol reagent.
D. Run a regular panel.

_____ **59.** Which of the following individuals is acceptable as a blood donor?
A. A 29-year-old man who had hepatitis B at age 14
B. A 21-year-old woman who had her ears pierced last week
C. A 30-year-old woman who had a rubella vaccination 6 weeks ago
D. A mental patient released from a state hospital 6 months ago

_____ **60.** What reagent/procedure is used to distinguish Kidd and Kell antibodies?
A. Ficin enzyme panel
B. Chloroquine
C. Low ionic strength solution (LISS) media
D. 2-Aminoethylisothiouronium bromide (AET)

_____ **61.** An antibody is detected in a pregnant woman and is suspected of being the cause of fetal distress. The antibody reacts at the indirect antiglobulin test (IAT) phase and causes *in vitro* hemolysis. What is the most likely antibody specificity?
A. Anti-Le^a
B. Anti-Lu^a
C. Anti-Lu^b
D. Anti-Xg^a

62. Which statement applies when preparing FFP or cryoprecipitate for transfusion?
    A. FFP and cryoprecipitate do not need to be the same Rh type as the patient.
    B. No antigen typing is required for transfusion of plasma products.
    C. Antibody screening of plasma products is not required.
    D. All blood components must be matched for both ABO group and Rh type.

63. Six units are crossmatched. Five units are compatible, one unit is incompatible, and the recipient's antibody screen is negative. Identify the problem.
    A. Patient may have a high frequency alloantibody.
    B. Patient may have an abnormal protein.
    C. Donor unit may have a positive direct antiglobulin test (DAT).
    D. Donor may have high-frequency antigens.

64. What is the disposition of a donor unit that contains an antibody?
    A. The unit must be discarded.
    B. Only the plasma may be used to make components.
    C. The antibody must be adsorbed from the unit.
    D. Label the unit indicating that it contains antibody; release into inventory.

65. Given a situation where screen cells, crossmatch, autocontrol, and DAT (anti-IgG) are all positive, what procedure should be performed next?
    A. Adsorption using rabbit stroma.
    B. Antigen type the patient's cells.
    C. Elution followed by a cell panel on the eluate.
    D. Selected cell panel.

66. Which physical examination result is cause for rejecting a blood donor?
    A. Weight of 105 pounds
    B. Pulse of 75
    C. Temperature of 99.3°F
    D. Diastolic pressure of 110 mm Hg

67. What is the *first* step in the laboratory investigation of a transfusion reaction?
    A. DAT on the posttransfusion sample.
    B. Check for a clerical error.
    C. Repeat ABO and Rh typing of patient and donor unit.
    D. Antibody screen on the posttransfusion sample.

68. A unit of packed RBCs is split using the open system. One of the half units is used. What may be done with the second half unit?
    A. Must be issued within 24 hours
    B. Must be issued within 48 hours
    C. Must be discarded
    D. Retains the original expiration date

69. SITUATION: A cancer patient recently developed a severe infection. The patient's hemoglobin is 8 g/dL due to chemotherapy with a drug known to cause bone marrow depression and immunodeficiency. Which blood products are indicated for this patient?
    A. Liquid plasma and cryoprecipitate
    B. Crossmatched platelets and washed RBCs
    C. Factor IX concentrate and FFP
    D. Irradiated RBCs, platelets, and granulocytes

70. Which immunization has the longest deferral period?
    A. Hepatitis B immune globulin (HBIG) injection
    B. Rubella vaccine
    C. Flu vaccine
    D. Yellow fever vaccine

Body Fluids

71. Urine that is dark red or port wine in color may be caused by:
    A. Lead poisoning
    B. Porphyria cutanea tarda
    C. Alkaptonuria
    D. Hemolytic anemia

72. The presence of tyrosine and leucine crystals together in a urine sediment usually indicates:
    A. Renal failure
    B. Chronic liver disease
    C. Hemolytic anemia
    D. Hartnup disease

73. Urine with a specific gravity (SG) consistently between 1.002 and 1.003 indicates:
    A. Acute glomerulonephritis
    B. Renal tubular failure
    C. Diabetes insipidus
    D. Addison's disease

74. SITUATION: What is the most likely cause of the following cerebrospinal fluid (CSF) results?

    CSF glucose = 20 mg/dL; CSF protein = 100 mg/dL; CSF lactate = 50 mg/dL
    A. Viral meningitis
    B. Viral encephalitis
    C. Cryptococcal meningitis
    D. Acute bacterial meningitis

_____ 75. Given the following data calculate the creatinine clearance.

Serum creatinine = 2.4 mg/dL; urine creatinine = 105 mg/dL; urine volume = 1.4 L/day; surface area = 1.80 m^2
A. 41 mL/min
B. 78 mL/min
C. 87 mL/min
D. 110 mL/min

_____ 76. Given the urinalysis below, select the most appropriate course of action.

pH 6.5   Protein, Neg
Glucose, Neg   Ketone, Tr
Blood, Neg   Bilirubin, Neg
Mucus, Sm   Ammonium urate crystals, Lg
A. Recheck urine pH.
B. Report these results assuming acceptable quality control.
C. Repeat the dry reagent strip tests to confirm the ketone result.
D. Request a new sample and repeat the urinalysis.

_____ 77. What is the principle of the colorimetric reagent strip determination of SG in urine?
A. Ionic strength alters the pK_a of a polyelectrolyte.
B. Sodium and other cations are chelated by a ligand that changes color.
C. Anions displace a pH indicator from a mordant, making it water-soluble.
D. Ionized solutes catalyze oxidation of an azo dye.

_____ 78. Which of the statements below accurately describes HCG levels in pregnancy?
A. Levels of HCG rise throughout pregnancy.
B. In ectopic pregnancy serum HCG doubling time is below expected levels.

C. Molar pregnancies are associated with lower levels than expected for the time of gestation.
D. HCG returns to nonpregnant levels within 2 days following delivery, stillbirth, or abortion.

_____ 79. Which condition below is associated with the greatest proteinuria?
A. Acute glomerulonephritis
B. Chronic glomerulonephritis
C. Nephrotic syndrome
D. Acute pyelonephritis

_____ 80. Which of the following results on a serous fluid is most likely to be caused by a traumatic tap?
A. An RBC count of 8000/μL
B. A WBC count of 6000/μL
C. A Hct of 35%
D. A neutrophil count of 45%

_____ 81. A routine urinalysis gives the following results:

pH 6.5   Protein, Neg
Glucose, Tr   Ketone, Neg
Blood, Neg   5–10 blood casts/LPF
Mucus, Sm   Amorphous crystals, Lg

These results are most likely explained by:
A. False-negative blood reaction
B. False-negative protein reaction
C. Pseudocasts of urate mistaken for true casts
D. Mucus mistaken for casts

_____ 82. Oval fat bodies are often seen in:
A. Chronic glomerulonephritis
B. Nephrotic syndrome
C. Acute tubular nephrosis
D. Renal failure of any cause

Microbiology

_____ 83. The ortho-nitrophenyl-β-galactopyronoside (ONPG) test is most useful when differentiating:
A. *Salmonella* spp. from *Pseudomonas* spp
B. *Shigella* spp from some strains of *Escherichia coli*
C. *Klebsiella* spp. from *Enterobacter* spp
D. *Proteus vulgaris* from *Salmonella* spp

_____ 84. Lysostaphin is used to differentiate a *Staphylococcus* from which other genus?
A. *Streptococcus*
B. *Stomatococcus*
C. *Micrococcus*
D. *Planococcus*

_____ 85. Which of the following tests best differentiate *Shigella* spp from *E. coli?*

A. Hydrogen sulfide, Voges-Proskauer (VP), citrate, and urea
B. Lactose, indole, ONPG, and motility
C. Hydrogen sulfide, methyl red, citrate, and urea
D. Gas, citrate, and VP

_____ 86. A gram-negative rod is recovered from a catheterized urine from a nursing home patient. The lactose-negative isolate tested positive for indole, urease, potassium cyanide (KCN), ornithine decarboxylase, and phenylalanine deaminase. The most probable identification is:
A. *Ewardsiella* spp
B. *Morganella* spp
C. *Ewingella* spp
D. *Shigella* spp

87. A helminth egg is described as having terminal polar plugs. The most likely helminth is:
A. Hookworm
B. *Trichuris trichiura*
C. *Fasciola hepatica*
D. *Dipylidium caninum*

88. A leg culture from a nursing home patient grew gram-negative rods on MacConkey agar as pink to dark pink oxidase-negative colonies. Given the following results, which is the most likely organism?

TSI = A/A	Indole = Neg
Methyl red = Neg	VP = +
Citrate = +	H_2S = 0
Urea = +	Motility = Neg

Antibiotic susceptibility: carboxicillin- and ampicillin-resistant, all others sensitive
A. *Serratia marcescens*
B. *Proteus vulgaris*
C. *Enterobacter cloacae*
D. *Klebsiella pneumoniae*

89. A curved gram-negative rod producing oxidase-positive colonies on blood agar was recovered from a stool culture. Given the following results, what is the most likely identification?

Lysine = +	Arginine = Neg
Indole = +	KIA = Alk/Acid
VP = Neg	Lactose = Neg
Urease = ±	String test = Neg

TCBS agar = green colonies
A. *Vibrio cholerae*
B. *Vibrio parahaemolyticus*
C. *Shigella* spp
D. *Salmonella* spp

90. Which test group best differentiates *Acinetobacter* spp. from *Pseudomonas aeruginosa?*
A. Oxidase, motility, 42°C growth
B. MacConkey growth, 37°C growth, catalase
C. Blood agar growth, oxidase, catalase
D. Oxidase, triple sugar iron (TSI), MacConkey growth

91. A gram-negative S-shaped rod recovered from selective media for *Campylobacter* spp. gave the following results:

Catalase = +	Oxidase = +
Motility = +	Hippurate hydrolysis = +
Growth at 42°C = Positive	Naladixic acid = Susceptible
Cephalothin = Resistant	

What is the most likely identification?
A. *Pseudomonas aeruginosa*
B. *Campylobacter jejuni*
C. *Campylobacter fetus*
D. *Pseudomonas putida*

92. Which media is best for recovery of *Legionella pneumophilia* from clinical specimens?
A. Chocolate agar
B. Bordet-Gengou agar
C. New yeast extract agar
D. Buffered charcoal yeast extract agar

93. A small, gram-negative coccobacillus recovered from the CSF of a 2-year-old gave the following results:

Indole = +	Glucose = + (Acid)
X requirement = +	V requirement = +
Urease = +	Lactose = Neg
Sucrose = Neg	Hemolysis = 0

Which is the most likely identification?
A. *Haemophilus parainfluenzae*
B. *Haemophilus influenzae*
C. *Haemophilus ducreyi*
D. *Haemophilus aphrophilus*

94. Urine cultured from the catheter of an 18-year-old female patient produced greater than 100,000 col/mL on a colistin-nalidixic acid (CNA) plate. Colonies were catalase-positive, coagulase-negative by the latex agglutination slide method. The best single test for identification is:
A. Lactose fermentation
B. Urease
C. Tube coagulase
D. Novobiocin susceptibility

95. A gram-positive spore-forming bacilli growing on blood agar anaerobically produces a double zone of β-hemolysis and is positive for lecithinase. What is the presumptive identification?
A. *Bacteroides ureolyticus*
B. *Bacteroides fragilis*
C. *Clostridium perfringens*
D. *Clostridium difficile*

96. β-Hemolytic streptococci, not of group A or B, usually exhibit which of the following reactions?

	Bacitracin	Trimethoprim-sulfamethoxazole
A.	Susceptible	Resistant
B.	Resistant	Resistant
C.	Resistant	Susceptible
D.	Susceptible	Indeterminant

____ **97.** A mycobacteria recovered from a patient with AIDS gave the following results:

Niacin = Neg
T_2H = +
Tween 80 hydrolysis = Neg
Nitrate reduction = Neg
Heat stable catalase (68°C) = ±
Nonphotochromogen

What is the most likely identification?
A. *Mycobacterium gordonae*
B. *Mycobacterium bovis*
C. *Mycobacterium avium* complex
D. *Mycobacterium kansasii*

____ **98.** A germ tube-negative, pink yeast isolate was recovered from the respiratory secretions and urine of a patient with AIDS. Given the following results, what is the most likely identification?

Cornmeal Tween 80 Agar

Urease = +   Blastospores = +
Pseudohyphae = +   Arthrospores = Neg
A. *Candida albicans*
B. *Rhodotorula* spp

C. *Cryptococcus* spp
D. *Trichosporon* spp

____ **99.** Upon examination of stool material for *Isospora belli,* one would expect to see:
A. Cysts containing sporozoites
B. Precysts containing chromatoidal bars
C. Oocysts that are acid-fast
D. Sporozoites that are hematoxylin-positive

____ **100.** Which of the following viruses is implicated along with EBV as a cause of infectious mononucleosis?
A. CMV
B. Coxsackie A virus
C. Coxsackie B virus
D. Hepatitis B virus

Table of Specifications

Section	Taxonomy 1	Taxonomy 2	Taxonomy 3	Number of Questions
Clinical chemistry	2	10	5	17
Hematology	4	7	7	18
Immunology	4	9	2	15
Blood banking	7	6	7	20
Body fluids	2	8	2	12
Microbiology	4	7	7	18
Totals	25	46	29	100

Answer Key

Chemistry

1. C
2. B
3. B
4. C
5. C
6. B
7. B
8. C
9. A
10. A
11. C
12. A
13. A
14. C
15. D
16. A
17. A

Hematology

18. B
19. C
20. A
21. D
22. A
23. B
24. A
25. C
26. B
27. C
28. C
29. C
30. D
31. C
32. C
33. B
34. B
35. A

Immunology

36. B
37. A
38. D
39. A
40. A
41. C
42. A
43. C
44. D
45. C
46. B
47. B
48. B
49. C
50. B

Blood Banking

51. D
52. B
53. A
54. D
55. A
56. B
57. C
58. B
59. C
60. D
61. C
62. A
63. C
64. D
65. C
66. D
67. B
68. A
69. D
70. A

Body Fluids

71. B
72. B
73. C
74. D
75. A
76. A
77. A
78. B
79. C
80. A
81. C
82. B

Microbiology

83. B
84. C
85. B
86. B
87. B
88. D
89. B
90. A
91. B
92. D
93. B
94. D
95. C
96. C
97. C
98. B
99. C
100. A

The enclosed disk contains a 100-question computerized mock examination. This computerized exam will help you identify your levels of preparation and give you experience in taking an examination by computer.

To simulate a real examination, allow yourself $2\frac{1}{2}$ hours to complete the mock examination.